Chiropractic care of the older patient

Commissioning editor: Heidi Allen
Development editor: Caroline Savage
Production controller: Chris Jarvis
Cover designer: Fred Rose

Chiropractic care
of the older patient

Editor: Brian J Gleberzon DC

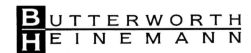

OXFORD   AUCKLAND   BOSTON   JOHANNESBURG   MELBOURNE   NEW DELHI

Butterworth-Heinemann
Linacre House, Jordan Hill, Oxford OX2 8DP
225 Wildwood Avenue, Woburn, MA 01801-2041
A division of Reed Educational and Professional Publishing Ltd

 A member of the Reed Elsevier plc group

First published 2001

© Reed Educational and Professional Publishing 2001

Disclaimer   The information and statements herein are believed to be reliable, but are
not to be construed as a warranty or representation for which the authors or publishers
assume legal responsibility. Users should undertake sufficient verification and testing
to determine the suitability for their own particular purpose of any information or
products referred to herein. No warranty of fitness for a particular purpose is made

British Library Cataloguing in Publication Data
A catalogue record for this book is available from the British Library

Library of Congress Cataloguing in Publication Data
A catalogue record for this book is available from the Library of Congress

ISBN 0 7506 4729 9

For information on all Butterworth-Heinemann publications
visit our website at www.bh.com

Produced by Gray Publishing, Tunbridge Wells, Kent
Printed and bound in Great Britain by The Bath Press, Avon

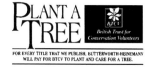

FOR EVERY TITLE THAT WE PUBLISH, BUTTERWORTH-HEINEMANN
WILL PAY FOR BTCV TO PLANT AND CARE FOR A TREE.

Contents

Foreword

When I get up in the morning I feel stiff and achy, so I go to the doctor who says it is just a little arthritis ... 'Take an aspirin'. When I don't feel well, I go to the doctor who says ... 'This is what being older feels like'.
Natasha Josefowitz,
Chronologically disabled, 1995

The ageing of the population is producing major shifts in the needs for the focus of health care professionals from young and middle aged to older persons. Much of medicine in the last century focused on technological advances aimed at prolonging life. Unfortunately, in the rush to embrace 'high tech' concepts there has been a tendency to forget that for most older persons 'high touch' concepts are as important in maintaining function and quality of life. In many cases physicians have moved their practices far away from holistic practices, resulting in the need for other health professionals to fill the void. Chiropractors are one such group, whose 'high touch' approach is focused on pain relief, functional improvement and prevention.

For sometime now the health care needs of the elderly have been looked after in parallel by a variety of practitioners. Thus, it represents an important event that a text on the health of the elderly is being published for chiropractors. Much of the development of frailty can be delayed with a focus on prevention. Resistance exercise has been shown to improve functional status. Balance exercises markedly decreased falls. Exercise also improves depression, congestive heart failure and chronic obstructive pulmonary disease. Appropriate muscle exercises can decrease arthritic pain and improve function in persons with osteoarthritis. Maintenance of good nutrition in older persons is key to promoting a healthy lifespan. Early recognition of anorexia and its reversal is a key. The appropriate replacement of vitamins and trace elements can prevent a variety of disturbances from cognition dysfunction to osteopenia. Pharmacological use of vitamin E may decrease coronary artery disease and prevent fee radical damage to a variety of tissues. These and other issues make the chapter on health promotion and illness prevention a key chapter.

Appropriate manipulation can produce dramatic relief in older persons. Being aware of the differences in the chiropractic technique as applied to older persons are key to successful manipulation. Understanding the different disease processes in older persons that may limit the form of manipulation is an absolute essential knowledge in providing care for the older person. This makes the chapter on chiropractic manipulation in the elderly an important section of this book.

Understanding the physiological changes with ageing allows the health professional to recognize the physiology/disease dichotomy associated with ageing. The extensive chapters that examine the diseases of the elderly provide essential information for the health professional to provide appropriate care and advice to their patient.

The recognition of the role of certain 'alternative medicines' such as St. John's wort for depression, ginger for dizziness, saw palmetto for prostate symptoms and phytoestrogens at the menopause, opens up a Pandora's box of therapeutic options to improve the quality of life of older persons. The South African biologist, Jan Smuts, first coined the term 'wholestic' medicine. This text represents a giant step forward in the field of holistic medicine.

Chiropractic Care of the Older Patient will play an important part in sensitizing the chiropractor and other

health professionals to the needs of individuals undergoing the last third of life's journey. This textbook will
play a key role in training health care professionals to
provide appropriate 'high touch' care for our elderly
friends as we enter this new millennium.

John E Morley
*Dammert Professor of Gerontology Saint Louis Univer-
sity Health Sciences Center and Director, Geriatric
Research, Education and Clinical Center St. Louis VA
Medical Center*

Preface

Thank you for purchasing *Chiropractic Care of the Older Patient*. It is my sincere hope that you will find it to be an excellent learning tool and reference when dealing with older persons. This textbook has been developed from the perspective of a chiropractic practitioner. It is for that reason that pharmacological and surgical interventions are discussed in general terms only, particularly focusing on how such treatments may necessitate a modification to chiropractic care. This textbook focuses on the characteristic diagnostic features of various disorders, and has emphasized the treatment options available to chiropractors. Preferential consideration has been given to those therapeutic interventions that are most supported by the literature, and an evidence-based approach is provided wherever possible. I have also included a brief appendix on human genetics. It has been my experience that many chiropractic students and practitioners have only a preliminary education in this area, and thus may benefit from a more detailed description of various concepts in the field of genetics.

This textbook has been divided into four sections, each section comprising of several chapters.

Brian J Gleberzon

Acknowledgements

A textbook of this magnitude requires the efforts of many individuals, many of whom are behind the scenes, and I would like to take this opportunity to thank them for their help. First and foremost, I must thank each of the contributing authors. It is with great humility that I can count these individuals as my colleagues, and can testify that each person demonstrated true professionalism in their contributions.

I must thank Dr Dave Waalen, who proof-read each of my chapters and offered many insightful suggestions. I have always held that he is an unsung hero in the chiropractic profession, an unselfish scholar, and the help and encouragement he has given me over the years has proven to be invaluable. I would also like to thank Dr Jane Mannington, who sadly died in October 2000, for giving me many of the opportunities I have enjoyed at the Canadian Memorial Chiropractic College. I hope I did not disappoint her.

I would like to thank Dr Howard Vernon for his encouragement and his efforts to facilitate my working relationship with the people at Butterworth Heinemann, who have proven to be a pleasure to work with. I would also like specifically to thank Drs Ayla Azad, Lisa Killinger and Robert Cooperstein, who have each helped me to become a better researcher, teacher and, I hope, scholar.

I must of course thank my parents, Billy and Ann Gleberzon, and my in-laws, Nathan and Shirley Rosenberg, for their lifelong support and love.

Last, but certainly not least, I would like to thank my wife, Anita, for her friendship and encouragement throughout my life. She is truly the better part of me. And if I may dedicate this book to anyone, I would dedicate it to my two sons, Jared and Andrew, who are the better part of both Anita and I. (I can only hope our kids don't use the kind of language I did when this $%#&! computer didn't do what I wanted it to do …)

Brian J Gleberzon

Contributors

Lori Albert MD
The Toronto Hospital,
Division of Rheumatology,
Toronto, Ontario, Canada

Robert Annis DC
Sudbury, Ontario, Canada

Ayla Azad
Canadian Memorial Chiropractic College,
Toronto, Ontario,
Canada

TA Bayley MD
Endocrinology & Metabolism and Nuclear Medicine,
University of Toronto,
Toronto, Ontario, Canada

David Byfield
Welsh Institute of Glamorgan,
Glamorgan, Wales,
UK

Paul Carey CD
President of the Canadian Chiropractic Protection
Association, and Associate Professor,
Canadian Memorial Chiropractic College,
Toronto, Ontario,
Canada

David Conn MD
Department of Psychiatry,
Baycrest Centre for Geriatric Care,
Toronto, Ontario, Canada

Robert Cooperstein DC
Palmer College of Chiropractic West,
San Jose, California,
USA

Marshall Deltoff
Images Radiology Consultants,
Toronto, Ontario,
Canada

Jodi B Dickstein PhD
Canadian Memorial Chiropractic College,
Toronto, Ontario,
Canada

Sheldon Freelan DPM
Mississuaga Podiatry Association,
Mississuaga, Ontario,
Canada

Allan M Freedman BA LLB
Professor, Canadian Memorial Chiropractic College,
Toronto, Ontario,
Canada

Brian J Gleberzon DC
Canadian Memorial Chiropractic College,
Toronto, Ontario,
Canada

William Gleberzon PhD
Canadian Association of Retired Persons,
Toronto, Ontario,
Canada

Jerry Grod DC
Los Angeles College of Chiropractic,
Whittier, California,
USA

Lisa Killinger DC
Palmer Center for Chiropractic Research,
Davenport, Iowa,
USA

Peter Kogan
Université du Québec à Trois-Rivières,
Trois-Rivières, Québec,
Canada

Sherryn N Levinoff Roth MD
Division of Cardiology, University of Toronto,
Toronto, Ontario,
Canada

Robert Mootz DC
Associate Medical Director for Chiropractic,
State of Washington, Department of Labor and
Industries, Olympia, Washington, USA

Joseph J Piccininni BA, BEd, MSc, Dip. ATM, CAT(C)
Professor, Sports Injury Program, Sheridan College,
Oakville, Assistant Professor, Canadian Memorial
Chiropractic College, Toronto, Ontario, Canada

Luba Plotkina DHM
Homeopathic College of Canada,
Toronto, Ontario,
Canada

Jaan Reitav PhD
Canadian Memorial Chiropractic College,
Toronto, Ontario,
Canada

Irving Rosen MD
Mount Sinai Hospital,
Toronto, Ontario
Canada

Michael Smith
Canadian College of Naturopathic Medicine,
Toronto, Ontario,
Canada

Susan St. Clair DC
Palmer College of Chiropractic-West,
San Jose, California,
USA

Odette Tunks DC
Hamilton,
Ontario,
Canada

Keith Wells DC
Los Angeles College of Chiropractic,
Whittier, California,
USA

Steven Zylich DC
Canadian Memorial Chiropractic College,
Toronto, Ontario,
Canada

Section I: The older person

On geriatrics: operational definitions, challenges and perspectives

Brian J Gleberzon

When Jeanne Calment was born, Ulysses S Grant was president and Queen Victoria sat on the British throne. The year was 1875. Slavery in America had been abolished only 9 years earlier and women would not be allowed to vote for almost another 50 years. Alexander Graham Bell had just invented the telephone. The phonograph, lightbulb and wireless radio were in early stages of development, but the automobile was still years in the future. General George C Custer would have his 'last stand' at Little Big Horn later that same year.[1] DD Palmer was practising spiritualism and had yet to begin his career as a magnetic healer; the concept of 'chiropractic' was still a generation away.[2]

In her native France, Jeanne remembered visiting a newly erected and impressive structure – the Eiffel Tower. She remembered Vincent van Gogh, whom she would later describe as ugly, bad tempered and reeking of alcohol buying paint in the store her family owned in Arles. At the age of 85 she took up fencing; at the age of 120 she gave up smoking because she was afraid it was becoming a habit.[3] She attributed her long life to a diet of olive oil, wine and humour. 'I have only one wrinkle', she said, 'and I'm sitting on it'.[3] At the time of her death in 1997, Jeanne Calment had the longest verifiable life span of any human being: 122 years, 5 months and 14 days.[3]

While Jeanne Calment may be an extreme exception, people are living longer, and generally better, now than ever before. The twenty-first century will witness a demographic phenomenon hitherto unknown: almost as many people alive will be over the age of 40 as under it. An ageing of the world's population will bring with it fundamental shifts in our cultural perception of 'old age', and changes in the issues germane to geriatric study. These include issues and concerns about retirement, social safety nets and health care. This textbook will primarily address issues surrounding health care, from the perspective of chiropractors and other complementary and alternative medicine (CAM) health-care providers. Topics discussed will focus on their clinical diagnosis, treatment, management and prevention.

Defining the topic

A simple but useful exercise to begin a study of geriatric care is akin to the free-association technique sometimes used in psychotherapy. Without any concerns for political correctness, the reader is asked to write down the words or phrases that come to mind when asked to define an older person. Descriptors can include any particular age, social roles, physical features, cognitive functions, behaviours, attitudes or impressions.

If the reader is like the typical fourth year chiropractic or naturopathic student, the list of adjectives and phrases associated with growing old will be, by and large, unflattering.

When asked to describe 'an older patient', these students used the following terms:

- frail
- stubborn
- obsolete
- osteoporotic
- demented
- slow
- forgetful
- incontinent
- poor driver
- 'old bag'

- cantankerous
- grandparent
- retired
- white-haired
- blue-haired
- impatient

- 'old fart'
- wise
- experienced
- knowledgeable
- rigid.

Most students cringe at the prospect of growing old and possibly becoming any of the people they have described. What becomes painfully obvious is that, even among students studying to become health-care professionals in what is typically their seventh year of tertiary education, ageism is rampant. This is no doubt a reflection of the overall negative attitudes associated with the process of growing old that are interwoven into the tapestry of our cultural fabric.

Operational definitions

Geriatrics is defined as 'the branch of medicine which treats all problems peculiar to old age and the aging, including the clinical problems of senescence and senility'.[4] Senescence, in turn, is defined as the 'process or condition of growing old, especially the condition resulting from the transition and accumulation of the deleterious aging process'.[4] This is quite different from gerontology, which is the 'scientific study of the problems of aging in all aspects – clinical, biological, historical and sociological'.[4] It is the author's opinion that older patients cannot be understood if they are removed from the societal structure in which they live, and so a gerontological approach is of greatest value. In fact, a truly anthropological approach, which considers a group of persons within their cultural context, is the most informative method for geriatric study overall. It is for this reason that clinical conditions described throughout this textbook do not merely recount a list of signs and symptoms, but also emphasize how each condition may impact a person's quality of life and overall well-being.

The World Health Organization differentiates between subgroups of older persons. The elderly are generally considered to be those between the ages of 65 and 75 years.[5] The old are those individuals between the ages of 76 and 90, and the very old or old old are those over the age of 90 years.[5]

For purposes of demographic study (see Chapter 2), a distinction must be made between life span and life expectancy. Essentially, life span is the length of the longest-lived member of a species.[5] It is generally agreed upon that the human life span is 120 years. Life expectancy, however, is the length of time an average particular individual can expect to live, depending on his or her current age.[5] Although usually calculated from birth, life expectancies can also be predicted from any other age point. For example, at birth, a women has a life expectancy of 79 years, a man about 73 years.[5] However, if a women lives to the age of 65, she can expect to live for another 20 years; a man, another 15.[5] It should be noted that life expectancies differ between different members of a population. Life expectancies for African-Americans from birth, for example, are only 74 years for women and 65 for men.[5] During the twentieth century, human life expectancy rose dramatically, whereas human life span remained relatively unchanged.

Diseases that are age caused must be differentiated from those that are age related. Age-caused diseases are those that primarily occur as the result of senescence, such as cardiovascular disease, or a decline in sensory abilities, such as diminished sight. Age-related diseases are those that are not necessarily attributable to the ageing process per se, but are a consequence of other deleterious changes. The classic example of an age-related disease is depression, which is more a result of other impairments or losses incurred while ageing, such as a loss of vision, as opposed to an actual biological or biochemical change in a person's brain.

Another anchor term of geriatric study is successful ageing. Successful ageing can be defined as the optimalization of a person's health while minimizing any physiological declines as the result of the ageing process.[5,6] Looked at another way, successful ageing can be thought of as how well an individual responds to those changes in their health that are due solely to the ageing process, uncomplicated by the damage from the person's environment, lifestyle or disease.[7] Therefore, healthy strategies such as proper nutrition, exercise, cessation of smoking, moderation of alcohol consumption, and social and intellectual stimulation can help to achieve successful ageing. This is in contrast to usual ageing, which is associated with the typical declines in physiological functions over time which reflect the combined effects of disease, adverse environmental conditions and poor lifestyle choices.[5–7]

A key concept underpinning geriatric study is the importance of conducting a comprehensive geriatric assessment (CGA).[5–8] A CGA is defined as a 'multidisciplinary evaluation in which the multiple problems of older persons are uncovered, described, and explained, if possible, and in which the resources and strengths of the person are catalogued, need for services assessed, and a coordinated care plan developed to focus interventions on the person's problem'.[8] A CGA is a systematic approach to the collection of patient data, which allows the evaluation of the patient's health status and functional abilities in multiple areas or domains.[5]

To continue with an introductory discussion of older patients, it is important to describe the major health challenges facing them.

The 'five Is'

Different segments of the population are preferentially affected by different clinical conditions. For example, the incidence of type II diabetes is much higher in Native Americans (Chapter 12), whereas hypertension is much more common in African-Americans (Chapters 15 and 16). Similarly, older patients are more commonly afflicted by certain specific clinical conditions. That is not to say that these conditions are unknown in younger patients, it is just that they are more likely to be encountered among the elderly. These conditions are best grouped under the mnemonic of the 'Five Is'.[9]

The first of the five 'Is' refers to *intellectual impairment*. This not includes not only diminished memory skills, decline in creativity, compromised learning abilities and slower behavioural responses to complex cognitive tasks (such as those involved while driving), but also intellectual impairments such as dementia, delirium and depression (the 'three Ds' of intellectual impairments; refer to Chapter 9).

Alzheimer's is the most common form of dementia, which is defined as the impairment of two or more intellectual or cognitive functions with a clear state of consciousness.[10] Dementia is identifiable by a patient exhibiting impaired concentration, forgetfulness, decreased attention span, loss of computational skills, problems maintaining personal hygiene and, most importantly, changes in personality. Change in personality is invariably a harbinger of serious pathology.[5,9]

Delirium is an acute state of confusion, characterized by a transient disturbance in the patient's ability to think clearly, concentrate and remember.[10] The patient will often suffer short-term memory loss, and may be disorientated. Unlike Alzheimer's cases, delirious patients exhibit a disturbance in consciousness. Delirium is a cardinal sign of serious physical illness or drug intoxication.[5,9]

Depression is an abnormality of mood or affect.[10] The patient is unable to initiate actions, or to experience pleasure or to sustain hope in the future. Thoughts of despair and suicide (which mandate an immediate referral to a psychiatrist) are common; 25–30% of hospitalized senior patients are clinically depressed.[5] A patient may be overwhelmed by challenges in their health status or personal lives, thus exhibiting depression. Some experts have suggested that the one word that best describes the challenge of growing old is loss. An individual may have lost their job, their physical or mental capabilities, their spouse, their home or their independence. These losses may culminate in a state of depression.

The second 'I' that preferentially affects older persons is *incontinence*. Defined as the inability to control bowel or bladder function, incontinence effects 10–20% of older patients, and its incidence increases with age.[5] It is important to remember that the psychosocial impact of incontinence is often more damaging then its physiological affects, and incontinence can lead to social withdrawal, diminished activities of daily living (ADLs) or even institutionalization. One study reported that 25% of patients with incontinence felt that their doctor or nurse was either embarrassed or unsympathetic, and 40% of patients thought that incontinence was a result of normal ageing[5] (see Chapter 18).

Immobility and *instability* are the next two 'Is' challenging the health of older persons (see Chapters 13 and 14, respectively). These can be discussed together because they are often interconnected. Instability, often the result of vertigo, orthostatic hypotension, diminished neck righting reflexes, altered proprioception or disturbances in gait, may lead to a patient becoming more sedentary (immobile). Just as importantly, the causes of instability are the major contributing risk factors to falls and fractures which are, in turn, a leading cause of mortality and morbidity in the elderly. Falls are the leading cause of death due to injury among older patients,[5] and 75% of persons who die as the result of a fall are over the age of 65 years.[11] Fourteen thousand deaths and 22 million hospitalizations are annually attributed to falls.[12] Falls account for 250 000 hip fractures a year in the USA and demographic projections predict that this number may rise to 650 000 by the year 2050.[5]

Causes of immobility are instability disorders as described above, pain syndromes resulting from arthritides or trauma, and other muscular disorders, the two most common being fibromyalgia and polymyalgia rheumatica. Prolonged immobility may exacerbate the various arthritides with which a patient may be afflicted. Immobility may further contribute to osteoporosis, and it may result in disuse atrophy and a decline in muscular strength. A worsening of these conditions further binds a person to a lifetime of immobility and compromised ADLs. It is for these reasons that exercise and strength training are essential for successful ageing[13] (see Chapter 28).

The last of the 'Is' for geriatric study is *iatrogenic drug reactions.* These are adverse drug reaction (ADRs) directly attributable to treatment by a physician, either in private practice or during hospitalization. ADRs are a major concern among older patients, since it is estimated that the number of prescription drugs, over-the-counter medications and self-selected supplements that the average older patient is taking is 12.[6] Thirty per cent of all prescription drugs and 40% of all over-the-counter drugs are purchased by patients over the age of 65 years.[11,14] More than two-thirds of Americans over the age of 65 years use at least one drug a day, with forty-five per cent of elderly patients taking several prescriptions daily.[14,15] As many as 70% of older patients use self-selected medications, usually without first consulting with their physicians.[15] Patients may contribute to the problem by obtaining prescriptions from multiple physicians, or they may be receiving medications from friends or family members who want to share the benefits of their prescriptions.[15] Two-thirds of all physician visits lead to a drug prescription, with 40% resulting in the prescription of two or more medications.[5] It has been estimated that almost 25% of older outpatients receive inappropriate medications.[5]

A recent article by Lazarou *et al.*[16] reported that, in 1994, 2 216 000 patients had serious adverse drug reactions, and 106 000 patients had fatal ADRs, making ADRs between the fourth and sixth leading cause of death in the USA, a ranking that is higher than either pneumonia or diabetes (see Chapter 22).

Complementary and alternative medicine and the 'five Is'

From the perspective of a field practitioner, what is most important about an understanding of the 'five Is'

of geriatric care is that chiropractors (and some other CAM providers) are well suited to manage each of these challenges. Chiropractors and other CAMs are able to diagnose each of the 'three Ds' of intellectual impairments, and can refer a patient to the appropriate health-care specialist. Disorders resulting in immobility and instability (vertigo, diminished neck-righting reflexes, fibromyalgia, pain syndromes) have been shown to respond favourably to manipulative therapies.[17–20] Theoretically, and often reported anecdotally, spinal manipulative therapy may positively influence incontinence. Acupuncture, botanical medicines, herbs and other supplements have been shown to provide positive therapeutic outcomes for a plethora of disorders, ranging from headaches to diabetes. Lastly, iatrogenic drug reactions are avoided owing to the drugless approach of chiropractic.

Taken as a whole, it becomes apparent that chiropractors are uniquely suited and well qualified for the successful management of those clinical conditions that preferentially affect older patients. As will be discussed throughout this textbook, the development of interdisciplinary networks, involving both traditional allopathic and CAM approaches, holds the best future for optimal geriatric care.

The challenges of assessing the older patient

Geriatricians, and other practitioners focusing on the care of older patients, must be made aware of the fact that older patients present with many clinical challenges.[21,22] While it is true that older patients are generally similar to younger adults and are simply at a different, older, stage of life, clinicians are faced with unique challenges when dealing with this group of people. By learning more about these challenges, many potential problems can be avoided, circumvented and managed appropriately.

Perhaps the most important challenge facing a clinician in the assessment of an older patient is that variability increases among individuals as they age. This is in stark contrast to the assessment of paediatric patients, who are expected to reach specific developmental milestones at a specific time.[22] If a child fails to reach an established milestone (walking by the age of 1 year, talking by 2 years, and so on), a referral for further investigation is warranted. When assessing older patients, however, the literature indicates that the range of normative values increases with age. The reader can undoubtedly think of examples of individuals they know who, although similar in age, demonstrate a wide margin of difference with regard to physical or cognitive abilities.

Although the majority of patients report that they are in good overall health, and this is often supported by objective measures, many older patients have multiple pathologies.[22] Many older patients have two or three coexisting problems, and often they have more, and for every one that is known to the clinician, there is another that is not.[21] The existence of multiple pathologies in an individual (termed comorbidity or coimpairment) creates further complications. First, it confounds the ability of the clinician to reach a definitive diagnosis. Secondly, a clinician may be unable to identify positive therapeutic outcomes in a patient.[22] The symptoms of one condition may mask the successful resolution of symptoms of another condition.[22]

Many older patients present with an atypical set of symptoms or presentation for a particular condition.[15] Many conditions that affect older patients are known for their slow onset and progression. McCarthy[15] reported the results of a survey of 'healthy' geriatric patients presenting to an outpatient clinic: 14% of these 'healthy' patients were found to have congestive heart failure, 4% had postural hypotension and 10% had a painful untreated arthropathy.[15] Other problematic conditions, such as pneumonia, often develop without fever, while vertebral fractures may occur in the absence of trauma.[15] For reasons that are not entirely understood, pain in older patients is often minimal or absent in many presenting chief complaints where its presence would usually be expected.[21] For example, myocardial infarcts in the elderly are often pain free.[21]

As previously described, adverse and iatrogenic drug reactions are a significant problem among older patients. Many symptoms may be the result of the side-effects of a medication or a supplement that a patient may be taking. In addition, many older patients suffer from a decrease in communicative abilities.[21] This may hamper both the interview and the physical examination processes.

There is often a tremendous variability in the response to therapy among older patients.[15] Older patients require a higher level or longer period of stimulation before the threshold for physiological response is reached.[15] Many clinicians report that the response to treatment is rarely as dramatic or as visible in older patients, and it is rarely as consistent as in younger persons.[15] Lastly, the range of safety for many therapeutic interventions is narrower in older patients than in younger patients.[15]

In some ways the last major challenge confronting a practitioner during the assessment of an older patient does not involve the patient at all. Ageism, the prejudicial assumption about a person based solely on their chronological age, or 'old appearance', can negatively influence an otherwise proficient clinical review.[22] A patient's symptoms may often be dismissed by a practitioner as simply the consequence of the normal ageing process, whereas the patient's presenting chief complaint may have nothing at all to do with their age.

The challenges facing a clinician when assessing an older patient may be daunting, but they are not insurmountable, especially if the practitioner is cognizant of their existence.

They include:[15,20,21]

- increase in variability between individuals
- comorbidity
- atypical presentation
- adverse drug reactions
- decrease in communication abilities
- variability in response to treatment.

As will be discussed throughout this textbook, there are many strategies to deal with these challenges. More importantly, the holistic approach advocated by CAM practitioners is especially well suited to manage the unique challenges with which older patients present.

Types of ageing

Historically, medical pedagogy preferentially explored geriatric health in terms of biological changes. In essence, geriatric medicine examined the ageing process from a physiological perspective, focusing on those conditions that affect older patients, perhaps to the exclusion of other components of the ageing process, such as historical and sociocultural contexts. This section will explore some of the other viewpoints from which the ageing process can be considered, providing examples of each.

Chronological ageing

While focusing on the number of years that a person has survived is certainly the simplest way to consider ageing, it is probably the least useful.[23] The chronological age of an individual provides only a poor approximation of the person's structural growth and decline, and his or her psychological or physiological status or abilities, and such an approach also provides little insight into the individual's social and emotional development.[21] Therefore, current thinking in geriatric pedagogy relies more heavily on the assessment of the functional abilities of a person, and the impact that the relative preservation or decline of a person's abilities has on their daily lives.[21,23] This distinction is made more important by the fact that, while underlying pathologies producing ill health in older persons are often irreversible, some degree of functional improvement is almost always possible.[21] It is for this reason that the functional assessment of the older patient is considered the cornerstone of geriatric health care.[21] Therefore, clinicians working with older persons must emphasize the importance of cognitive, physical and social status and abilities.

Biological ageing

As discussed previously, traditional geriatric education provided students with a laundry list of those clinical conditions that preferentially affect older persons. Although this approach must continue to be a significant component of any geriatric education, more and more geriatricians are emphasizing the importance of these biological changes within the context of the individual's overall lifestyle. For example, the loss of vision may in and of itself not be significant from a strictly biological perspective. However, visual impairment may result in the person no longer being able to read, or the person may no longer be able to operate an automobile, which in turn could result in social isolation. In either case, these limitations may adversely affect a person's quality of life. Moreover, social considerations such as stress or depression may accelerate the biological changes associated with ageing.

Psychological ageing

The study of 'normal ageing' also explores changes to an individual's intellectual and cognitive function. Areas of change include cognitive abilities, memory, learning, problem solving and creativity. These changes are often linked to changes in neurological structures. The psychopathologies preferentially affecting older persons are described in greater detail in Chapter 9.

Social ageing

Ageing can be considered as a social process.[24–26] In general, the theories proposed to explain ageing as a social process are divided into microlevel theories, which focus on the individual and their interactions with each other and society as a whole, and macrolevel theories, which explore social structure, social processes and problems, and their interrelationships.[24] An example of a microlevel approach would be a consideration of the relationship of a child to his or her parents, whereas the macrolevel approach would, for example, consider the effects of industrialization on the status of older persons.[24]

Dawe, a sociologist, proposed two contrasting perspectives of social ageing.[23] The normative perspective posits that established rules and status levels exist in a society in order to provide social order. This order is deemed necessary for the survival of a society. According to this perspective, individuals learn roles by internalizing shared norms and values by socialization. The majority of persons generally adhere to these rules. In the event of a transgression of these rules, varying types of sanctions may be imposed.[23]

In contrast, the interpretive perspective views individuals as social actors who define, interpret and control their institutionalized roles in society.[23] In essence, this approach examines how individuals create social order and define those situations in which they find themselves, and how each person ultimately relates to others in daily life.[24] According to Novak, social gerontologists have made the least use of this perspective, although it can provide useful insights into everyday interactions.[24]

Some authorities prefer to divide social theories of ageing into three different perspectives. Along with the interpretive perspective, some sociologists speak of a fundamentalist perspective.[24] This perspective posits that social order is based on co-operation, interdependence, shared values, and adjustment by the individual to society allowing for societal equilibrium.[24] The fundamentalist perspective is used in gerontology's most influential theories, the disengagement theory and the activity theory.[24]

Lastly, a few gerontologists use what is called the conflict perspective.[24] This perspective is employed by those investigating social inequalities and conflicts from a politicoeconomic approach. An example of this approach would be the work of Karl Marx.

Although a complete description of all the proposed social theories of ageing is beyond the scope of this textbook, a brief review of the more established theories is provided below.

Microlevel theories of ageing

These theories are based on certain assumptions. Among these are: (i) that individuals pass sequentially through stages of life while attempting to accomplish certain goals or tasks within each stage; (ii) that development is cumulative, orderly and hierarchical; (iii) that ageing is a lifelong process based on antecedent and subsequent events; (iv) that ageing is influenced by historical events; and (v) that social ageing also involves psychological and biological processes.[23]

The role theory proposes that society imposes expected behavioural patterns, rights and responsibilities. Thus, social roles are either ascribed at birth (the child is male or female, black or white, and so on) or acquired or achieved throughout a person's life (being a spouse, parent, widow, etc.).[23] With changes in a person's life, social roles change. In general, there is a progressive loss of, or reduction in, the number of major social roles (worker, parent, spouse). Moreover, there are role transitions throughout a person's lifetime, such as moving from the job market to retirement. From this perspective, old age is seen to be a time in a person's life that ends in physical, psychological and social losses, often resulting in a period of devalued status with few meaningful roles.[23]

Because role loss was thought to be an inevitable process, the role theory dominated the thinking within social gerontological circles for many years. However, because seniors in today's society often maintain or acquire new roles with high status, current thinking holds that, as a person ages, he or she experiences both gains and losses in a variety of interrelated roles. Ageing is seen as a period of role transition and change in which most individuals seek out, and adjust effectively to new role sets. For some older persons, the transition from one role to another may be stressful, difficult or confusing, while for others the change may be uneventful and successful.[23]

Similar to role theory, activity or substitution theory posits that individuals replace lost roles with new ones. First suggested by Neugarten, Havighurst and Tobin in 1968, this theory argues that individual adaptation in later life involves a continuing active lifestyle in order to achieve successful ageing, general well-being and life satisfaction.[23,24] This can only be achieved by replacing lost roles with appropriate new ones. The activity theory was the first theory that sought to explain the concept of successful ageing.[24]

For many years the activity theory was accepted without question, and was the basis for many of the social programmes and services provided to the elderly, based on the assumption that if older persons are kept busy with a range of activities and social roles from which to chose, they would age successfully.[23] In essence, older persons would be happiest if they were able to substitute previous roles for new ones. The activity theory was the paramount theory in sociological circles for many years until the development of the disengagement theory.

Disengagement theory

This theory proposes that the changes in social roles throughout a person's life are necessary and beneficial for both the individual and society. The disengagement theory argues that there is a disengagement of society from the individual and the individual from society which is inevitable, universal and satisfying to both parties.[23,24] This is necessary to allow younger persons (with newer skills) to enter the workforce, and to allow the retirement and withdrawal of the older person which makes their death less disruptive to a society.[23,24] The disengagement of the older individual from the society is of benefit because it provides a release of responsibilities, and accords a greater amount of freedom to the individual, without any social sanctions.[23] Hence, for the benefit of the individual and of the society, normal ageing should involve a voluntary process of disengagement by both parties.[23] Unfortunately, events such as mandatory retirement or the loss of a spouse are often involuntary and unpredictable, and are thus very damaging to a person's emotional well-being.

Many studies have questioned the validity of the disengagement theory, in terms of both its methods of development and content.[23,25] Indeed, some social gerontologists have called it a myth.[25] Critics attack the theory because it relies on the stereotypes that older persons are weak, frail or incompetent, and that older persons generally perform less well than younger persons; and the theory also assumes that all older people have the same desire to disengage from the society in which they live.[24] Still others question why some of the aged choose to disengage and others do not.[25] Nevertheless, the disengagement theory appears to be useful when explaining an individual's behaviour as opposed to a universal, inevitable behaviour.[23]

The activity theory and the disengagement theory also help to explain a potential problem of great consequence associated with growing old; the roleless role.[23,25] A concept first proposed by Burgess in 1960, a roleless role refers to the retired senior men and women who find themselves having no vital function to perform.[23,25] Similarly, Wood suggested that there is an ambiguity in the norms concerning the behaviour of older persons and that those norms are generally vague, incomplete or simply non-existent.[24] Similar to the concept of *anomie* purposed by Dunkheim, older persons are seen as having no support or guidance from their society.[25] However, recent involvement by older persons in social programmes and renewed political activism suggests that many older adults to not succumb to this potential social problem.

Continuity theory

Continuity theory argues that as individuals age, they strive to maintain continuity in their lifestyle. That is, people feel most satisfied and adapt most successfully to ageing if they are able to continue their roles and activities throughout their lives.[23,24] Thus, a person who is mildly active in their youth will seek to remain only mildly active in their old age.[24] This theory does not predict an absence of change, but rather that an individual must meet the challenges imposed by internal features (attitudes, values, beliefs and temperament) and external features (role relationships and environment change), as well as coping with discontinuity resulting from illness, disability, role loss or loss of skill.[23]

Research exists to support and refute elements of each of these theories.[24] In large part, a person's quality of life and life satisfaction depends on what kinds of activity decline with age, and how this loss is perceived by the individual.[24] As Gerin *et al.* emphasize, 'an individual's personal experience is the only realistic reference for use in subjective quality of life assessment ... it is the person himself who is best qualified to make the assessment'.[26]

Summary

This chapter sought to provide the reader with the key definitions used in the field of geriatrics, the most common challenges facing a practitioner when assessing an older patient, and the different perspectives used by social scientists to study this group of persons. It was also the author's intent to demonstrate to the reader that, in many respects, the definition of a 'geriatric' person is both arbitrary and capricious. Now equipped with this lexicon of terms and concepts used in geriatric health care, the reader is better able to understand many of the concepts explored in greater depth throughout this textbook.

References

1 Hux A, Jarman F, Gleberzon W. America – A History. Toronto: Globe/Modern Curriculum Press, 1987.
2 Morgan L. Innate intelligence: its origins and problems. J Can Chiropractic Assoc 1998; 42: 35–41.
3 Shulman P. Design for living. Sci Am 2000; 11(2): 19–21.
4 Elliot M. Dorlan's Illustrated Medical Dictionary. 28th edn. Philadelphia, PA: WB Saunders, 1994.
5 Ferri F, Fretwell M, Watchel T. Practical Guide to the Care of the Elderly Patient. 2nd edn. St Louis: Mosby-Year Book, 1997.
6 Killinger L, Azad A. Chiropractic Geriatric Education: An Interdisciplinary Resource Guide and Teaching Strategy for Health Educators. US Health Resources and Services Administration Contract, 1997.
7 Abrams W, Beers M, Berkow R. The Merck Manual of Geriatrics. 2nd edn. Whitehouse Station: Merck and Co., 1995.
8 Hawk C, Killinger L, Zapotocky B. Chiropractic training in the care of the geriatric patient: an assessment. J Neuromusculoskeletal Syst 1997; 5: 15–25.
9 Lonergan E. Geriatrics. A Lange Clinical Manual. 1st edn. Stamford, CT: Appleton & Lange, 1996.
10 American Psychiatric Association. Diagnostic and Statistical Manual of Mental Disorders, 4th edn, 1994.
11 Tibbits M. Patients who fall: how to predict and prevent injuries. Geriatrics 1996; 51(9): 24–31.
12 Hoskin AF. Fatal falls: trends and characteristics. Stat Bull Metrop Insur Co 1998; 79(2): 10–15.
13 Gleberzon B, Annis R. The necessity of strength training for the older patient. J Can Chiropractic Assoc 2000; 4: 99–103.
14 Cohen J. Avoiding adverse reactions. Effective lower-dose drug therapies for older patients. Geriatrics 2000; 55(2): 37–43.
15 McCarthy KA. Management consideration in the geriatric patient. Top Clin Chiropractic. 1996; 3(2): 66–75.
16 Lazarou J, Pomeranz B, Corey P. Incidence of adverse drug reactions in hospitalized patients. JAMA 1998; 279: 1200–1205.
17 Van de Velde GM. Benign paroxsymal positional vertigo. Part I: Background and clinical presentation. J Can Chiropractic Assoc 1999; 43(1): 31–39.
18 Douglas F. The dizzy patient: strategic approach to history, examination, diagnosis, and treatment. Chiropractic Technique 1993; 5: 5–16.
19 St. Clair S. Diagnosis and treatment of fibromyalgia syndrome. J Neuromusculoskeletal Syst 1994; 2: 101–111.
20 Blunt K, Rajwani M, Guerriero R. The effectiveness of chiropractic management of fibromyalgia: a pilot study. J Manipulative Physiol Ther 1997; 20: 389–399.
21 Bowers L. Clinical assessment of geriatric patients: unique challenges. Top Clin Chiropractic 1996; 3(2): 10–22.
22 Gleberzon BJ. Chiropractic geriatrics: the challenges of assessing the older patient. J Am Chiropractic Assoc 2000; 4: 36–37.

23 McPherson BD. Aging as a Social Process. An Introduction to Individual and Population Aging. 3rd edn Toronto: Harcourt Brace & Co., 1998.

24 Novak M. Aging & Society. A Canadian Perspective. 3rd edn. Toronto: ITP Nelson, 1997.

25 Barrows GM. Aging, the Individual, and Society. 3rd edn. St Paul, MN: West Publishing Co., 1986.

26 Gerin P, Dazord A, Boissel J, Chifflet R. Quality of life assessment in therapeutic trials: rationale for and presentations of a more appropriate instrument. Fundam Clin Pharmacol 1992; 6: 263–276.

2

Geriatric demographics

Brian J Gleberzon

Why the special concern for older persons? Why is it necessary for educational institutions to devote time in an already-crowded core curriculum for a course specific to geriatrics? Are older persons expected to comprise a significantly large proportion of a practitioner's patient portfolio? Are the concerns of older patients any more important or different than the concerns of younger persons? Do trends in utilization rates of complementary and alternative medical (CAM) practices provide any guidance? These pedagogical questions are best answered by the powerful tool that is demographics.

According to some authorities who specialize in the field, demographics can explain two-thirds of everything.[1] That is to say, if one understands the study of human populations (demographics), in terms of both growth and change, one can explain past events, understand current trends and accurately prognosticate changes yet to come in areas as diverse as health care, education, real estate, employment, retail sales and recreation.[1]

According to David Foote, an economist at the University of Toronto, there are two fundamental principles that empower the field of demographics. The first is the general rule that, every year a person ages, they become 1 year older. Using this rule, one can follow groups as they ascend up population 'pyramids', and thus better understand any changes in societal structure. The other general concept is that people in certain age groups, in general, share common concerns, beliefs and attitudes, despite some individual variability.[1] For example, people in their twenties are, as a rule, more preoccupied with establishing themselves in their chosen vocation, concerned about the financial commitments associated with purchasing a new home, less interested in long-term investments and much more likely to be concerned about issues relating to child welfare, education and daycare. By contrast, older individuals are more established in their jobs and are preparing for retirement, able to spend more time and money on recreational activities (which may explain the current popularity of cruises) and particularly concerned with issues relating to health-care accessibility, cost and quality and the availability of long-term care facilities.[1]

Current and future demographic trends

One of the most important demographic changes in the twentieth century has been the increase in human life expectancy. In 1900, the average life expectancy in the USA was 47 years; in 1990, it was 75 years.[2] This is reflected in the changes in the leading causes of death in the USA between these 2 years (Table 2.1).

Currently, in Canada and the USA, those over the age of 65 years represent about 12% of the total population.[1,4,5] However, by the year 2030, the number of those over the age of 65 is expected to increase to 20% (Figure 2.1).[5,7] In real numbers, this calculates to a total projection of 70 million American seniors by the year 2030,

Table 2.1 Leading causes of death in the USA in 1900 vs 1997[3]

1900	1997
Pneumonia and influenza	Heart disease
Tuberculosis	Cancer
Diarrhoea and intestinal ills	Stroke and brain lesions
Heart disease	Lung disease
Stroke and brain lesions	Accidents
Kidney inflammations	Pneumonia and influenza
Accidents	Diabetes
Cancer	Suicide
Senility	Kidney inflammations
Diphtheria	Liver disease

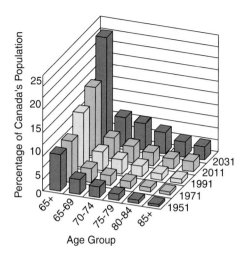

Figure 2.1 Growth of population aged 65+ in Canada between 1951 and 2031. Source: Statistics Canada.[6]

more than twice the number seen in 1990.[8] These numbers may not be apocalyptic, but they are sobering.

Even though they constitute only 12% of the current population, American seniors account for 37% of all hospitalizations and 21% of all visits to physicians, they purchase 31% of all prescription medications and require 36% of total health-care expenditures (about $162 billion).[7,9] This amounts to roughly $5360 per year for each elderly person, compared with $1290 per person per year for younger Americans.[7] However, those numbers are based on data compiled in 1987. Rupert *et al.* estimated the average annual health-care costs for Americans aged 65 years and older in 1994 to be $10 041.[10] In any event, Killinger *et al.* accurately stated that: 'Our nation must recognize that health-care *is* becoming primarily *geriatric* health care and will remain so for quite some time'.[8] This explains the nation-wide, government-funded initiatives in geriatric pedagogy in all areas of health-care delivery.[8] As their numbers rise, it can be prognosticated with confidence that the disproportionately larger percentage of health-care resource utilization by seniors will continue to increase.

Of greatest significance, the fastest growing segment of the population is the 'old' old; those over the age of 85 years.[5] Indeed, as predicted, the number of persons over the age of 85 doubled between the years 1990 and 2000,[5] and the number of those over the age of 100 is expected to increase 11-fold by the year 2050, when the number of American centenarians is predicted to exceed 800 000.[11] Given that these groups of people are

more likely to experience multiple health problems concurrently, the potential economic impact on health-care costs is enormous.

The baby boomers

The demographic reality that the population is ageing in countries such as Canada, the USA, the UK and Australia is primarily due to the confluence of two events: an increase in life expectancy (primarily due to advances in technology) and the ageing of the demographic group known as the baby boomers. Born in the years following World War II, from 1947 to 1966, the baby boomers represent the largest cohort group in many industrialized countries.[1] In Canada, the baby boomers represent 34% of the population, or 10 million persons (Figures 2.2 and 2.3).[1,5] The USA, Australia, New Zealand and the UK all have a similar baby boomer group, but none is proportionately as large as Canada's.[1]

There is one principal feature of this segment of the population that makes it so powerful and influential: its size. Because there are so many of them, and because they generally share similar attitudes and concerns, the impact that baby boomers have on all areas of political, social, cultural and economic life cannot be understated. The attention bestowed on many 'issues of the day' can be directly attributed to the boomers. For example, in the 1960s, when many of the boomers were in universities, issues related to that milieu were at the forefront of the American agenda. In the 1980s, when the boomers were more settled and now had children of their own (the so-called echo generation, the children of the boomers), the political arena turned its collective attention to child welfare and education. Today, with the leading edge of the boomers having turned 50 in 1996, concerns have shifted to issues related to social security, health reform and long-term nursing care. Throughout their progression along the demographic continuum, because they constitute such a large cohort, the concerns of the boomers have dominated the industrial world.[1]

Demographers have developed a new term to describe the distinctive profile of the boomers' population growth: rectangularization.[1] The visual concept is fairly easy to understand.

A chart depicting population numbers is typically in the form of a pyramid because there are usually more children alive than there are older people. Such

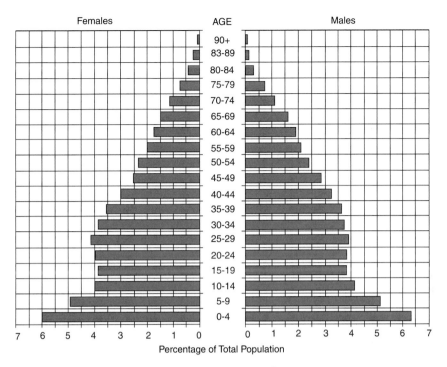

Figure 2.2 Canada's population pyramid, 1951. Source: Statistics Canada.[6]

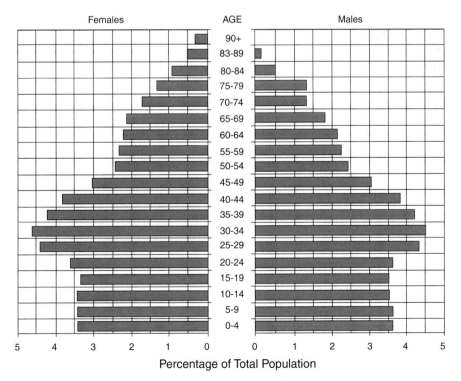

Figure 2.3 Canada's population pyramid, 1991. Source: Statistics Canada.[6]

population pyramids exist currently in countries such as Mexico and India. However, the baby boomers produce a rectangular 'bulge' that progresses up a population pyramid as they age (remember demographic rule no. 1: every year a person lives they become 1 year older). Thus, we have a rectangular baby boomer bulge migrating up the population pyramid.

The dependency ratio

The dependency ratio is the ratio of the number of persons in economically dependent segments of the population to the number of persons in economically productive segments of the population.[5] For the discussion here, the old-age dependency ratio is of particular importance. This ratio is the number of those aged 65 years and older compared with the number of individuals in the 'working age' range of 18–64 years:[5]

$$\text{Old-age dependency ratio} = \frac{\text{65 and over age group}}{\text{18–64 age group}} \times 100$$

In countries such as Canada and the USA, the dependency ratio increases as the population becomes proportionately older. In Canada, the dependency ratio increased from 14.3% in 1961 to 18.3% in 1991, an increase of 28% (Figure 2.4).[5] In essence, over a 30-year span, 28% more older adults are now being supported by the 'working population'.

The dependency ratio is often cited as a significant source of intergenerational strife in countries such as Canada and the USA. On the one hand, older people maintain that they have contributed to social security and health care programmes (Medicare and the like)

during the years they were working by paying taxes, and are therefore entitled to access these programmes now that they need them in their old age. In essence, older persons see themselves as withdrawing moneys and resources that they contributed during their youth, and are not economically relying on the younger generation's altruistic hand-outs. On the other hand, working adults maintain that the funds contributed by older persons were not proportional to the current costs of health care and other resources. This is because people are living substantially longer than in the past and are doing so with chronic illnesses that require expensive technological interventions to manage.

Trends in CAM utilization

Utilization rates of CAMs have surged since the late 1980s. A demographic study conducted by Eisenberg et al. in the USA and published in 1998 revealed that almost 50% of respondents had been to a CAM practitioner, an almost 50% increase from his original study of a decade earlier.[13,14] The researchers calculated that this represented an increase from 427 million total visits in 1990 to 629 million visits (by 22 million people) in 1997, a number that exceeded the total visits to all US primary-care physicians.[13] The total cost for CAM providers was conservatively estimated at $21.2 billion in 1997, with $12.2 billion paid for by the patient out-of-pocket.[13] This exceeded the 1997 out-of-pocket expenditures for all American hospitalizations.[13] The total out-of-pocket expenditure of alternative therapies of all kinds was conservatively estimated to be $27 billion.[13]

Certain therapies, such as the use of herbal medicines, massage, megavitamins, self-help groups, folk medicine, energy healing and homoeopathy, increased the most in the decade between the two studies by Eisenberg et al..[13] The average demographic profile of a CAM user was Caucasian, age 25–49 years, and of higher education and higher income than non-users of CAM services.[13] Thus, the age group of highest utilization of CAMs encompassed the baby boomer. Women were more likely to use CAMs; African-Americans were the least likely to use CAMs. Utilization of CAM providers for individuals over the age of 50 years remained at 35% during the two different studies, which represented the largest demographic age group of users.[13] A more recent study by Shua-Haim and Ross[15] also reported that utilization rates of CAM by

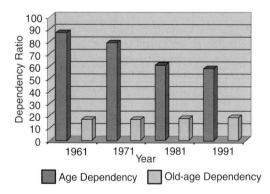

Figure 2.4 Age and old-age dependency ratios for Canada, 1961–2001. Source: Statistics Canada.[12]

older persons were increasing. According to their study, the most common forms of alternative and unconventional therapies used by older persons include relaxation therapy, chiropractic, acupuncture, massage therapy and herbal, vitamin and mineral supplementation.[15]

The pattern of use for unconventional providers was more common than for conventional providers for five of the 10 most frequently cited medical conditions.[13] The most common chief complaints that prompted patients to consult a CAM provider were, in descending order, chronic low back and neck pain, anxiety, depression, headaches, fatigue, insomnia, arthritis, and sprains and strains.[13] One-third of patients presented with more than one of these problems. Patients with back problems, neck problems, headaches, and sprains and strains were most likely to seek out chiropractic care.[13] Of particular interest, in both studies, was that 50% of those who utilized a CAM practitioner did not tell their medical doctor that they were doing so.[13,14]

National surveys conducted outside the USA suggest that CAMs are popular throughout the industrialized world. Studies have estimated that utilization rates of CAM providers were 10% in Denmark, 33% in Finland and 49% in Australia, and public opinion polls and consumers' associations suggest high prevalence rates throughout the rest of Europe and the UK.[13] The percent age of the Canadian population who sought out the services of CAMs was estimated at 15% in 1994.[13]

Visits to chiropractors and massage therapists accounted for nearly half of all visits to CAM practitioners in 1997.[13] Roughly 11% of respondents in the study sought out chiropractic care, and visits to a chiropractor accounted for 30% of CAM total visits.[13] Others have estimated that 27 million Americans sought chiropractic care in 1999.[16] Patients with back problems, neck problems, headaches, and sprains and strains were most likely to seek chiropractic care.[11] Visits to a naturopath accounted for about 0.7% of total CAM use.[13]

Older patients with problems other than spinal pain may also seek out CAM care. In a prospective study of patients with prostatic carcinoma undergoing radiation therapy, 39% were found to rely also on complementary health practices not prescribed by their medical practitioners.[17] In contrast, physicians believed that only 4% of their patients reported to these practices. CAM treatment was continued even after initiation of definitive treatment for prostatic carcinoma. Patients seeking out CAM care tended to have higher education and income. Herbal remedies were the most frequently used CAM (60%), followed by traditional remedies (47%), high-dose vitamins (41%), chiropractic, massage and relaxation techniques (18% each) and special diets (12%).[17] More recent studies of rheumatology patients reported between 40.7% and 66% use of CAM.[18] Similarly, a survey of 103 patients referred for rehabilitation outpatient care revealed that 29.1% had used a CAM in the past 12 months.[19] The most common CAMs used were massage therapy, chiropractic, vitamins and mineral supplementation, and acupuncture.[18]

A survey by Austin[20] found several variables to be predictive of CAM use, including higher education, slightly poorer health status, a holistic orientation towards health care and a personal transformation experience. CAM users tended to identify with cultural values that included a commitment to environmentalism, feminism, and an interest in spirituality and personal growth psychology.[20,21] As Meeker noted, contrary to popular opinion, dissatisfaction with conventional medicine was not prevalent and was not predictive of CAM use.[21] Please also refer to Chapter 27 for a more detailed description of homoeopathy, podiatry and naturopathy.

Attitudes about health care

A recent poll conducted by the National Coalition on Health Care in Washington DC revealed some intriguing attitudes held by Americans.[22] Of the 1011 respondents, 79% reported that they lacked confidence in the US health-care system, with only 15% of respondents expressing 'complete confidence' in the American health-care system.[22] Moreover, in spite of the fact that the major chronic diseases (heart disease, cancer, diabetes, obstructive pulmonary disease and liver disease) are in large part preventable, the US health-care system spent only 0.07% of its total budget on prevention, an average of $1.21 per person.[22]

A study by Lee and Kasper sought to assess the level of satisfaction with medical care reported by older patients in the USA.[23] Overall, elderly patients reported very high levels of satisfaction with the general quality of medical care that they received from their family physician. Respondents reported satisfaction rates exceeding 90% in areas of overall quality of care, follow-up care and information provided. Perceived satisfaction of physicians' qualities in specific areas was also very favourable. Reported satisfaction rates exceeded 90% in areas such as levels of competence, understanding of the patient's medical history, diagnostic abilities ('understands what is wrong') and thoroughness ('checks everything'). Quite surprisingly, older patients placed greater importance on a physician's technical skills than on the physician's interpersonal skills. There were some areas in which older patients were less satisfied with the care they received. Some older patients in this study felt that physicians seemed to be in a hurry, that they did not explain or discuss the patient's problem with them, and some patients felt that the doctor was 'doing them a favour' by examining them.[23] One potentially important finding of the study was that there appears to be a negative association between the patient's age and favourable assessment of medical care.[23] Compared with elderly white people, elderly black people were much less likely to be highly satisfied with access, global quality or the technical skills of their physician.[23]

Medical attitudes towards complementary and alternative medicine

Studies indicate that there has been an increased interest in and acceptance of CAM within the medical community. For example, of the 117 (of 125) medical schools in the USA that responded to a survey documenting information about CAM education within their curricula, 64% offered some type of CAM instruction.[21] Most classes offered were electives, although some institutions provided information within required courses. Common topics included chiropractic, acupuncture, homoeopathy, herbal therapies and mind–body techniques. In another study, when asked, 39% medical physicians described chiropractic as a 'legitimate medical practice'.[21]

A practice pattern analysis by Ko and Berbrayer sought to describe the attitudes and behaviour of Canadian physicians with respect to CAM.[18] In this study, 98 Canadian physiatrists were surveyed: 72% reported referring to a CAM therapist (12.5% often) and 20% had training in and 20% practised some form of alternative medicine. The therapists most highly rated in terms of usefulness were acupuncture (85%), biofeedback (81%) and chiropractic (80%). Sixty-three

per cent of respondents thought that alternative medicines had ideas and methods that would be beneficial to physiatrists. Less than 38.8% of respondents believed that CAM worked by the placebo effect and only 9% of this group thought that CAMs were a threat to public health. This contrasts with an earlier 1990 study of Canadian family physicians, which found that 21% felt CAM to be a threat.[24] CAM referrals and utilization appeared to be higher in younger, more recently graduated physiatrists.[23]

Utilization rates of chiropractic care by older patients

As mentioned, the largest group seeking CAMs comprised those over the age of 50 years. The incidence of low back complaints among older patients, although less than in those aged 45–65, is significantly high. A study of the rural elderly in Iowa reported that 22% of the subjects had experienced back pain during the past year.[2] A larger review of the literature on low back pain among the elderly was conducted by Bressler *et al.*[25] They concluded that, while there is a general underrepresentation of the older population in the back-pain literature, the prevalence of back pain in the elderly is between 13 and 49%.[25] Again, these numbers are important when one remembers that neuromusculoskeletal impairments are the most common chronic condition causing activity limitation in the USA[9] and increasing age has been associated with an increase in musculoskeletal symptoms.[25] For persons under the age of 45 years, back pain is the most common cause of activity limitation; for those between the ages of 45 and 65, it ranks fourth.[9]

Coulter *et al.* reported that older persons are overrepresented among chiropractic patients.[9] In Canada (in 1994), the over-65 population comprised 14.1% of chiropractic patients, while this group was only 8.7% of the total population.[9] A survey conducted by the American Chiropractic Association reported that, in the USA, the over-65 population constitutes between 15 and 17% of a chiropractor's patient portfolio, while representing 12% of the total population.[9] If this relationship between population numbers and chiropractic utilization were to remain constant, when older patients comprise 20% of the total population, they could represent 25% of a chiropractor's patient profile.

Demographic features of older patients seeking out chiropractic care

A recent article by Hawk *et al.* sought to characterize patients over the age of 55 years who presented for chiropractic care.[26] This practice-based research study involved 121 chiropractors in Canada and the USA. A total of 8312 patients participated in the study, 805 of whom were over the age of 65 years. The investigators reported that those patients in the study group (age 55+) were predominately female (60.1%), white (94.7%), married (66.3%), high-school graduates (54.0%) and retired (68.0%).[26]

Height and weight information was available from 656 of the study patients. From this information, the body mass index (BMI) was calculated (see Chapter 5): 20% of patients were obese and 38.6% were overweight. Overall, 50% of the study patients reported taking regular exercise and 71% reported using vitamins and food supplements. Over half of the patients reported never smoking. Blood-pressure information was available for 590 patients (73.3%). Of these, almost 10% had hypertension.[26]

Not surprisingly, the most common chief presenting complaint was back pain: 32.9% of patients cited back pain in a single location only and 35.5% of patients cited multiple locations (such as 'back and leg' or 'neck and shoulder').[26] Most complaints were chronic, with 54.9% of patients having onset of symptoms more than 6 weeks before presenting to the practitioner. Forty-six per cent of patients reported that had seen another provider for their current complaint. Using a Pain Disability Index scale, most patients reported their pain to be only mild or moderate in intensity.[26]

In this study 56.6% of patients were treated using an Activator, a mechanical manually assisted instrument that generated a low-amplitude, high-velocity force (this finding is undoubtedly related to the participation of chiropractors who use Activator technique in this study, which was the only professional organization that responded to the researcher's recruitment efforts). Spinal manipulative therapy was the next most commonly used therapeutic intervention, with 23.5% of patients receiving this type of treatment. In addition to spinal adjustments, the most commonly administered procedures were recommendations for exercise at least 20 min three times per week (41.0% of patients), instruction on the use of heat or cold application at home (24.5%) and recommendations on food supplements (24.5%). Other procedures used less often included ice packs in the office (13.5%), ultrasound (12.3%), hot packs (11.3%), electrical stimulation, massage therapy, corrective exercises and diet (each used on under 10% but over 5% of patients). Procedures used on fewer than 5% of patients were acupressure, traction, orthotic fitting, recommendation of bed rest, acupuncture, recommendations for weight loss and homoeopathy. An important finding in this study was that pain medication use decreased after 4 weeks of care among the group of patients who were discharged by the clinician, but not among those who patients who either self-discharged or were continuing with care.[26]

The researchers concluded that musculoskeletal complaints composed nearly the entire case load of the chiropractors in this study, a finding consistent with other demographic studies. Moreover, the researchers concluded that, based on the data collected, many patients (66.6%) seek only chiropractic care for complaints related to mild to moderate musculoskeletal complaints, whereas patients with more severe pain were more likely to seek out both chiropractic and medical treatment.[26]

Chiropractic maintenance care and the older patient

Although the literature indicates that older patients primarily seek out chiropractic care for spinal pain, there is evidence to suggest that patients may continue with care for reasons other than symptom relief. For example, surveys by Rupert *et al.* sought to investigate the primary care health promotion activities associated with what has been historically termed 'maintenance care' in both chiropractors and chiropractic patients over the age of 65 years.[10,27] Maintenance care can be defined as periodic visits that seek to prevent disease, prolong life, promote health and enhance quality of life.[27] Specific schedules of treatment are theoretically designed to provide for a patient's well-being or to maintain their optimum state of health.[28] In contrast to crisis care (during which symptoms are present) and supportive care, symptoms need not be present during a maintenance care appointment. Supportive care is for those patients who have reached maximum therapeutic benefits but who fail to sustain this benefit and progressively worsen when there are periodic trials of treatment withdrawal.[28] In the absence of supportive care, symptoms re-emerge.

In this study, 658 chiropractors were surveyed and their attitudes relating to the importance of maintenance care compiled. Notwithstanding the absence of any scientific support, the majority of American chiropractors who responded to the survey believed in the value of maintenance care for patients of all ages for a variety of conditions ranging from stress to musculoskeletal and visceral conditions, with 79% of chiropractic patients receiving recommendations to enter a maintenance care programme.[27] Ninety per cent of respondents (chiropractors) agreed or strongly agreed with the statement that the purpose of maintenance care was to optimize health, 88% stated that it was to prevent conditions from developing, 86% reported that they were providing palliative care and 95% believed that they were minimizing recurrences or exacerbations.[27] It was estimated that 23% of all chiropractic income in the USA was generated from maintenance care, and similar studies conducted in England and Australia found that chiropractors in those countries also suggested maintenance care for a significant portion of their patients.[27]

In a companion study, Rupert *et al.* sought to investigate information regarding multiple health issues of those chiropractic patients aged 65 years and over who have had a long-term regimen of maintenance care.[10] The study reported that elderly patients receiving maintenance care did not rely solely on chiropractic care but instead utilized both medical and chiropractic services. The average number of visits to a medical doctor by patients aged 65 and older under chiropractic maintenance care was 4.8 visits per year, which is approximately half the national average of nine visits per year.[10] This differs from previous studies by Coulter *et al.* which concluded that chiropractic care complemented rather than replaced medical care.[9]

According to the study by Rupert *et al.*, most chiropractors used diversified techniques (70.4%) for older patients receiving maintenance care.[10] Other named techniques utilized, in descending order, were Activator (28.3%), Thompson terminal point (21.9%), Nimmo/soft-tissue techniques (20.6%), applied kinesiology (16.1%) and sacro-occipital technique (13.5%).[10] Thirty-eight per cent of elderly patients were treated for chronic health problems, while 61.7% were not.[10] Eighty-three per cent of older patients were treated to control or prevent musculoskeletal conditions, 31.2% visceral problems and 73.3% subluxations.[10] The need for hospitalization was markedly reduced for patients receiving maintenance care.[10] The total annual cost of health-care services for older patients receiving maintenance chiropractic care was conservatively estimated at only one-third of the expenses required by American citizens of the same age who did not receive maintenance care. Lastly, there was a significant positive correlation between a reduced use of non-prescription drugs and the number of years under maintenance chiropractic care.[10]

One of the most interesting findings in this study was the response by patients to the question: 'How important do you feel chiropractic treatment has been in maintaining and promoting your health?' An overwhelming 95.8% patients believed that maintenance care was either considerably or extremely valuable.[10]

With the exception of total annual visits to medical doctors, the studies by Rupert *et al.* closely paralleled earlier studies by Coulter *et al.*[9] In their study, Coulter *et al.* reported that chiropractic patients were less likely to have been hospitalized, less likely to have used a nursing care facility, more likely to report a better health status, more likely to exercise and more likely to be mobile in their community.[9] In addition, chiropractic patients were less likely to use prescription medication.[9] Of course, this may reflect more the general behaviour of people who seek out chiropractic care than any benefits directly attributable to chiropractic treatment.

Future trends in health care

If CAM providers wish to position themselves strategically at the forefront of health-care, there must be an emphasis on developing interdisciplinary networks.[4,8] An interdisciplinary approach allows for a collaborative effort to provide optimal patient care.[8] This can only be achieved by nurturing respect among different health-care providers.[8] This means that all providers, both allopathic and drugless, should put aside and lay to rest any historical differences each may have, which are often based on stereotypical prejudices. Regrettably, there are those in all camps who would oppose collaborative networking. Daunting though the process may be, it becomes incumbent upon those with the foresight and wisdom to pursue and establish this network of interdisciplinary teams to do so, in order to achieve the highest level of patient care.

An ageing population may have a cataclysmic impact on the economics of both managed care (in the

USA) and socialized medicine (in Canada and the UK). However, the baby boomers are nothing if not impatient. It is unlikely they will sit back idly as health-care changes reduce coverage and accessibility, causing long delays in diagnostic tests and therapeutic procedures. Given the baby boomers' size, clout and historical audacity, issues relating to health-care reform will undoubtedly stay at the forefront of the political agenda. One solution (for good or bad), even in countries with socialized medicine such as Canada, is the development of a two-tiered health system.[1] Others solutions for health-care cost containment may be an integrated health-care system.[1,29] Those in charge of deriving solutions for the health-care systems in baby boom countries will, like Odysseus, have to choose between the Scylla of providing the ageing population with the best health care that technology can provide and the Charybdis of its mounting cost.

References

1 Foote D. Boom, Bust & Echo. Profiting From the Demographic Shift in the New Millennium. Toronto: Macfarlane, Walter & Ross, 1998.

2 Hawk C, Killinger L, Zapotocky B, Azad A. Chiropractic training in care of the geriatric patient: an assessment. J Neuromusculoskeletal Syst 1997; 5: 15–25.

3 Brandstrader JR. From baby boomer to geezer glut. Sci Am 2000; 11(2): 23–29.

4 US Bureau of the Census, Statistical Abstracts of the United States. 1994 data.

5 Elliot G, Hunt M, Hutchison K. Facts on Aging in Canada. Office of Gerontological Studies, McMaster University, Hamilton, Ontario, Canada, 1996.

6 Population and Elderly. Ottawa: Statistics Canada, 1993.

7 Department of Health and Human Services. A Profile of Older Americans. Administration on Aging and the Program Resources Department, American Association or Retired Persons, 1996.

8 Killinger L, Azad A, Zapotocky B, Morschhauser E. Development of a model curriculum in chiropractic geriatric education; process and content. J Neuromusculoskeletal Syst 1998; 6: 146–153.

9 Coulter I, Hurwitz E, Aranow H et al. Chiropractic patients in a comprehensive home-based geriatric assessment, follow-up and health promotion program. Top Clin Chiropractic 1996; 3(2): 46–55.

10 Rupert R, Manello D, Sandefur R. Maintenance care: health promotion services administered to US chiropractic patients aged 65 and older, Part II. J Manipulative Physiol Ther 2000; 23: 10–19.

11 Brown K. How long have you got? Sci Am 2000; 11: 9–15.

12 Kerr D, Ram B. Focus on Canada – Population Dynamics in Canada. Ottawa: Statistics Canada, 1994.

13 Eisenberg D, Davis R, Ettner S et al. Trends in alternative medicine use in the United States, 1990–1997. JAMA 1998; 280: 1569–1575.

14 Eisenberg D, Kessler R, Foster C et al. Unconventional medicine use in the United States. N Engl J Med 1993; 328: 246–252.

15 Shua-Haim JR, Ross JS. Alternative medicine in geriatrics: competing with or complementing conventional medicine. Clin Geriatrics 1999; 7(6): 37–40.

16 Presented at the Association of Chiropractic Colleges, San Antonio, Texas, March 16–19, 2000.

17 Ko GD, Devine P. Use of complementary health practices by prostate carcinoma patients undergoing radiation therapy. Cancer 2000; 88: 615–619.

18 Ko GD, Berbrayer D. Complementary and alternative medicine: Canadian physiatrists' attitudes and behavior. Arch Phys Med Rehabil 2000; 81: 662–667.

19 Wainapel SF, Thomas AD, Kahan BS. Use of alternative therapies by rehabilitation outpatients. Arch Phys Med Rehabil 1998; 79: 1002–1005.

20 Austin JA. Why patients use alternative medicine. JAMA 1998; 279: 1569–1575.

21 Meeker WC. Public demand and the integration of complementary and alternative medicine in the US health care system. J Manipulative Physiol Ther 2000; 23: 123–126.

22 Anonymous. 79% lack confidence in US Health Care. Alternative Medicine, 1997; 19: 112–117.

23 Lee Y, Kasper J. Assessment of medical care by elderly people: general satisfaction and physician quality. Health Serv Res 1998; 32: 741–758.

24 Verhoef MJ, Sutherland LR. Alternative medicine and general practitioners: opinions and behavior. Can Fam Physician J 1995; 41: 1005–1011.

25 Bressler H, Keyes W, Rochon P, Badley E. The prevalence of low back pain in the Elderly. A systematic review of the literature. Spine 1999; 24: 1813–1819.

26 Hawk C, Long CR, Boulanger KT et al. Chiropractic care for patients aged 55 years and older: report from a practice-based research program. J Am Geriatr Soc 2000; 48: 534–545.

27 Rupert R. A survey of practice patterns and the health promotion and prevention attitudes of US chiropractors. Maintenance care; Part 1. J Manipulative Physiol Ther 2000; 23: 1–9.

28 Henderson D, Chapman-Smith D, Mior S, Vernon H. Clinical guidelines for chiropractic practice in Canada. J Can Chiropractic Assoc 1994; 38(1), Supplement.

29 Manga P. Trends in health care economics and their impact on chiropractic practice. Top Clin Chiropractic 2000; 7(1): 48–52.

3

Elderly people and their concerns

William Gleberzon

Elderly people, or seniors, are human beings at another, older, stage of life, rather than a separate species. Understanding this truth will make better chiropractors, health-care professionals – and human beings. The purpose of this brief study is to present the concerns that seniors have so that chiropractors can treat the whole person holistically, rather than just the physical complaint or an 'old person'. This chapter will set the context of the great ageing revolution, explore who seniors are and what characterizes them, and explore some of their common concerns such as ageism, financial issues, health and health care, sexuality, retirement, housing, crime and transportation.

Context: the great revolution

The world is on the cusp of one of the greatest revolutions in human experience. For the first time in recorded history, more human beings than ever will live into advanced old age. According to the Bible, the allotted life span of human beings is 'three score and ten' or 70 years. As described in Chapter 2, the fastest growing segment of the North American population is among people 85 years of age and older.[1] By 2050, 25% of the elderly will be over 85, compared with about 15% today[2–4] By the end of the second decade of the twenty-first century, millions of people will live to be over 100 years of age.[5] This is more than double the life expectancy of white males only 100 years ago.[5] In addition, as scientific knowledge of the genetic map of human beings, ongoing medical technology and pharmaceutical innovations progress exponentially over the next decades, coupled with improved hygiene, nutrition and disease prevention, the prolongation of life may increase even more. Old age on this magnitude is a totally new phenomenon for society.

As this new century dawns, there are about 3.5 million seniors in Canada and about 34 million in the USA.[4,6,7] By 2030, the number of seniors in Canada will more than quadruple, representing about 25% of the population, and number about 70 million in the USA, or 20% of the population.[2–4,6,7] These older people will remain a dominant and obvious part of the social landscape until at least the ninth decade of the century.

Given the right genetic inheritance, a good lifestyle and luck, not only will older people be living longer, but they will be healthier for a longer period of their lives. They will be better educated than previous generations of seniors and higher education is one of the key determinants of good health. They will be more aware of how to prevent disease and to maintain a high quality of health. Exercise, better medical care and greater use of alternative medicines and of health-care professionals (such as chiropractors) will provide the possibility of a better standard of well-being. These new seniors will be wealthier, which is another key determinant of good health, than their ancestors owing to the existence of public pensions systems in the USA, particularly social security, and in Canada, particularly old age security (OAS), guaranteed income supplement and the Canada pension plan (CPP). Many of them will also have saved for their retirement. The new generation of seniors will be likely to be computer literate, and using innovative telecommunications linkages older people will be able to remain independent and active for longer periods.

Despite this rosy picture, older people have a number of concerns. However, before we look at these concerns, we have to answer the following questions.

Who are seniors?

The answer to that question is linked to a specific age. Today, seniors are generally defined as anyone in their mid-sixties because that is the age at which they begin to receive public pension. In turn, public pensions commence because it is assumed that people stop working for pay at this time. Thereafter, seniors are assumed to be retired. In the USA, the age at which the public pension, that is social security, begins to be paid is increasing over the next 20 years, a month at a time, to 67. In Canada, OAS is provided from the public treasury, that is, paid for by general income taxes, to everyone from the age of 65. The CPP, the equivalent of US social security, was designed to be accessed at age 65. However, it can be claimed at the age of 60, with a life-long penalty, or 70, with a life-long bonus.

Today, the traditional definition of a senior may be in need of revision. An older worker, sometimes described as an 'experienced worker', is defined at the age of 45 and North Americans are retiring from work at an average age of 61–62 years. Mandatory retirement at any age does not exist legally in Canada, although corporations can determine retirement policies. In the USA, a mandatory retirement policy can be adopted by companies with over 20 employees. Nevertheless, 6% of Canadians and about 9% of Americans aged over 65 years are still in the workforce.[4,8] Some analysts believe that these percentages of working seniors will increase over the coming years as they experience better health, desire to keep active and engaged, require more money to sustain themselves or are needed by their industry or professions, especially when employees may have been downsized too vigorously.

What characterizes seniors?

Many gerontologists, those who study seniors from a non-medical perspective, characterize seniors on the basis of their common 'normative history-graded events' or generational experiences.[9] According to this view, the current generation of seniors was shaped by the unifying experience of the roaring 'twenties, the crash of the stock market in 1929 and ensuing great depression and World War II. Those born during World War II may have been shaped by the absence of their fathers who had gone overseas to fight in the war. World War II babies are considered the forgotten generation, eclipsed by the depression babies, who preceded them, and the baby boomers, who succeeded them. However, some sociologists suggest that the World War II babies might actually represent the first wave of the baby boomers, rather than a distinct generation.

In turn, the baby boomers, who are those people born between 1946/1947 and about 1965, were the first generation to have had their early formative years shaped by television, rock-and-roll music, the atomic bomb and the cold war, although these novel experiences probably had a similar impact on the slightly older World War II babies. In any event, the sheer number of baby boomers also affected their experiences because of how society accommodated or, some have said, pampered and spoiled them by building more schools and universities when the baby boomers needed them.

Another way in which seniors are characterized is on the basis of age bands: pre-seniors, 55–64 years; young-seniors, 65–74; middle-seniors, 75–84; and old seniors, 85-plus.[9,10]

However, this characterization has to be treated gingerly because its broad sweep can easily shade into stereotyping. It infers that all people born during a certain period and, consequently, of a generally similar age, are somehow identical in their thoughts and behaviour. It disregards individual differences as well as intragenerational differences and similarities within any and all generations, regardless of age.

In reality, people who are the same general age do not all adopt the same ideological or political beliefs. All of them do not enjoy the same economic status, whether rich, middling or poor. All of them do not have the same tastes in music, books, sports, dress or styles. All of them are not frail, nor are they all active.

Therefore, within the population over 65, people differ about as much as people under 65 and people do not magically change because of their age. It is important to reiterate that people over 65 are not a different species of human being from those under 65. Rather, they are the same people at a different stage in their life. Nor do their personalities or behaviour patterns necessarily change from what they had been when they were younger.

At the same time, however, despite individual differences, people over 65 have many basic concerns in common.

What are some of the common concerns of seniors?

Ageism

Many seniors feel that they are not respected and are even discriminated against on account of their age. Prejudicial attitudes and behaviours against older people on account of their age are called ageism.

Ageism manifests itself through a variety of misconceptions about seniors, such as:

- all seniors are alike and predictable
- all seniors live in institutions
- all seniors are frail, sick, dependent or senile
- all seniors are rich
- all seniors cannot learn new things (such as how to operate computers)
- all seniors are useless and waiting to die
- all seniors feel isolated and lonely
- all seniors feel lost in retirement and die soon after they retire
- all seniors are more easily victimized than younger people
- all seniors are devoid of sexual feelings

and so on.

All of these myths and stereotypes are both nonsense and ageist. First, any perception about any people, regardless of age, that states 'all those people are …' usually reflects personal prejudice. Secondly, none of the propositions above is true. For example:

- Those 65 and older and those under 20 years are the fastest growing users of computers and the internet.
- Studies demonstrate that seniors do not spend their days thinking about death.
- If individuals have prepared for retirement, they are not lost once they retire. In fact, they enjoy it.
- Younger people are more victimized by crime than are seniors.
- Many seniors continue to pay back society through volunteering for a host of causes and services. They provide financial and other support for children and grandchildren, such as babysitting.
- In 1999, about 17% of Canadian seniors and about 10% of American seniors lived in poverty.[4,7,8] Many more lived just above the poverty line.
- Other Canadian seniors winter in the southern USA. Dubbed 'snowbirds', these seniors are assumed to personify all seniors, as being wealthy enough to afford this expensive pleasure. In reality, they represent about 5–10% of seniors at most and many of them do not spend an extended period there. Even this number is dwindling as the value of the Canadian dollar relative to the American dollar decreases and the cost of out-of-country health and travel insurance, which is a must for Canadians visiting the USA, increases with the onset of age and pre-existing health conditions, even though venturing to warmer climates is good for health and general well-being, regardless of age.
- Seniors do have sexual feelings, a topic which will be dealt with in more detail later.

The essence of ageism is captured in the following sad and bad joke: An old woman goes to her doctor to complain about her painful knee. 'What do you expect?' the doctor says, 'You're old and wearing down.' 'Well,' responds the old lady, 'My other knee is old too and it doesn't hurt!'

There is a great deal of anecdotal evidence about second-class care being given to seniors in hospitals, although offsetting evidence suggests that this may not reflect reality. Nevertheless, doctors receive only a few hours of training on geriatrics. Geriatricians, doctors who specialize in the illness of seniors, are not being graduated, while those already in practice are being advised to take up another specialty. Indeed, more geriatricians may be needed to deal with the concurrence and complexity of multiple diseases that afflict many older people.

Ageism is at the heart of many of the predictions about the future crisis in health care and public pensions due to the ageing population. It also accounts for the common greater difficulty for people aged over 45 in the job market. It underlies the rationale for downsizing employees when they reach their fifties. It creates intergenerational conflict.

What causes ageism? In part it is a manifestation of cultural attitudes in North American and elsewhere which venerate youth as the new and improved and denigrates the old, which is associated with decline and decay. This perception is reflected in the saying, 'you can't teach an old dog new tricks'. However, some research suggests that mental decline in humans amounts to 5–15% of mental capability over a lifetime, starting at about the age of 26.[11]

In part, of course, ageism arises from the conceptual link between old age and death. The antidote for ageism is knowledge about the realities of ageing and interacting with older persons as people.

Gender and race

The majority of older seniors are women since, statistically, women outlive men.[2,7,8] Therefore, ageism may also have an underlying sexist bias. In fact, of all seniors, older men who are married and living with their spouses are healthiest and happiest, according to studies.

In the USA, life expectancy is lower and poverty is higher among black and Hispanic Americans than among Caucasian Americans.[8] Nevertheless, the percentage of Hispanic American seniors will triple from 4% today to about 12% by 2040.[8] This racial/ethnic pattern may also apply in Canada. In both countries, First Nations or Native people generally live shorter and poorer lives.

North America is still a land of immigrants, a melting pot in the USA and a mosaic in Canada. Unfortunately, deficiency in English can be a barrier to information about entitlements and services, especially for non-English–speaking seniors. At the same time, many native-born seniors are also unaware of entitlements and services because of the lack of proper information from governments and the authorities.

Financial issues: retirement income

Retirement income is a major concern for seniors, regardless of their age, socioeconomic status, gender, geographical location or any other factor.

The distribution of income among seniors is about the same as that among the non-senior population but, since women outlive men, a minority of wealthy widows are balanced by a majority of poor widows. In the USA, about 10% of seniors and in Canada about 17% of seniors have incomes below the poverty line.[8] The percentage of seniors, males and females, singles and couples, who live in poverty has greatly declined over the last few decades because of the existence of public pensions in both countries. Still, about 40% of Canadian seniors receive guaranteed income supplement, which the federal government pays to poor seniors.[9] In both countries, the current generation of older women, about 42% of older women in Canada, is particularly blighted by poverty,[7] because a large number of these women were not gainfully employed and therefore they did not contribute to social security or the CPP. However, they can receive a survivor's benefit from these plans after their husbands have died as, of course, do men who survive their wives. In Canada, all women over 65 also receive OAS, independently from their husbands, who also receive this public pension.

In Canada, the retirement income system has three parts:

- The public pension system consists of OAS, which is received by all Canadians who reach the age of 65. As noted, those who are below the poverty line are also eligible for guaranteed income supplement. This universal pension is paid by the federal government through public taxes. Some provinces will also top up the retirement incomes of poor seniors.
- The CPP, to which all employees and their employers pay an equal share, is administered by the federal and provincial governments on behalf of the contributors.
- Corporate pension plans, including private companies and public service, are becoming scarcer Retirement savings plans (RSPs) or registered retirement savings plans (RRSPs) are available, to which everyone can contribute up to a certain amount of their earned income which is designated by the federal government.

In the USA, the retirement income system consists of:

- social security: poorer seniors can receive supplementary social insurance (SSI) and food stamps
- public or private corporate pensions
- savings plans, e.g. defined contribution plans such as 104(k) and individual retirement accounts (IRAs).

All pensions in both countries are taxed. During the 1980s, taxes on social security were increased 14 times.[12] A recent bill now allows recipients of social security between the ages of 65 and 69 to continue to receive the pension if they work, no matter how much they earn. As noted, the age at which social security could be accessed is gradually being raised to 67, which will affect younger baby boomers. It is interesting to note that seniors who opposed these changes were castigated in the media as 'greedy geezers'.

During the 1990s, debates erupted over the future solvency of social security. It was predicted that, since social security (like the CPP) was a 'pay-as-you-go system', in the future there would not be enough workers to contribute to social security in order to continue paying the pensions of retirees. However, most recent federal government actuarial reports affirm that social security will be able to pay 100% of benefits until 2037 and 72% thereafter.[6,8,13] The issue was also raised over whether the federal government should continue to administer social security or whether its administration should be privatized or even personalized. Proposals have been floated to enable individuals to detach their entitlements from the general social security fund in the form of personal retirement accounts in order to invest them in the marketplace. This sort of procedure has occurred in Chile and the UK. These conflicting opinions and debates ratchet up the level of uncertainty and fear among seniors, and young people, about whether social security will even exist in the future.

At the same time in Canada, clawbacks were introduced on the public pensions. For poor seniors, these clawbacks, that is, an additional tax on these pensions, amounted to 50% for guaranteed income supplement, based on family income.[13] For wealthier seniors, the clawbacks on OAS came into force, based on individual income, beginning at about $53 000 per year, until the pension evaporated at about $83 000 per year.[13] The government unsuccessfully tried to reduce public pensions, during the mid-1980s and again in 1996–1998. This latter effort, coupled with the doubling of contribution rates to the CPP, mobilized seniors to oppose it, raised the spectre of intergenerational conflict and left a legacy of fear among younger Canadians that neither the public pension system nor the CPP would be available when they retired. In both countries, the debates over the public pension system created a sense of insecurity among seniors.

In Canada, the federal government scrapped its plans to revise the public pension system. Indeed, its most recent pronouncements have assured Canadians that the OAS/guaranteed income supplement pensions and the CPP are sustainable into the future. Nevertheless, seniors are still rankled by the existence of clawbacks.

In the UK, as noted previously, the government allowed retirees to transform their public pension into individual pension accounts to be invested in the general stock market under strict regulations. However, many problems arose with this experiment, including heavy losses through bad or risky investments, outright fraud and high management fees. The British government is in the process of rectifying this situation.

In both Canada and the USA, registered retirement savings plans were introduced to make individuals more financially self-reliant so as to reduce their dependence on the public pension system. It has been estimated that, in the USA, retirement income derived from 104(k) will eventually exceed income from social security.[8,14] In Canada, the federal government reduced the age at which individuals have to withdraw funds from their retirement savings plans and, correspondingly, can no longer contribute to them, to 69 from 71. Federal and provincial governments will earn

a great deal of money from these changes since this retirement income is taxed.

Many senior persons are concerned about having sufficient income for their retirement years. For many of them, public pensions (social security in the USA and in Canada, OAS/guaranteed income supplement and CPP) are a major source of income. Some were able to save additional money or to have work-related pensions, but most current seniors retired before registered savings plans, such as RSPs or RRSPS or 104(k) or IRAs, were in existence. The great changes in employment patterns during the first 5 years of the 1990s may have a long-term impact on future seniors. If they have not been able to contribute sufficiently to social security in the USA or the CPP in Canada, to have saved for their retirement or to have received a sufficient 'golden handshake' when downsized, they may indeed find it difficult financially to bridge the years before accessing their pension entitlements, and may still face a bleak old age even after they do so.

Increased life span may necessitate additional health-care expenses. Many are fearful that they could outlive their savings and be reduced to depending solely on income from their public pensions. Social security will replace about 25% of preretirement income and accounts for about 50% of seniors' incomes.[8] In Canada, OAS and the CPP were designed to replace 35–40% of preretirement income.[12] For poorer seniors, adding guaranteed income supplement into the mix replaces between 70 and over 100% of retirement income.[12]

Inflation and taxes, including income taxes and property taxes, if they own a house, also erode seniors' savings and, of course, increase their costs. The rising costs for telephone service, utilities, petrol/gasoline, entertainment and food impact adversely on seniors with fixed incomes.

However, if they own a house and have lived in it for a long time, the chances are that they have been able to pay off the mortgage, although since they probably live in an older house, it is likely to be in need of repair and, in any event, normal maintenance. One of the myths about seniors being rich stems, in part, from the fact that many of them live in mortgage-free houses.

If seniors live in an apartment, unless protected by rent control, the rent that they pay will increase annually and sometimes substantially. If they live in a rural area, on a farm for example, they may be 'land rich and money poor', that is, their land may be worth more money than their savings and cash flow.

Low interest rates have created a great deal of consternation, confusion and fear among current seniors. They are not sure where to invest their funds, as the interest on traditional sources for investment, such as government bonds, decreases. If seniors live on fixed income from investments, their lifestyle is dependent on the prevailing interest rates. If the rates are relatively low, their income decreases; if relatively high, it increases. Many are very reluctant to place their funds in riskier, but higher yielding, investments. If they lose their savings, they have very limited opportunities, if any, to recoup the loss. Similarly, if they purchased annuities, their lifelong income will be totally dependent on the prevailing interest rates when they made the purchase.

Employment as well as financial choices and decisions made during younger years have a profound impact on a senior's well-being, level of stress and quality of life during retirement years.

Health and health care

For many seniors, maintaining good health is a major goal and often a preoccupation. As noted previously, today's older adults are frequently more engaged in an active lifestyle, practise good nutrition, use vitamins, minerals, herbs and supplements, and turn more frequently to alternative medicine, such as chiropractic and other alternative health-care modalities. Many are turning to cosmetic surgery and other non-surgical cosmetic antiageing aids to preserve their youthfulness and youthful appearance.

After retiring, many seniors stay socially connected through sports such as golf or tennis, paid work or volunteerism; intellectually stimulated through continuing education courses, surfing the internet or hobbies; and stay independent by evading dehabilitating diseases as much as possible through wellness and prevention.

In turn, health-care practitioners promote a regime of active living, healthy lifestyle, disease prevention and wellness, what gerontologists call 'successful ageing'. However, these health experts recognize that the maintenance of good health also depends on what has been called 'the determinants of health', such as a good income, higher education, good diet, exercise and not smoking. As noted previously, the right parentage or genes and just good luck also play an important role in good health. Seniors fear catastrophic diseases that can result in the loss of independence, as their ability to perform activities of daily living (ADL) or instrumental activities of daily living are sapped by ill health, or their cognitive skills become impaired in some way. Serious illness can also deplete their savings.

With regard to their health, according to Statistics Canada, about three-quarters of Canadian seniors aged 65–74 and two-thirds of those aged 75 and older rated their health as good, very good or excellent.[7] Approximately one-half of seniors reported that they were physically active for 15 min or more at least 12 times a month.[7] The most common popular physical activities in which they engaged were walking, gardening, home exercise, swimming and dancing.

About 5–7% of seniors are directly engaged in the health system at any given time.

Health care is expensive throughout North America, although its delivery is organized differently north and south of the 49th parallel. In the USA, the health-care system is complex and confusing, as politicians try to maintain a balance between a public and private system. Hospital and medical care for seniors is covered by Medicare, which is delivered through fee-for-service or through managed-care organizations (HMOs). Medicare is divided into two parts: part A primarily finances inpatient hospital services and part B pays for the costs of physician services, outpatient hospital services and medical equipment. Part B is optional but most seniors take it. There is no premium for part A, which is financed out of general federal government revenues. Part B, however, has a premium as well as deductibles and co-payments which amount to 20% of health-care expenses. Payment is a source of great concern for seniors.

American seniors seek to reduce out-of-pocket health-care expenses, which can be financially ruinous. If they can afford it individually or can arrange to receive it through a former or current employer, seniors will purchase additional coverage from a third-party insurer, such as AARP or private insurance companies. This type of insurance is called medigap insurance, because it fills in the gaps in Medicare, especially for prescription drugs, which are not currently covered by Medicare. However, there is a movement afoot in Congress to extend Medicare to include prescription drugs. Unfortunately, poor or unattached seniors can face serious economic hardship if illness strikes them or a spouse because they may have to make up the extra costs out of their own pockets. Many seniors are not aware of federal pro-grammes such as the Qualified Medicare Beneficiary (QMB), the Specified Low-Income Medicare Beneficiary (SLMB) and the Qualifying Individuals-1 (QI-1) programmes, which provide subsidies for low- and some middle-income seniors unable to pay all of their Medicare premiums, coinsurance or deductibles. Some low-income seniors can also qualify for Medicaid to obtain prescription drugs and other care not covered by Medicare. Still, half a million Americans, including seniors, declared personal bankruptcy in 1999 because of the high costs of treatment for serious illnesses.[8]

Health care is organized differently in Canada. The Canada Health Act, passed by the federal government in 1984, is the foundation for the current Canadian health care system, which is based on the principle of a single payer, that is, the federal government. The Canada Health Act ensures universal coverage for all hospital and physician services for Canadians, regardless of age, socioeconomic status and geographical location. No user fees or extra billing are permitted. In other words, basic medical coverage in Canada is based on a one-tier, single-payer system. The other principles incorporated in the Canada Health Act decree that services be comprehensive, portable, accessible and administered on a public or non-profit basis throughout Canada. Seniors receive medications at no cost within hospitals or doctor's offices. However, dental services are not covered by the plan. It is also interesting to note that quality of care is also omitted.

Funding for the plan was to be shared on a 50–50 basis between the federal and provincial and territorial governments. The delivery of services was under the jurisdiction of the provinces and territories.

Major revisions to the Canada health plan began to occur during the early 1990s as the federal government strove to reduce its deficit. Federal transfer payments from the federal government to the provincial and territorial governments were greatly reduced, and the share of federal funding declined. In turn, the provinces and territories reduced funding to hospitals, downsizing the number of hospitals, including staff, especially health-care professionals and particularly nurses. Many health-care and other services provided in hospitals were outsourced. Other services, such as chiropractic, which were covered, even minimally, by provincial health plans, came under severe scrutiny and were reduced. Numer-ous medications for seniors previously covered by provincial health plans or formularies were delisted. Each province and territory began to charge seniors premiums, co-payments and deductibles for prescription drugs still covered by the provincial health plans. User fees varied by province and territory, and in some provinces greatly increased during the second half of the 1990s. Needless to say, many seniors became alarmed by the new and growing costs that they would have to bear on their fixed incomes.

The need to reduce health-care costs, coupled with new medical technologies and pharmaceutical therapies, enabled governments to direct hospitals to send patients home more quickly and, often, sicker. Health-care strategy shifted from institutional care to care at home. Home care, which had always been on the periphery of the Canadian health-care system, as a supplement to hospital care, especially for frail seniors, moved into its centre. Home care became a substitute for institutional care, including postacute and chronic care.

Home care was not specifically or directly covered by the Canada Health Act, although provinces did endeavour to provide some services at no or minimal charge to patients who were recuperating at home. Care has shifted to families, who became known as 'informal caregivers', especially spouses, many of whom were elderly, and children, other relatives, friends and neighbours. Most of them are women. Their participation was assumed to be available and direct. They are the backbone of the home-care system, but they also fill the gaps in personal care created in hospitals or long-term care institutions by fiscal cut-backs. Not only are many informal caregivers on call 24 h a day, 7 days a week, and suffering from 'the burden of caregiving', that is, a syndrome of physical, psychological and emotional stress as well as social isolation, but they also pay for a great deal of the direct costs for providing care with no direct and very little indirect compensation. There is often an adverse impact on their future job prospects and retirement income: if they are not earning money, they cannot contribute to the CPP or a RSP and, therefore, the financial foundations of their retirement years are weakened. The federal government calculated that as of 1999, Canadians are paying about one-third of the costs for health care out of their own pockets, especially in regard to home care, either directly or through the purchase of supplemental medical, dental and prescription drug insurance, which usually did not reimburse full costs.[13]

Many American states and the British government have recognized the pivotal role that informal caregivers (or carers as they are also called) play in the health-care system. Many states have provided them with direct compensation and the British government has announced its intention to do so. The Canadian government has been silent on this issue.

While seniors prefer to remain in their own homes rather than recuperate in hospitals or enter long-term care facilities, there is a growing recognition that the baby boomers may not have children nearby, or at all, to fill the role of informal caregivers. Many seniors also feel guilty about the burden that their recuperation places on their families. They are also concerned about having sufficient savings to pay for the increasing costs of care at home. Long-term care insurance for institutional care, such as nursing homes and/or home care, is a new product. Relatively few American and even fewer Canadian seniors have purchased it, although many supplemental medical insurance policies provide some coverage.

At the same time, the costs for resident care in a nursing home have also greatly increased. American and Canadian seniors are concerned that they will not have sufficient savings to pay for it, when required. In the USA, some nursing homes will continue to provide residency and care even after the individual has no more money to pay for it, whereas others force the resident to make other arrangements. However, about 10% of nursing homes in the USA have become bankrupt,[8] taking a serious toll on their elderly and vulnerable residents. In Canada, there is usually a two-tiered long-term care system, one for those who can afford payment and the other for those who cannot afford it. The first group can enter for-profit nursing homes, while the second group is accepted at non-profit homes for the aged. The problem lies in the lack of sufficient long-term care beds across the country to meet the needs of an ageing population.

In the USA, debate has raged over the sustainability of Medicare and Medicaid, along with, as noted previously, that of social security. However, the most recent statements affirm that part A of Medicare is solvent until at least 2023, and plans are underway to extend its longevity. Others still believe that Medicare and Medicaid need major reforms. Like conflicts over the viability of social security, the debate over

Medicare shakes certainty and arouses fear among both seniors and seniors-in-waiting.

In Canada, the tides of change in the organization of health care have not yet settled. The federal government has promised more funding to the provinces for health-care, but only if they work together to develop a grand national health care plan, incorporating home care and prescription drugs. Many provinces respond that the federal government should give them more money and let them work out their own individual health-care plans, including more health-care services in private clinics. Seniors, many of whom remember the days before the universal health system, are alarmed at the movement towards privatization and the spectre of a two-tiered health-care system based on wealth.

Health care politics in North America is fraught with irony. Many Americans are demanding the reform of Medicare and Medicaid along the lines of the Canadian-style single-payer health-care system which would afford universal coverage to all Americans, including the estimated 42 million Americans, a large percentage of whom are children, without health-care coverage.[8] The effort by President Clinton during his first term in office to adopt this policy met with failure. At the same time, many Canadians are pressing that the Canada Health Act should be replaced by a two-tiered American style system, based on payment for service.

Some analysts argue that health-care policy in North America may converge as the two systems adopt similar principles and practices. In part, this coming together may be the result of the North American Free Trade Agreement (NAFTA), which many Canadians feared may reshape the Canadian health-care system in the American image. Others attribute potential convergence to better communications and knowledge about each other because of more visits to Canada by Americans (because of the relatively low value of the Canadian dollar) and the internet. As always with predictions, only time will tell what will happen.

In the UK, during the 1980s, the public system was increasingly starved for funding, although from time to time money was pumped into it for short bursts. An anomaly was created that a service or procedure was done more quickly in the private health-care system than in the public system, often by the same doctor and staff, using the same equipment, in the same medical facility. The private system thrived as the public system deteriorated. By the end of the 1990s, the British government announced that it would invest £50 billion into the public-health system in recognition of its threadbare condition.

Seniors with severely debilitating diseases have grave concerns over a dignified and pain-free end of life. On the one hand, there are greater demands for increased palliative care, especially at home. Achieving this goal will necessitate, among other things, a transformation in the training of doctors and nurses, who are taught to prolong life rather than ease its departure. On the other hand, the ethical issues raised by palliative care may be extended to embrace euthanasia. Palliative care may include the application of various types of pain-killing drug which, while easing pain, will reduce the cognitive awareness of patients and even shorten life.

Euthanasia, from the Greek, meaning 'a good death', has stimulated a host of concerns. Who has the right to decide whether another individual, or even oneself, should die? Are motives unsullied? Who will actually 'pull the plug'? At the time of writing, only The Netherlands has declared euthanasia legal. In North America and the UK euthanasia is illegal, although surreptitiously and indirectly practised in various ways. Occasionally a case of 'mercy killing' is reported in the media and generates a great deal of public debate, including within the judicial system.

Today, men can look forward to a life expectancy of about 77 years of age and woman to about 83 years of age.[7] This means that if they retire at 65 (in Canada) or 67 (in the USA), men may live in retirement for abut 12 years before they die and women for about 18 years.[7] However as noted previously, fewer people are actually retiring at the 'official' age of retirement in Canada or in the USA, so their retirement years may even be longer. In addition, for a part of their retirement years, particularly after about the age of 75, almost two-thirds of women will live alone because their husbands will have died, a percentage that increases greatly for women after 90. Increasingly, many women today have never married or are divorced.

Regardless of gender, people who live alone, especially if they do not have children, other family or friends, can become very lonely and isolated. Depression can increase as friends and family die. These social conditions, in turn, can adversely affect their health and general well-being, both directly, through deterioration, and indirectly, in that they may have no one to care for them if their health collapses.

The health-care issues of the current generation of seniors will probably become of even greater concern after 2030 as the baby boomers reach retirement age because of the sheer numbers. Many of today's concerns may be eradicated, especially as medical innovations prolong life and, perhaps, an even healthier long life. A recent study by the World Health Organization (WHO) predicts that Canadian children born in 1999 can on average look forward to 72 years of good health, ranking Canada 12th among the nations of the world in this category.[13] By comparison, American children born in 1999 will enjoy 2 years less than Canadians, ranking 24th. According to the study, the top 2.5% of Americans have among the highest healthy life expectancies in the world, while the health expectancy of 50% of that nation's population, inner-city poor, rural southern blacks and natives on reservations, pull its ranking down to among the mid-50s. The Japanese rank first for healthy life expectancy.[13] An even more recent WHO study ranking health-care systems in the world placed Canada 30th and the USA 37th.[13]

Will medical breakthroughs continue apace as the genetic mapping of human beings unfolds? Will new medical discoveries and innovations prolong life, including healthy long life, even further? How will society in the future cope with 120 or 150-year-old people?

More immediately, how will the baby boomers deal with prevailing health-care concerns when they become seniors? Will they easily accept the uncertainty and fears that they witnessed in their parents' ageing process? In both the USA and Canada, will they demand greater public expenditure on health care, reminiscent of the vast public expenditure on education during their youth? Or, will they live up to their reputation as the 'me generation' and, selfishly self-centred, insist that health care should become even more privatized, especially in Canada, to enable quicker access to those who can afford it? Finally, what impact will they have on the health-care system, when all of them have turned 65 after 2030 and they account for roughly one out of every four North Americans?

Sex

Sex is one of the last taboo areas in exploring issues of ageing. For some young people, it is hard enough to imagine their parents having sex. It is even more of a stretch to thinking of grandparents in sexual relations.

The pejorative term 'dirty old men' is applied to older males who exhibit interest, implying that there is something wrong about their behaviour. There does not seem to be an equivalent term for older women, suggesting that it is still not even conceivable that they would have an interest in sex. Or, perhaps, this lack of sexual association with older women is a continuation of the gender-based and gender-biased double standard.

The stereotypical image of seniors is that they are asexual, that is, disinterested in sex. For some of them, sexual feelings may pose a serious problem because they seem to be at odds with the myth of seniors' lack of interest in sex. Others may be plagued by a lack of knowledge about the physical and biochemical changes, for example the decrease in testosterone in men and oestrogen in women or the increase in ailments such as osteoporosis, that accompany ageing. However these changes affect an individual's body, they may not necessarily reduce or end sexual impulses. Seniors may, however, have to adjust to different methods of sexual relations and a longer period to accommodate these bodily changes or ailments of various sorts such as arthritis, back pain, heart disease or stroke. New medication may also help male erection problems. Nor is age a damper for exchanges of affection and intimacy, such as hugging, holding hands and kissing. Others may sublimate sexual passions into other interests.

According to a 1999 study sponsored by a US seniors organization, half of the people between 45 and 59 years old are sexually active, as are one out of three men and one out of four women aged 60–74.[13] An earlier study reported that men and women between the ages of 80 and 102 reported sexual interest and behavior.[13] That is why Viagra has enjoyed such a boom. It also appears that an individual's sexual drive after 50 years of age is about the same as it was before that age.

For older women loss of a partner can become a serious impediment to sexual relations and can end a woman's sexual relations since women outlive men generally. For residents in nursing homes the absence of privacy and misunderstanding about the realities of human sexuality can also create obstacles to sexual intimacy. However, more nursing homes are setting aside privacy rooms for couples who want to use them.

The prevailing myths about seniors' sexuality has given rise to a disturbing phenomenon: the increase in infection by the human immunodeficiency virus (HIV) and other sexually transmitted diseases (STDs) among older people. According to one Canadian study, HIV has grown rapidly among women over 65.[13] Another study demonstrated that 14% of women with HIV were over 50 and it was estimated that 58% of them were infected through heterosexual relations.[13] After menopause, women may believe that their sexual partner no longer has to use a condom because there is no need for birth control. Nevertheless, women and men should use protection regardless of age.

As more people age, the generally held myths about the lack of sexuality among older people may be stripped away. Seniors may become more aware of the realities concerning ageing and sex because of their numbers and previous interest in the subject, as may non-seniors.

Retirement

It may seem ironic that retirement can be fraught with concerns when the prevailing goal for many people is to retire early. However, pre-retirement planning is still not that common. If it does occur, it frequently focuses on financial considerations, with little serious thought about non-financial or lifestyle issues. Pre-retirement planning should encompass both facets since they are of equal importance during the ensuing 20–40 years of life of retirement.

Recent studies have demonstrated that retirement can be very unsettling, especially for those who have not prepared for it or had it suddenly thrust on them, through downsizing, for example. It can even have a devastating impact on those who were given some advanced notice. It can cause consternation for married women who work outside the home, since they are frequently expected to retire because their spouses have retired, and for those women who have stayed at home suddenly to have their spouses around full time.

Of course, for those with sufficient income, retirement can bring freedom to travel, to engage in hobbies, learn new skills, pursue new interests or devote more time to old ones, play golf, and the like.

Many current seniors, especially over 75, are embracing the new computer technology to e-mail friends and family, to make new friends and to keep connected with knowledge and the world, both figuratively and literally.[13] Baby boomers are generally computer literate as part of their work experience. However, although costs for desk-top computer systems have been drastically reduced, many still cannot afford to buy them, although they may be able to turn to public libraries or senior and community centres to access them.

Volunteering is a popular option for retired people which can provide both personal satisfaction and great benefit to society.

Many seniors may not be able to afford to retire before being eligible to collect their pensions although, as noted, the average age of retirement today is about 62 and, in some cases, their pensions may be inadequate to sustain them. These seniors have to continue working to support themselves or to supplement their income and, for some of them, looking for a job may be difficult because of ageism.

In Canada, CPP can be accessed at the age of 60 but there is a 6% penalty for each year it has been taken prior to the age of 65. Seniors after 65 can receive CPP and still earn income up to a specified amount. As noted, in the USA, seniors between 65 and 69 can now receive social security and earn an unlimited income.

A growing segment of seniors comprises people too active to 'sit around'. They represent the new face of retirement. Seniors are retiring younger but living longer and healthier lives. Therefore, they still have many active years left after they 'retire'. Some may opt for full-time work of some sort, while others may chose to work part-time work. Depending on their work experience, still others may become consultants with former employers, or in their field of employment or on their own, using their expertise.

Some may decide on creating a new career, perhaps their second, third or fourth career. Indeed, people have even been advised for some time now to prepare for several careers over their working life. It is not uncommon for retired persons to start a business in which they 'do what they've always wanted to do'. Others work their hobbies for profit.

People should spend as much time on planning for lifestyle in retirement as on preparing the financial foundations for this phase of life. However, as John Lennon reminded us, 'life is what happens to you while you're making plans!' Balance is needed.

Housing

Fear of outliving their savings haunts seniors in regard to housing arrangements.

The majority of seniors live independently in the community. Only about 7% of seniors live in institutions, such as long-term care facilities and retirement homes. Most of these people are women who have outlived men.

Living in care-assisted communities, or depending on home-based live-in or visiting attendants, can be quite expensive. In the USA, Medicare expenditures for these support services is limited by differing state policies, although 35 states either provide some reimbursement or plan to reimburse some costs. Many seniors move to nursing homes that are funded by Medicare because they cannot afford to pay for the support services necessary to remain in their own homes. About 10% of American seniors live in age-restricted communities, of whom about 7% live in communities without care.[8] 15% of them receive special care at home, while 10% reside in shared accommodation, such as 'granny flats', and 5% dwell in supportive housing.[8]

Although throughout North America 90% of seniors live in conventional housing, only about half of the homes owned by seniors with disabilities have had the necessary modifications to accommodate their problems. Many seniors find it too expensive to fund such improvements.[8]

Seniors who live in houses frequently own them free and clear, having paid off the mortgage over the 30 or 40 years for which they possessed them. This fact contributes to the myth that seniors are wealthy. Although they may be wealthy collectively, when all the value of all of the property they own is added up, they are not necessarily rich individually. As noted, many seniors who own houses worry about paying property tax and about the general upkeep of the house which, if it is old, probably requires a great deal of maintenance or modifications, which can be beyond the financial ability of the owner. In the USA, some states and municipalities, and in Canada, some municipalities provide subsidies for middle- and low-income seniors in the form of property tax rebates or freezes, which have to be repaid when the property changes hands. Nevertheless, many seniors fret that they will not be able to leave their houses to their heirs. In turn, the heirs may be in for a big surprise, when they sell inherited property, only to discover that they have to reimburse property taxes with interest which did not have to be paid during the seniors occupant's ownership. Some seniors take out a reverse mortgage on their house, that is, take out a mortgage on their property, which only comes due (with accumulated interest) when the property is sold, thereby allowing them to maintain themselves in their house in the meantime.

Many seniors could find themselves living in run-down neighbourhoods because they have not been able to sell their properties as their surroundings change or deteriorate. At the other end of the socioeconomic spectrum, there are those who move into gated communities because of their fear of crime.

For the approximately 20% of seniors who rent accommodation, there is the concern that they could be evicted from their homes if they cannot pay the rent, which may continue to rise annually, unless under rent control. As stated earlier, in general, seniors who rent have a much lower income than those who own their own accommodations.

Poorer seniors suffer from the lack of subsidized housing of any kind and the chances are that they may not be able to maintain a house or to pay rent for an apartment.

Predictions abound that when the baby boomers age, they will downsize their living spaces, especially if they own a house. They will opt to rent apartments or purchase condominiums, especially in age-related or age-restricted communities. Some may move away from big cities into smaller or rural communities. If this happens, it is estimated that the ensuing glut on the market and lack of purchasers will result in a decrease in the value of houses.

However, with the current high rate of divorce and cost of living, many children are returning home to live with their parents. Many of these 'boomerang kids' are themselves parents, so they and their own children create special housing needs, as well as the potential for increased stress for seniors.

More and more American seniors are moving to the warmer climates of places such as California, Texas, Arizona and Florida. Canadian 'snowbirds' who can afford it winter in these states. Such a move may cut off, or at least cut down, interaction with children and relatives. As seniors age and neighbours and friends die, this may lead to greater social isolation, increased depression and the lack of informal caregivers when needed.

Crime

Seniors are extremely fearful of becoming the victims of crime. Many live alone and feel vulnerable as they grow older. Many believe, based on what they see on television and in the movies, that crime is rampant. Statistically, however, most forms of crime have declined over the past few years. Nevertheless, the concern over crime should not be minimized or dismissed.

Some seniors become victims of frauds and scams. It has been estimated that telemarketing fraud alone is responsible for $4 billion in stolen revenue across North America.[13] This form of fraud transcends borders, since many telemarketing scammers operate out of Canada and prey on Americans. Various con games operate on the local level, such as fraudulent repairs to older houses or the 'bank inspector' scam.

People of all ages are open to being fleeced by a scam-artist. However, for seniors, aside from the normal embarrassment and humiliation at having been bamboozled, the loss of savings can be devastating. Little, if any, of the stolen money may be recovered and replacing it is extremely improbable. For people on fixed incomes this loss can be catastrophic. In recognition of this crisis, several jurisdictions in the USA, such as the state of Illinois, have decreed increased penalties for crooks who are found guilty of defrauding seniors.[13,14] This policy has not yet been introduced in Canada.

A particularly heinous form of crime perpetrated on seniors is elder abuse, which is manifested in the forms of financial, physical, mental or emotional abuse, and direct or indirect neglect (please also refer to Chapter 6). What makes elder abuse especially pernicious is that it is frequently committed by family members, including spouses and children. Indeed, some experts maintain that spousal abuse among elderly couples is a common form of elder abuse.

It has been estimated that about 4% of seniors are the victims of elder abuse,[9,16] but the exact number is not known and is probably higher. Many abused elderly spouses are unwilling to bring charges against the offending mate or child. Even when the pattern of abuse may be longstanding, the abused person may be either in denial or fearful of the consequences. Similarly, many parents do not want their abusing children punished, for fear that they may be completely abandoned. Some familial abusers may not even be aware that their threats or shouts shade into elder abuse. Often, the victim does not know what to do or where to go to escape the abuser. Indeed, a 'safe house' in which to take refuge may not be available in their community. Some persons with dementia who are cared for at home violently act out against their informal caregivers, who do not want to send loved ones to a nursing home.

Exposés of outright elder abuse, from theft to physical or verbal abuse, in nursing homes are not uncommon, including the use of restraints and other controversial forms of control of patients. In addition, some informal caregivers might lash out at their loved ones as a consequence of the frustration, exhaustion and stress caused by the 'burden' of caregiving.

An insidious form of elder abuse that has been recognized recently is denying grandparents access to grandchildren as a result of divorce.

Although many states and the four maritime provinces in Canada have passed laws against elder abuse, initiating legal proceedings for the crime is still difficult, for the reasons noted previously. In San Diego, frauds and scams against seniors are prosecuted as a form of elder abuse.

Elder abuse is another taboo subject that cries out for exposure. The legal responsibility of health-care professionals and social service providers to notify law enforcement varies from jurisdiction to jurisdiction across North America. Nevertheless, as front-line health-care professionals, chiropractors should accept the responsibility of monitoring their elderly patients for such abuse.

Transportation

Transportation is essential to seniors for, without it, they can be reduced to social isolation.

Seniors who are dependent on public transportation find that it is not always convenient, accessible or even available. Although many communities offer subsidized rates for seniors, some seniors are still too poor to afford even the reduced cost. Perhaps consideration should be given to free transportation at certain hours. Others are too frail and require specialized public transit which, unfortunately, is not always available.

In many jurisdictions, doctors or other authorities can order the withdrawal of a senior's right to drive an automobile on the grounds of mental or physical impairment as a safety measure to protect both the senior and the general public. Although necessary, the loss of a driver's licence can have a profound psychological impact on the senior, as it would on anyone, regardless of age, because it represents the curtailing of independence and freedom. Accordingly, it is important to make sure that the individual's condition warrants the loss of a driving licence and the decision is not based solely on age.

Summary

Longevity is a new reality, as is good health for a longer period of life. New medical breakthroughs may enable people to live longer with life-threatening diseases, even such as the acquired immunodeficiency syndrome (AIDS).

Will the future witness a reversal or slowing down of the ageing process, and an even greater extension of the life span? How will society cope in the future with a greater percentage of older people, potentially millions over 100 years of age? How will the new generation of seniors adapt to ageing? Will young people ape all of the seniors they see around them by painting artificial lines and liver spots on their own bodies, while seniors try to prolong their youthful appearance by plastic surgery or non-medical methods? The answers to these questions are still a mystery, although only a few years away.

The issues of seniors explored in this chapter are not always in the forefront of their minds. Seniors do not necessarily dwell on them at the same time or, for some, even at any time, nor at the same age. Nor do all seniors encounter all of them. Some seniors experience some or all of them more acutely than other seniors. Therefore, generalities about the concerns of seniors must be balanced by individual experience.

Nevertheless, the more these issues are appreciated, the better the relationship and interaction, both professionally and personally, between older and younger people will be. The process of understanding must start with the truism that ageing is an integral and normal part of life.

Acknowledgement

My thanks to Judy Cutler for editing this material.

References

1   Elliot G, Hunt M, Hutchison K. Facts on Aging in Canada. Office of Gerontological Studies, McMaster University, Hamilton, Ontario, 1996.
2   US Bureau of the Census, Statistical Abstracts of the United States, 1994 data.
3   Department of Health and Human Services. A Profile of Older Americans. Administration on Aging and the Programs Resources Department, American Association of Retired Persons, 1996.
4   Moore EG, Rosenberg M, McGuiness D. Growing Old in Canada. Statistics Canada and ITP Nelson, Toronto, Ontario, 1997.
5   Brown K. How long have you got? Sci Am 2000; 11(2): 9–15.
6   www.ssa.gov
7   A Portrait of Seniors in Canada. Statistics Canada, 1997.
8   Housing America's Senior. Joint Center for Housing Studies of Harvard University, 1999.
9   Novack M. Aging and Society: A Canadian Perspective. Toronto: ITP Nelson, 1997.
10 Ferri F, Fretwell M, Watchel T. The Care of the Geriatric Patient. 2nd Edn. St Louis, MO: Mosby-Year Book, Donnelly and Sons Co., 1997.

11   Buzan T, Keene R. The Age Heresy. London: Ebury Press, 1996.
12   MacPherson BD. Aging as a Social Process: An Introduction to Individual and Population Aging. Toronto: Harcourt Brace Canada, 1998.
13   www.fifty-plus.net The Website of CARP, the Canadian Association of the Fifty-Plus.
14   www.aarp.org/pbo

Additional references

www.medicare.gov
www.hcfa.gov/medicaid/mcaicnsm.htm
Clark PG. Canadian–American Policy: The Moral Economy of Health and Aging in Canada and the Unites States. Canadian–American Center, University of Maine, Orono, Maine, 1995.

4

Theories of ageing

Brian J Gleberzon

The story of Tithonus

Tithonus was a handsome young prince with whom Eros, goddess of the dawn, fell in love. Unable to marry a mortal, Eros pleaded with Zeus to grant Tithonus eternal life. He did so, and Eros and Tithonus wed, living happily together for many years. But Eros had forgotten to also ask Zeus to grant her lover eternal youth as well. So it came to pass that Tithonus' fate was to forever age. He grew weaker and smaller, shrinking and shriveling over the years. He lost strength in his limbs and his voice grew ever weaker. As he became more and more frail, his voicing becoming little more than a squeak, Eros placed him in a basket. Tithonus' aging continued unabated. Eventually, he turned into a grasshopper, ignored in Eros' basket chirping away for all eternal.

Recounted by Henig.[1]

It would seem that Tithonus is not alone in his plight. Comparative anthropology teaches us that human cultures are remarkably similar. As far back as palaeolithic times, people have shared common fears, values and aspirations. All cultures share a mythology about the afterlife, they emphasize the importance of kinship, the necessity of social order, the powers of shamanistic healing, and a common folklore about immortality. Deities are often portrayed as all-knowing, venerable and eternal. Indeed, legendary heroes are often bestowed immortality as an ultimate reward for exemplary courage. According to the Old Testament, after his expulsion from the Garden of Eden, Adam fathered a son, Seth, at the age of 130 years, and lived to the age of 930 years. Small wonder, then, that the quest for immortality has been inculcated into modern times.

In today's society, restoring a youthful appearance by cosmetics and cosmetic surgery is a multi-billion dollar business. Modern approaches to postpone ageing or to restore youthfulness include macrobiotic diets, 'new age' practices using megadoses of vitamins and minerals, ginseng, melatonin and other hormone-replacement therapies and various Hindu health practices. All these attempts have one thing in common: their failure to achieve any results. While the mean human life expectancy has been remarkably extended over the past century, maximum life span has not. This has resulted in what demographers describe as the 'rectangularization' of human ageing demographics, in which longevity is compressed against a fixed end-point, the maximum life span of no more than 120 years.[2,3]

Some authorities consider the ageing process to be a disease which can be combated and conquered. It is only since the 1990s, however, that science has begun to unlock the mysteries of the ageing process, to understand the mechanism by which ageing may occur, and to provide a foundation upon which the restoration of youthfulness may actually be achieved.

Hayflick[4] in the 1960s was the first to propose that fibroblasts have a finite replicative capacity which is unique to each organism and that accounts for the process of senescence. Currently, there are over 300 different theories that attempt to explain the ageing process, many of which question the fatalism attached to the Hayflick constant concept. The two major theories of ageing can be categorized as: (i) programmed theories and (ii) damage theories. In many cases, these theories are not contradictory, but complementary.[5]

At present, the predominant programmed theories of ageing include: genes, genetic clocks and immunity; evolutionary process theory; and chromosomal degradation telomere shortening. The damage theories include: the accumulation of detrimental biochemical and oxidative agents; mitotic misregulation; and caloric restriction.

This chapter will also discuss the anti-ageing effects of meditation, stem cell therapies and cloning.

Programmed theories of ageing

Genes, genetic clocks and immunity

Age, *clk* and *daf* genes

Primitive nematode worms, such as *Caenorhabditis elegans*, are ideal test subjects for research into ageing, since they have a life span of only 20 days. Over the latter half of the 1990s, researchers throughout North America have been able to extend the life span of *C. elegans* by a factor of five. That is to say, mutant strains of *C. elegans* with particular genomes (notably *clk-1* and *daf-2*) live nearly five times as long as their wild-type cohorts.[6–8] Researchers have independently, and yet consistently, identified particular classes of genes that seem to convey longevity, primarily by slowing down the physiological rate of metabolism. This is often referred to as the 'rate of living' theory.[6] In essence, the rate of living theory posits that certain genes have as their phenotypic effect the slowing down of cellular metabolism. This results in a decreased production of detrimental metabolic byproducts (such as oxidative biochemicals) which ultimately conveys longevity.[6,7] Those organisms that do not have such genes have a higher rate of living, produce a larger amount of oxidative byproducts, are more vulnerable to the deleterious effects of such metabolites, experience earlier senescence and die.

The first class of genes identified to convey longevity in *C. elegans* was called *age-1(hx546)*.[9] This class of genes is thought to be involved in oxidative stress reactions (see Oxidative stress and caloric restriction theory). Other mutant strains that convey longevity are *daf-2, daf-12, daf-18, daf-23, daf-28* and *spe-26*.[9–12] All of these 'age' mutant strains tested to date convey resistance to oxidative stress, thermal stress and ultraviolet radiation, with the degree of resistance often proportional to the extension of the organism's life span.[9] Researchers have demonstrated this extension of longevity by genetic manipulation in yeasts, fruit flies and mice.[10,11]

Currently, another class of age genes, the genes *clk 1-4* (for 'abnormal function of biological clocks') has also been correlated with longevity in *C. elegans*.[7–9] Of particular importance, the *clk-1* protein has been identified in many eukaryotes, including humans.[7] Of equal interest, mutant *clk-1* genes demonstrate a maternal effect in *C. elegans*.[7,9] That is, only homozygous mutants from a homozygous mother exhibit the *clk-1* phenotype and subsequent longevity. This gene controls the worm's embryonic and postembryonic development, growth rate, cell-cycle time, swimming abilities and feeding cycles.[9]

Other genetic markers have been identified as possibly being related to ageing. Studies examining French centenarians have revealed a lower frequency of apolipoprotein (apo) E_4 alleles, which is correlated to increased susceptibility to coronary heart disease and Alzheimer's disease.[2,12]

Immunity

In every mammalian organism, the thymus undergoes a genetically programmed shrinkage called involution, which begins in humans after the age of 1 year. T-cells, which play a key role in maintaining the effectiveness of the immune system, are developed and matured in the thymus.[13] It should not come as a surprise that researchers, working with mammals such as mice, have determined that high immune responsiveness is correlated with increased life span.[12] This has further led to studies into the human leucocyte antigen (HLA) locus, which is involved in immune function. Taken as a whole, some researchers conclude that the preservation of a high rate of immunological function, perhaps achieved by continued thymus function, can allow for a greater life span.[8]

Ageing as an evolutionary process

Proponents of the theory of ageing as an evolutionary process remind us that, despite tremendous improvements in health-care delivery, sanitation and disease prevention, people who survive today into their seventies are only slightly more likely to enjoy a robust old age than were their cohorts of a millennium ago.[2] Life expectancies have increased mostly through a decline in infant mortality, while few strides have been made in the retardation of the physiological processes seemingly linked to ageing. To some authorities, this is not only not surprising but expected, and can be explained by the fundamentally simple principles of evolutionary survivability. In fact, researchers such as Dr Michael Rose, an evolutionary biologist at the University of California, posit that ageing is best understood from the evolutionary perspective of natural selection.[2]

The concept of natural selection was first proposed by Darwin over a hundred years ago.[14] Generally speaking, the theory of natural selection states that heritable traits persist and become prevalent in a population, that is, they are selected for, if the trait allows the bearer successfully to reach reproductive age.[2,14] The more advantageous the trait, the more offspring the organism will produce. The offspring will generally be more robust, live longer and propagate in greater numbers compared with less successful members of the group, and hence the frequency of those genetic traits most advantageous to the organism increases in the population.[14]

In contrast, those traits that diminish survivability are selected against, because the bearers of those genes do not survive long enough to reproduce. Moreover, there is not the same degree of selective pressure against those genes that result in deleterious physiological manifestations later in life, after the reproductive age. Such genes, then, would accumulate: in genetic terms, their genetic frequency would increase.[2] In fact, Rose argues that the later the gene caused its deleterious effect, the more likely it would increase in frequency because the bearer of the genes would live longer and theoretically produce more offspring.[2] The evolutionary theory of ageing, therefore, is based on the observation that the efficacy of natural selection decreases with age or, looked at another way, ageing in general, and senescence in particular, can be considered the normal result of natural selection.[2,15] In essence, ageing is the result of an evolutionary attempt to optimize fitness early in life[15] (Figure 4.1).

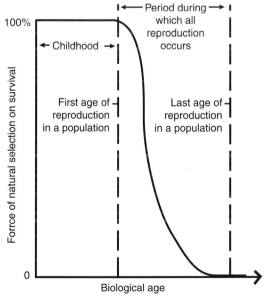

Figure 4.1 The evolutionary theory of ageing. Source: Scientific American.[1]

This theory accounts for the relative rarity of diseases that afflict children and are fatal before normal reproductive age. Such diseases include progeria, a genetic disorder caused by a single genetic mutation that is characterized by the rapid deterioration of all biological systems.[2] Progeria typically causes death by the age of 15 from heart disease or stroke. In contrast, diseases such as Huntington's chorea, a neurological disorder that typically manifests after the age of 40, is relatively common. This fits well into the evolution theory of ageing. Specifically, this theory would predict the established observation that, since those individuals with the genes for Huntington's chorea could produce an average number of children, the genes for Huntington's chorea are not selected against, but rather are preserved and propagated in the population.[2]

Lithglow and Kirkwood question the validity of an evolutionary theory of ageing.[9] They point out that few species achieve maximum life expectancy in a natural world (owing to natural diseases, predation and so on), and are thus unable to demonstrate observable signs of senescence.[9] It is their opinion that natural selection cannot plausibly explain the evolution of a temporal control system of ageing whose primary function is to bring about senescence and death in a handful of survivors, especially since this action is detrimental to the individuals in which it occurs.[8] However, it could be counter-argued that ageing and death do serve an important biological function: population control.

Chromosomal degradation: telomeric shortening and ageing

In 1990, Calvin Harley, a researcher at McMaster University in Hamilton, Ontario, demonstrated a phenomenon in human fibroblasts first observed only in yeasts: the successive loss or shortening of the terminus of chromosomal tips called telomeres with each replicative generation (or serial passage) during ageing.[16] Since that time, the inhibition of this successive shortening of DNA has been observed to result in the immortalization of cell lines.[17–22] This theory has been so successfully defended that one author concluded that the telomeric degradation hypothesis is perhaps the best explanation of a cellular division 'counting' mechanism.[23]

In eukaryotic cells, chromosomes end in repetitive DNA sequences called telomeres. It has been postulated that the finite doubling capacity of normal mammalian cells (the Hayflick constant) is the result of the loss of telomeric DNA, which leads to the deletion of essential genetic sequences. Researchers have observed that 200 base pairs of DNA are lost with each cellular division.[24]

Of possible importance, telomeric loss seems to be greater in chromosome 17 than in other chromosomes.[8] Telomeric loss does not pose an immediate threat to cellular integrity because of the highly redundant nature of the telomeric DNA.[24] However, over time, a sufficient amount of chromosomal content is lost, which ultimately proves fatal to cellular survivability (Figure 4.2).

As a corollary to this reasoning, if telomeric loss acts as a cellular divisional clock, any process that inhibits telomere degradation would have as a result the retardation of the ageing process. In 1998, researchers at Geron Corporation (Menlo Park, CA, USA) demonstrated the validity of this theory by linking telomere shortening to cellular senescence by the inhibition of telomeric loss.[24] The Geron team extended the life span of normal human fibroblasts and epithelial cells by genetically engineering these cells to express telomerase, an enzyme that protects chromosomal telomeres from degradation.[22,24] In those cells in which telomerase is expressed, telomeres do not shorten during cell division.[22,24] These cells break through the 'senescence barrier', continuing to divide beyond the Hayflick limit, essentially achieving immortality. In the study at Geron, cells which normally senesce at 50–55 divisions, instead divide over 100 times.[24] Moreover, according to Geron vice-president Calvin Harley, 'the cells are staying youthful'.[24] That is, the cells do not accumulate lipofuscin pigments or increase in size.[24]

Telomerase activity has also been strongly linked to tumour cells. In one study, telomerase expression was identified in 98 of 100 immortalized cell lines, and 90 of 101 primary tumours, while being absent from 22 normal somatic cell cultures and 50 normal or benign tissues.[25] Expression of telomerase activity in almost all advanced malignancies tested has led researchers to conclude that immortal cells are likely to be required to maintain tumour growth.[25–29] Could increasing life span by telomerase administration therefore lead to an increase risk in cancer development? Harley opines that this may not be the case: his interpretation of the data is that telomerase has a permissive, rather than causative role in cancer.[24] Moreover, Harley suggests that, for therapeutic uses, telomerase activity may only have to be temporarily upregulated in order achieve a transient increase in cellular longevity, thus avoiding immortalization and possible tumour development.[24] However, Camprisi[23] counters this opinion by suggesting that replicative senescence may in fact be a powerful tumour-suppressive mechanism, while having the unselected effect of contributing to ageing and age-related pathologies.

It should be noted, however, that the telomere hypothesis appears to be more complex than originally thought, and telomeric loss alone may not account for the ageing process. Researchers have identified telomerase-negative immortal cell lines, and some normal somatic cells have been found that express telomerase activity.[29] These data suggest that telomerase activity alone may not account for telomere length maintenance, or that telomeric activity may effect ageing via an intermediate process.[17,29] For example, DePinho, a researcher at Harvard Medical School, recently suggested that 'telomere attrition does not precipitate a classical premature aging syndrome. But we do believe it influences an absolutely critical aspect of getting old – the ability of organisms to counteract acute and chronic stress'.[22] Other researchers believe that the intermediate process between telomeric loss and cellular senescence is oxidative stress.[12,30,31]

Cellular damage theories

Oxidative stress and stress-related mechanisms

Of the more than 300 theories of ageing, the free-radical theory, first postulated by Harman in 1956, is

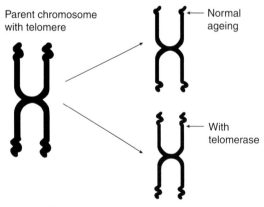

Figure 4.2 Telomeric degradation and replicative senescence.

possibly the most popular and widely tested.[1,32–35] In its most simplistic form, oxidative stress can be considered analogous to the rusting of metal in damp weather.[33] In both cases, 'oxidation' causes a fundamental loss of the inherent strength and stability of the structure and function of its target. The use of oxygen by cells in aerobic organisms generates potentially deleterious reactive oxygen metabolites, first observed in laboratory animals as early as 1878.[32,36] A balanced state therefore usually exists between pro-oxidants and antioxidants. The degree or extent of oxidative damage increases as an organism ages, and it is postulated to be a major cause of senescence. This theory is based on three observations: (i) overexpression of antioxidative enzymes retards the age-related accumulation of oxidative damage and subsequently extends the maximum life span in *Drosophila melanogaster*; (ii) variation in longevity in different species is inversely related to rates of mitochondrial generation of superoxide anion radicals and hydrogen peroxide (powerful oxidative chemicals); and (iii) caloric restriction lowers levels of oxidative stress and damage, retards age-associated changes and extends life span in mammals.[32,37]

The basic tenet of the oxidative stress hypothesis is that senescence and loss of cellular function are due to the progressive and irreversible accrual of metabolic oxidative damage.[32] Oxygen, although essential for the survival of aerobic organisms, is a potentially toxic substance and poses a risk to their long-term existence. This has often been described as the 'oxygen paradox'.[32] Molecular oxygen can generate superoxide anion radicals (O_2^-, H_2O_2 and $-OH$), as well as an array of other reactive oxygen metabolites (ROMs) that can cause extensive oxidative damage to macromolecules and cellular function. Cellular damage includes peroxidation of membrane polyunsaturated fatty acid chains and modification to DNA (including base-pair alterations, single-strand breaks, chromotid exchanges and DNA–protein cross-changes). Other changes include carbonylation and loss of sulfhydryls in proteins.[28] The mitochondrial genome is especially vulnerable to oxidative damage.[12] Several researchers believe that it is the damage to the mitochondrial genome (mtDNA) by oxidative stress that leads to senescence; this is due to the fact that mtDNA lacks the excision and recombination repair mechanisms of the nuclear genome.[33,38,39] This is often referred to as the oxygen stress–mitochondrial mutation theory.[38,39]

Taken as a whole, the emerging consensus is that oxidative damage by oxyradicals to nuclear and mitochondrial DNA (including telomeres) during ageing is ubiquitous, substantial and increases exponentially with age.[12,30–32] Furthermore, it seems that during ageing there is an increase in the rate of ROM generation and a concomitant increase in tissue susceptibility to oxidative damage.[32] To combat these ROMs, 'stress-response' genes are required to shift cellular physiology towards maintenance.[9,12]

In humans, a great deal of research has pointed to the importance of metabolic capacity and stress response in ageing. Oxidative stress appears particularly important, especially since oxidative damage increases with age.[12] Lithgow and Kirkwood posit that those genes that are responsible for the proper regulation of the stress-response system are the *age-1 (hx546)* genes.[9] They base this model on the experimental findings that, compared with wild-type, *age-1* mutant strains of *C. elegans* are more resistant to hydrogen peroxide (H_2O_2) and paraquat, accumulate fewer mitochondrial genome deletions and have elevated levels of the antioxidant enzymes Cu,Zn-superoxide dismutase and catalase.[9,12,33] The *age-1* mutant strains also have increased intrinsic thermotolerance and are more resistant to ultraviolet radiation.[8]

Several researchers have focused their attention specifically on superoxide dimutase (SOD) and catalase.[37] Orr and Sohol,[33] for example, found that test animals (fruit flies) with extra copies of the genes for SOD and catalase production survived on average one-third longer than their normal life span. Other researchers, such as Tower, found their SOD and catalase-producing enhanced test flies lived on average 48% longer than normal. Said Towers: 'That's pretty convincing evidence that overexpression of SOD extends life'.[33] Similar results were reported by Phillips working at the University of Guelph, who said, 'we didn't just delay dying so that we had geriatric flies living longer. The extended time of life was youth'.[33]

One of the problems, however, is that some researchers achieve these results by selecting *daf-2* mutant worms which, while demonstrating an enhanced resistance to oxidative stress, display a simultaneous plummet in their metabolic rate, resembling hibernation.[1] Sohol opined that: 'It's just like going to sleep for three years and calling those three extra years of life'.[1]

As mentioned previously, telomeres seem to be especially sensitive to oxidative stress, and telomeric degradation may reflect the cumulative amount of oxidative damage to an organism.[30,31] The oxidative stress theory of ageing is further strengthened by the accumulated evidence of the benefits of antioxidants, such as vitamin E, which act as free-radical scavengers (please see Chapter 26, Clinical nutrition).[31,33,35,40]

Genetic instability

Recent studies coming out of California suggest that ageing may be the result of the impairment of the machinery needed for normal separation of chromosomes during cellular division.[41] This genetic impairment could lead to genetic instability and a variety of disturbances in gene function.[41] As one of the researchers concluded, 'aging is predominately a disease of mismanagement of cell division checkpoints'.[41]

A study by Ly *et al.* sought to measure the messenger RNA levels in actively dividing fibroblasts of young, middle-aged and older persons and compared them with those isolated from people with progeria, which is a rare genetic disorder characterized by accelerated ageing.[42] The data suggested that an underlying mechanism of the ageing process may involve increased errors during mitosis. The authors proposed that this dysfunction in cellular division could lead to chromosomal pathologies that result in the misregulation of genes involved in the ageing process. They believe that such misregulations cause an increased rate of somatic mutations, leading to numerical and structural chromosomal aberrations, and that these mutations manifest themselves as an ageing phenomenon.[42]

An important finding in this study was that those genes involved in inflammation were upregulated only in the progeria group.[41,42] This same group of genes is thought to be linked to Alzheimer's and heart disease.[41] Conversely, mitochondrial genes are downregulated, which is consistent with age-related mitochondrial dysfunction, as described previously.[42]

A team of researchers from Wisconsin found that the genes involved in the production of stress-response proteins, which are needed to repair or eliminate damaged DNA or proteins, were activated in aged animals' muscles.[43] More importantly, the Wisconsin team found that many of the changes observed in aged animals fed a normal diet did not occur in mice on a calorie-restricted diet, a finding that provides a possible explanation for how caloric restriction extends life spans.[41,43]

Caloric restriction

Currently, caloric restriction is the only widely accepted and validated manner in which to extend life span and postpone senescence in mammals (lowering of ambient temperature and/or a decrease in physical activity in cold-blooded animals can also increase maximum life span).[12,44–47] In research animals, caloric restriction causes an unambiguous, robust and reproducible extension of maximum life span and delays many biochemical, physiological and behavioural changes associated with ageing.[32,46] Possible mechanisms by which caloric restriction may extend maximum life span are: retardation of growth, reduction of body fat, delay of neuroendocrine and immunological changes, increase in DNA repair capabilities, alteration of gene expression, enhanced apoptosis, reduced body temperature, depression of the metabolic rate and reduction of oxidative stress.[46,47] However, most of these explanations lack any supportive evidence and experiments have refuted many of these theoretical models, with the notable exception of oxidative stress reduction.[46,47] Caloric reduction seems to allow the preservation of the oxidative stress response, perhaps by inhibiting the formation of free radicals and thus limiting oxidative damage.[12,30,46]

If the hypothesis that caloric reduction conveys a decline in oxidative stress, then it would be predicted that caloric reduction would be shown to lower the steady-state level of oxidative stress, retard the age-associated accrual of oxidative damage and increase metabolic potential.[46] Experimental results tend to support these predictions and thus validate the caloric reduction–oxidative stress relationship.[45,46] It should be noted that the highest degree of oxidative damage, as well as its attenuation by caloric reduction, occurs in the tissues of the brain, heart and skeletal muscles.[12,44,45]

For caloric restriction to have any effect on human longevity, it has been calculated that an individual would have to reduce their dietary intake to 1500 calories a day or less. It would further require an individual to achieve 'undernutrition without malnutrition',[1] ensuring an adequate consumption of vitamins and minerals.

A unified theory of ageing

It is readily apparent that the various theories of ageing are not mutually exclusive, but are instead complementary. For example, it seems most likely that the accumulation of free oxyradicals (the formation of which can be limited by caloric restriction) results in damage to both nuclear and mitochondrial DNA. The extent of damage may depend on the genetically determined stress-maintenance abilities of an individual, with those individuals who possess a genome similar to the *age-1* allele being at a comparative advantage. Telomeres appear to be especially sensitive to oxidative stress and accelerated telomeric degradation may act as a replicative clock that leads to senescence. Accrual of oxyradicals may also result in an increase in mitotic misregulation. This process may be inhibited by either antioxidants, telomerase or caloric restriction.

The antiageing effects of meditation

Techniques of meditation and relaxation have been reported to prevent or reverse changes associated with old age, including cognitive declines, compromised cardiovascular function and diminished quality of life.[48–51] Studies have indicated that transcendental meditation was twice as effective as a placebo to lower anxiety[52,53] and was the most effective relaxation method to lower blood pressure.[53,54]

Stem cells

Stem cells are undifferentiated cells collected from either a fertilized egg or the inner cell mass of a blastocyte.[55] In either case, stem cells maintain the ability to differentiate into the other types of specialized cellular types, such as nerves, blood or muscle. In 1998, two groups of researchers were each able to isolate human stem cells.[55] Since that discovery, researchers have successfully utilized stem cells in animal experiments to repair cellular structures, such as neural regeneration in mice.[55] For example, experiments on Parkinson's-induced mice injected with neural stem cells achieved normal movement patterns in 75% of test animals in less than 3 months.[55] Some researchers hope that the use of stem cells may repair damaged cellular tissue and ultimately reverse diseases such as Parkinson's, amyotrophic lateral sclerosis and dementia.[55]

The most versatile stem cells originate from embryonic tissue, which are able to differentiate into any other cell type, but have yet to undergo immunological changes. That is, embryonic stem cells are less likely to be rejected by a recipient. However, ethical concerns about the use of human foetal tissue in research has led to a ban on federal funding by the United States Congress. The National Bioethics Advisory Committee concluded that 'The Commission believes that federal funding for the use and derivation of [embryonic stem] cells should be limited to two sources of such material: cadaveric fetal tissue [from naturally aborted fetuses] and embryos remaining after infertility treatments'.[55]

Cloning and the extension of life

When news of the cloning of a sheep (named Dolly) was released in 1997,[56] the accolades bestowed on the researchers were overshadowed by the ethical concerns and implications of such technology. However, when researchers examined the DNA of Dolly,[57–59] they found that her telomeres were shorter than normal.[60] This was an indication that cloned animals such as Dolly might age prematurely. Over the next 2 years, researchers proposed methods to overcome this telomeric loss,[61,62] and in April 2000 the telomeres of cloned mammals (cows) were discovered to be not only preserved, but extended.[60]

Lanza *et al.* successfully cloned six calves derived from a population of senescent cells.[60] They reported that the nuclear transfer extended the replicative life span of these senescent cells (zero to four population doublings remaining) to greater than 90 population doublings.[60] Early population doubling levels of complementary DNA expression in cells from the cloned animals were 3.5–5-fold higher than those in cells from age-matched controls.[60] Lastly, examination of the telomeres of the cloned calves indicated that they were extended in length beyond those of newborns.[60] The authors state that 'the potential of cloning depends in part on whether the procedure can reverse cellular aging and restore somatic cells to a phenotypically youthful state'.[60] The results reported suggest that cloning may convey the ability to regenerate animals and cells, and that this may ultimately have important implications in the study of mammalian ageing.[60]

Summary

If researchers are ultimately able to identify the genetic basis of ageing, it may be subsequently possible to develop a 'cure' or 'treatment' for senescence. For example, let us assume that researchers definitively establish that a particular set of genes (such as the *clk-1* gene) controls telomeric loss, and that telomeric loss is the biological clock that leads to senescence and ageing (perhaps by diminishing immune effectiveness or oxidative-stress maintenance). It has already been shown that telomerase can prevent telomere degradation. Alternatively, perhaps scientists will achieve longevity by reissuing an individual's stem cells to him- or herself once the need arises, thus circumventing the moral dilemma of using human foetal tissue. Or perhaps a calorie-restricted diet can be developed that is actually palatable, using early activation of satiety receptors. If antiageing elixirs are developed and marketed, assuming that such elixirs could avoid the tumorigenic effects of cellular immortalization, imagine the social ramifications. Consider the change to every aspect of any culture if life span is no longer measured in terms of decades, but in centuries. Assuming that such an elixir would be available and affordable to all who desired it (a very large assumption) or that its lack of universal availability did not lead to serious civil unrest, obvious pressures would be placed on demographic and population growth, food resources, living space, work opportunities and vocational choices (would the reader want to engage in the same occupation for centuries?). With near-immortal life spans, it would seem necessary to repeal the age of forced retirement from age 65 years, but to what age? 650? 6500? How would this effect marriage and procreation (my wife and I get along well, and we hope to one day celebrate our 50th anniversary, but our 500th?). How would this affect a couple's decision to have children, and would governments enforce regulations that would prevent couples from having children at a particular age, considering that a women might be able to reproduce between the ages of 13 and 1300? How would this affect criminality, when life imprisonment might last from one millennium to the next?

To paraphrase noted science fiction writer Arthur C Clarke, the future would not only be more fantastic than we imagine, it would be more fantastic than we *can* imagine. . . .

References

1 Henig RM. Living longer: what really works? Sci Am 2000; 11(2): 31–37.
2 Rose M. Can human aging be postponed? Sci Am 1999; 281(6): 106–111.
3 Foote DK, Stoffman D. Boom, bust & echo 2000. Profiting from the Demographic Shift in the New Millennium. 1st end. Toronto: Macfarlane, Walter & Ross, 1998.
4 Hayflick L. The limited *in vitro* lifespan of human diploid cell strains. Exp. Cell Res 1965; 37: 614.
5 Banks D, Fosse M. Telomeres, cancer and aging. JAMA 1997; 278: 1345–1348
6 Lakowski B, Hekimi S. Determination of life-span in *Caenorhabditis elegans* by four clock genes. Science 1996; 272: 1010–1013.
7 Ewbanks J, Barnes T, Lakowski B *et al.* Structural and functional conservation of the *Caenorhabditis elegans* timing gene *clk-1*. Science 1997; 275: 980–983.
8 Riabowol, K. Biological aging research in Canada: past, present and future. *Can J Aging* 1999; 18(1): i–vii.
9 Lithglow G, Kirkwood T. Mechanisms and evolution of aging. Science 1996; 273: 80.
10 Brown K. How long have you got? Sci Am 2000; 11(2): 9–15.
11 Strauss E. Of hyperaging and Methuselah genes. Sci Am 2000; 11(2): 69–71.
12 Jazwinski S. Longevity, genes and aging. Science 1996; 273: 54–59.
13 Guyton AC, Hall JE. Textbook of Medical Physiology. 9th edn. Toronto: WB Saunders, 1997.
14 Havilland W. Anthropology, 8th. edn. Fort Worth: Harcourt Brace College Publishers, 1997.
15 Zwaan BJ. The evolutionary theory of ageing and longevity. Heredity 1999; 82: 589–597.
16 Harley C, Futcher B, Greider C. Telomere shorten during ageing of human fibroblasts. Nature 1990; 345: 458–460.
17 Reddel R. A reassessment of the telomere hypothesis of senescence. Bioessays 1998; 20: 977–984.
18 Johnson F, Marciniak R, Guarente L. Telomeres, the nucleolus and aging. Curr Opin Cell Biol 1998; 10: 332–338.
19 Harley C, Sherwood S. Telomerase, checkpoints and cancer. Cancer Surv 1997; 29: 263–284.
20 Bryan T, Reddel R. Telomere dynamics and telomerase activity in in vitro immortalised human cells. Eur J Cancer 1997; 33: 767–773.
21 Mera SL. The role of telomerases in ageing and cancer. Br J Biomed Sci 1998; 55: 221–225.
22 Strauss E. Counting the lives of cells. Sci Am 2000; 11(2): 51–55.
23 Camprisi J. The biology of replicative senescence. Eur J Cancer 1997; 33: 703–709.
24 Finkel E. Telomeres: keys to senescence and cancer. Lancet 1998; 351: 1186.
25 Kim N, Piatyszek M, Prowse K *et al.* Specific association of human telomerase activity and immortal cells and cancer. Science 1994; 266: 2011–2015.
26 Shay J, Bacchetti S. A survey of telomerase activity in human cancer. Eur J Cancer 1997; 33: 787–791.
27 Nakamura, T, Morin G, Chapman K *et al.* Telomerase catalytic subunit homologs from fission yeast and human. Science 1997; 277: 955–959.
28 Meyerson M, Counter C, Eaton E *et al.* hEST2, the putative human telomerase catalytic subunit gene is upgraded in tumor cells and during immortalization. Cell 1997; 90: 785–795.
29 Smith J, Smith O. Replicative senescence: implications for *in vivo* aging and tumor suppression. Science 1996; 273: 63–67.
30 Bunout D, Cambiazo V. Nutrition and aging. Rev Med Chile 1999; 127: 82–88.
31 Saretzki G, von Zglinicki T. Replicative senescence as a model of aging; the role of oxidative stress and telomere shortening – an overview. Z Gerontol Geriatrie 1999; 32(2): 69–75.
32 Sohol R, Weindruch R. Oxidative stress, caloric restriction and aging. Science 1996; 273: 59–63.
33 Brown K. A radical proposal. Sci Am 2000; 11(2): 39–43.
34 Ashok BT, Ali R. The aging paradox: free radical theory of aging. Exp Gerontol 1999; 34: 293–303.

35 Knight JA. Free radicals: their history and current status in aging and disease. Ann Clin Lab Sci 1998; 28: 331–346.

36 Beckman KB, Ames BN. The free radical theory of aging matures. Physiol Rev 1998; 78: 547–581.

37 Orr W, Sohol R. Extension of lifespan by over expression of superoxide dismutase and catalase in *Drosophila melanogaster*. Science 1994; 263: 1128.

38 Miquel J. An update on the oxygen stress–mitochondrial mutation theory of aging; genetic and evolutionary implications. Exp Gerontol 1998; 33(1–2): 113–126.

39 Wei YH. Oxidative stress and mitochondrial DNA mutations in human aging. Proc Soc Exp Biol Med 1998; 217: 53–63.

40 Yu BP, Kang CM, Han JS, Kim DS. Can antioxidant supplementation slow the aging process? Biofactors 1998; 7(1–2): 93–101.

41 Marx J. Chipping away at the causes of aging. Science 2000; 287: 2390.

42 Ly DH, Lockhart DJ, Lerner RA, Schultz PG. mitotic misregulation and human aging. Science 2000; 287: 2486–2491.

43 Lee CK, Kloop RG, Weindruch R, Prolla T. Gene expression profile of aging and Its retardation by caloric restriction. Science 1999; 285: 1390–1392.

44 Weindruch R. Caloric restriction and aging. Sci Am 1996; 274(1): 32–38.

45 Taubes G. The famine of youth. Sci Am 2000; 11(2): 45–49.

46 Lane M, Ingram D, Roth G. Beyond the rodent model: calorie restriction in rhesus monkeys. Age 1997; 20: 45–56.

47 Masoro EJ. Influence of caloric intake on aging and on the response of stressors. J Toxico Environ Health B Crit Rev 1998; 1: 243–257.

48 Alexander CN, Langer EJ, Newman RI et al. Transcendental meditation, mindfulness and longevity: an experimental study with the elderly. J Pers Soc Psychol 1989; 57: 950–964.

49 Alexander CN, Schneider RH, Staggers F et al. A trail of stress reduction for hyertension in older African Americans (Part II): sex and risk subgroup analysis. Hypertension 1996; 28, 228–237.

50 Schneider R, Staggers F, Alexander C et al. A randomized controlled trial of stress reduction for hypertension in older African Americans. Hypertension 1995: 26: 820–827.

51 Orme-Johnson D. Medical care utilization and the transcendental meditation program. Psychosom Med 1987; 49: 493–507.

52 Eppley K, Abrams A, Shears J. The differential effects of relaxation techniques on trait anxiety: a meta-analysis. J Clin Psychol 1989; 45: 957–974.

53 Orme-Johnson DW, Walton KG. All approaches to preventing or reversing effects of stress are not the same. Am J Health Promotion 1998; 12(5): 297–299.

54 Eisenberg DM, Delbanco TL, Berkey CS. Cognitive behavior techniques for hypertension: are they effective? Ann Intern Med 1993; 118: 964–972.

55 May M. Mother Nature's menders. Sci Am 2000; 11(2): 57–61.

56 Wilmut I, Schnleke AE, McWhir J et al. Viable offspring derived from fetal and adult mammalian cells. Nature 1997; 385: 810–813.

57 Ashworth D, Bishop M, Campbell K et al. DNA microsatellite analysis fo Dolly. Nature 1998; 394: 329.

58 Signer EN, Dubrova YE, Wilde C et al. DNA fingerprinting Dolly. Nature 1998; 394: 329–330.

59 Solter D. Dolly is a clone – and no longer alone. Nature 1998; 394: 315–316.

60 Lanza RP, Cibelli JB, Blackwell C, Cristofalo VJ. Extension of cell life-span and telomere length in animals cloned from senescent somatic cells. Science 2000; 288: 665–669.

61 Shiels PG, Kind AJ, Campbell KHS et al. Analysis of telomere lengths in cloned sheep. Nature 1999; 399: 316–317.

62 Cibelli JB, Stice SL, Golueke PJ et al. Cloned transgenic calves produced from nonquiescent fetal fibroblasts. Science 1998; 289: 1256–1258.

5

Normal ageing

Brian J Gleberzon

All physiological systems display morbific changes to some degree during the process of growing old. These changes are normal and unavoidable, being the result of genetic programming; however, many deleterious changes may be exacerbated by the environment in which a person lives or, conversely, they may be mitigated by salutary lifestyle strategies. It is imperative for a clinician to be able to differentiate between those changes that occur normally with ageing and those changes that are pathological, as many of these pathological changes necessitate modifications to treatment strategies or referral to another health-care specialist, or both.

In general, the ageing process involves the gradual decline or loss of the reserve capacity of organs or systems; there is a progressive decline in the body's ability to respond to environmental stressors.[1] Ageing processes are defined as having the following four common characteristics:[1]

- They must be deleterious to the organism.
- They must be progressive over a period of time.
- They must be intrinsic to the organism.
- They must be universal, occurring in all members of the species.

This chapter will review the normal changes in biological and cognitive systems that are associated with senescence. Those changes considered to be pathological are discussed in greater detail throughout the textbook.

Intellectual functions

Cognitive changes

Despite normal losses in neurological structure and function, many components of intellectual performance, which can be defined as those underlying mental abilities that can be applied across many general categories or situations, tend to be maintained well into the eighth decade of life.[2,3] Moreover, the degree of cognitive decline is often a function of the instrument used for its measurement, or the context in which intelligence is defined. For example, one of the most widely used tests to measure the intelligence of older adults is the Wechsler Adult Intelligence Scale (WAIS-R).[4,5] The WAIS-R measures two of types of intelligence: (i) verbal intelligence, which is comprised of comprehension skills, computation abilities, similarities, vocabulary and the ability to recall digits, and (ii) psychomotor intelligence, aspects of which involve task completion, block design and assembly of objects. In general, using this scale, psychomotor speed has been shown to decline with age. However, critics of the WAIS-R argue that the test only emphasizes those skills learned in school and not those skills acquired during everyday life.[4] Another drawback of this test is that the speed in which a psychomotor skill is performed is measured, a bias that tends to favour younger persons. Current research indicates that older persons, although typically requiring a longer period to complete a psychomotor task, tend to compensate for this by a concomitant increase in accuracy.[4]

Other authorities favour differentiating between what is colloquially termed crystallized intelligence and fluid intelligence, a concept first proposed by Horn and Cattell in the early 1960s.[2,5] Fluid intelligence is influenced by neurological and physiological capabilities, and represents incidental learning not based on culture.[2,5] Furthermore, fluid intelligence represents the ability to adjust one's thinking to the demands of a specific situation, and to organize information for the purposes of problem solving. It makes little use of knowledge gained through reading, schooling or work.[5] Fluid intelligence is measured by performance tests (novel or new problem-solving challenges, inductive reasoning, matching symbols to numbers) and is scored according to accuracy and speed. Not surprisingly, based on the results gathered from cross-sectional and longitudinal studies, fluid intelligence declines with age after reaching a peak in adolescence.[2] By some estimates, fluid intelligence declines by 3–7 intelligence (IQ) units per decade between age 30 and 60 years.[2] This may be related to a decline in cerebral blood flow and a general deterioration of neurological structures.[2]

The performance of cognitive tasks, especially those that involve complex, decision-making processes such as driving a car, may take longer and may indicate a slowing in central processing.[1,3] The characteristic slowing of behavioural speed observed in older persons during activities such as driving has been termed cautiousness.[3]

In contrast to the decline in fluid intelligence, crystallized intelligence increases with age.[2,3,5] Crystallized intelligence, often measured using verbal-comprehension tests, is thought to be preserved or even increased throughout a person's lifetime because this knowledge is acquired during education, acculturation, learning and personal experience.[2,4,5] However, because crystallized intelligence is in large part a reflection of an individual's education and learning opportunities, there is tremendous variability based on the person's level of education obtained, socioeconomic status and race.[2]

Verbal skills are often well maintained into a person's seventies, as evidenced by the preservation of vocabulary stores.[3] However, other changes in mentation occur, including increased difficulty in learning a new language, as well as non-critical forgetfulness.[3]

Given that certain aspects of intelligence appear to decline less rapidly than previously assumed, researchers have sought an explanation as to the measurable difference in intellectual functions during an individual's middle and later life. Recent evidence suggests that measured intellectual decline is not simply a reflection of chronological age.[2] Instead, investigators suggest that various environmental factors may interact, resulting in intellectual declines. These factors include age-graded influences (specific socialization practices and events unique to each individual), historical influences (economic depressions and wars that may necessitate early school-leaving) and personal life events that create crisis for an individual (such as the death of a spouse, unemployment, divorce or trau-

matic medical illness).[2] Similarly, other researchers have linked cognitive declines in older persons to mandatory retirement.[2]

Many clinicians have observed that a sudden, severe decline in cognitive abilities, termed terminal drop, is often a harbinger of the individual's death.[4] Many geriatricians maintain that an abrupt decline in cognitive functioning may be related to the individual's distance from death rather than his or her chronological age.[4]

A useful concept when considering the degree to which an individual may experience intellectual decline is cognitive reserve.[5] As the name implies, a person with a greater cognitive reserve may be better able to withstand physiological impairments to neurological structures than an individual with a lesser cognitive reserve.

Wisdom

The difference in types of intelligence emphasizes an important cognitive asset seen in older persons: wisdom. Wisdom can be defined as 'expert knowledge about the important and fundamental matters of life, their interpretation and management'.[5] Baltes *et al.* compiled a list of criteria pertaining to the acquisition of wisdom.[5] These are: (i) a rich factual knowledge about life matters, (ii) a rich procedural knowledge about problems, (iii) knowledge about the contexts of life and their temporal relationships (referred to as life-span contextualism), (iv) knowledge about differences in values and priorities (relativism), and (v) knowledge about the relative indeterminacy and unpredictability of life and ways to manage it.[5]

Learning and memory

Learning and memory are complementary processes. Although both learning and memory are affected by age, the degree of change is highly variable. Learning, which can be defined as the ability to acquire knowledge or understanding, is a cognitive process.[4] Research indicates that older persons can learn new skills provided specific criteria are met. One of these criteria is that older individuals are allowed to pace themselves at their own speed.[4] In general, older people need to pace themselves slower than their younger cohorts.[2,4] In addition, older persons perform better if they are given a lengthened period in which to respond to questions. Lastly, a recurrent finding among cognitive researchers is that older persons can master new skills if the acquisition of these skills is perceived to be relevant; that is, the learning objective must have concrete value to an older individual's daily life.[2] Some authorities have suggested this may be more problematic for women as they are more likely to attend to irrelevant stimuli.[2] Within these parameters, older persons can learn as well as younger persons. Moreover, this age-related change in attentional selectivity also affects other cognitive processes, such as problem solving.[2] Therefore, it is important to eliminate distractions in the learning environment for older adults.

There are other non-cognitive factors that influence the ability of an older person to learn. Of particular importance is that the person must be motivated and willing to use his or her physical and cognitive capacities.[2] Researchers have also determined that an individual must have a sufficient level of intelligence to acquire the new information.[2] Previous experience in learning environments, which may convey learning strategies and skills, has also been shown to be advantageous to potential learners. Thus, older adults who have been involved in learning and education throughout their lives are not only more likely to want to learn, but are better able to do so efficiently.[2]

There is a relationship between memory and learning. This is because learning requires the ability to retain, store and retrieve the information previously demonstrated. As a general rule, the more one learns, the more one can remember. Cognitive researchers divide memory into three components: sensory, short term and long term[5] Research has demonstrated that short-term memory (recalling events that happened seconds or minutes before) or recent memory (recalling events that occurred hours or days before) is compromised in older individuals to a greater extend than long-term memory.[4] It is for this reason that many older people are able to recall events that occurred in their youth (episodic memory), but may not remember what they had for breakfast that morning.[2] Moreover, studies indicate that not only do older persons require a longer period to learn new information, but it also takes longer for them to search for it in their memories and longer to use it when they need it.[5] Lastly, some studies indicate that explicit memory, in which a person intends to remember something, decreases more with age than implicit memory, in which memory occurs without intention.[5]

Similar to learning in general, researchers believe that if incoming information is perceived to be relevant, it is less likely to be interrupted by competing stimuli, and is transferred to short-term memory.[4] Again, if it is considered important, the information may be repeated or rehearsed and thus ultimately transferred to long-term memory. As with learning, however, the older person requires more time to retrieve information from both short- and long-term memory, especially when faced with many stimulus–response alternatives.[4]

Thinking, problem solving and creativity

The specific manner or characteristic way in which an individual conceptually organizes their environment, manipulates the knowledge they possess and makes decisions or approaches problems that have to be solved is termed the person's cognitive style.[2] Two contrasting cognitive styles have been labelled 'field-dependent' and 'field-independent'.[2] An individual who uses a field-dependent cognitive style appears to be more perceptive of social milieu, more people orientated, and generally more conventional in dress and behaviour. In contrast, an individual who uses a field-independent cognitive style is more analytical, more internally directed, and less constrained by current behaviour or tradition.[2]

With respect to their cognitive styles, research has indicated that older persons tend to be more rigid and cautious in their thinking, and they are sometimes more reluctant to make difficult decisions (especially if the situation is ambiguous or requires great speed, or when they have a fear of failure).[2] Thus, as previously mentioned, older persons tend to substitute accuracy for speed in the form of cautiousness in these circumstances. In other instances, they may rely on previous experience, even if it is no longer applicable to the problem at hand.

With further respect to problem solving, there appears to be a decline in this ability with age that is attributable to a slowing of this behaviour and, more importantly, an unwillingness or inability to incorporate newer, more efficient cognitive styles. This tendency is a great impediment in the twenty-first century society that can be classified as a technocracy; that is, a society that changes quickly as new technological advances are developed.

Creativity can be defined as the total productivity (quantity) throughout an individual's career, or it may be the point in an individual's career at which the highest quality work was completed.[2] According to some authorities, creativity generally peaks at the age of 40 years, with a decline appearing at 50 years.[2] However, there are many notable exceptions to this belief. For example, Grandma Moses did not start her painting career until she was in her sixties, and Linus Pauling won his second Nobel Prize at the age of 70 years.

Personality

Personality is an amalgam of a person's traits, characteristics, moods, cognitive styles, and lifestyles, and is heavily influenced by societal and cultural factors.[2,4] In general, the preponderance of literature supports the conclusion that an individual's personality traits, such as presentation of self, attitudes, values and temperament, do not normally change as a consequence of ageing. Current opinions hold that, with age, an individual merely exhibits those characteristics that they demonstrated in their youth to a greater or lesser extent. For example, a person who has a negative outlook as a young adult is more likely to have a similar outlook as a senior. However, a significant life change (bereavement, mandatory retirement, chronic illness) may manifest itself as a change in an individual's personality, but such a change is usually restricted to change along a consistent continuum. In general, a significant change in an individual's personality is considered to be a harbinger of serious illness.[3]

Pathological cognitive impairments (dementia, delirium, depression and neuropsychiatric disorders) are discussed in greater detail in Chapter 9.

Neuromusculoskeletal system

Neurological system changes (see also Chapter 11)

Central nervous system

Unlike other organ systems, cells in the nervous system cannot reproduce, and damaged cells simply wither and die.[3] With normal ageing, the brain undergoes shrinkage of cerebral sulci and enlargement of the gyri, especially in the frontal region.[1] This shrinkage leaves an older person more susceptible to subdural haematoma, even after minor head trauma.[1] There is typically fibrosis of the meninges and the blood vessels become atherosclerotic, with the deposition of amyloid.[1,3] This results in a decrease in cerebral blood flow and an associated loss of neurons.[1] This loss of neurons occurs primarily in the cerebral and cerebellar cortices, with as much as 45% of neurons lost over a lifetime, resulting in an overall decline in brain weight of 10% from the second or third decade to the age of 90 years.[1,3] In the areas of degenerative change there is an accumulation of lipofuscin.[1] Lastly, the cerebral ventricles increase in size by as much as three or four times in cross-section, with the appearance of granulations.[1,3]

It is important to note that the clinical implications of these degenerative changes are difficult to judge, since brain weight and ventricular size are not correlated with intelligence.[3] Moreover, ventricular size has been observed to be unaffected even in those individuals with severe dementia.[3]

In some individuals, normal senescence results in the accumulation of neurofibrillary tangles and, less frequently, the appearance of neuritic plaques.[1,3] When these histological structures are rampant throughout the cortex, they are the hallmark of Alzheimer's disease. According to some experts, neurons may be completely lost in many regions of the brain, with senile plaques accumulating in the hippocampus and limbic cortex.[1]

Research indicates that there is a significant decrease in the cross-sectional area of the spinal cord after the age of 80, particularly at the level of C6; however, the length of the spinal cord was found to have no correlation with ageing.[1]

Other neurophysiological changes include a depletion of neurotransmitters, and a reduction in the concentration of enzymes, coenzymes and catecholamine precursors.[1,3] The alteration in the regulation, formation and degradation of acetylcholine results in the loss of dopamine, noradrenaline and acetylcholine receptors, which eventually leads to the death of neurons.[1] Conversely, the activity of other enzymes, such as monoamine oxidase (MAO), may increase, and some authorities believe that inhibitors of MAO may forestall the onset of disabilities in patients with Parkinson's disease.[1]

The brain possesses certain properties that mitigate these adverse physiological changes. First, many more neural cells in the brain exist then are needed. This is called redundancy.[3] For example, symptoms of diabetes insipidus do not appear until there is a loss of 85–90% of the nerve cells in the supraoptic and paraventricular nuclei.[3] However, because the number of cells required for certain functions is not known, the extent of redundancy is difficult to estimate.[3]

Secondly, compensatory mechanisms may appear in the brain if it is damaged. For example, if the speech centres in the dominant hemisphere are damaged, the non-dominant hemisphere may compensate, allowing for the gradual return of speech function.[3] Likewise, large areas of the cerebellum may be destroyed or injured, and recovery is often observed as other motor systems take over.[3] Compensatory mechanisms are more evolved and effective in the higher centres, so that the spinal cord, for example, has less ability to recover after injury than the brain.[3]

Lastly, it is now believed that more neural plasticity exists than was previously suspected.[3] For example, recent studies have revealed that the deterioration and death of nerve cells are partially compensated for by the lengthening and increase in dendritic connections remaining in the brain. This may be a biological attempt to preserve cerebral function.[3]

The senses

In general, there is an impairment in positional sense and light touch perception with ageing.[1,3] These changes result in instability and a general sense of difficulty with regard to navigating around one's environment, especially in dimly lit rooms, which partially accounts for the increase in the risk of falls and fractures associated with ageing. Loss of vibrational sense is common (especially below the knees), although joint position sense is relatively preserved.[3] However, a loss of somatosensations (proprioception and cutaneous sensation) may result in a loss of the ability to detect body sway.[6] This may further hamper an individual's ability to initiate balance-correcting responses, especially when walking in areas of changing surface terrains.[6]

Hearing loss is often evident in older persons. Significant hearing loss occurs in as many as 25% of older persons over the age of 65 years.[1] The most common diagnosis is presbyacusis, which is the bilateral loss of hearing, especially of sounds of higher frequencies. Changes also occur in the labyrinthine system of the middle ear. This is a major contributing cause of benign positional paroxysmal vertigo in older persons (see Chapter 14).

Vision loss is very common in older persons, with one in six people over the age of 75 and one in four over the age of 85 years demonstrating significant visual impairments.[1] Opacification of the ocular lens is very common in older persons, as is macular degeneration.

Macular degeneration is not necessary considered to be an aspect of normal ageing, but there is a high prevalence of this disorder in the elderly. With ageing, the pupils become smaller, decreasing the amount of light that reaches the retina. This makes it harder for an older person to see in a dimly lit room.[6] Moreover, the eyes take longer to adjust to darkness and to glare.[6] Taken as a whole, diminished peripheral vision, depth perception, visual discrimination and visual acuity deficits may culminate in an increased difficulty for an older person to discriminate environmental obstacles, leading to an increased risk of falls and subsequent fracture.[6] However, most age-related changes to vision can usually be successfully managed by corrective lenses.

It is important for the clinician to be cognizant of the fact that loss of hearing and vision often results in social isolation and a depressive mood. These social constraints are often more detrimental to a person's quality of life than the sensory impairments themselves.

Taste sensation often diminishes with age, but this is usually a result in a decline in olfactory function rather than to the ability of taste itself.[3] However, the number of taste buds diminishes with age, along with some taste-bud sensitivity.[3,6] This may result in an older person complaining of a loss of appetite.[6]

It is still unclear whether pain sensation changes with ageing. The majority of research at this time, however, tends to support the opinion that pain perception does not diminish with age.

Peripheral nervous system

In general, there is a slowing of transmission speed along peripheral nerves, with a concomitant decrease in reaction time.[1,3] It is imperative for a clinician not to interpret normal changes in the peripheral nervous system as pathological. Although the Achilles' reflex is often normally diminished or absent, other muscle stretch reflexes (deep tendon reflexes) are typically unaffected.[3,6] There is also a reduction in motor coordination, due to changes in central mechanisms.[3]

There is a normally a gradual decline in the total number of myelinated fibres in the dorsal column of the spinal cord.[7] With ageing, the there is a decrease in the density of myelinated fibres (particularly those of large diameter), as well as an increase in the number of degenerated myelinated and unmyelinated fibres.[7] Peripheral polyneuropathy is suspected if a patient presents with progressive sensory and motor symptoms that begin in the feet and lower legs, and later affect the hands. In these cases, sensory loss spreads proximally.[7]

Muscular system changes

In general, ageing results in a loss of bone mass and a concomitant increase in fat.[1] By the eighth decade, 30% or more of skeletal muscle mass may have been lost.[8] This decline is the result of many different complex factors, including biochemical changes in muscle metabolism, changes in neurological control, nutrition, immobility and psychological disorders such as depression.[1]

Muscle strength is considered to be the most physiological limiting factor of the older person, and a determinant of their health status.[9,10] With ageing, there is a loss of lean body mass, particularly of the skeletal muscle compartments.[3,11] This loss of muscle mass and strength is accompanied by a decrease in the number of muscle fibres, and a decrease in muscle fibre size.[11] Moreover, a decrease in motor neuron units results in the remodelling of the neuromuscular junction. This decline in motor neuron units is partially compensated for by an increase in the collateral reinnervation of adjacent muscle fibres by neighbouring neurons. This results in an increase in motor neuron size but a decrease in muscle control.[11,12]

This sacropenic effect does not occur uniformly throughout the muscular system.[11,13,14] Certain muscle, such as the quadriceps, atrophy to a much lesser extent than other muscles, such as the biceps of the upper limb and the tibialis anterior of the lower limb.[12,13] This finding is attributed to the fact that muscles such as the quadriceps are involved in many more activities of daily living (ADLs) than the biceps. Diminished strength in the biceps can seriously hamper a person's ADLs, because of its involvement in such activities as lifting, cleaning and manipulating household objects.[12,14] Similarly, a weakened tibialis anterior muscle has been associated with an increase in the risk of falling and subsequent fracture.[13,14] As will be discussed in Chapter 14, falls and fractures are a leading cause of morbidity and mortality among older patients, and place an enormous financial burden on health-care systems. It is important for a clinician to be aware of the fact that these changes in muscle strength are reversible with strength-training exercises, even among the frail elderly.[15]

The deposition of fat into muscle fibres increases in older patients. This is clinically important because lipophilic drugs have more uptake potential, and therefore a prolonged pharmacological action.[1]

The decline in muscle (and bone) mass results in older patients being less able to tolerate trauma, and those practitioners performing high-velocity, low-amplitude (HVLA) manipulations must do so with extra caution.[16] The modifications to chiropractic treatment necessitated by changes to the musculoskeletal system will be described in further detail in Chapter 25.

When assessing the motor system, the clinician must remember that older persons, especially women, often appear weak on routine examination.[3] If the weakness is symmetrical, it is most likely to be non-pathological.[3] There is normally a slight increase in muscular tone with ageing, but arm movements should not be jerky or demonstrate cogwheel rigidity (the later is indicative of Parkinson's disease).[3]

Skeletal system changes (see also Chapter 10)

The osseous mass tends to decline with age. There is a decline in the conversion of 25-hydroxyvitamin D to the more active 1,25-hydroxy D_3, with a diminished intestinal absorption of calcium.[8] Parathyroid hormone secretion increases with lower levels of serum calcium, resulting in a release of calcium from bone.[8] Moreover, oestrogen levels drop during menopause, further contributing to a reduction in bone mass.[8]

In cortical bone, the rate of loss is 2–3% per year after menopause, whereas trabecular bone, found in vertebral bodies and the ends of long bones, is lost at a rate of 1–2% per year in men and women.[3,8] The loss of trabecular bone begins a decade earlier than does the loss of cortical bone.

Throughout their lives, women lose about 35% of cortical bone and up to 50% of trabecular bone; men lose about 20% of cortical bone and 30% of trabecular bone.[1,3,8] Overall, women tend to lose 0.75–1% of their total bone mass per year, starting between the ages of 30 and 35 years, whereas men lose only about 0.4% of their total bone mass per year, starting as late as 50 years of age.[1]

Not only is there a loss of the amount of bone, but the bone itself is adversely affected. The bone mineral content and comprehensive tensile strength of trabecular bone decrease with age.[1]

With ageing, the intervertebral discs become more dry, generally lack proteoglycans and possess no nucleus pulposus after the age of 40.[1] The uncinate processes become flat and may project either laterally or posterolaterally, where they may impinge neurological structures.[1] The dural root sleeves often become fibrotic and rigid, which may also lead to neurological impingement. Lastly, the ligamentum flavum of the spinal canal becomes hypertrophied and may, along with osteophytes that typically develop, compromise the spinal canal space.[1]

Postural and gait changes

Older people display characteristic postural stances with ageing. Typically, an older person is flexed with their head and neck held forward and the dorsal spine becoming kyphotic.[1] The upper limbs are bent at the elbow and wrist joints, and the hip and knee joints are usually slightly flexed.[1] These changes are the result of the ankylosis of ligaments and joints, the atrophy of tendons and muscles, and degenerative changes in the extrapyramidal nervous system.[1]

With age, gait changes. In general, older men display a wide-based gait; older women adopt a narrow-based, waddling gait.[3] Gait speed tends to diminish, and older persons display a reduction in stride length, force of push-off, toe-clearance, arm swing, and hip and knee rotation.[1,6,14] A more detailed description of gait changes and their impact on the incidence of falls and fractures is described in Chapter 14.

Coronary and cardiovascular system changes

The heart, great vessels and peripheral vascular system typically experience degenerative changes to their respective structure and function, usually as the result of artherosclerosis.[1] These changes are described in detail in Chapter 15, and hypertension and stroke are covered in Chapter 16.

Pulmonary system changes

Ageing adversely affects both the physiological function of the lungs, since the they are less able to move air in and out, and the lungs capacity to defend themselves against infection and other diseases.[3,17] The lungs lose their inherit elasticity, with an associated decline in vital capacity and an increase in residual volume.[3,17]

Thus, less of the air breathed is properly oxygenated, and the air previously used is inadequately cleared.[3,17]

The defence mechanisms of the lungs decline with age.[3] The clearance mechanism, humoral immunity response and cellular immunity response are all compromised as the individual ages.[3] This results in older persons being more susceptible to infections, such as pneumonia.[3] Pulmonary disorders, such as the chronic obstructive lung diseases, are discussed in detail in Chapter 23.

Gastrointestinal system changes

The gastrointestinal system, comprised of the oral cavity, oesophagus, stomach, and the small and large intestines, undergoes major changes with age. These changes are described in detail in Chapter 17.

Endocrine system changes

Thyroid function tends to be preserved during the ageing process.[1] However, various pathologies often target the thyroid gland. These are described in detail in Chapter 20.

Similarly, although pancreatic function tends to be unaffected with normal ageing, there tends to be a decrease in peripheral response to the effects of insulin.[1] Moreover, disorders of the pancreas, such as diabetes, are very common. Please see Chapter 12 for a complete description of the epidemiology of diabetes.

Genitourinary changes

The kidneys, ureter and sex organs undergo several important normal changes with ageing. These changes may ultimately result in sexual dysfunction or incontinence. These changes are described in Chapter 18.

Menopause

Menopause is defined as the physiological cessation of menses of greater than 1 year due to decreased ovarian function.[3] Menopause may be classified as natural, artificial or surgical.[3,18] Menopause is often diagnosed retrospectively after 6–12 months of amenorrhoea in women aged 55 years or older. It may also be diagnosed in a women who has had a hysterectomy or oophorectomy.[18] With a life expectancy of 81 years and the average onset of menopause being

51 years, a women can expect to live more than a third of her life after the menopause.[19]

It must be emphasized that menopause is not a clinical condition, but a normal biological change. Each woman will experience menopause differently. The age of onset can be anywhere from the age of 40 to 60 years, and associated symptoms experienced vary widely.[3] Symptoms include:[3,17,18]

- hot flashes: defined as the subjective sensation of intense warmth in the upper body lasting from 30 s to 5 min, approximately 75% of American women experience hot flashes, but they are severe in only 10–15% of women. Hot flashes may persist for more than 4 years in 85% in menopausal women;
- psychoemotional changes including fatigue, irritability, insomnia, inability to concentrate, depression, memory loss, headache, anxiety and nervousness;
- sleep disturbances;
- intermittent dizziness, paraesthesia, arthralgia, myalgia and a cold feeling in the extremities;
- weight gain;
- thinning, drying and epithelial atrophy of the vaginal mucosa, and atrophy and los of elasticity of vulvar skin. This may make the person more prone to infection and cause sexual intercourse to be uncomfortable or painful;
- urinary problems such as urgency, burning, frequency and stress-type incontinence.

These physiological and psychological changes may be concurrent with other changes in a woman's life such as her children leaving home, change in body image, widowhood, retirement, increased in anxiety about illness or death, bereavement over loss of friends or loved ones, concerns about financial security, increased responsibility for ageing parents and other morbific health changes.[20] These life changes may amplify menopausal symptoms.

There is evidence that men also experience a less pervasive change at this age, manifested by such symptoms as a degree of lethargy, depression, increased irritability, mood swings, changes in libido and sexuality, difficulty attaining and sustaining an erection, weight gain and a loss of interest in life.[21]

The major concerns associated with these changes in both men and women are the increased risk of osteoporosis and cardiovascular disease. This is because of the rapid decline in levels of oestrogen in women and testosterone in men.

Menopause does not require 'treatment' in the conventional sense. A chiropractor can provide information to a patient concerned with the changes that they are experiencing, and can suggest referrals to self-help groups, medical physicians or psychologists as needed.

Vaginal dryness may require lubricants, while Kegel exercises may help in the management of stress incontinence (see Chapter 18). Hormone-replacement therapy (HRT) is also often recommended to combat the symptoms of menopause. Oestrogen therapy is considered to be the only effective treatment for genital atrophy.[3] In the past, there has been concern over the association between HRT and breast or endometrial cancer. However, a newer group of HRT drugs, the selective oestrogen-replacement drugs such as Evista, provides the benefit of oestrogen therapy without the associated increase in risks. Moreover, the selective (o)estrogen receptor modulator (SERM) drugs have also been demonstrated to provide some protection from cardiovascular disease.

Other alternative therapies for the management of menopausal symptoms and the associated diseases include a low fat, high-fibre diet. It is also recommended that a women avoid caffeine, spicy foods and alcohol, as these foods have been known to trigger hot flashes and aggravate mood swings and urinary incontinence. To counter the risk of osteoporosis, a person can shift to a diet consisting of foods rich in sources of calcium or calcium supplements. The cessation of smoking and increase in weight-bearing exercises will also inhibit the osteoporotic process. Botanical medicines considered to diminish the unpleasant consequences of menopause include alfalfa, black cohash, chaste tree and dong quoi.[22]

Benign prostatic hyperplasia

It is estimated that one in every four men in the USA will be treated for symptoms related to benign prostatic hyperplasia (BPH).[8] A recent study among normal volunteers found a 51% prevalence of BPH among men aged 60–69 years.[8]

As men age, the prostate increases in size owing to hyperplasia of the prostatic epithelium.[3] Symptoms of BPH may be thought of as being either obstructive or irritative.[18] Obstructive symptoms of BPH include difficulty in initializing urination (hesitancy), incomplete emptying of the bladder and postvoid dribbling.[3,8] Irritative symptoms of BPH include increased frequency of urination and nocturia.[8,18] The American Urological Association (AUA) has developed a symptom index for BPH (Table 5.1).[3,18]

Physical examination of the prostate includes rectal examination, which is beyond the scope of chiropractic in many jurisdictions. Additional tests include urinalysis, uroflowmetry, ultrasonography and advanced imagining techniques.[8]

Treatment options are divided into surgical, medical and watchful waiting.[3,8] The surgical procedure of choice is a transurethral resection of the prostate (TURP), whereas medical management includes the use of α-adrenergic blockers and hormonal manipulation.[8] Other non-pharmacological suggestions include relaxing before urination, minimizing fluid intake before bedtime and avoiding caffeine, unnecessary diuretics and anticholinergic agents.[3] Some practitioners have also found the use of saw palmetto or nettle to be beneficial for patients with BPH.[22]

Table 5.1 AUA Symptom Index[3,18]

Question No.	
1	Over the past month, how often have you had a sensation of not emptying your bladder completely after you finished urinating?
2	Over the past month, how often have you to urinate again less than 2 hours after you finished urinating?
3	Over the past month, how often have you found you stopped and started again several times when you urinate?
4	Over the past month, how often have you found it difficult to postpone urination?
5	Over the past month, how often have you had a weak urinary stream?
6	Over the past month, how often have you had to push or strain to begin urination?
7	Over the past month, how many times did you most typically get up to urinate from the time you went to bed until the time you got up in the morning?

Patients are asked to rank each question from not at all (0), less than 1 time to 5 (1), less than half the time (2), about half the time (3), more than half the time (4) to almost always (5).
The scores recorded from each question are added. A score of 0–7 indicates mild incontinence, 8–19 moderate incontinence and 20–25 severe incontinence.

Although current scientific evidence suggests that BPH and prostatic cancer are independent entities, some authorities now question whether the two conditions are related.[8] Experts in this field note that the two conditions not only occur more commonly and with increased frequency with advanced age, but often coexist in the same person.[8]

Dermatological changes

Normal changes to the skin, such as drying and wrinkling, are quite typical. However, several other important dermatological changes may also occur, predisposing a person to several clinical conditions, such as eczema or cancer. These changes are described in detail in Chapter 19.

Sleep changes

Sleep patterns change with age, but authorities disagree as to which changes are the result of normal ageing and which are pathological.[3] Moreover, individual variability as to the amount of sleep required in order to feel adequately rested further complicates the differentiation between normal and abnormal changes.[3]

The most striking age-related change in sleep physiology is the reduction in the amount and amplitude of delta sleep, although rapid eye movement (REM) sleep is generally unaffected by ageing.[8] In general, studies indicate that older persons spend less time asleep at night, awakening more frequently and staying awake longer, although other studies indicate that the total amount of sleep time does not change with ageing.[3,8] Daytime napping and redistribution of sleep throughout the day may compensate for poor nocturnal sleep.[3] Older persons demonstrate a general tendency to fall asleep and awaken early, and are less tolerant of shifts in the sleep–wake cycle.[3]

Nevertheless, according to one study of non-institutionalized seniors, 45% of those over the age of 65 reported having at least some trouble with sleep during the previous year, and 25% reported having serious difficulties.[8]

A poorly understood phenomenon associated with changes in sleep patterns is the sundowning effect.[3] Often associated with dementia, the sundowning effect involves an exacerbation of disruptive behaviour at night. Agitation is a prominent feature of this effect.[3] About 12–14% of patients with dementia in nursing homes demonstrate agitated behaviour more often at night than during the day.[3]

In addition to dementia, many medical illnesses can result in a disturbance of sleep or, conversely, are detrimentally affected by sleep.[8] These clinical conditions will be described in further detail in Chapter 21.

Summary

The physiological changes observed during the ageing process occur along a continuum that has, at one end, those changes that are considered normal and, at the other end, those changes that are pathological. A clinician must be able to differentiate between these two poles, in order to determine whether a patient's physiological changes require the therapeutic intervention of other health-care specialists. It is also important for field practitioners to encourage their patients to choose those lifestyle habits that deter the development of pathological conditions as opposed to the normal changes that can be achieved with ageing. These choices include adopting such preventive strategies (see Chapter 30) as seeking a spinal check-up, maintaining a regular exercise routine, proper nutritional choices and keeping socially active within a community.

References

1 Souza T, Soliman S. Normal aging. Top Clin Chiropractic 1996; 3(2): 1–9.

2 McPherson BD. Aging as a Social Process. Toronto: Butterworth & Co. (Canada), 1983.

3 Abrams W. The Merck Manual of Geriatric Patients. 2nd edn. Whitehouse Station: Merck & Co., 1995.

4 Barrows GW. Aging, the Individual and Society, 3rd edn. St Paul, MN: West Publishing Co., 1986.

5 Novak M. Aging and Society: A Canadian Perspective. 3rd edn. Scarborough, ON: International Thomson Publishing, 1997.

6 Morgenthal AP. The geriatric examination: general principles and examination procedures. Top Clin Chiropractic 2000; 7(3): 19–27.

7 McCarthy KA. Peripheral neuropathy in the aging patient: common causes, assessment, and risks. Top Clin Chiropractic 1999; 6(4): 56–61.

8 Lonergan E. Geriatrics. A Lange Clinical Manual. 2st edn. Stamford, CT: Appleton & Lange 1996.

9 Bracewell DD et al. Muscular strength changes in women ages 75–80 after six weeks of resistive training. Presented at the Active Living Coalition for Older Adults (ALCOA) Conference, 14 May 1999.

10 Brill PA et al. The value of strength training for older adults. Home Care Provide 1999 4(2): 62–66.

11 Hicks A. Loss of strength in old age: is it aging or disuse? Presented at the ALCOA Conference, 14 May 1999.

12 Porter M, Vandervoort A, Lexell J. Aging of human muscle: strength, function and adaptability. Eur J Appl Physiol and Occup Physiol 1997; 76: 62–68.

13 Jakobi J, Rice C. Differential neuromuscular changes with age in limb muscle. Presented at the ALCOA Conference, 14 May 1999.

14 Rantanen T, Guralnik J. Disability, physical activity and muscle strength in older women: the women's health and aging study. Arch Phys Med Rehabil 1999; 80: 130–135.

15 Gleberzon BJ, Annis RS. The necessity of strength training for the older patient. J Can Chiropractic Assoc 2000; 44(2): 99–103.

16 Bowers L. Clinical assessment of geriatric patients: unique challenges. Top Clin Chiropractic 1996; 3(2): 10–22.

17 McCarthy KA. Management considerations in the geriatric patient. Top Clin Chiropractic 1996; 3(2): 66–75.

18 Ferri F, Fretwell M, Watchel T. Practical Guide to the Care of the Elderly Patient, 2nd edn. St. Louis: Mosby-Year Book, 1997.

19 National Institute on Aging. Menopause. www.nih.gov/nia/health/pubs/menopause

20 Planned Parenthood. Menopause, Another Change in Life. www.plannedparenthood.org/WOMENSHEALTH/menopause

21 Introduction to Male Menopause. www.midlife-passages.com/impotence:htm.

22 Boon H, Smith M. The Botanical Pharmacy. The Pharmacology of 47 Common Herbs. Kingston: Quarry Press, 1999.

Section II: Assessment of the older person

6

Patient history and interview suggestions

Brian J Gleberzon

A comprehensive geriatric assessment begins with the history or patient interview. The majority of information about the patient is obtained during the interview process. It remains the primary investigative tool, providing diagnostic yields of up to 90%, although this figure may be lower in the older patient.[1] In many ways, it is useful to compare oneself, as the doctor, to a detective. In this instance, however, the patient is both the victim and the scene of the 'crime'. It is the practitioner's mission to determine the events preceding the problem, to deduce the most likely cause of the patient's presenting concerns and to decide upon the best course of action for the patient's benefit. This may include accepting the patient for treatment under your care, referring the patient to a specialist, or co-managing the patient with other members of the healthcare team.

Challenges to the interview of an older patient

Although that of an older patient is very similar to that of a younger individual, the interview of an older patient presents many unique challenges to a clinician:[1,2]

- underreporting of illnesses
- overestimation of cognitive abilities
- atypical presentations
- symptoms of different disorders may overlap.

One significant problem is the underreporting of illnesses.[1] Many older patients have a tendency to assume that particular symptoms are just the result of old age. The patient's cultural upbringing may influence their willingness to admit his or her state of health, or the patient may be embarrassed to admit the extent of their problems. This is especially true for those patients experiencing incontinence, sexual dysfunction or dementia.[1] Moreover, a patient may wish to avoid the appearance of frailty, especially if they are concerned about the prospect of institutionalization.

A second problem is that older patients may overestimate their cognitive abilities.[1] Again, many patients may either be unaware of, or do not want to admit, the extent to which their cognitive faculties have diminished or been compromised. There is also a tendency for older patients' spouses to underestimate any cognitive loss.[1]

The third major challenge that a practitioner may be faced with when interviewing an older patient is that the symptoms of many different conditions may overlap.[1,2] For example, arthritic conditions, fibromyalgia and stress-related muscular hypertonicity may all present with morning stiffness. It may therefore be difficult for the clinician to differentiate between each of these disorders and determine which condition is contributing to the patient's presenting symptoms. According to Bowers, the average older patient has at least three identified health disabilities and, for every one of these that is known to the practitioner, there is another that is not.[1] Moreover, the apparent non-resolution of a patient's condition may be due to the manifestations of a completely different, identified or unidentified condition.[3] This diagnostic challenge of overlapping of symptoms is more likely to occur in those patient who are afflicted with multiple pathologies (called comorbidity).[1–3]

For reasons that are not completely understood, the perception of pain due to illness or trauma is often diminished or absent in an older patient.[1] This may confound the diagnosis of those clinical conditions that present primarily with pain.

Another challenge facing a clinician during the interview process is the atypical presentation of many illnesses in the older patient.[2] This can be the most daunting obstacle to the development of an accurate diagnosis. Cancers, heart disease and other life-threatening conditions may be clinically silent, or the presentation of symptoms in a patient may not be 'textbook normal'. Typically, incontinence, gait disturbances, dementia and depression go unreported.[1]

Adverse drug reactions are a serious problem in the older patient (see Chapter 22, Iatrogenic drug reactions). Many presenting chief complaints may be the result of prescription medications or self-prescribed or self-selected medications.[2,4,5]

Augmenting the interview process

A clinician can use many strategies to augment the information obtained from the patient interview:[1,2,5]

- Make more than one visit for the interview (or follow up questions on a subsequent appointment).
- Schedule appointments in the mid-morning or late afternoon.
- Send a history form home with the patient prior to the appointment.
- Ask the patient to bring in any prescription medications, over-the-counter drugs or supplements.
- Speak clearly and move slowly, facing the patient.
- Ask the patient to wear glasses, hearing aid, dentures, etc.
- Keep the examination room quiet, warm, well lit and uncluttered.
- Augment the interview with the patient's caregiver if required.
- A reverse stethoscope may be us for hearing-impaired patients.
- The previous health-care provider may be contacted.

If a barrier exists that prevents easy communication between the clinician and the patient, the help of a third person may be necessary. The caveat here, however, is that because the dynamics between the patient and doctor are altered when a third person acts as an interpreter, the meaning of various statements may become significantly transformed during the translation from the question to the answer.[1]

Because the history-taking process of an older patient typically takes longer than the interview of a younger person, the clinician should set aside more time for older patients.[1] This can be achieved by scheduling a new patient during mid-morning or early after-

noon, periods in a practitioner's day which may be less busy.[1] The older patient may also be more alert at these times of day.[1] Alternatively, more than one appointment may be scheduled in order to complete the history and physical examination.[1] New patient forms can be sent home with older patients before their appointment, allowing patients to complete them at their own pace.[1]

Often, a patient may not know the name, dose or physiological rationale for a prescribed medication they are taking. Therefore, the patient should be asked to bring in all their current medications, over-the-counter remedies, vitamins, minerals or other supplements.[1]

The clinician's office should be well lit, uncluttered and free from any obstacles or hazards that may cause a fall, such as magazine tables, area rugs or extension cords.[1] During the interview itself, the practitioner should speak slowly and clearly while facing the patient.[1,4] If the patient is hearing impaired, the doctor could recommend that patient wear a stethoscope, and the doctor could talk into it. The patient should be encouraged to wear their dentures, eyeglasses and hearing aids during the interview.[1]

The chief complaint

Typically, a patient will present with a specific problem, most often pain. This is called the chief complaint. In a recent practice-based study by Hawk *et al.*, for example, the researchers reported that, among patients aged 55 years and older seeking chiropractic care, the presenting chief complaint was pain related in 72% of the 805 cases examined.[6] However, the patient may present with a more vague sense of discomfort. The general reason for the appointment should therefore be determined.[1] It is common for an older patient to recount a constellation of symptoms unrelated to a particular disorder, a process that can be very time consuming and uninformative for the clinician.[1,5] To avoid this, there are certain, specific questions that can be asked in order to identify the cause of the presenting chief complaint. The basic questions that need to be asked during a patient interview are the same for any new patient, irrespective of his or her age.

The history-taking process should begin with the clinician introducing him or herself to the patient, and the clinician should then briefly describe the sequence of events to follow. The clinician should explain that, following the interview, a physical examination will be conducted in order to reach a diagnosis, and that X-rays may or may not be taken. Lastly, the patient should be told that the practitioner will explain the diagnosis to the patient and that the patient's permission will be obtained before any treatment is rendered.

The opening question should be non-judgemental. Asking a new patient 'what seems to be the trouble' may appear to the patient as if the clinician is questioning whether a true problem exists. A more appropriate question would be 'what brings you in today?' This open-ended question allows the patient to describe their chief complaint without feeling that they are either malingering or imposing on the doctor's time. This question may also be more appropriate for patients who are not seeking symptom relief. This approach is especially useful for those patients who present with concerns about their posture, their general health or for a spinal check (general assessment). This approach allows the practitioner to determine the general reason for the office visit.

It is usually best to allow the patient the opportunity to detail fully and explain the reason that he or she has sought out care. Interrupting the patient is not advisable as it may hinder the development of a rapport between the doctor and the patient. In spite of this seemingly obvious fact, some studies have revealed that clinicians provided only 50 s to the patient before they interrupted with questions.[4] A similar study conducted by the Canadian Chiropractic Association revealed that the average amount of time that elapsed before a doctor interrupted a patient during the interview was 12 s.[7] Of particular interest, the same study revealed that the longest amount of time for which a patient spoke continuously was 2.5 min[7] and the average was only 90 s.[7]

When performing a history, it is best to divide the questions into two categories: those that specifically detail the chief complaint, and those that address the general status of the patient. In order to detail the chief complaint, a useful mnemonic is LO DR FICARA:

- Location
- Onset

- Duration
- Radiations

- Frequency
- Intensity
- Character of pain
- Associated symptoms
- Relieving factors
- Aggravating factors.

The key questions to be asked during the interview of an older patient should cover:[1]

- significant previous surgeries, falls, accidents or hospitalizations
- prior occurrence of chief complaint
- family history of diseases (including chief complaint)
- system review in functional terms [activities of daily living (ADLs) and instrumental activities of daily living (IADLs)]
- general reason for appointment
- lifestyle.

Although the specific order of questions that need to be asked is not especially important, the first question that should be asked is the *location* of the chief complaint. This question should be asked first because many patients have a limited knowledge of anatomy and they may identify a particular region of the body erroneously. Therefore, the patient should be asked to point to the area of chief complaint. For example, among the most common presenting chief complaints is low back pain emanating from the sacroiliac region. A patient with sacroiliac dysfunction will often describe this as hip pain. If the clinician does identify the difference between what the patient described and what they meant, the clinician may spend considerable time formulating questions specific to the (incorrectly) identified region. In the example above, the clinician may ask questions that serve to elicit information about pathologies of the hip that do not exist in the sacroiliac joint, such as bursitis. The clinician may even go so far as begin to form a clinical impression based on the location of the chief complaint, along with certain treatment protocols, which in fact may be completely unnecessary or inappropriate. Lastly, the manner in which the patient identifies the area of chief complaint may be informative. For example, the patient may use a single finger to identify the painful area, indicating a specific, focal problem. Alternatively, the patient may use a broader contact, indicating a more diffuse area of discomfort.

When transcribing the location of the patient's chief complaint, is it imperative to use appropriate anatomical nomenclature. This ensures that, in the event that another health-care provider wishes to consult the chiropractor's files for guidance, the clinician will know where the problem was reported to be. A novice clinician may only record the chief complaint as 'back pain'. This term is clearly too vague to be of any diagnostic value. Instead, the clinician should indicate whether the problem is central, bilateral or specific to one side or the other. A chief complaint recorded as '(R) sacroiliac pain', for example, provides much more useful clinical information. Lastly, as mentioned above, the clinician should record whether the problem is in a specific, focal location or whether it is diffuse and widespread.

Following the order of the LO DR FICARA mnemonic, the next question would enquire as to the *onset* of the chief complaint. In general, problems are acute (occurring within the past 10 days or less), subacute (meaning that the problem has existed for the past 10 days to 7 weeks) or chronic (occurring over 7 weeks ago).[8] A chief complaint may also be recurrent, indicating that episodes of symptoms are interrupted by periods when there is symptom remission.

The period over which symptoms have developed may be particularly informative. For example, forgetfulness that has been gradually increasing over the past 2 or 3 years suggests Alzheimer's disease, whereas a sudden onset of confusion may indicate delirium (see Chapter 9, Cognitive impairments).[1] The sudden onset of headaches may indicate stroke (Chapter 16) or giant cell arteritis (Chapter 13). The sudden loss of bowel and bladder function is considered a medical emergency.[1]

Eliciting information related to the onset of the chief complaint emphasizes an important aspect of the interview process. Certain responses can provide guidance as to the treatment protocols that will ultimately be employed. For example, acute problems are typically treated with ice to limit or reduce inflammation, and acute problems may require a higher frequency of patient visits initially. Prognosis is often good, in that the patient may recover within a short period. By contrast, chronic conditions may benefit from the application of heat to promote blood flow. Patients may require fewer treatments over a longer period (over many weeks or months) before any improvement occurs. For chronic conditions, the prognosis is generally more guarded.

The patient should be asked whether they know what may have caused the problem to develop. The patient may be aware of a particular activity that caused the problem (e.g. shovelling snow, gardening), or the onset of symptoms may have no known cause (insidious onset). If the injuries were sustained as the result of a motor vehicle accident, a specific set of questions needs to be asked:

- How much time has elapsed since the accident?
- Was the patient driving the car?
- Was the patient prepared for the accident (did they brace)?
- What was the mechanism of impact (rear-ended, side-swipe, front-end impact)?
- Was the patient's headrest up and was their seatbelt on?
- Do they remember striking a part of the car's interior?
- Did they lose consciousness?
- Did they have any immediate symptoms?
- Was there an ambulance on site? Were they sent to hospital? If so, what did they have done (X-rays, prescriptions, etc.)?
- What are their current symptoms?

The time of the day, week or year that symptoms occur can provide significant information as to the aetiology of a chief complaint. For example, if symptoms are worse in the morning, this may indicate a problem with sleeping position, whereas symptoms that appear predominantly later in the day may indicate that postural considerations, work habits or leisure activities may be causative. Symptoms that occur only during weekdays but not weekends may indicate a work-related aetiology. Some symptoms may be seasonal. Other conditions, such as the arthritides, are often identified by their onset during transitional times of the year (spring and autumn) or during damp weather. Episodes of low back pain may be related to a women's menstrual cycle. If a women's low back pain is aggravated during her menstrual periods, office appointments and treatments may be timed to anticipate this association.

The *duration* of the chief complaint can be determined next. Symptoms can be continuous or intermittent and the presence and intensity of symptoms may vary throughout the day. Symptoms can be described as constant continuous, indicating an unabated pattern of symptoms, or constant and intermittent, indicating an ebb and flow of symptoms that never completely disappear. Conversely, symptoms may be truly intermittent, indicating periods when symptoms are absent.

The presence of any *radiations* can be determined next. In an example of low back pain, this can include any radicular pains down the patient's extremities, which often (but not necessarily) follow specific dermatomal patterns. The identification of any involved dermatome can provide an aetiological location for the chief complaint and may suggest where treatment will be ultimately directed. An unusual or bizarre symptom presentation that does not follow a standard anatomical pattern may indicate a systemic illness or a problem of non-organic origin.[8]

The *frequency* of symptoms is then ascertained. Exploration into the frequency of symptoms highlights another important element of the interview process: detailing subjective descriptions provided by patients. For example, if a patient presents with a chief complaint of headaches and is asked how often the headaches occur, the patient may reply 'once in a while' or 'all the time'. Such descriptions are clearly subjective. Delving into what the patient meant by 'once in a while' may reveal that the patient was actually referring to a frequency of headaches of three times a week, indicating a severe problem.

A similar situation exists when enquiring as to the *intensity* of the chief complaint. Simply asking about the extent or severity of the symptoms may elicit responses such as 'really bad' or 'so-so', which are somewhat uninformative. As with questions about the frequency of the chief complaint, the subjective nature of such answers, heavily influenced as they are by a patient's ethnicity, gender or cultural upbringing, may provide information of limited value. Instead, a skilled clinician will provide a patient with a scale to grade his or her symptoms (typically pain). A 10-point scale, with 1 being no pain and 10 the worst pain the patient has experienced, provides a useful parameter to which a patient can respond. There are many pain-rating and visual analogue pain scales that can be used to quantify the extent of a patient's pain.[8]

Asking for a description of the *character* of the pain is similarly fraught with dangers, but in this case the dangers lie with the clinician. Because the primary treatment used by chiropractors is spinal manipulative therapy (SMT; adjustments), a clinician may inadvertently guide or edit the patient's responses in such a way that validates a therapeutic selection of SMT. This can be compared to the carpenter who only has a hammer. After a while, everything starts to look like a nail.

It is imperative that clinicians pose their questions in such a way as to allow patients to describe their pain accurately without any prompting by the practitioner. For example, a clinician should avoid such biased questions as: 'The pain is sharp with movement, isn't it?'. Instead, the clinician should provide the patient with an oral list of descriptors from which to choose, such as 'sharp, dull, achy, numbing, tingling or burning'. There is a general association between a pain description and its anatomical origin (Table 6.1). For example, sharp pains are generally associated with facet joint dysfunction (subluxation), whereas dull, achy pains often indicate muscular disorders.[8] This relationship between a description of the character of pain and an anatomical etiology, albeit a general association, further emphasizes the link between the information gathered during the interview and the treatment plan. Using the example of low back pain, if the pain was described as sharp in character, especially with motion, the chiropractic practitioner may diagnose a facet irritation (or subluxation) what would be amendable to SMT.

Any *associated* symptoms must be identified. Some associated symptoms may constitute a medical emergency. In the example of low back pain, loss of bowel or bladder control would indicate severe neurological compromise and must be aggressively investigated by allopathic methods. Cervical pain may be accompanied by headaches, changes in vision, dizziness, nausea or vomiting. If a patient presents with neck pain accompanied by all of these associated symptoms, the clinician must be wary that the patient may be experiencing a transient ischaemic attack (see Chapter 16). Associated symptoms may not by themselves be severe enough to prompt the patient to seek care. Such symptoms are often of secondary importance and may resolve with treatment of the chief complaint.

Table 6.1 Descriptions of pain and related structure[8]

Type of pain	Structure
Cramping dull, aching	Muscle
Sharp, shooting (especially with motion)	Nerve root
Sharp, lightening-like	Nerve
Throbbing, diffuse	Vascular

Relieving and aggravating factors must also be identified. The patient may describe which activities or motions aggravate the symptoms, but they need not perform them at this time; that would be done during the physical examination. If the patient is unsure which activities may influence the chief complaint, the clinician can ask whether such activities as walking, sitting, standing, changing position or lying prone modify the symptoms in any way. As with enquiries into the character of the pain, the clinician must refrain from attempting to elicit answers that may validate the diagnosis that the clinician may be formulating.

The last question that should be asked pertaining to the chief complaint is *prior occurrence.* Depending on the response, this can be the most informative question asked during the interview. Certain responses can lead to other branch-point questions that can, in turn, provide volumes of information.

If the patient indicates that he or she has had the chief complaint in the past, the clinician can enquire whether the episode of symptoms was the same then as now (same symptoms, similar cause). If it was, the practitioner can then ascertain what, if any, treatment the patient may have sought. If treatment was sought, the nature of the treatment must be described. Has the patient been to another chiropractor? If so, the methods employed by the other practitioner must be identified. One should never assume that the other chiropractor used the same method of treatment that the reader, as the current clinician, may want to use. For example, if the reader was planning to use high-velocity low-amplitude (HVLA) adjustments during the treatment, but the previous practitioner used an Activator (a hand-held, spring-loaded, manually manipulable device), the patient may be unprepared for any audible noises that may emanate from their facet joints. Based on their experience with other health-care providers (medical physicians, dentists), the patient may erroneously assume that the treatment approaches of different chiropractors are identical. Given the fact that chiropractic is arguably the least standardized of all health-care disciplines, the patient's assumption of the profession's uniform approach to treatment is misplaced.

It is possible that the patient discontinued care with the other chiropractor because he or she did not like the other chiropractor's method of treatment. In the example above, perhaps the patient did not believe that the Activator was having any therapeutic effect. Conversely, the patient may dislike the audible noise elicited during manual adjustment, and would benefit from a non-manipulative adjustment. Either way, if the reader (as the 'new' chiropractor) was planning on utilizing the same or a similar technique used by the first practitioner, and the patient has indicated that they disliked that type of approach, the therapeutic options should be reconsidered. This scenario, which could quickly dissolve the doctor–patient relationship, can easily be avoided only if the clinician is astute enough to look for it.

A great deal of information can be gathered from a previous health provider. If X-rays were taken, and if they are recent and of adequate quality, the acquisition of those X-rays may preclude the need to X-ray the patient again and expose them to additional radiation unnecessarily. A synopsis of the other health-care provider's diagnosis, treatment plan, treatment methods and prognosis may all be of clinical assistance.

If the patient has been treated by another health-care provider for this condition in the past, the diagnosis that they provided must be identified. It may serve as a guide or confirmation of the diagnosis that you are forming as to the cause of the patient's symptoms. However, it is also possible that the patient has been given a different diagnosis, one with which the chiropractor adamantly disagrees. This may be especially true if the patient has been to a medical doctor, who is unlikely to suggest that a 'subluxation' is the aetiology of the chief complaint. The chiropractor is now faced with an ethical dilemma: should the reader, as the current clinician, disagree with the opinions of another health-care provider? This may not seen like a major issue, but often the patient may have a strong rapport with, and confidence in, another practitioner such as their medical doctor, a relationship that they have not yet built with the chiropractor. It may therefore be a wise approach to envelop the previous diagnosis into the newly formulated diagnosis, in order to avoid confusing the patient. Criticizing another health-care provider is rarely beneficial, and in most cases will be viewed as being unprofessional by both the patient and other practitioners.

If the patient has had a similar problem in the past and it was successfully treated by another chiropractor, several important questions logically follow. The time frame required for the resolution of the symptoms may provide a guide as to the patient's prognostic outcome. As mentioned previously, techniques that resulted in successful outcomes should be emulated (if possible) and techniques that had no significant positive outcome are best avoided.

The last question in this algorithmic chain is possibly the most important: if the patient has had this problem in the past and was successfully treated by another chiropractor, why has the patient not returned to the other chiropractor? The answer may be as simple as the patient and doctor have moved a significant distance from each other, or perhaps the doctor has retired. However, if the patient is very vague as to why they have not returned to the previous chiropractor, it may be a good idea to call the other practitioner. Perhaps this patient was dismissed for disruptive behaviour. Perhaps they left behind a large, unpaid outstanding balance. In any event, a call to the other provider, especially if specifically asked by the patient not to call, may allow the reader to avoid the same difficulties experienced by the previous practitioner.

General health status of the patient

General information about the patient must be gathered. This includes any medications that the patient may be taking, any allergies that they may have, and their overall general health (systems review). Any recent changes in health status or behaviour must be explored. For example, recent episodes of polyuria, polyphagia and polydipsia may raise suspicions of diabetes (Chapter 12). Unexplained weight loss can indicate serious pathologies such as cancer or depression (see Nutritional assessment of the older patient, below).

A systems review is a list of questions that asks the patient about each of their physiological systems. It is most expeditious simply to list each system and ask the patient to elaborate if applicable. For example, the clinician can ask: 'Any problems with your vision? Hearing? Breathing? Heart or circulation? Going to the toilet?' and so on. For the older patient, the practitioner should focus on problems of confusion, memory loss, falls, incontinence, immobility, instabilities, insomnia and sensory loss.[1] The leading causes of morbidity among older patients are:[2]

- arthritis
- hypertension
- hearing impairments
- heart disease
- cataracts
- orthopaedic deformities
- chronic sinusitis
- diabetes
- visual impairments
- varicose veins.

The leading causes of mortality are:[2]

- heart disease
- malignancies
- cerebral vascular accidents
- respiratory conditions
- accidents
- diabetes
- suicide
- liver disease.

During the interview, certain clinical conditions may be identifiable by characteristic descriptions. For example, if a patient relates a cycle of neurological impairments with episodes of remission and exacerbations which cannot be accounted for by one neurological lesion, multiple sclerosis should be suspected. Other examples are provided in Table 6.2.

Of particular importance, significant previous surgeries, falls, accidents and hospitalizations must be explored.[1] It may be necessary to guide the patient away from a full account of every mishap and injury

Table 6.2 Examples of serious pathologies identified by characteristic description from the patient interview[5,8]

Sign/symptom	Associated clinical condition
Cachexia, night pain	Cancer
Mental confusion	Acute delirium, urinary tract adverse drug reaction
Personality change	Dementia
Transient ischaemic attack	Stroke
Resting tremor, shuffling gait mask-like facial expression	Parkinson's disease
Polyuria, polyphagia, polydipsia	Diabetes
Cycle of neurological impairments with episode of remissions and exacerbation not attributable to one neurological lesion	Multiple sclerosis

they have ever experienced in their lifetime, and instead ask them to elaborate on their more serious injuries and surgeries, especially those that may have affected the area of chief complaint. Along the same lines, information about significant past illnesses (including childhood diseases) should be obtained. In the older patient, significant past illnesses may include influenza, tuberculosis and meningitis.

The patient's family history should be explored along two main paths. The first is an exploration of a family history of the chief complaint, and the other is to determine a family history of those diseases that have a strong familial association. Such diseases include heart disease, high blood pressure, certain cancers and diabetes (both types I and II).

Functional assessment of the older patient: the key to the geriatric interview

Determining the level to which a patient can participate in their ADLs,

- ambulation
- bathing
- continence
- dressing
- feeding
- using the toilet
- transfer,

and (IADLs),

- money management
- shopping
- cooking
- cleaning
- using a telephone
- doing laundry,

is arguably the most important element of the interview of an older patient.[1,2,5] The patient should be asked whether they are able to perform each of the ADLs and IADLs. Observing patients for their personal grooming, general appearance and how they manoeuvre themselves in the office provides a clinician with a rough guide as to the patients' ability to perform these activities.

Many authors consider the cornerstone of a geriatric assessment to be the determination of a patient's ADLs, which in turn is a reflection of their functional abilities. The current literature discussing outcome measures in both allopathic medicine and chiropractic care

emphasizes the importance of quality of life, or health-related quality-of-life measures. In the parlance of chiropractic, this is often encompassed in the term 'wellness' (see Chapter 24).

Older patients often have multiple chronic conditions that may not completely resolve with any treatment, allopathic or otherwise. Focusing on the resolution of an older patient's symptoms, such as pain, may be futile, misguided and frustrating for both the patient and the doctor. Instead, the astute practitioner should emphasize the preservation of ADLs and IADLs, the reacquisition of lost functions and the adaptability and development of different coping strategies in the face of often unavoidable health adversity. As Killinger has recently written: 'Whereas a provider must be desirous of facilitating the patient's progress in improved score on outcome assessments and return to normal ranges of motion, the patient's goal may be much more straightforward – independence'.[9] The inability to perform their ADLs may have a tremendous impact on the individual's self-esteem, pride and will to survive.[9]

One word that may best describe an older patient's fears is *loss*. Older patients must cope with the potential loss of their physical abilities, cognitive functions, the loss (death) of a spouse and friends, loss of financial independence, loss of their jobs through forced retirement and often the loss of their self-esteem. Moreover, older patients fear that their losses will mount, perhaps to a point where they are no longer in control of their own lives.

Lifestyle

Questions about the lifestyle of the patient should be asked. These include questions about alcohol consumption, smoking, general level of physical activity, frequency and extent of exercise, levels of stress and sleep patterns. A clinician must also be vigilant with respect to the possibility of elder abuse.

Sleep patterns

Sleep disorders are very common in the elderly: 45% of older patients report a problem with sleeping, and 25% of patients report the problem to be serious.[5] Sleep patterns should be investigated not only in terms of the position in which the patient sleeps, but also the total amount of time for which the patient sleeps, and whether or not the patient wakes up refreshed (non-restful sleep may indicate fibromyalgia). Certain pathological conditions may affect a patient's sleep pattern and some clinical conditions result in characteristic sleep manifestations. For example, a deep, boring, severe pain that wakes the patient from sleep may indicate a neoplasm, whereas numbing or tingling sensations during sleep that are relieved by the patient 'walking it off' may raise suspicions of spinal stenosis. The type of bed in which the patient sleeps must be assessed. Inexplicably, some patients sleep in a bed that is decades old. Age-related disturbances of sleep include spending more time in bed and less time asleep, being easily aroused from sleep, experiencing daytime fatigue and napping, and the patient may be less tolerant of phase shifts in the sleep–wake cycle.[5] For the treatment of sleep disorders, sleeping pills are considered the treatment of last resort and other non-pharmacological suggestions should be considered (see Chapter 21, Sleep and the elderly).

Alcoholism

Older persons are more sensitive to the effects of alcohol, and alcohol abuse is much more common among older patients than previously suspected.[1] The prevalence of alcoholism in the elderly is estimated to range between 6 and 53%.[1] One out of three chronic alcoholics develop the problem after the age of 60[1] and one-third of the individuals in Alcoholic Anonymous are over the age of 60 years.[5] Up to 20% of the elderly living in long-term institutions are alcoholic.[1] Alcoholism is four times more common in elderly men than elderly women.[5]

Many presenting complaints may be secondary to alcoholism. These include insomnia, anxiety, falls and a decline in cognitive function.[1] If a practitioner is concerned that the patient may be abusing alcohol, the practitioner can ask the patient the CAGE questions:[1,5]

- Have you ever felt you should *cut* down?
- Have people *annoyed* you by criticizing your drinking?
- Have you ever felt bad or *guilty* about your drinking?
- Have you ever had to drink first thing in the morning to steady your nerves or to get rid of a hangover (*eye-opener*)?

Treatment involves overcoming the patient's denial. This may require enlisting the help of other family members.

Table 6.3 Prevalence of lifestyle choices among older patients[1]

Lifestyle choice	Prevalence among older patients (%)
Smokes	16
Drinks 10–12 alcoholic beverages every 2 weeks	12
Sedentary	71
Overweight	20
Sleeps less than 7–8 h per night	41
Does not use a seatbelt regularly	50
Stress affects their health	11

Smoking

Older patients who smoke should be encouraged to quit, as they have a 52% higher risk of coronary heart disease and death than non-smokers.[1] This risk rapidly declines after smoking cessation, increasing life expectancy by 2–4 years.[1] The author has heard tobacco described as the only legal substance which is harmful when used in its intended manner.

Sedentary lifestyle

A sedentary lifestyle can lead to deconditioning and disuse atrophy.[1] Older patients are particularly susceptible to deconditioning, although strength training has been shown to be an effective means of preventing it in older patients.[10] The health benefits of regular exercise include: a reduced risk of coronary heart disease, a decline in hypertension, increased bone mineralization, improved joint flexibility, increased ranges of spinal motion, reduced body fat and improved mental health, and it is also a vital component in the management of type II diabetes[1,10] (see Chapter 12). The prevalence of various harmful lifestyle choices among older patients is shown in Table 6.3

Elder abuse

It is estimated that there are 1 million cases of elder abuse annually in the USA.[5,11] Forms of abuse include physical, mental and financial.[11,12] Among older patients, physical abuse is not the most common type: 45% of cases of abuse in older patients are due to neglect, whereas 20% of cases are physical abuse.[11]

There are five major risk factors for abuse. These can be remembered with the mnemonic SAVED: Stress, Alcoholism, Violence, Emotions and Dependency.[11]

The most common cause is a cycle of violence or abuse. Social and emotional stressors increase the likelihood of abuse, although elder abuse is common in all socioeconomic, racial and religious populations.[5,11]

The most common victims of abuse are mentally competent, isolated females.[5] The most common abuser is a family member. In 60% of cases, the abuser is the spouse.[5]

The victim of abuse may not report the abuse for many different reasons. The victim may be fearful or ashamed, they be under the control of the abuser, they may not know where to turn for help and the victim may think that no one can offer any help. Lastly, the victim may be fearful of reprisals by the abuser if they report the abuse. Unlike child abuse, there are no legal obligations on a practitioner to report suspected cases of elder abuse. However, most jurisdictions provide a 'good faith' immunity for the reporter.[12] Immunity is offered to the practitioner because this information is technically confidential. Thus, a clinician contacting the authorities about an abusive relationship might otherwise place themselves at risk of prosecution for breach of patient confidentiality (see Chapter 31).

Living arrangements

An exploration of the patient's living arrangements should be conducted, as well as an assessment of the psychosocial environment.[2] Is the patient a widow or widower? Does the patient live alone? Do they have family living nearby? All of these factors may influence a patient's state of mind to a greater extent than the symptoms that they may experience from the chief complaint.

Life history

It may be valuable to ask the patient about their personal experiences during the depression or World War II. For many older patients, this time in their life may have been devastating. Some patients may be Holocaust survivors. Some older persons may have lived through the air raids of cities such as London or Berlin. Still others may have served in the military, where they may have been wounded or imprisoned in prisoner-of-war camps, or they may suffer from postcombat stress disorders. For many patients, the experiences that they lived through during these stressful times may influence their expression of pain, attitudes about doctors and illnesses, and potentially complicate their compliance with treatment.

To manage successfully many challenges originating from a patient's life history, a practitioner may suggest that a patient seek out a self-help group. Members of self-help groups are experiencing the same problem as the patient (widowhood, coping with a family member who has Alzheimer's disease, cancer patients and so on), and may therefore be better able to understand what the patient is going through. Self-help groups, and other community organizations, offer support, guidance and a safe place for people to share and voice their fears, doubts, concerns and triumphs.

Nutritional assessment

Assessing the nutritional status of an older patient is very important. Malnutrition is a state of too few macronutrients (protein-energy malnutrition, or vitamin and mineral deficiencies) or too many macronutrients (obesity), or the consumption of excessive amounts of inappropriate substances (such as alcohol).[13] Poor clinical outcomes have been linked to each of these nutritional states.

Studies have shown that undernutrition increases the risk of respiratory and cardiac problems, infection, deep venous thrombosis, pressure ulcers, perioperative mortality and multiorgan failure.[13] Undernutrition can also result in severe immune dysfunction.[13]

Obesity has been linked to an increased risk of hypertension, type II diabetes, hypercholesterolaemia, respiratory impairments and degenerative joint disease.[13] In the USA, the prevalence of obesity in persons aged 65–75 years old is 25% in men and 40% in women.[13] Older black women living below the poverty line have the highest rate of obesity.[13]

The key question to ask during the interview in order to assess the patient's nutritional status is: have you experienced unexplained weight loss? Weight loss after the age of 50 is associated with longer stays in hospital, an increase in medical expense requirements and an increase in mortality.[13]

Unexplained weight loss is often related to depression. Ninety per cent of depressed older patients experience significant weight loss, compared with only 60% of younger depressed persons.[13] Unexplained weight loss may also be related to a decline in cognitive abilities.

There are many different treatable causes of malnutrition, as listed in the mnemonic MEAL ON WHEELS:[13]

- Medications
- Emotional problems (depression)
- Anorexia tardive (nervosa) or alcoholism
- Late-life paranoia

- Oral problems
- No money

- Wandering and other dementia-related behaviour
- Hyperthyroidism, hyperparathyroidism, hypoadrenalism
- Enteric problems (malabsorption)
- Eating problems (inability to feed self)
- Low-salt, low-cholesterol diets
- Social problems.

Evaluation of nutritional status

There are many different tools available for a clinician to evaluate the nutritional status of a patient. These include a food record diary (usually recorded over a period of 4–7 days), a food-frequency questionnaire and a mini-nutritional assessment.[13]

Body mass index

The most accurate indicator of the health of an older patient as related to his or her nutritional status can be calculated using a body mass index (BMI).[13] The BMI is the ratio of the patients weight to their height, which can be expressed mathematically as:

$$BMI = \frac{Weight\ (kg)}{Height\ (m)^2}$$

Normal and optimal values for a patient's BMI are between 22 and 27. Both extremes of the BMI value scale are associated with an increased risk of mortality (Figure 6.1).[13]

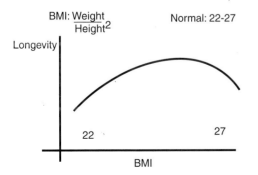

Figure 6.1 Graphic depiction of risk of mortality as related to body mass index (BMI).[13]

Other screening tools are available to determine a patient's nutritional status. Laboratory examinations focus on levels of serum proteins (albumin, transferrin), urine creatinine, total lymphocyte count and serum cholesterol.[14] General tools for nutritional screening are:

- Sadness
- Cholesterol
- Albumin
- Loss of weight
- Eating problems
- Shopping problems.

The nutritional status of older patients is described in more detail in Chapter 26, Clinical nutrition for the geriatric patient.

Completing the interview

To complete the interview, the clinician should ask the patient whether they would like to add any information. It is possible that the patient may have a concern that you have not asked about. If the patient has other areas of concerns, called secondary complaints, the practitioner can ask the patient about those now, following the same list of questions that enquired about the chief complaint.

A list of differential diagnoses may have been developed during the interview. Differential diagnoses are a list of possible aetiological causes for the patient's chief complaint, in order of probability. The purpose of the physical examination is to attempt to identify which of the possible diagnoses is the correct one, best accounting for the patient's chief complaint.

The clinician is now ready to proceed to the physical examination. It is important to inform the patient of your intentions before commencing this next stage of the patient examination.

References

1 Bowers L. Clinical assessment of geriatric patients: unique challenges. Top Clin Chiropractic 1996; 3(2): 10–21.
2 McCarthy KA. Management consideration in the geriatric patient. Top Clin Chiropractic 1996; 3(2): 66–75.
3 Gleberzon B. Chiropractic geriatrics: the challenges of assessing the older patient. J Am Chiropractic Assoc 2000; April: 36–37.
4 Lonergan E. Geriatrics: A Lange Clinical Manual. Stamford, CT: Appleton & Lange, 1996: 1–9, 560–561.
5 Ferri F, Fretwell M, Watchel T. The Care of the Geriatric Patient, 2nd Edn. St Louis, MO: Mosby-Year Book, 1997: 19–25, 461–463, 468–471.
6 Hawk C, Long CR, Boulanger KT et al. Chiropractic care for patients aged 55 years and older: report from a practice-based research program. J Am Geriatr Assoc 2000; 48: 534–545.

7 Study by the Canadian Chiropractic Protective Association, Toronto, Ontario, 1996.

8 Magee DJ. Orthopedic Physical Examination. 3rd Edn. Philadelphia, PA: WB Saunders Co. 1997: 1–6.

9 Killinger LZ. Trauma in the geriatric patient: a chiropractic perspective with a focus on prevention. Top Clin Chiropractic 1998; 5(3): 10–15.

10 Gleberzon BJ, Annis R. The necessity of strength training for the older patient. J Can Chiropractic Assoc 2000; 4(2): 98–102.

11 Marshall CE, Benton D, Brazier JM. Elder abuse: using clinical tools to identify clues to mistreatment. Geriatrics 2000; 55(2): 42–53.

12 Cammer Paris BE, Meier DE, Goldstein T *et al.* Elder abuse and neglect: how to recognize warning signs and intervene. Geriatrics 1995; 50(4): 47–51.

13 Omran ML, Morley JE. Assessment of protein energy malnutrition in older patients, Part I: History, examination, body composition and screening tools. Nutrition 2000; 16: 50–63.

14 Omran ML, Morley JE. Assessment of protein energy malnutrition in older patients, Part II. Laboratory examination. Nutrition 2000; 16: 131–140.

7

Physical examination

Ayla Azad

The physical assessment of the geriatric population poses its own unique set of challenges for the clinician. Normal procedures need to be modified because of the physiological and mental changes associated with the ageing process.[1,2] Older patients usually have at least two existing problems and often they have more.[3] According to Bowers, the average older patient has at least three disabilities and, for every one known to the practitioner, there is another that is not.[2] This results in a complex interaction among physical, psychological and emotional factors. Older people are often hesitant to speak about their problems because their symptoms are vague or they accept that their health declines as part of old age.[4] It is therefore imperative that an organized approach be applied during the physical examination of a geriatric patient, as this will result in a more accurate diagnosis and appropriate plan of management.[5] Owing to the complexity of the conditions that can be present in a geriatric patient and the need for thoroughness, the physical examination may seem to be a daunting task to both the doctor and patient.

It is imperative that the doctor be efficient yet thorough and at the same time keep the patient's comfort in mind.[2,6] A 'routine' is usually recommended to cover all areas during the physical examination. That said, some authorities have suggested that an approach different to the traditional 'head-to-toe' routine be used during the physical examination of an older person. For example, Wright has suggested starting with the back. However, this deviation from the normal may result in missing vital areas for examination. Therefore, the traditional head-to-toes approach is usually recommended for the physical examination of an older person, and it is the approach most often followed.[7,8]

Hurwitz outlined a suggested sequence for physical examination in the frail elderly (Table 7.1). This system avoids frequent changes in position by the patient, which he or she may find exhausting.[3,5] Although this chapter will outline the traditional head-to-toe approach, it is important to remember that a physical examination is both an art and a science, and should be adapted to meet individual patient needs.[5]

Table 7.1 Suggested physical examination sequence in the elderly

Patient position	Examination
Standing	Weight and height
Standing	Gait, 'timed get-up-and-go' test (see Nervous system review and Chapter 11), proximal leg strength, posture, agility and Romberg's test
Standing	Blood pressure (after 2 min)
Sitting on examination table (facing examiner)	Visual fields and acuity, eye movements, funduscopy, hearing and otoscopy and oral examination and upper limb musculoskeletal testing
Sitting, legs on examination table	Spine, lung fields and thyroid gland
Reclining at 45 degrees	Precordium, jugular vein pulse, breasts, lymph nodes and upper limb neurological
Supine	Abdomen, lower limb neurological, range of movement, pulses, supine blood pressure, rectal and/or pelvic examination

Source: adapted from Hurwitz.[5]

General guidelines

It is extremely important to establish a rapport with the elderly patient. Sometimes an older person will have difficulty communicating with the doctor because of visual or hearing problems. Older people are often slow to bring their troubles to the doctor because their symptoms are vague, or because they believe, often erroneously, their disability to be the result of the normal ageing process.[7] When examining an older patient, the doctor should strive to avoid patient discomfort and maintain patient dignity at all times.[1] Conveying sincere interest and respect for the patient will help to establish a comfortable rapport with him or her, and gain the trust of the patient.[6,7] A quiet, private and undisturbed setting is important for the physical examination. Clear explanations before performing any procedure should be provided to the patient, as this will help to reduce nervousness and keep the patient comfortable.[7] This can also be considered a form of informed consent. The doctor should be positioned close to the patient and maintain eye contact. This will allow for lip reading, if necessary, and will improve attention and concentration. A slow and clear tone of voice, at a comfortable pitch for the patient, should be used. Unnecessary shouting can irreparably destroy patient rapport.[7] Some tips to provide a safe and comfortable environment for examining the older patient are as follows:[1,2]

- The examination room should be quiet and at a comfortable temperature.
- Chairs should have arm rests and be of adequate height for easy arising.
- The examining table should not be too high, so that patients with mobility disorders can easily mount the table. The table should also be of adequate width so that patients are in no danger of falling off. A wide footstool facilitates mounting and dismounting. Assist the patient on and off the examining table.
- Provide a pillow under the patient's head.
- Grab bars should be near the scale to steady patients with balance problems.
- Examining gowns should be short enough to prevent tripping.
- Positional changes should be minimized for patients with mobility disorders.
- Sound amplification should be used for hearing-impaired patients.
- Never leave an older patient alone because a fall from the examining table could be devastating.

General appearance

This aspect of the physical examination can be performed throughout the procedure. The process of observation can provide tremendous amounts of information on functional ability in the elderly. Watching the patient rise from a chair can provide information about his or her level of strength, balance and mobility. Helping the patient to undress can assess self-care and one can observe any inappropriate articles of clothing. For example, a lot can be said about function in a patient who wears thermal underwear in August.[1] Nutritional state, grooming, facial expressions, posture and involuntary movements can also be observed.[7] Muscle atrophy and loss of subcutaneous tissue may cause a normal elderly patient to appear somewhat wasted and malnourished. However, more severe generalized wasting and cachexia raise the possibility of an underlying chronic or malignant disease.[7]

Skin

Age-related changes cause a decrease by about 20% in total body water and an increase in overall body fat.[1,9] It is important to check skin turgor to assess hydration.[2] As a result of the usual degeneration of collagen and elastin, atrophy of epidermal structures, loss of subcutaneous fat and increased vascular fragility it is common to find conditions such as dryness, thinning and wrinkling of skin, senile purpura (commonly found on the dorsum of the hand and forearm), and loss of hair on the scalp, axillae and pubic regions.[2,7] Other abnormal findings include small papular lesions (cherry angiomas), hyperpigmented macular lesions called lentigines or 'liver spots'.[1,7]

It is also important to check sun-exposed areas for active keratoses. These are premalignant lesions and are usually multiple and scaly, enlarging slowly.[1] In immobile patients (bed or wheelchair bound), it is important to check the buttocks, sacrum, trochanters and heels for pressure sores[1,7,10] (see also Chapter 19).

Vital measurements

Height and weight should be measured and recorded in the standard manner, i.e. dressed in underwear with no shoes. Unexplained weight loss may indicate malnutrition, whereas unexplained weight gain may indicate fluid retention.[2] A loss in height is a late sign of osteopenia.[11]

Baseline temperature measurements are important to detect any changes and improve the recognition of fever.[2] Any rise of 1.33°C (2.4°F) over baseline is significant.[11] If the oral temperature is less than 98°F, it should be rechecked with a low-reading rectal thermometer to rule out hypothermia.[1] Thermoregulatory responses are impaired as one ages as a result of disordered autonomic function.[6]

Normal ageing causes some degree of atherosclerosis and thickening in blood vessels. This creates aortic stiffening and results in an increase in blood pressure.[12] Because an individual's blood pressure fluctuates considerably throughout the day, multiple measurements under resting conditions are required to diagnose hypertension[2] (see Chapters 15 and 16).

Ageing causes a decreased sensitivity in baroreceptors and therefore a decreased response to pressure changes.[12] Postural hypotension is common in the elderly and therefore their blood pressure and pulse should be measured both while seated and standing. A rise of less than 10 beats per minute with a drop in blood pressure suggests baroreceptor impairment.[1,2,13] Postural hypotension with an unchanging pulse rate indicates autonomic dysfunction (see also Chapter 15 and 16).

Orthostatic hypotension consists of a drop in systolic blood pressure of at least 15 mmHg or a fall in diastolic blood pressure of at least 10 mmHg, on being seated after a supine measurement or on standing after a seated measurement.[2,11] Common causes of orthostatic hypotension include antihypertensive and antianginal medications.[3]

A seated blood pressure of greater than 160/90 mmHg is considered elevated in the elderly.[1,2,6] Hypertension may be distinguished from pseudohypertension (due to non-elastic, atherosclerotic arteries) by performing Osler's manoeuvre.[1,2,11,14] Osler's manoeuvre is performed by inflating the blood-pressure cuff above the systolic pressure. The radial or brachial pulse is then palpated. The arteries should be pulseless. If they can still be palpated the intra-arterial pressure may be lower than the blood pressure obtained by auscultation, which may indicate that there is sufficient arteriosclerosis to produce some degree of pseudohypotension.[1,2,15]

Blood pressure should be routinely recorded in the geriatric patient. It is important to obtain a baseline value to detect any changes and note fluctuations over time. A palpatory systolic pressure should be taken each time to avoid the auscultatory gap and minimize the risk of a reading that is too high or too low.[16]

Checking respiration is also an important aspect of the vital signs examination. This can be easily performed while taking the pulse of the patient. It is important not to tell the patient while measuring breaths per minute since this can make the patient conscious of the test, altering his or her breathing pattern. The normal respiratory pattern is 12–20 breaths per minute in the older patient. A rate above 22 breaths per minute suggests the possibility of a lower respiratory tract infection even prior to the appearance of other clinical signs.[2,11]

Head and neck

Eyes

A visual disability is common in the geriatric patient. It is estimated that 8% of older Americans are severely visually impaired. It is therefore imperative that visual acuity is checked.[1,2,17] This can be accomplished by using a Snellen's eye chart or a hand-held Jaeger chart.[1,2,18] Since it is also important to assess a geriatric patient's functional capacity, a newer instrument, the Activities of Daily Vision Scale, has been devised to evaluate visual function.[19] Patients should also be asked about problems with their vision during normal daily activities such as driving, sewing, watching television and reading the newspaper.[20]

A sunken appearance of the eyes is normal due to the loss of orbital fat and senile ptosis. Degenerative changes in the muscles of accommodation and the iris may result in constricted, irregular, unequal pupils. This can also cause a sluggish response to light.[7] External examination of the eyes may reveal arcus senilis. This is a grey, opaque ring surrounding the margin of the cornea and is usually seen bilaterally after the age of 50. This is not of pathological significance and is a sign of normal ageing.[1,2]

Lens opacification may indicate cataracts and this makes the funduscopic examination difficult in the geriatric patient.[1,2] Decreasing the intensity of the light from the ophthalmoscope will help to decrease pupillary constriction, therefore allowing a larger pupil for easier viewing. Increased cupping can indicate glaucoma. The US Preventive Services Task Force does not recommend routine performance of tonometry by primary-care physicians as a screening test for glaucoma.[1,21] Periodic referral to an ophthalmologist for this test is recommended.[21]

Other problems in this area may include entropion, ectropion, cataracts, diabetic retinopathy, retinal detachment and senile macular degeneration.[7]

Ears

Impaired hearing increases with age and can contribute to poor health, social isolation, depression and paranoid psychosis.[2,6] Prevalence of hearing loss is high in the geriatric population and therefore routine tests are important.[2] A hand-held audioscope has been shown to be both a valid and reliable screening test, with 90% sensitivity.[1,2] The audioscope is an otoscope that automatically generates tones ranging from 500 to 4000 Hz at 40 dB hearing level.[1,22] If an audioscope is not available, whisper tests in a quiet room have been shown to approximate the results of an audio examination. Weber and Rinne tests can be conducted in the routine manner to localize bone and air conduction hearing loss, respectively.

Impaired hearing due to problems with the external ear may include fully impacted cerumen.[1] Routine examinations of the ear drum for wax should be performed. External otitis may result as an allergic reaction to a hearing aid.[1]

Mouth

Patients who wear dentures should first be examined with the dentures in their mouths to check the general fit, and also to check for bacterial plaque and food debris. Once the dentures have been removed, areas of reversible local irritation caused by excessive dental pressure or a bone spicule beneath the mucosa should be noted.[1]

Dentate patients should be checked for periodontal disease by looking for erythematous, oedematous, gingival, bleeding gums, exposure of the root surfaces of the teeth or lost teeth. Patients with these symptoms should be referred to a dentist.[1]

The tongue should also be checked for colour and mobility. The area under the tongue is a common site for early malignancies and should also be examined.[1] The sensitivity of taste buds and olfactory receptors declines with age, causing a decrease in sweet and salt tastes and an increase in bitterness.[4]

Head

The examination of the head should include gentle palpation of the scalp for any nodules or depressions in the skull.[16] The temporal arteries should also be pal-pated for tenderness, nodularity and thickening.[1,2] Patients with temporal headaches, jaw pain, earache or unexplained fever should be screened for temporal arteritis.[1]

Neck

The examination of the neck includes cervical ranges of motion (see Musculoskeletal examination), thyroid palpation and examination for any nodules or supra-clavicular lymphadenopathy. The presence of carotid artery bruits should be assessed by auscultation.[1,7]

While performing the cervical range of motion it is important to check for dizziness and ensure that the patient is supported to prevent falling. Uncinate processes in the cervical region are flattened and project bone laterally and posterolaterally in the older patient. While this prevents disc herniations, it results in a decrease in the intervertebral foramina space.[12] Ranges of motion are normally decreased in the elderly person.

Between 40 and 70% of arteries with asymptomatic bruits do not have major significant compromise in blood flow.[1] Similar sounds can be created by anatomical variations and tortuosity, goitre, venous hum and transmitted cardiac murmurs.[1] A carotid bruit is more likely to be due to generalized athero-sclerosis and coronary insufficiency than to cere-brovascular symptoms. Noise transmitted from a heart murmur will diminish as the stethoscope is moved up the neck, whereas a bruit from carotid artery stenosis will increase.[1]

With time, the aorta and its branches stretch and lose their elasticity. Unilateral jugular distension may be caused by a dilatation of the subclavian artery obstructing venous return on the left side of the neck.[7]

Thorax

Respiratory system

Ageing results in chest-wall stiffening and a weakness in the muscles of the thorax wall. There is also a reduction in costal cartilage elasticity and coalescence of alveoli.[7,12] Normal ageing also causes a loss of capillaries in the area, as well as calcification of the bronchi.[12] These changes culminate in a decrease in chest expansion, with a concomitant reduction in various measures of airflow and an increase in residual volume. This leaves the geriatric patient more susceptible to conditions such as pneumonia.[7,12] The continuous exposure to environmental pollutants throughout life causes the lung to develop structural and functional deterioration with ageing.[12,23] The older lung has a decrease in base-to-apex length with an increase in anteroposterior diameter. This will be apparent during percussion in the thorax.

Other causes of respiratory difficulty may be caused by kyphoscoliosis, chronic obstructive pulmonary disease or bronchial carcinoma.[7] Basilar rales are common and may be found in the absence of any pathology. These crackles should disappear after the patient takes a few deep breaths.[1]

Cardiovascular system

Normal ageing causes ventricular thickening in response to increased peripheral resistance, a decrease in pacemaker cells and a decreased response to sympathetic stimulation. This results in a decrease in stroke volume.[12] Sclerotic changes occurring in the valves of the heart lead to nodular thickenings that occur along the closure lines of the valves. This most commonly affects the mitral and aortic valves, which accounts for the common systolic murmurs heard in the elderly. These are of little clinical significance.[7,12] An S4 murmur in the elderly is also of little clinical significance, whereas an S3 gallop indicates an overloaded ventricle due to congestive heart failure. Diastolic murmurs are always abnormal in the elderly.[1]

The progressive decline of reserve organ function that occurs with ageing has been termed 'homeostenosis' by Resnick.[24] An example of this is heart failure in the elderly. Changes in heart function that occur with ageing lead to an increase in diastolic dysfunction. This may be abrupt in onset and deterioration may be rapid. An older patient may appear perfectly normal while under no physiological stress; however, if a stress is applied, the heart is less able to respond appropriately because it has lost physiological reserve. This physiological change may cause a domino effect, and other organs with less physiological reserve may also be stressed and fail, leading to renal failure, decreased brain perfusion and other pathological consequences.[9]

Breast examination

This is a very important aspect of the physical examination of the older woman. Older women compose a relatively high risk group for breast cancer and advanced tumours are not uncommon in women who have been reluctant to seek care in the past or to under-

go routine physicals.[1,7] Annual clinical breast examination and mammograms are recommended for all older women every 1–2 years[21] (see also Chapter 23).

Breast lumps become more apparent in the elderly owing to atrophy of overlying tissue.[7] The axillae should be checked for metastatic lymphadenopathy while doing a breast examination. Age-related changes can cause retraction of the nipple but gentle pressure around the nipple will cause it to evert. Retraction due to an underlying growth will not be everted.[1] The skin under large, pendulous breasts should also be checked for maceration from perspiration and fungal infection.[1]

Abdomen

The abdomen should be assessed in the following order: (i) inspection, (ii) auscultation, (iii) percussion, and (iv) light and deep palpation.[1,16] Any distension or scars from previous injuries or surgery should be noted. Transverse abdominal skin creases could be caused by collapsed vertebrae due to osteoporosis or severe kyphosis.[1,7]

Percussion may reveal abdominal masses of scybala (firm faeces) in the transverse or descending colon. These should be reassessed after an enema.[7] Percussion should also include the suprapubic area for urinary retention in the bladder.[1,7] The borders of the liver and spleen should also be determined by percussion, since the presence of hepatomegaly or splenomegaly could indicate occult malignant disease.[7]

Owing to the loss of subcutaneous tissue, most elderly people have a relatively thin abdomen, making palpation easier than in a younger person.[1,7] The normal sized aorta is commonly palpable as a pulsatile mass and is more apparent in the elderly.[7] This should be checked for an abdominal aortic aneurysm. Normally, an aneurysm may have lateral as well as anteroposterior pulsations, is wider than 3 cm and may have an associated bruit.[1]

Normal ageing of the gastrointestinal tract causes a decreased peristaltic response of the oesophagus which may cause dysphagia and food regurgitation.[12,23] Reflux oesophagitis and a corkscrew oesophagus (presbyoesophagus) are also common since the lower oesophageal sphincter becomes incompetent.[12] Ageing also results in a reduced gastrointestinal mucosal surface area and relative achlorhydria.[9]

A rectal examination should be routinely performed on the elderly patient.[7] Faecal impaction and rectal carcinoma should be screened for. In elderly men, the prostate should be routinely examined for benign prostatic hypertrophy or prostatic carcinoma, although this procedure is often beyond the scope of chiropractic practice in many jurisdictions.[7,25] Benign prostatic hypertrophy, the most common tumour-like condition, is characterized by enlargement of prostatic nodules, although the prostate itself should feel soft and smooth.[25] Tumours often occur in portions of the prostate (medial and anterior) that cannot be felt by the examining finger: Therefore, measurement of the prostate specific antigen (PSA) is also recommended on a regular basis.[25]

Genitourinary system

Bladder capacity and elasticity decrease with age.[23] These changes, combined with a decrease in normal inhibitory corticol control of the bladder, may lead to incontinence.[12] Incontinence occurs in as many as 20–40% of individuals aged 65 or over, and nocturia occurs in as many as 60–70% of older individuals.[23] A simple 'pad test' can be performed for individuals suspected of having stress incontinence. This test is performed by instructing the patient to place a sanitary pad over the urethral orifice and cough forcefully three times in the standing position. Leakage of urine with this manoeuvre confirms the presence of stress incontinence[1] (see Chapter 18).

Routine gynaecological examinations are recommended for all elderly women. Normal findings may include some degree of atrophic vaginitis, atrophic uterus and non-palpable ovaries.[1,7] Note should also be made of any cystocele, rectocele or uterine prolapse that may occur as the pelvic musculature becomes lax with age.[1]

Musculoskeletal system

Musculoskeletal disease is the leading cause of functional impairment in the older patient.[26] Studies have shown that until humans are 60–70 years old, age-related changes in muscle function and structure are relatively small. However, after the age of 70 these alterations are accelerated considerably.[12] Muscular wasting in older adults is characterized by a decrease in the number of muscle fibres, particularly in the small muscles of the hands.[12] There is also a decline in muscle strength and muscle mass, which makes the older person less able to tolerate trauma.[3,12]

The primary complaint of a patient with musculoskeletal disease is pain. It is important to determine the location of pain (regional or diffuse), its pattern (articular or non-articular), its time course (when it occurs) and its association with other symptoms.[26] A detailed examination of the involved area must be performed and an examination of asymptomatic joints is also of importance. Painless swelling or loss of motion in several joints may indicate a systemic or generalized inflammatory process, which may not have been elicited during the patient interview.[26]

The posture of an older person is usually flexed with the head and neck held forward. The dorsal spine becomes kyphotic and the upper extremities are bent at the elbows and wrists. The hips and knees are also slightly flexed.[12] This forward flexed posture can become the primary cause of many cervical, cranial and shoulder dysfunctions. These dysfunctions can include cervical degenerative joint disease, radiculopathies, shoulder impingement syndromes, headache and craniomandibular dysfunction.[27,28] Sudden onset of a kyphosis may be indicative of a compression fracture. This is often accompanied by pain, although the patient may recall little or no trauma. A pathological fracture should also be considered because of the higher incidence of cancer in the older patient.[12]

The loss of passive range of motion in older persons is often progressive and subtle, occurring usually at the extremes of a joint's potential movement.[3] Females tend to lose the range of motion at a slower rate than males, and joints of the upper extremities remain more flexible than those of the lower extremities.[3,29] Range of motion should be assessed in all regions of the spine in the normal manner; however, care must be taken to provide support due to a loss of balance or sudden onset of dizziness. To discover the mechanical origin the patient's problem the clinician should look for: (i) any differences in active versus passive range of motion, (ii) specific movements that are painful, (iii) a painful arc, (iv) a capsular pattern, (v) restricted accessory motion, and (vi) the type of end-feel (bone-to-bone, capsular, empty, etc.).[30] Muscle testing should also be completed in all extremities.

Functional assessment is a very important aspect of the musculoskeletal examination. This can be defined as 'the measurement of a patient's ability to complete functional tasks and fulfill sound roles'.[5] Functional abilities are more important in the elderly to overall health, well-being and may guide the clinician towards areas of potential treatment.[5] Functional abilities are assessed in two general levels of function: (i) activities of daily living (ADLs) and (ii) instrumental activities of daily living (IADLs).[5,20]

ADLs include dressing, eating, ambulating, using the toilet and hygiene. IADLs are aspects of patients' personal independence, including shopping, housework, food preparation and transportation.[20] The Modified OARS Multidimensional Functional Assessment Questionnaire can be used to collect this information.[20,31]

The feet deserve special attention in the elderly patient, as they may produce severe pain and impair function. The insoles of the shoes may reveal points of weight-bearing and indicate the need for corrective orthotics or footwear. Common problems in the feet include corns, calluses, bunions, ingrown toenails and fungal infections.[7]

Nervous system

Sensory signs of ageing are characterized by impairment of position sense, light touch reception and pain. These changes explain why accidents and falls are more common in the elderly than in younger individuals.[12] All geriatric patients should have their muscle strength, cranial nerves, sensation and reflexes assessed. Age-related changes in the nervous system may include decreased vibration sense (especially in the lower extremities), absence of deep tendon reflexes and the release of some primitive reflexes such as glabella, snout and palmomental.[1] The presence of primitive reflexes should be documented, as their presence is suggestive of frontal lobe dysfunction (most commonly found in senile dementia of the Alzheimer type).[7]

Cranial nerve deterioration may include an absence of the upward conjugate gaze and convergence, deterioration in pupillary constriction in response to light, and slow irregular movements of the eye.[12]

The slow movement of an older patient might be attributed to the 10–15% reduction in conduction velocity of peripheral nerves; however, it should be emphasized that the extent of age-related changes varies from muscle to muscle and from one person to another.[12] Motor signs of ageing may reveal

decreased speed of movement and impaired co-ordination with or without tremors.[12] Motor tone is often increased. Rigidity can be classified into three different types: (i) spasticity, (ii) lead-pipe stiffness (as found in Parkinson's disease), and (iii) paratonia or gegenhalten.[1] Another relatively common finding is that of tremor. This may be due to Parkinson's disease, cerebellar dysfunction, hyperthyroidism or benign senile tremor.[1,7]

Balance and mobility tests are an essential aspect of the neurological assessment in the elderly. Older patients often lose some or all of their proprioceptive strength as well as quadriceps strength.[20] This can lead to difficulty in standing erect, rising unaided from a chair, using the bath and rising from a toilet seat.[20] A good test for balance and proprioception is the Romberg's test. Balance can be thought of as either static (unsupported sitting or standing) or dynamic (balance while reaching or bending or ability to withstand an external force such as a sternal nudge) and both should be assessed independently.[32]

Mobility and balance can be tested efficiently using the timed 'get-up-and-go' test. A wealth of information can be obtained by simply asking the patient to rise from a chair, walk 3 m, turn, walk back and sit down in the chair as quickly as is comfortable.[5,20] In the frail elderly, this is normally completed in less than 20 s.[5] Patients who have weak quadriceps muscles compensate with increased use of their arms, therefore using chairs with armrests and raised seats.[20]

Normal ageing causes a more waddling and narrow-based gait in women and a wide-based, smaller stepped gait in men. Arm swing decreases in both genders.[1] In observing a patient's gait, attention should be paid to the height, length and symmetry of steps, width of stance, movement at the ankle, knee and hip, arm swing, deviation of path and trunk sway.[32] Abnormal gait patterns provide diagnostic clues to underlying diseases such as the parkinsonian gait which is characterized by short steps, shuffling feet, stooped trunk, decreased or absent arm swing, festination and the tendency to fall backwards.[1] Balance and gait can be assessed using the Tinetti Balance and Gait Evaluation assessment instrument.[33] Tinetti et al. have developed a series of gait manoeuvres that mimic obstacles in everyday life and can point towards specific corrective interventions.[1,33] Other tests are discussed in Chapter 11.

Assessment of mental status is another vitally important aspect of the geriatric examination.

Approximately 5% of persons aged 65 or older suffer from dementia.[34] The Folstein Mini-Mental state Examination is routinely used to assess cognitive function.[35,36] Any limitation in language skills (such as aphasia, non-native speaker) or in hearing ability invalidates the results of mental status testing. Such factors should be removed before the test is given.[20] Depression occurs in 10–30% of the elderly population.[5] Screening with the Geriatric Depression Scale is a useful tool for assessment and can easily be administered in less than 10 min[20,35] (see Chapter 9).

Summary

Although the assessment of the geriatric patient is challenging and time consuming, it is often very informative if performed systematically. If performed in an organized and efficient manner, an accurate diagnosis can be reached, resulting in appropriate interventions and therefore leading to enhanced quality of life for the patient. Practitioners are encouraged to develop specific checklists or forms to facilitate the assessment procedure.[5] Demographic trends indicate that the percentage of individuals over the age of 65 years is rising and is expected to reach 23% by the year 2031.[37] Practitioners will find that a large percentage of their patients will be comprised of this age group and therefore must become familiar with, and learn how to overcome, the challenges that they will encounter during the assessment of an older patient.

References

1 Fields SD. Special considerations in the physical exam of older patients. Geriatrics 1991; 46(8): 39–44.

2 Bowers LJ. Clinical assessment of geriatric patients: unique challenges. Top Clin Chiropractic 1996; 3(2): 10–22.

3 McCarthy KA. Management considerations in the geriatric patient. Top Clin Chiropractic 1996; 3(2): 66–75.

4 Morgenthal P. The geriatric examination: general principles and examination procedures. Top Clin Chiropractic 2000; 7(3): 19–27.

5 Hurwitz JS. Geriatric assessment: a manageable approach. Can J Continuing Medical Education. 1996: 111–122.

6 Souhani RL, Moxham J, eds. Textbook of Medicine. New York: Churchill-Livingstone; 1990.

7 Skrastins R, Merry GM, Rosenberg GM et al. Clinical assessment of the elderly patient. Canadian Medical Journal 1982; 127: 203–206.

8 Wright WB. Geriatrics is medicine – how to examine an old person. Lancet 1977; i: 1145–1146.

9 Troncale JA. The aging process. Postgrad Med 1996; 99: 111–122.

10 Aldman RM. Pressure ulcers among the elderly. N Engl J Med 1989; 320: 850–853.

11 Schneiderman H. Physical examination of the aged patient. Conn Med 1993; 57: 317–324.

12 Souza T, Shahihaz S. Normal aging. Top Clin Chiropractic 1996; 3(2): 1–9.

13 Lipsitz LA. Orthostatic hypotension in the elderly. N Engl J Med 1989; 321: 952–957.

14 Miller DK, Kaiser FE. Assessment of the older woman. Clin Geriatr Med 1992; 9: 1–31.

15 Messerli FH, Ventura HO, Amodeo C. Osler's maneuver and pseudohypertension. N Engl J Med 1985; 312: 1548–1551.

16 Seidel HM, Ball JW, Dains JE et al., eds. Mosby's Guide to Physical Examination. St Louis, MO: Mosby-Yearbook, 1991.

17 Nelson KA. Visual impairment among elderly Americans: statistics in transition. J Vis Impair Blind 1987; 81: 331–334.

18 Ochs M. Selecting routine outpatient tests for older patients. Geriatrics 1991; 46: 39–50.

19 Beck JC, Freedman ML, Warshaw GA. Geriatric assessment: focus on function. Patient Care 1994: 10–32.

20 Paist SS, Jafri A. Functional assessment in older patients key to improving quality of life. Postgrad Med 1996; 99: 101–108.

21 Report of the US Preventive Services Task Force Guide to Clinical Preventive Services: An Assessment of the Effectiveness of 169 Interventions. Baltimore, MD: Williams & Wilkins, 1989.

22 Ventry L, Weinstein B. Identification of elderly people with hearing problems. ASHA 1983; 25: 37–42.

23 Arking R. Biology of Aging: Observations and Principles. Englewood Cliffs, NJ: Prentice Hall, 1991.

24 Resnick NM. Geriatric medicine In: Isselbacher KJ, Braunwald E, eds. Harrison's Principles of Internal Medicine. 13th edn. New York: McGraw Hill, 1994: 30–36.

25 Bakshi S, Miller DK. Assessment of the aging man. Med Clin North Am 1999; 83: 1131–1149.

26 Ettinger WH. Joint and soft tissue disorders. In: The Merck Manual of Geriatrics. Rahway, NJ: Merck & Co., 1990.

27 Bergmann TF, Larson L. Manipulative care and older persons. Top Clin Chiropractic 1996; 3(2): 56–65.

28 Paris SV. Cervical symptoms of forward head posture. Top Geriatr Rehabil 1990; 5: 11–19.

29 Bell RD, Hoshizaki TB. Relationship of age and sex with range of motion of seventeen joint action in humans. Can J Appl Physiol 1989; 58: 353–360.

30 Goldstein TS. Geriatric Orthopaedics: Rehabilitative Management of Common Problems. 2nd edn. Gaithersburg, MD: Aspen, 1999.

31 Fillenbaum GG. Screening the elderly: a brief instrumental activities of daily measure. J Am Geriatr Soc 1985; 33: 698–706.

32 MacKnight C, Rockwood K. Mobility and balance in the elderly. Postgrad Med 1996; 99: 269–276.

33 Tinetti ME. Performance-orientated assessment of mobility problems in elderly patients. J Am Geriatr Soc 1986; 34: 119–126.

34 Morgenthal P. The geriatric examination: neuromusculoskeletal system and mental status examinations. Top Clin Chiropractic 2000; 7(3): 50–57.

35 Folstein MF, Folstein SE, McHugh PR. Mini-mental state: a practical method for grading the cognitive state of patients for the clinician. J Psychiatr Res 1975; 12: 189–198.

36 Rockwood K, Silvius JL, Fox RA. Comprehensive geriatric assessment. Postgrad Med 1998; 103: 247–264.

37 Gleberzon BJ. Chiropractic geriatrics: The challenges of assessing the older patient. J Am Chiropractic Assoc 2000; 4: 36–37.

8

Geriatric radiology

Peter Kogan and Marshall Deltoff

The adage 'growing old gracefully' hardly applies for those familiar with the diagnostic images of the aged. In fact, quite the contrary is true. Our senior citizens probably represent the largest group of individuals most frequently imaged. Unfortunately, the ravages of time take their toll on all aspects of the human frame. Those amongst us who take responsibility for diagnosing the images of the aged encounter ample testimony to these ravages.

Without doubt, the senior part of our patient population not only demonstrates the cumulative effects of the wear and tear of advanced years, but also becomes the target of many sinister conditions which favour this age group. Experience teaches us that seniors are prone to a wide variety of skeletal and non-skeletal pathologies. Although there are exceptions to the above rule, older people frequently harbour the most dreaded diseases for which one must always be on the alert.

It should be remembered that any congenital anomaly or skeletal dysplasia can persist into adulthood and beyond. When evaluating the images of the aged, this fact must be continuously borne in mind. It is not within the scope of this chapter to include even a partial list of these conditions. It is sufficient to note, however, that some of these pre-existing conditions may be responsible for the premature development of other phenomena, for example osteoarthritis. The practitioner is advised to consider appropriate imaging procedures, particularly when contemplating the implementation of active chiropractic therapy.

Of course, a proper diagnosis is best formulated after obtaining an optimum radiographic exposure. With respect to seniors, certain special imaging considerations and challenges must be endured. Included is the fact that an elderly patient may be difficult to stabilize while conducting a study. In addition, altered patient postures, such as hyperkyphosis associated with

marked anterior head carriage, may make axial skeletal imaging virtually impossible. It is also noteworthy that, particularly in the case of older women, practically without exception, they suffer from some degree of acquired osteoporosis. This fact will necessitate a significant alteration in technical exposure factors, principally, a reduction in the mAs (milliAmpere-seconds). Lastly, it is essential to obtain informed consent, either directly from the patient or from his or her guardian.

It is also important to realize that most conditions, such as fractures, are much slower to resolve in the aged than in their younger counterparts. There is a generally slower physiology in the geriatric patient and therefore, a delayed healing process. Altered circulation and nutritional considerations may also contribute to this delay.

The purpose of this chapter is to familiarize the reader with some of the more frequent ailments of senior citizens, brought to light by diagnostic imaging. These conditions are reviewed in a pictorial format, as the images will speak volumes about the diseases. Informative captions are included to assist readers in their appreciation and understanding of the presented cases.

The images that follow (Figures 8.1–8.74) are in no way intended to represent a comprehensive examination of geriatric pathology; rather, they constitute an overview of a variety of conditions that commonly afflict the elderly and may play a central role in chiropractic case management. An attempt has been made to categorize or classify these diseases into the CATBITES (Congenital, Arthritides, Tumour, Blood, Infection, Trauma, Endocrine, Soft tissue) mnemonic. It is sincerely hoped that the reader will enjoy this brief account of these assorted conditions in this atlas format, and that the sharing of this experience will assist him or her in everyday geriatric practice.

Since this atlas is only meant to serve as a brief overview of some of the more common conditions afflicting our elderly patient population, the reader is invited to explore more specialized radiographic texts for a more comprehensive and detailed explanation of the pathophysiologies of these various diseases. A list of references is provided to facilitate your search for additional information.

Further reading

Berquist TH. Diagnostic Imaging of the Acutely Injured Patient. Baltimore, MD: Urban & Schwarzenberg, 1985.

Chapman S, Nakielny R. Aids to Radiological Differential Diagnosis. 3rd edn. London: Baillière Tindall, 1995.

Daffner RH. Clinical Radiology: The Essentials. Baltimore, MD: Williams & Wilkins, 1993.

Deltoff MN, Kogon PL. The Portable Skeletal X-ray Library. Baltimore, MD: Mosby-Year Book, 1997.

Eideken J, Hodes J. Roentgen Diagnosis of Diseases of Bone, Vol. I–II, 3rd edn. Baltimore, MD: Williams & Wilkins, 1981.

Epstein BS. The Spine: A Radiological Text and Atlas. Philadelphia, PA: Lea & Febiger, 1976.

Francis KC, Hutter RVP. Neoplasms of the spine of the aged. Clin Orthop 1963; 26: 54–66.

Gehweiler JA, Osborne RL, Becker RF. Radiology of Vertebral Trauma. Philadelphia, PA: WB Saunders, 1980.

Krishnamurthy GT et al. Distribution pattern of metastatic bone disease. JAMA 1977; 327: 2504–2506.

Lester PN. The Essentials of Roentgen Interpretation, 3rd end. London: Harper & Row, 1972.

Paul LH, Juhl JH. Essentials of Roentgen Interpretation, 4th edn. New York: Harper & Row, 1981.

Reeder M, Felson B. Gamuts in Radiology. Cincinnati, OH: Audiovisual Radiology of Cincinnati, 1975.

Resnick D, Niyawama G. Diagnosis of Bone and Joint Disorders. Philadelphia, PA: WB Saunders, 1996.

Schaberg J, Gainor BJ. A profile of metastatic carcinoma of the spine. Spine 1985; 10: 1.

Weissman BNW, Sledge CB. Orthopedic Radiology. Philadelphia, PA: WB Saunders, 1986.

Yochum TR, Rowe LJ. Essentials of Skeletal Radiology, 2nd edn. Baltimore, MD: Williams & Wilkins, 1996.

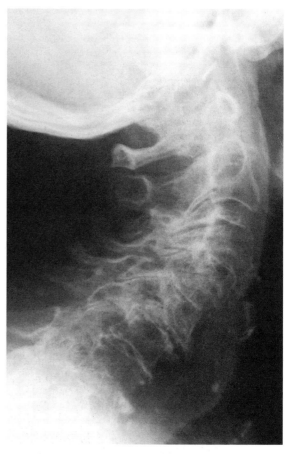

Figure 8.1 Advanced osteoarthritis of the cervical spine may be characterized by varying degrees of intervertebral disc space narrowing, irregularity and subchondral sclerosing of the endplates, and excrescences of the margins of the opposing vertebral endplates. Non-uniform joint space narrowing, roughening and sclerosing of the opposing facet surfaces may be seen. The uncinate processes are likely to be asymmetrical, blunted and hypertrophied. Hyperlordosis of the cervical spine may also exhibit vertebral segmental degenerative spondylolisthesis.

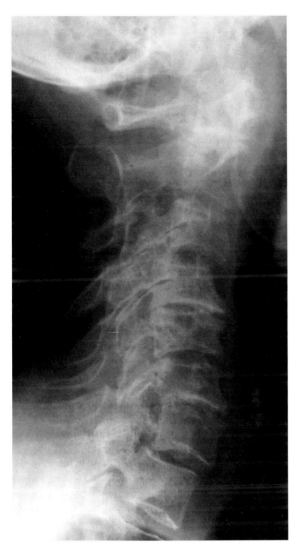

Figure 8.2 Cervical kyphosis in this 77-year-old woman accompanied by degenerative spondylolistheses at C2 and C3, as well as grade 1 retrolistheses at C5 and C6. Advanced facet arthrosis is noted from C3–C4 caudad, and marked degenerative disc disease at C4–C5 and C6–C7. (Courtesy of Michael Prendergast, DC, Toronto, Ontario, Canada.)

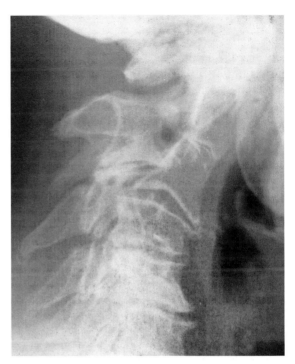

Figure 8.3 Significant curve reversal accompanied by a congenital block vertebra of C2–C3, and marked degenerative disc disease from C3–C4 to C5–C6 inclusive.

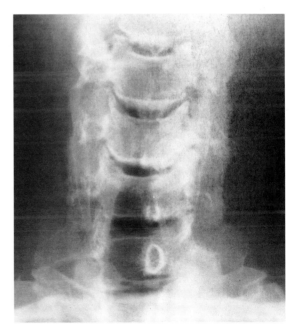

Figure 8.4 Advanced osteoarthritic changes, including marked sclerosis, asymmetry and spurring of the C6 uncinate process on the reading right and its corresponding articular surface on C5.

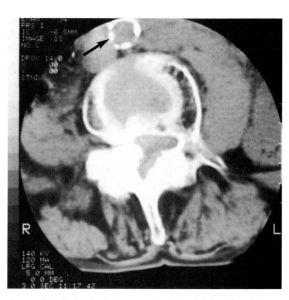

Figure 8.6 Computed tomographic examination demonstrating extensive right facet arthrosis causing marked spinal stenosis and deformity in an 81-year-old woman. Of additional note is marked sclerosis of the descending abdominal aorta (arrow).

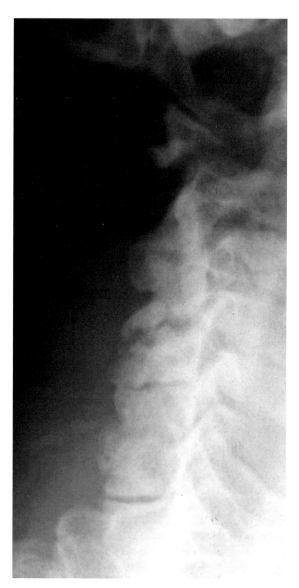

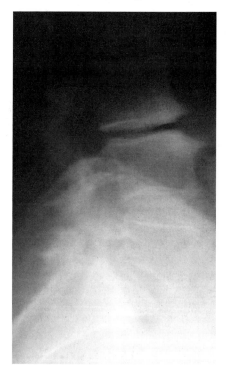

Figure 8.5 Right pillar projection demonstrating severely advanced facet osteoarthrosis at all cervical levels. Note the sclerosis, marked surface irregularity, osteophyte formation, and absence or marked non-uniform diminution of all joint spaces. (Courtesy of George Gale, MD, Toronto, Ontario, Canada.)

Figure 8.7 A 56-year-old woman demonstrating a classic Knuttson's vacuum phenomenon, indicating marked degeneration of the nucleus pulposus of the L3–L4 disc. Osteophytosis, subchondral sclerosis, endplate irregularities and posterior joint changes complete the picture of advanced osteoarthritis at this level.

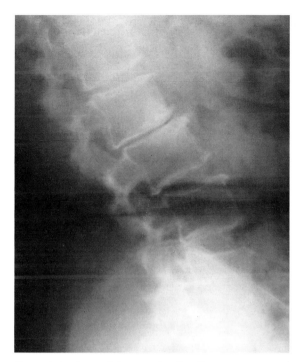

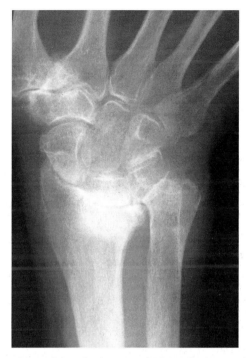

Figure 8.8 Advanced degenerative disc disease at L2–L3 and L3–L4 has resulted in a grade 1 retrolisthesis of the L2 vertebral body. (Courtesy of Sid Sheard, DC, FCCR(C), DACBR, Burnaby, British Columbia, Canada.)

Figure 8.10 Advanced wrist osteoarthritis manifesting as subarticular sclerosis with diminution of the radiocarpal articulations in a 74-year-old woman. Note also the degenerative resorption of the distal ulnar styloid. (Courtesy of James Clark, MD, Toronto, Ontario, Canada.)

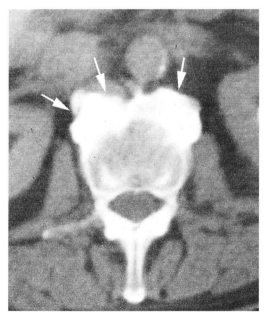

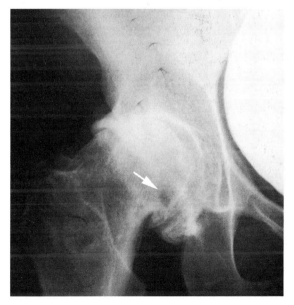

Figure 8.9 Extensive anterior osteophytosis (arrows) in the axial plane on computed tomographic examination of a lumbar vertebra in this 72-year-old man.

Figure 8.11 Subchondral sclerosis, selective diminution of the superior joint compartment, osteophytosis and a subarticular geode (arrow) denoting advanced osteoarthritis of the hip in a 57-year-old woman.

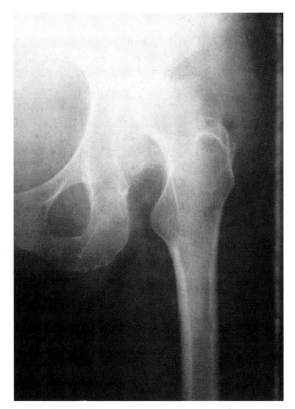

Figure 8.12 Advanced osteoarthritis of the hip. The usual radiographic features include irregular joint space narrowing, particularly the superior compartment, roughening of the opposing articular surfaces, subchondral sclerosis, subchondral pseudocystic formation (geodes) and marginal articular spur formation. In advanced conditions (mala coxa senilis), articular cortical collapse and hyperaemic bone resorption may result in apparent deformity of the affected femoral head, as observed in this case.

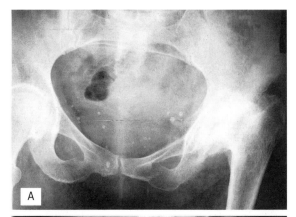

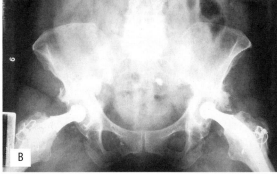

Figure 8.13 Serial study consisting of two views of the pelvis. (A). The initial study exhibits significant osteoarthritis of the iliofemoral articulations bilaterally. Although both hips are implicated, degenerative arthritis does not occur in a symmetrical fashion, as do certain types of inflammatory systemic arthropathy. (B). This subsequent image reveals corrective bilateral hip prostheses.

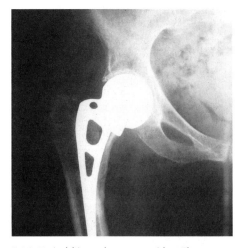

Figure 8.14 Typical hip replacement with a Thompson prosthesis. Note that other forms of instrumentation may be used to accomplish the same effect.

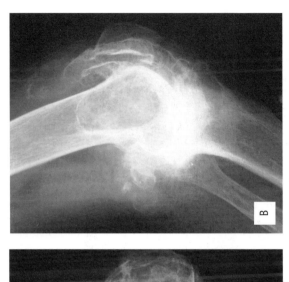

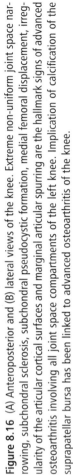

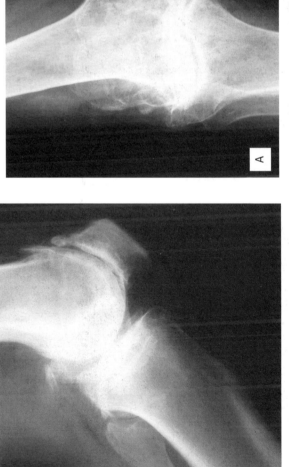

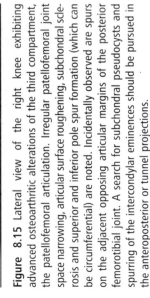

Figure 8.15 Lateral view of the right knee exhibiting advanced osteoarthritic alterations of the third compartment, the patellofemoral articulation. Irregular patellofemoral joint space narrowing, articular surface roughening, subchondral sclerosis and superior and inferior pole spur formation (which can be circumferential) are noted. Incidentally observed are spurs on the adjacent opposing articular margins of the posterior femorotibial joint. A search for subchondral pseudocysts and spurring of the intercondylar eminences should be pursued in the anteroposterior or tunnel projections.

Figure 8.16 (A) Anteroposterior and (B) lateral views of the knee. Extreme non-uniform joint space narrowing, subchondral sclerosis, subchondral pseudocystic formation, medial femoral displacement, irregularity of the articular cortical surfaces and marginal articular spurring are the hallmark signs of advanced osteoarthritis involving all joint space compartments of the left knee. Implication of calcification of the suprapatellar bursa has been linked to advanced osteoarthritis of the knee.

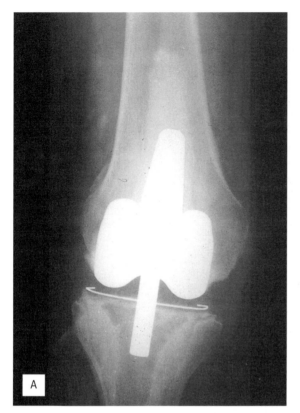
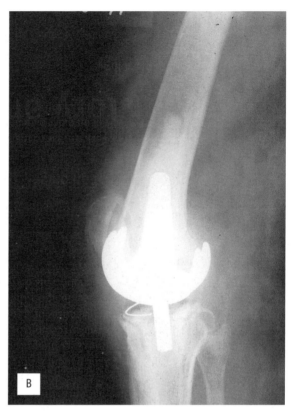

Figure 8.17 (A) Anteroposterior and (B) lateral views of the knee demonstrating a femorotibial prosthesis. This elderly woman suffered from advanced osteoarthritis of the knees, and received a metallic replacement of the femoral condyles and a prosthetic tibial plateau. She was contemplating similar intervention in the equally affected contralateral knee.

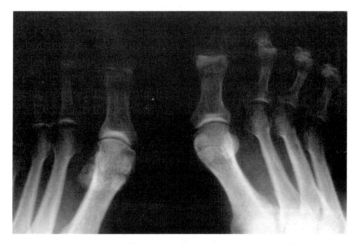

Figure 8.18 Hallux valgus deformity may be principally observed in both younger and elderly women alike. A medial deflection of the first metatarsal associated with a lateral deflection of the first ray is classic. A form of osteoarthritis of the great toe, the condition may be bilateral, but not often symmetrical. A familial tendency has been noted.

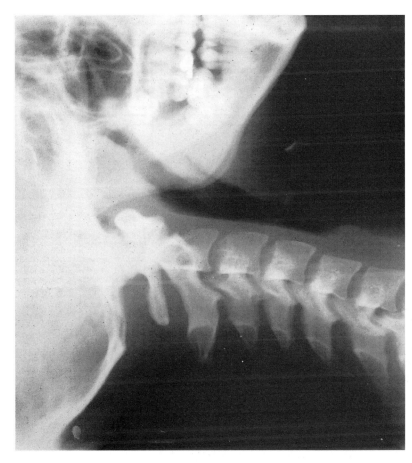

Figure 8.20 As with all inflammatory arthropathies, seropositive or seronegative, it is essential to evaluate the stability of the upper cervical spine complex. It is imperative to note that, in the evaluation of the atlantodental interval in the neutral posture, the space should not exceed 3.5 mm in adults and 5 mm in children under the age of 12 years. Manipulation of an unstable atlas–axis mechanism can portend the most clinically sinister of consequences. This patient suffered from a chronic form of rheumatoid arthritis. Note the markedly increased atlantodental interspace.

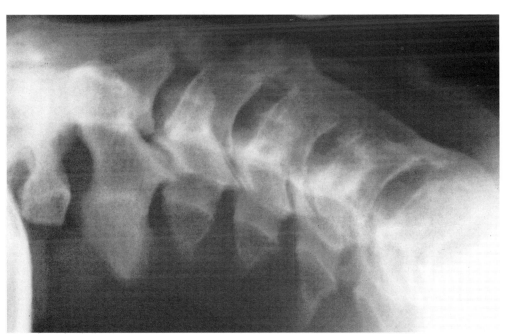

Figure 8.19 Advanced diffuse idiopathic skeletal hyperostosis (DISH) is seen throughout the cervical spine of this 55-year-old man. Note the anterior osseous vertebral body bridging, with the relative preservation of the intervertebral discs and facet joints, aiding in the differentiation of this condition from that of severe cervical spine osteoarthritis.

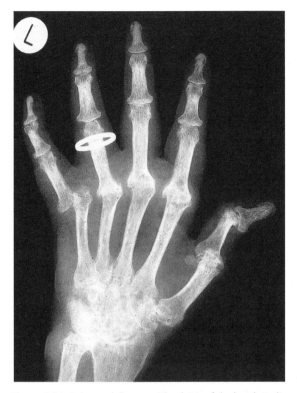

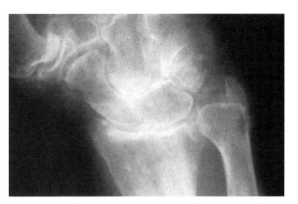

Figure 8.22 Since rheumatoid arthritis favours the small joints of the hands and wrists, this case features a rather classic example of carpal coalition. This phenomenon is characterized by uniform pancompartmental joint space narrowing which may progress to a state of frank ankylosis. Resorption of the distal ulna in varying degrees and locations frequently accompanies the carpal fusion. A bilateral and symmetrical involvement can be anticipated.

Figure 8.21 Advanced rheumatoid arthritis of the hand. Radiographically, this seropositive inflammatory arthropathy is characterized by fusiform soft-tissue oedema adjacent to the proximal interphalangeal joints, juxta-articular osteoporosis, marginal articular erosions (due to pannus production eroding the periarticular bare bone), ulnar deviation, subluxations (boutonniere and swan-neck deformities), and zig zag or 'hitchhiker's' thumb. Rheumatoid arthritis of the hand generally favours the proximal interphalangeal joints and metacarpophalangeal articulations. Osteoarthritis of the hand tends to favour the distal interphalangeal joints and first carpometacarpal articulation. Similar radiographic changes may be expected within the small articulations of the feet and ankles. Hips, knees, shoulders and elbows may also be affected. Clinical note: one is cautioned to evaluate the atlantoaxial stability before contemplating manual or mechanical manipulation of the upper cervical complex in a patient with known rheumatoid arthritis. As this is regarded as a systemic arthropathy, one may anticipate bilateral and symmetrical joint involvement. A positive sheep cell agglutination or rheumatoid factor serological assay is noted in 80% of cases.

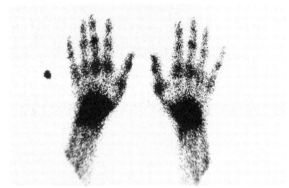

Figure 8.23 Radioisotopic bone scan demonstrating the bilateral and symmetrical uptake particularly noted in the regions of the carpus, metacarpophalangeal and proximal interphalangeal articulations. This represents a graphic appreciation of the systemic nature of rheumatoid arthritis.

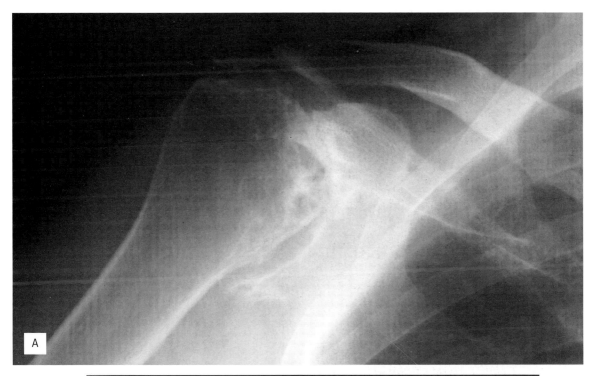

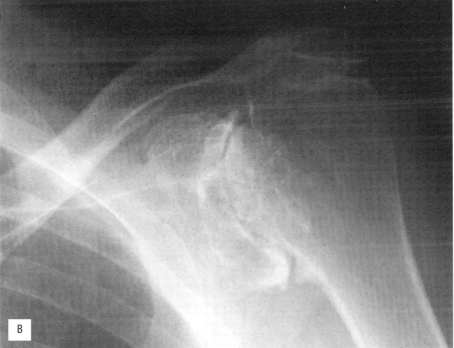

Figure 8.24 Rheumatoid arthritis of the shoulders in a 77-year-old man. (A) Right shoulder; (B) left shoulder. Note the character-istically bilateral symmetrical involvement. Marked symmetrical joint space diminution is present. Significant subchondral pseudo-cystic formation is noted. Observe the superior subluxation of the right humerus in the glenoid due to inflammatory ligamentous and joint capsule laxity. (Courtesy of Bryan Sher, DC, Toronto, Ontario, Canada.)

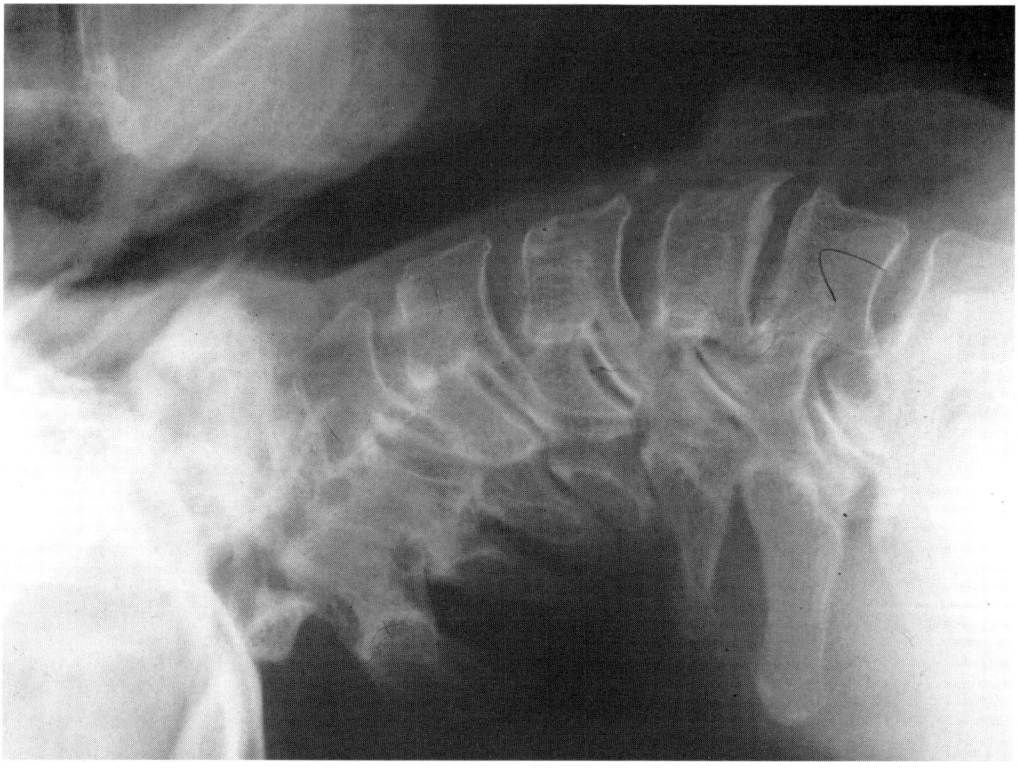

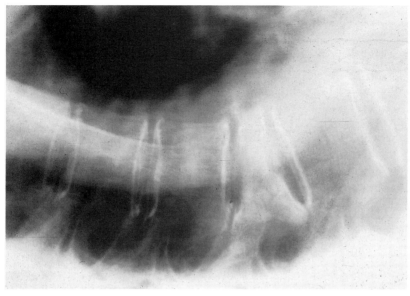

Figure 8.26 Significant collapse of a lower thoracic vertebral body. Because the entire superior endplate has been implicated, one must suspect an underlying osseous pathology. Post-traumatic compression vertebral body fractures tend to involve, principally, the anterior one-third or two-thirds of the superior endplate. This patient demonstrates a complete superior endplate compression fracture secondary to a malignant metastatic involvement.

Figure 8.25 Lytic metastasis has virtually obliterated the body and dens of the axis in this 71 year-old woman. Note the lytic appearance of the C3 vertebral body. (Courtesy of Shane Fainman, MD, Toronto, Ontario, Canada.)

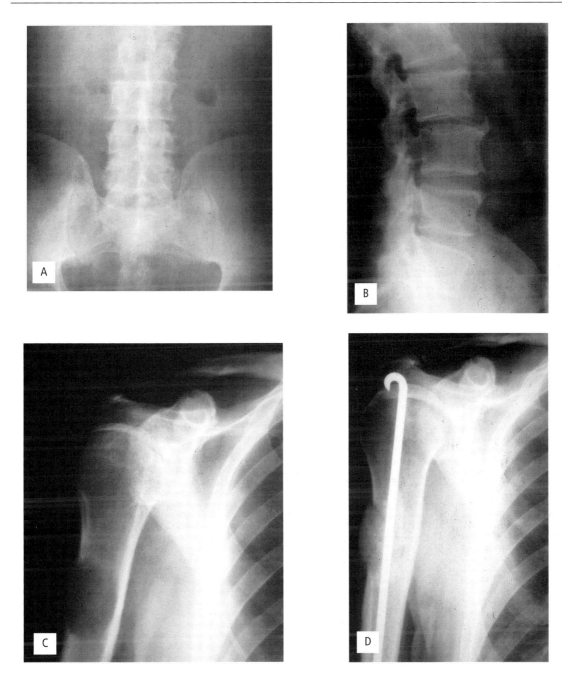

Figure 8.27 Series of four views of a 64-year-old man who presented with a complaint of generalized low back pain. (A, B) Antero-posterior and lateral studies of the lumbopelvic region demonstrating an absence of the left L3 pedicle. The contralateral pedicle remains intact, with no evidence of compensatory hypertrophy or sclerosis. This is a particularly ominous sign, known as the 'wink-ing' vertebra. Should both pedicles of a segment be implicated, this would then be regarded as a 'blind' vertebra. (C, D) Addition-al plain film studies revealing a rather significant, solitary, ill-marginated lesion within the lateral aspect of the proximal diaphysis of the humerus. This lesion was subsequently stabilized by a surgically implanted intramedullary Rush pin and osteotomized bone chips. This patient was diagnosed with primary bronchogenic carcinoma, which had metastasized to multiple skeletal sites. The patient died from the disease within 6 months. Metastatic disease favours the pulmonary parenchyma the hepatic parenchyma, and skele-tal tissue. Haematopoietic red bone-marrow sites are preferred and, next to the skull, the axial skeleton is a predilectory target.

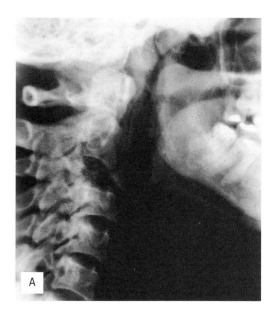

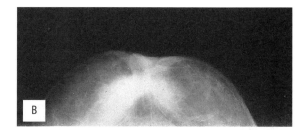

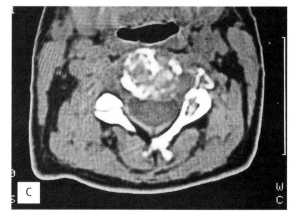

Figure 8.28 Sequence of representative studies including plain film, mammography and computed tomographic (CT) scan. (A) Initial plain film exhibiting a subtotal osteolysis of the C3 vertebral body. (B) Mammography demonstrating a large radiopacification within the breast parenchyma, which was diagnosed as a primary breast carcinoma. (C) Accompanying CT revealing only remnant fragments of bone in the vertebral body. The trained observer will also note an extension of the lytic lesion into the left pedicle. The patient was diagnosed with primary breast carcinoma with osteolytic metastasis to the upper cervical spine. She died from her condition within 6 months.

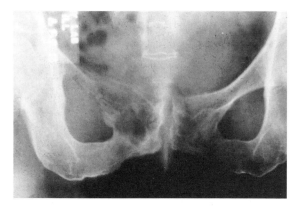

Figure 8.29 Significant osteolysis within the superior and inferior rami of the reading left pubis bone. The overlying cortex has thinned to the point of rupture. The adjacent symphysis pubis articulation has remained intact, aiding in the differentiation of this condition from that of focal infection. This elderly woman was diagnosed with an osteolytic metastatic neoplastic bone disease. Seventy-five per cent of metastases are osteolytic in nature, are haematogenously spread and predispose the affected bone to pathological fracture.

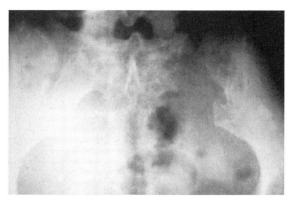

Figure 8.30 A large, ill-marginated osteolytic lesion has completely infiltrated this elderly woman's sacral ala on the right. The adjacent sacroiliac joint and opposing innominate remain uninvolved. Typically, hyalin and fibrocartilage serve as a natural barrier to the spread of this disease. This is in direct contrast to infectious organisms which demonstrate no respect for the aforementioned cartilaginous barriers. This condition was diagnosed as an osteolytic metastatic carcinoma which had metastasized from a primary carcinoma of the breast.

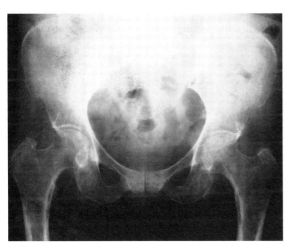

Figure 8.31 Widely disseminated lytic metastasis manifesting as a 'moth-eaten' to permeative pattern throughout the pelvis and proximal femora.

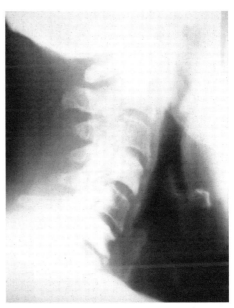

Figure 8.33 The C4 and C5 vertebral bodies are characterized by a dense, homogeneous sclerosis. This phenomenon is, generally, the hallmark of osteoblastic metastatic neoplastic bone disease. Osteoblastic metastases account for 15% of osseous metastases. The primary sources for osteoblastic metastasis are carcinoma of the breast in females and of the prostate in males. Note that Paget's disease (phase 3) and Hodgkin's lymphoma may also produce the 'ivory' vertebra. This case reveals no bone expansion, eliminating Paget's disease, or anterior osseous erosive scalloping due to adjacent neoplastic lymphadenopathy secondary to Hodgkin's lymphoma. This senior-aged man was diagnosed with primary prostatic carcinoma with spinal metastasis.

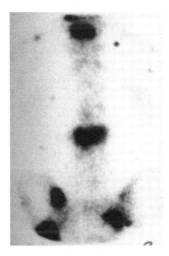

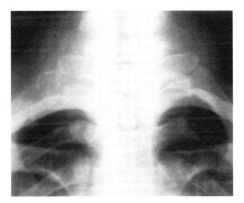

Figure 8.32 Technetion-99m radioisotopic bone scan demonstrating the typical alterations in size, shape, density and distribution of isotope intake. This lack of pattern has been termed the 'Christmas tree' effect and, when present, is highly indicative of a skeletal metastatic phenomenon.

Figure 8.34 Reading left first costal element revealing a focally expansile, large, solitary lesion with an ill-defined, 'moth-eaten' matrix. This elderly woman suffered from a primary breast carcinoma which had metastasized to the ribs. Metastasis to the thoracic cage ranks third, after the skull and axial skeleton, in incidence of involvement.

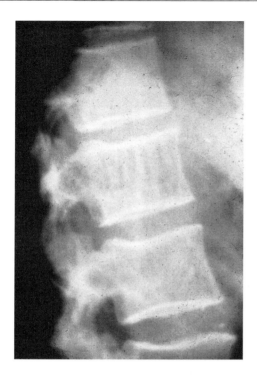

Figure 8.35 Coarsened vertical trabecular formation known as the 'corduroy cloth' appearance, observed in a single vertebral body, is indicative of an haemangioma, which is the most common primary benign tumour of the spine. When observed in flat bones such as the skull, scapula and ilium, the 'wagonwheel' sign may be seen. A selective resorption of the transverse trabecular pattern, observed in multiple vertebral bodies, has been termed 'pseudohaemangiomas' and is associated with advancing osteoporosis. Note that there is no vertebral body expansion in the presented case, helping to distinguish this benign tumour from Paget's disease, which is generally characterized by accompanying osseous expansion.

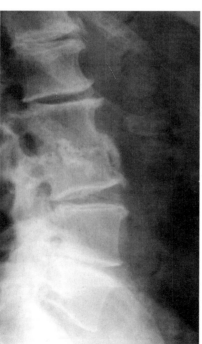

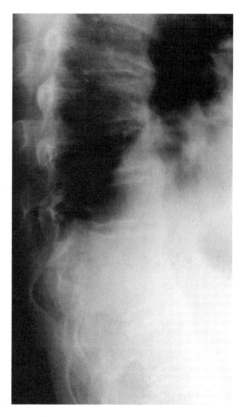

Figure 8.36 The L2–L3 intervertebral disc demonstrates subtotal destruction. Marked irregularity, sclerosing and anterior spurring of the adjacent vertebral endplates suggest the presence of a resolving infectious discopathy. No soft-tissue abscess is noted in this study.

Figure 8.37 This elderly patient had an antecedent pulmonary tuberculosis infection. The lower thoracic region demonstrates osseous ankylosis of two adjacent vertebral bodies as a consequence of the infection. The thoracolumbar spine is a favoured site for this phenomenon. (Courtesy of Andre Robidoux, DC, Montreal, Quebec, Canada.)

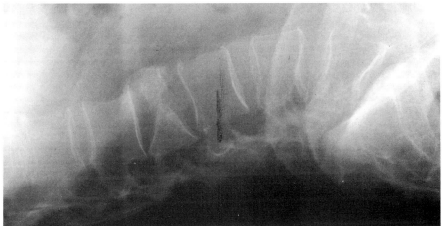

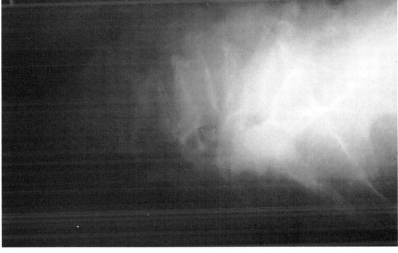

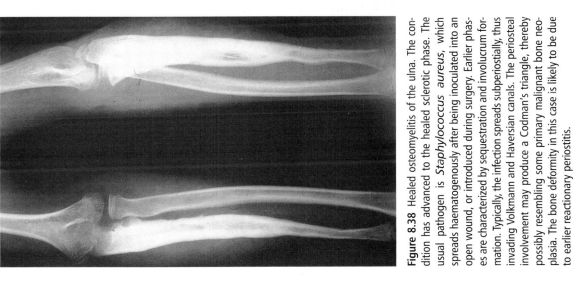

Figure 8.40 Osteoporotic compression fracture of the L2 vertebral body in a 70-year-old man. Note the universal osteopenia. (Courtesy of Robert Bacon, DC, FATA, Toronto, Ontario, Canada.)

Figure 8.39 Typical post-traumatic vertebral body compression fracture of L3 in a severely osteoporotic lumbar spine. Note the trapezoidal shape of the body, sloping anteriorly, indicative of a compression fracture secondary to a traumatic event.

Figure 8.38 Healed osteomyelitis of the ulna. The condition has advanced to the healed sclerotic phase. The usual pathogen is *Staphylococcus aureus*, which spreads haematogenously after being inoculated into an open wound, or introduced during surgery. Earlier phases are characterized by sequestration and involucrum formation. Typically, the infection spreads subperiostially, thus invading Volkmann and Haversian canals. The periosteal involvement may produce a Codman's triangle, thereby possibly resembling some primary malignant bone neoplasia. The bone deformity in this case is likely to be due to earlier reactionary periostitis.

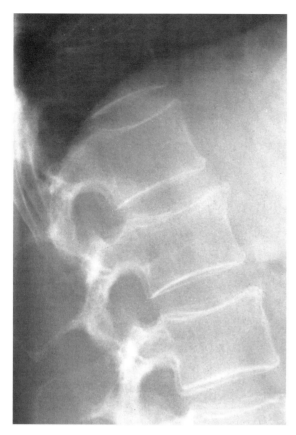

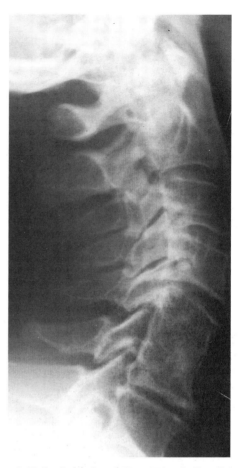

Figure 8.41 T11 lytic metastatic compression fracture. Note the decrease in posterior body height which helps to distinguish this vertebral collapse from one due to osteoporosis, wherein the posterior body height tends to be maintained. (Courtesy of Bryan Sher, DC, Toronto, Ontario, Canada.)

Figure 8.42 Surgical fusion of C5 to C6 has facilitated the progression of degenerative disc disease at C6–C7 in this 57-year-old man. (Courtesy of Kumar Kelkar, MD, Toronto, Ontario, Canada.)

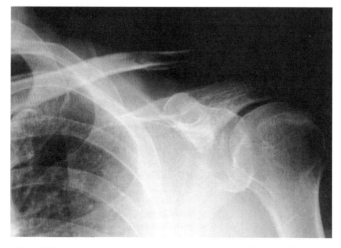

Figure 8.43 Shoulder separation. This acromioclavicular joint space measures 11 mm; the maximum normal limit is 7 mm. (Courtesy of Robert Bacon, DC, FATA, Toronto, Ontario, Canada.)

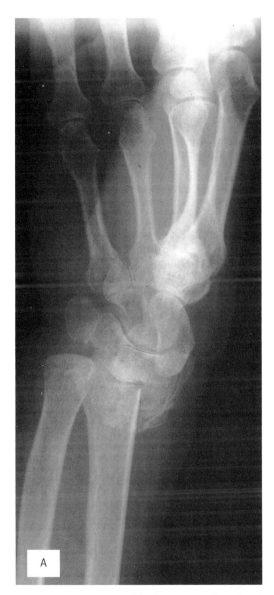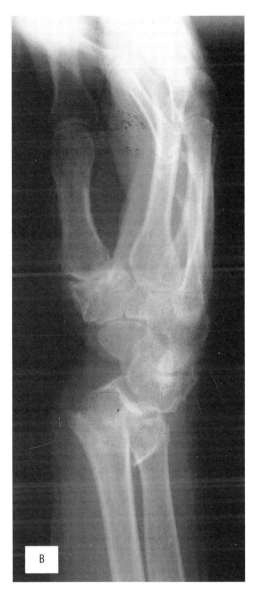

Figure 8.44 (A) Oblique and (B) lateral views of a Colle's fracture of the distal radius in a 78-year-old woman. The lateral depicts the classic 'dinner-fork' deformity caused by volar displacement of the distal fragment and hand. The fracture usually occurs at least 25 mm from the articular surface, with a volar angulation of at least 10 degrees.

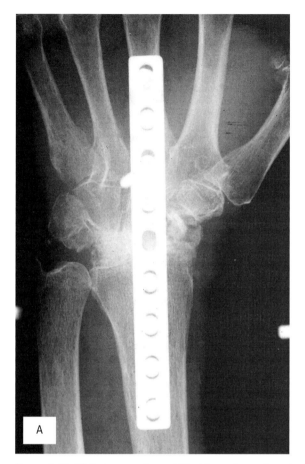
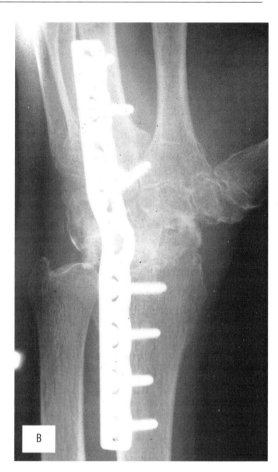

Figure 8.45 (A) Posteroanterior and (B) oblique views of proximal carpal row fractures and distal radius fracture with metal fixation plate and screws. (Courtesy of Henry Clark, DC, Toronto, Ontario, Canada.)

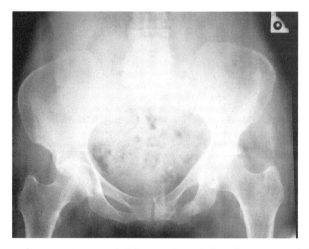

Figure 8.46 An 80-year-old woman demonstrating a vertical fracture through the inferior ramus of the left ischium. The production of an osseous callus has begun, suggesting that the fracture is more than 3 weeks old. A fracture of this type is generally sustained by the direct force of a fall upon underlying osteoporotic bone.

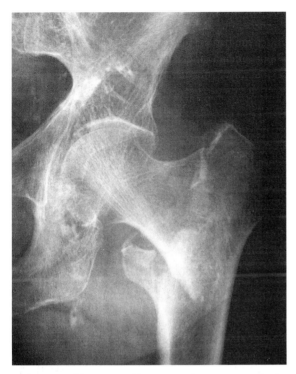

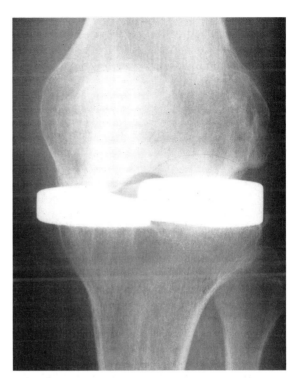

Figure 8.47 This 84-year-old osteoporotic woman sustained a fracture to the lesser trochanter and intertrochanteric region after a fall.

Figure 8.48 Tibial plateau prosthesis in a 61-year-old woman. Of incidental note is atherosclerotic calcification of arteries superimposed over the interosseous membrane.

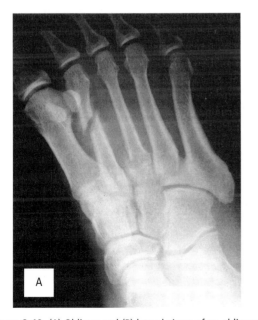

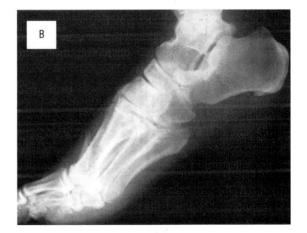

Figure 8.49 (A) Oblique and (B) lateral views of an oblique fracture through the mid-diaphysis of the second metatarsal in a 66-year-old man. Note how the angulation of the distal fragment is only appreciated on the lateral projection. (Courtesy of Eric Shrubb, DC, DACBR, FCCR(C), Scarborough, Ontario, Canada.)

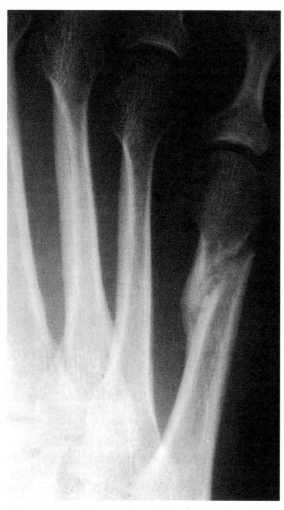

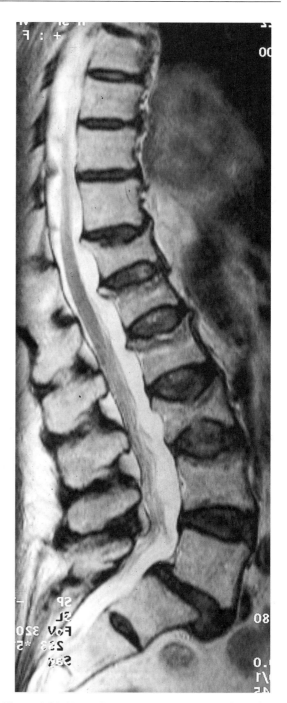

Figure 8.50 Spiral fracture through the mid-diaphyseal portion of the fifth metatarsal. This is a recent fracture, as there is no evidence of bone resorption noted along the opposing fracture surfaces. The practitioner must consider any long-term effects of altered biomechanics that may result from the fracture.

Figure 8.51 Magnetic resonance imaging reveals multiple osteoporotic vertebral body compression fractures (T12 to L3, as well as the L4 superior endplate) in a 56-year-old woman. The L4–L5 disc exhibits a bulging annulus, resulting in mild canal stenosis. L5 demonstrates bilateral pars defects with a grade 2 spondylolisthesis. Moderate canal stenosis is present at this level. (Courtesy of Buffalo MRI, Amherst, NY, USA.)

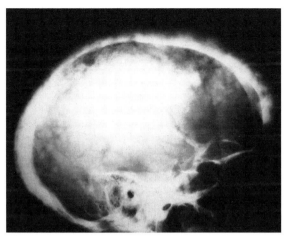

Figure 8.52 Lateral view of the skull exhibiting the multiple focal regions of osteoporosis, typically associated with the initial phase of Paget's disease. This radiographic appearance has been termed osteoporosis circumscripta.

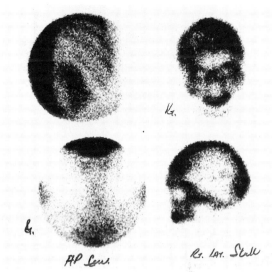

Figure 8.53 Technetium phosphate radioisotopic bone scan exhibiting a homogeneous uptake of isotope principally limited to the occipital bone of an elderly man's skull. This pattern is consistent with Paget's disease. As this ia a bone-softening ailment, it is imperative to evaluate the skull for the presence of basilar invagination. If this disease is found to be polyostotic in nature, an extremely elevated alkaline phosphatase and urinary hydroxyproline should be anticipated.

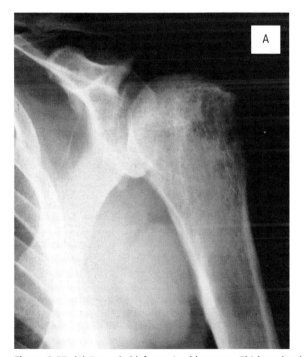
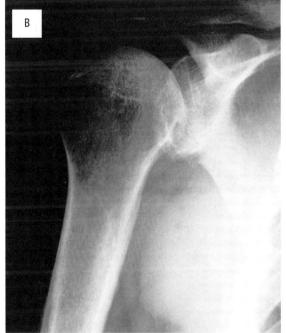

Figure 8.55 (A) Expanded left proximal humerus. Thickened trabeculae and widened intertrabecular spaces principally involving the subarticular bone can be noted. Paget's disease, stage 2, is the most probable diagnosis. (B) The right proximal humerus is offered for comparison.

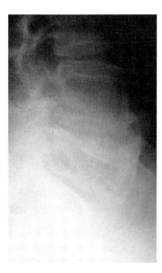

Figure 8.55 The L5 vertebral body is characterized by an expansion associated with marked sclerosis of both the superior and inferior endplates ('picture-frame' vertebra). This appearance is consistent with phase 3 Paget's disease.

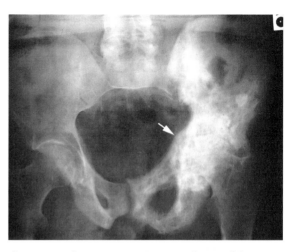

Figure 8.56 Phase 3 monostotic Paget's disease of the innominate in a 60-year-old man, manifesting as marked expansion, coarse, irregular trabeculation and cortical thickening. Note the protrusio acetabulum (arrow) due to the bone-softening nature of this pathology.

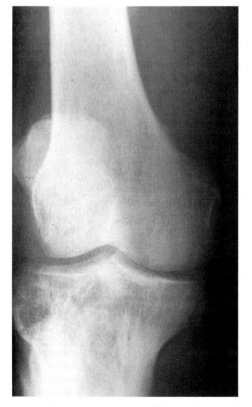

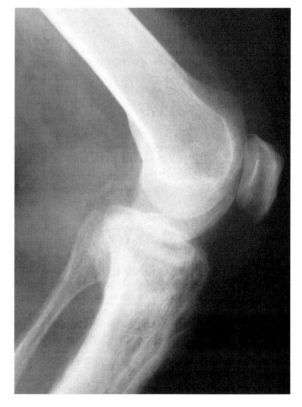

Figure 8.57 (A) Anteroposterior and (B) lateral views of Paget's disease of the tibia in a 71-year-old man. Note the typical cortical thickening, osseous expansion and coarse, irregular trabeculation. (Courtesy of Cecil McQuoid, DC, Brighton, Ontario, Canada.)

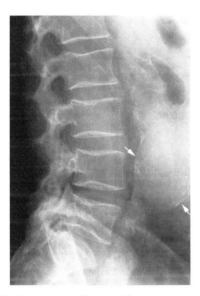

Figure 8.58 Expanded curvilinear calcification anterior to L3–L4 outlining a 6 cm balloon aneurysm (arrows) of the abdominal aorta in a 75-year-old man. (Courtesy of J Stephen Gillis, DC, Saint John, New Brunswick, Canada.)

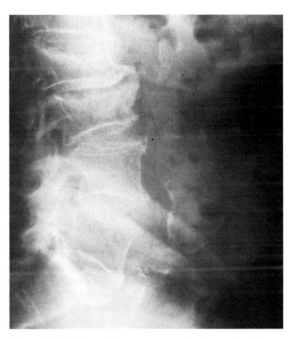

Figure 8.60 A 7 cm balloon aneurysm is observed anterior to the L3 vertebral body in this man. Note the severe osteoporotic compression fractures of the L2 and L3 bodies; the long-standing nature of these fractures is suggested by the marked attendant osteophytosis. Advanced lower lumbar facet arthrosis is present. (Courtesy of Dominique Dufour, DC, Quebec City, Quebec, Canada.)

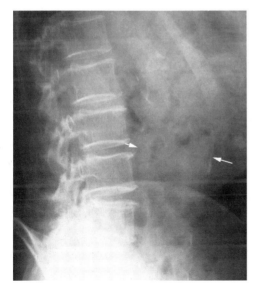

Figure 8.59 Marked expansion of the curvilinear calcification of atherosclerotic plaquing (arrows) denoting a 7 cm aneurysm of the descending abdominal aorta. (Courtesy of Bryan Sher, DC, Toronto, Ontario, Canada.)

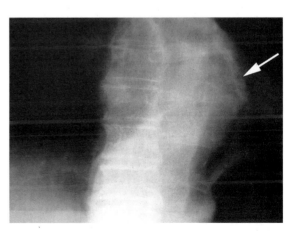

Figure 8.61 This 80-year-old man presented with left chest and shoulder pain. Note the marked curvilinear expansion of the thoracic aorta (arrow) indicative of a thoracic aorta aneurysm. (Courtesy of Ed Lubberdink, DC, Willowdale, Ontario, Canada.)

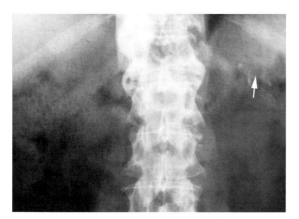

Figure 8.62 Splenic artery calcification in a 75-year-old male. Note the serpiginous, tortuous curvilinear sclerosis (arrow).

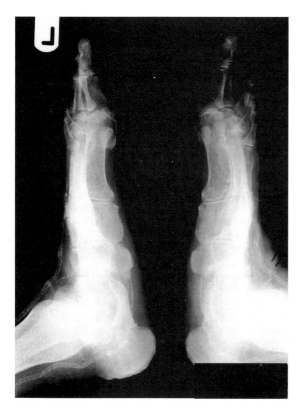

Figure 8.63 Bilateral lateral foot projections demonstrating marked arterial calcification. Known as Monckeburg's sclerosis, this process involves calcium deposits in the tunica media of arteries and arterioles, and is commonly seen in diabetic patients, such as this 68-year-old woman. Of incidental note are osteoarthritic changes at the first metatarsophalangeal joints bilaterally.

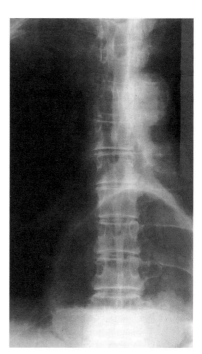

Figure 8.64 Hiatal hernia in a 75-year-old man. Observe the air–fluid meniscus level in the stomach which is superimposed over the thoracic spine and faint cardiac silhouette. (Courtesy of Richard Collis, DC, Toronto, Ontario, Canada.)

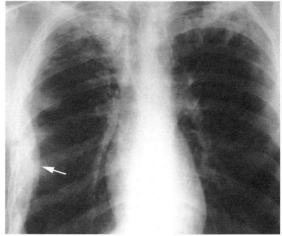

Figure 8.65 Posteroanterior view of the chest demonstrating multiple, confluent radiopacifications in both lung apices. A blunting of the right costophrenic angle, along with an 'extrapleural' sign (arrow) at the lateral aspect of the midportion of the right thoracic wall are also observed. Although many conditions may produce this complex, the two most likely are primary tuberculosis and primary bronchogenic carcinoma associated with costal metastases. This patient was diagnosed with primary pulmonary tuberculosis, which was in an infectious stage.

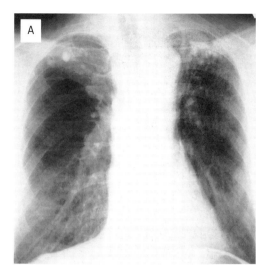
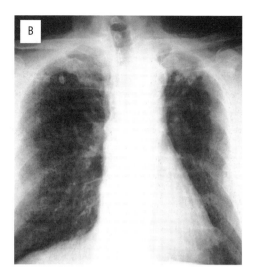

Figure 8.66 (A) Posteroanterior and (B) apical lordotic views of an aged man's chest demonstrating the presence of multiple discrete and coalescing radiopacification, principally contained within the apex of each lung. Often termed 'coin' lesions, this appearance is most closely associated with pulmonary tuberculosis. The fibrocaseous lesions must be differentiated from those associated with such mycotic diseases as histoplasmosis and coccidioidomycosis. Note that the apical view permits a more advantageous appreciation of the parenchyma of the apical and middle lobes. Of incidental note is the presence of the 'thumbnail' sign, signifying calcified atherosclerosis in the aortic arch.

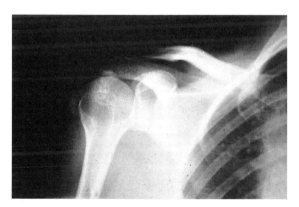

Figure 8.67 The large, homogeneous calcific lesion paralleling the head of the humerus was diagnosed as calcific tendinitis. Deposition of hydroxyapatite crystals into tendons, ligaments and bursae is not uncommon. The supraspinatus and infraspinatus tendons, as well as calcific deposits into the subacromial and subdeltoid bursae of the shoulder, are frequent conditions observed in the aged.

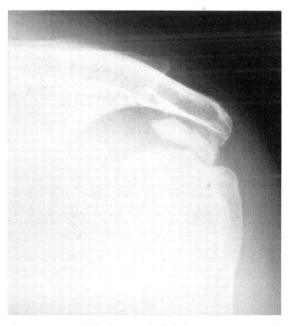

Figure 8.68 Marked subacromial calcific bursitis in a 59-year-old man. (Courtesy of Paul Charlton, Scarborough, Ontario, Canada.)

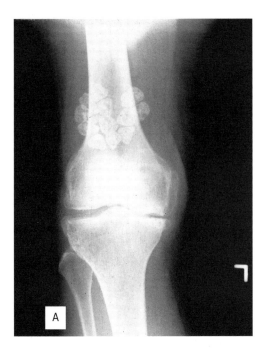

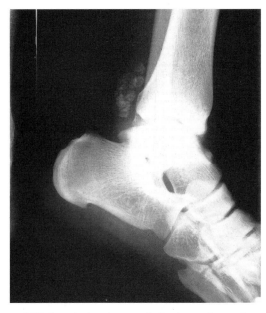

Figure 8.70 Synoviochondrometaplasia observed posterior to the terminal ends of the left mortise joint. This represents the second most frequent site of involvement of this condition.

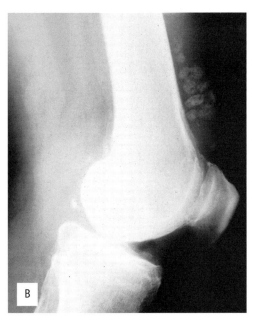

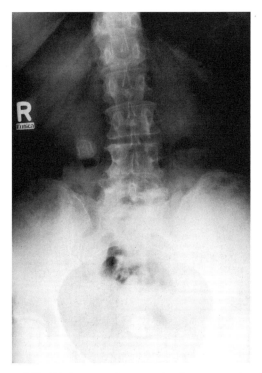

Figure 8.69 (A) Anteroposterior and (B) lateral views of the right knee demonstrating multiple, well-circumscribed radiopacities within the region of the suprapatellar pouch. This condition is known as synoviochondrometaplasia or osteochondrometaplasia. It may arise *de novo* or has been associated with advancing osteoarthritis. This case demonstrates the condition in its most typical location.

Figure 8.71 Elderly woman demonstrating the presence of a solitary, mixed cholelithiasis on the right side, adjacent to L4, as well as the appearance of a 2.5 cm calcified uterine fibroma.

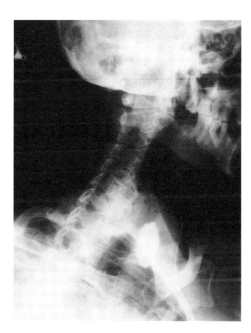

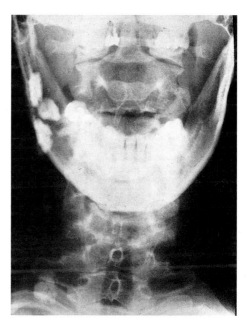

Figure 8.72 Well-marginated, solitary radiopacification at the medial clavicular level. This condition was diagnosed as a benign, calcified thyroid adenoma. This 75-year-old woman complained of a chronic, persistent, non-productive cough. This was probably due to a local mechanical irritation of the vagus nerve. Thyroid hormonal titre studies were determined to be normal. Because of the haemorrhagic nature of thyroid gland surgery, it was decided to leave the lesion in situ.

Figure 8.73 Multiple, oval, discrete, homogeneous radiopacifications superimposed over the right superior ramus of the mandible. These lesions are said to have a 'popcorn' appearance, and are indicative of calcific lymphadenopathy. A single acute or chronic upper respiratory tract infection may elicit a corresponding lymphadenopathy; this may subsequently proceed to ensuing calcification. These are regarded clinically as benign and insignificant incidental findings on X-ray.

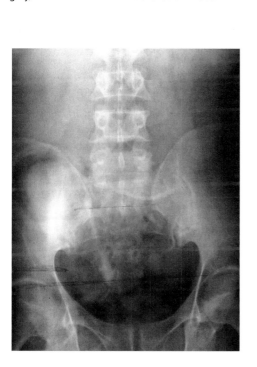

Figure 8.74 Large, radiolucent, circular shadow superimposed over the right ilium, indicative of a surgical stoma. (Courtesy of Andre Robidoux, DC, Montreal, Quebec, Canada.)

Section III: Clinical conditions affecting the older person

9

Mental disorders in the elderly: an overview of diagnosis and management

David Conn

The proportion of elderly individuals in the population is rapidly rising, as described elsewhere in this book. This applies especially to the group aged 80 years and older. A further acceleration in the 'greying' of the population will take place in approximately 2010 as the baby boom generation enters their senior years. This has important implications for those planning mental health services for the elderly. The disorders that most commonly require treatment include the dementias and their associated psychiatric complications, delirium, mood and psychotic disorders. The resources required to treat elderly persons with mental disorders must also grow rapidly if the needs of this population are to be met.

Arie and Jolley[1] and, more recently, Shulman[2] have outlined fundamental principles with regard to the delivery of psychiatric services for the elderly. These principles include: comprehensiveness, defining the target population, community outreach, availability and flexibility, and support for caregivers. Shulman[2] has described the essential components of a regional programme. When a geriatric psychiatry service wishes to provide programmes for a region, it must be comprehensive to the extent that it will ensure the provision of care for a full range of mental disorders in later life. It is particularly important to ensure that the psychiatric needs of the most severely ill are met. Such services are generally provided by a multidisciplinary group of mental health-care workers. In addition, the service must take on responsibility for an all-inclusive primary geographical catchment area. In a fully regionalized system, these boundaries must be prop-

erly co-ordinated with other services. Such programmes have been developed in Britain based on a population range of between 20 000 and 40 000 individuals over the age of 65 per service. Geriatric services have pioneered the development of domiciliary visiting, that is community outreach services which provide care for people in their own homes. This is especially important in the elderly, many of whom are unable or unwilling to leave their homes. As a result, it is important to note that community outreach is an essential component of any regional geriatric psychiatry service. This service must be available, accessible and responsive, and collaborative relations must exist with both the community at large and with other health-care services, such as hospital and geriatric medical services. In addition, links must be established with community agencies and with long-term care and residential facilities within the catchment area. Ideally, hospital-based psychiatric services should be integrated with geriatric medical services. The ideal components of a hospital-based service include a community outreach team, a day hospital, an inpatient assessment and treatment unit, outpatient clinics, consultation and liaison with medical and surgical services within the hospital, and access to chronic care beds. There is often a need to improve co-ordination among community-based services, which generally consist of a large number of health and social agencies, both private and public. It is important for community-based services to screen individuals who may be at high risk and thus help to identify individuals who are in need of mental health services at an early stage of their illness.

Because such services manage frail elderly who are at very high risk, it is important that hospital-based services provide adequate and responsive back-up. Day-care programmes, which are generally run using a social model, can provide considerable support and respite for families caring for individuals with dementia. Such programmes can allow individuals to remain in the community rather than resorting to premature institutionalization.

Epidemiology of mental disorders

The prevalence of various mental disorders varies considerably depending on the living situation of the population. Studies of the elderly generally focus on community residents, residents of nursing homes or psychiatric inpatients. With regard to the elderly living in the community, it appears that clinical depression which conforms to diagnostic criteria occurs in between 2 and 4% of the population. However, if all patients with depressive symptomatology are included, the rate rises to between 10 and 15%. The prevalence rate for all anxiety disorders in individuals over the age of 65 is reported to be 5.5%. The most common form of anxiety is phobic disorder.

Most anxiety in later life can be accounted for by generalized anxiety disorders and phobias. Between 6 and 8% of the elderly population residing in the community suffer from a progressive dementia. The most common form is Alzheimer's disease, followed by vascular dementia. The prevalence of dementia rises dramatically in those over 80 years of age. In the nursing-home setting, studies suggest that approximately 80% of residents suffer from some kind of psychiatric or behavioural disorder. One large study found that 27% of new admissions to nursing homes suffered from dementia complicated by depression, delusions or delirium.[3] Forty per cent suffered from uncomplicated dementia, 10% suffered from a mood disorder and approximately 2% were diagnosed as having schizophrenia.

Studies of patients with dementia report that a high proportion exhibit one or more behaviour problem. Common problems include physical and verbal aggression, anger, wandering, insomnia and incontinence. Between 15 and 25% of nursing-home residents have symptoms of major depression and another 25% have depressive symptoms of lesser severity.

Diagnostic classifications

The diagnoses used in this chapter are based on the diagnostic system of the American Psychiatric Association (APA), entitled DSM-IV (APA, 1994).[4] It is a multiaxial system, with axis I containing the major psychiatric diagnoses, axis II personality traits and disorders, axis III the medical disorders, axis IV the level of psychosocial stress and Axis V the level of functioning of the individual.

In attempting to understand the aetiology of psychiatric illness, a biopsychosocial model is more helpful than the traditional biomedical model and is the model of choice in both geriatrics and psychiatry. In formulating a clinical problem, it is generally helpful to categorize aetiological factors into biological (physical), psychological and social categories. These are further broken down into predisposing, precipitating, perpetuating and protective factors. The category 'social' includes both cultural and environmental factors. This model allows for the design of treatment interventions which are aimed at a variety of aetiological factors.

The diagnostic assessment

The first component of an assessment regarding a geriatric mental health problem is the history. Many patients can give a clear account of their problem, but in other cases it is essential to obtain collateral history from family or other caregivers. It is important to ascertain the reliability of the patient's history during the early stages of the interview. The following categories of information make up the complete history: chief complaint, history of presenting illness, past psychiatric history, family history, personal history, past medical history, current medications, drug and alcohol history, and a history of functional status, in particular, the activities of daily living (ADLs). The ADLs include the basic functions as well as more complex tasks, which are referred to as instrumental activities of daily living (IADLs) (Table 9.1). Following the history, it is important to assess the patient's mental status. The components of the Mental Status Examination include behavioural observations, mood and affect, thinking processes, perception and cognition. During the history, it is possible to obtain a significant amount of information with regard to the mental status. One observes appearance, general behaviour, speech, attitude, the patient's affect (displayed emotions), as well as any unusual beliefs and a general sense of the individual's memory, on the basis of the details and accuracy of the history. It is important to ask the patient about their current emotional state. Simple questions such as 'how would you describe your feelings?' can be an important starting point. During an assessment, one should always ask patients whether they have suicidal thoughts. The elderly are at high risk for suicide and, although it can be somewhat uncomfortable to ask a person about suicidal ideation, the vast majority of patients do not have a problem with this question. Individuals who have feelings that life is not worth living or active suicidal thoughts often welcome the opportunity to share and discuss these feelings. Useful questions include, 'have you ever felt that your life was not worth living?' and, subsequently, 'have you ever felt so depressed that you wanted to end your life?' If the individual does express some feelings that life is not worth living, it is important to ask whether they have any specific thoughts or plans with regard to killing themselves.

In assessing the patient's thinking, it is important to assess both thought processes, that is, how an individual actually thinks, as well as thought content. With regard to thought process, there may be abnormalities in the rate, quantity and form of speech. There may be excessively slow or fast speech or a lack of spontaneous speech, or there may be circumstantial speech, which refers to a pattern of responding to questions in an overinclusive manner. When thinking is tangential, it means that the person's responses do not relate to the actual question and the individual ends up talking about a completely different topic. Thinking may be disorganized to the point where speech makes little sense. With regard to thought content, a number of disturbances may be seen. The patient may become preoccupied with a particular subject. They may have obsessions, which are repetitive unwanted thoughts, or phobias, which are irrational fears. Delusions are fixed false beliefs which the individual does not recognize as being irrational. These delusions may be persistent and highly structured or disorganized and brief. The most common delusions are paranoid delusions in which the person believes that they are in danger or that other people want to harm them. Before determining whether a belief is actually delusional, it is important to remember that belief systems vary from one culture to another. Perceptions are also assessed and abnormalities include illusions when there are misinterpretations of a real stimulus, for example, when a person hears others talking and imagines that what they are saying refers to him. Hallucinations are perceptions that occur in the absence of any external stimulus. These can involve any of the sensory systems, but the most common are auditory or visual.

With regard to the assessment of cognitive functions, the major components are listed:

- attention and concentration
- language
- memory
- abstraction
- constructional ability
- praxis
- insight and judgement.

Cognition means the mental processes involved in the acquisition, processing and utilization of knowledge or information. Depending on the clinical situation, the cognitive evaluation may be quite brief or may be detailed. In some cases it is helpful to obtain a full neuropsychological battery of tests, carried out by a psychologist. The most commonly used screening instrument is the Folstein Mini-Mental State Examination (MMSE; see Table 9.2), which allows clinicians to determine quickly whether there might be a significant problem.[5] It is useful to have a standardized instrument that can be used by individuals in different settings, or even different countries. It is important to note, however, that an instrument such as the MMSE is only a screening instrument and cannot be used to make a diagnosis.

Table 9.1 Activities of daily living, for functional assessment

Physical (self-care) activities of daily living	
Bathing	Eating
Dressing	Transferring
Grooming	Using the toilet
Instrumental activities of daily living	
Using the telephone	Doing household chores
Shopping	Driving
Preparing food	Travelling
Using tools	Managing medication
Doing laundry	Managing money

Table 9.2 The Mini-Mental State Examination

Patient   _____

Max. Score _____

Score   _____

Orientation

5 ☐ What is the (year) (season) (date) (month) (day)?
5 ☐ Where are we? (state) (country) (town) (hospital) (floor)

Registration

3 ☐ Name 3 objects: 1 second to say each.
      Then ask the patient all 3 after you have said them.
      Give 1 point for each correct answer.
      Then repeat them until he learns all 3.
      Count trials and record.
      Trials _____

Attention and Calculation

5 ☐ Serial 7s. 1 point for each correct. Stop after 5 answers. Alternatively, spell 'world' backwards.

Recall

3 ☐ Ask for the 3 objects repeated above. Give 1 point for each correct answer.

Language

9 ☐ Name a pencil, and watch (2 points).
      Repeat the following 'No ifs, ands or buts' (1 point)
      Follow a 3-stage command:
        'Take a paper in your right hand, fold it in half, and put it on the floor' (3 points).
      Read and obey the following:
        Close your eyes (1 point).
        Write a sentence (1 point).
        Copy design (1 point).

Total score

Instructions for Administration of the Mini-Mental State Examination

Orientation

Ask for the date. Then ask specifically for parts omitted, e.g. 'Can you also tell me what season it is?' One point for each correct.
Ask in turn 'Can you tell me the name of this hospital?' (town, country, etc.) One point for each correct.

Registration

Ask the patient if you may test his memory. Then say the names of 3 unrelated objects, early and slowly, about one second for each. After you have said all 3, ask him to repeat them. The first repetition determines his score (0–3), but keep saying them until he can repeat all 3, up to 6 trials. If he does not eventually learn all 3, recall cannot be meaningfully tested.

Attention and calculation

Ask the patient to begin with 100 and count backwards in 7s. Stop after 5 subtractions (93, 86, 79, 72, 65). Score the total number of correct answers.
If the patient cannot or will not perform this task, ask him to spell the word 'world' backwards. The score is the number of letters in correct order, e.g. dlrow = 5, dlorw = 3.

Recall

Ask the patient if he can recall the 3 words you previously asked him to remember. Score 0–3.

Language

Naming: Show the patient a wrist watch and ask him what it is. Repeat for pencil. Score 0–2.

Repetition: Ask the patient to repeat the sentence after you. Allow only one trial. Score 0 or 1.

3-Stage command: Give the patient a piece of plain blank paper and ask him to carry out the command. Score 1 point for each part correctly executed.

Reading: On a blank piece of paper print the sentence 'Close your eyes' in letters large enough for the patient to see clearly. Ask him to read it and do what it says. Score 1 point only if he actually closes his eyes.

Writing: Give the patient a blank piece of paper and ask him to write a sentence for you. Do not dictate a sentence, as it is to be written spontaneously. It must contain a subject an verb and be sensible. Correct grammar and punctuation are not necessary.

Copying: On a clean piece of paper, draw intersecting pentagons, each side about 1 inch, and ask him to copy them exactly as they are. All 10 angles must be present and the 2 pentagons must intersect to score 1 point. Tremor and rotations are noted. Estimate the patient's level of sensorium along a continuum, from alert on the left to coma on the right.

Source: Folstein et al.[5]

Tests of attention and concentration are very important. If a person is unable to concentrate, it is likely that they will have difficulty in other areas of the cognitive examination as well. Some simple tests of attention include digit recall, in which the interviewer recites a series of random numbers at a rate of one number per second, and asks the individual to repeat the numbers back. The series of numbers is increased following a correct response, with different numbers being used each time. Subsequently, a more difficult task is to attempt to repeat a series of numbers backwards. Other tests might include repeating the months of the year forwards and then in reverse. One popular test is serial sevens, in which the individual must subtract 7 from 100 and continue to subtract 7 from each successive answer. This is also, of course, a test of simple arithmetic. When testing language, it is important to note the individual's spontaneous speech, to test the ability to repeat simple phrases, to name objects, to comprehend simple information, and to assess the ability to read and write. Memory can be classified simply into three types: immediate, recent and remote. Immediate memory is tested by asking a person to repeat a series of words. Recent memory can be tested by asking a person to remember three or four words and then to retest after a period of 2–20 min. If the person has difficulty, then it is helpful to provide a cue which can be either a category, such as 'that word was a colour', or a sound, e.g. 'the word began with the sound bl'. Remote memory involves recalling information that has been known for a long period and might include birthdays, key dates, names of grandchildren, famous political figures or important historical events. In order to test abstraction, patients are often asked to give similarities between items, for example an apple and an orange, a table and a chair, a statue and a poem. The interpretation of proverbs is also used to test abstraction. Constructional ability, which relates to visuospatial functioning, can be tested by asking the individual to copy a two- or three-dimensional figure, or by drawing a clock, which is a helpful and simple screening instrument. The resident is asked to place the numbers in the correct position in a circle and then set the hands for a particular time, such as 3 o'clock (an easy task) or ten minutes after 11 (a more difficult task). Praxis is the ability to perform voluntary purposeful movements and the inability to carry out such movements is called apraxia. This can be tested by asking the individual to pretend that they are carrying out a particular activity, such as 'pretend you are holding a toothbrush, show me how you would brush your teeth'. Assessing insight and judgement is important in developing an overall management plan. It is often helpful to ask the patient how they understand their current problem and how they are planning to deal with the problem at this time.

Common psychiatric disorders in late life

The dementias

In the vast majority of patients suffering from dementia, there is a persistent and progressive illness that causes functional impairment. These patients suffer from cognitive impairment, which refers to a loss of the various mental abilities that have been described above in the mental status examination. Patients demonstrate impaired functioning with primarily a loss of the ability to perform the ADLs, also described above. Initially, the individual may present with problems in occupational functioning or inappropriate social behaviour, but ultimately he or she may develop an inability to perform basic ADLs, such as feeding, grooming, dressing and using the toilet. Patients with dementia always demonstrate some memory impairment and must also be experiencing difficulty in at least one other cognitive area. The diagnostic criteria for dementia according to the DSM-IV (APA) are listed in Table 9.3. The diagnosis of dementia remains primarily clinical and is made on the basis of both the history and the clinical examination. When dementia is suspected, various laboratory investigations are carried out to rule out potentially reversible causes of dementia, such as vitamin B_{12} deficiency, thyroid disease and chronic drug use. It should be noted that some patients with severe depression can present with significant cognitive impairment which is often reversible with the treatment of depression. This disorder is referred to as the dementia syndrome of depression or 'pseudodementia'.

In addition to memory disturbance, many patients with dementia demonstrate behavioural problems.[6] This is a common reason for families ultimately to decide on the need for institutionalization. Common behavioural disturbances include agitation, aggression, wandering, repetitive or bizarre behaviours, hallucinations, delusions, shouting, disinhibited behaviours, sleep disturbance and sexually inappropriate behaviour.

Table 9.3 Diagnostic criteria for dementia

(A) 1. Memory impairment, AND
    2. At least one of the following:
        (a) disorder of language (aphasia)
        (b) inability to carry out motor activities (apraxia)
        (c) inability to recognize objects (agnosia)
        (d) impairment of abstract thinking, judgement, planning (executive functioning)

(B) The disturbance in (A) 1 and 2 significantly interferes with work or usual social activities or relationships with others, and represents a decline from a previously higher level of functioning.

Adapted from DSM IV, American Psychiatric Association.[4]

The common causes of dementia are listed in Table 9.4. At least 50% of the dementias are related to Alzheimer's disease, with vascular dementia being the second most common cause. A significant number of patients suffer from mixed dementias in which there are features of Alzheimer's and vascular dementia. Although at this time there is no specific laboratory test or imaging technique that can result in a definitive diagnosis of Alzheimer's disease, it is useful to obtain brain scans, such as a computed tomographic (CT) or magnetic resonance imaging (MRI) scan to ensure that

Table 9.4 Causes of dementia

Alzheimer's disease
Vascular dementia
Dementia with Lewy bodies
Alcoholic and other toxic dementias
Frontotemporal dementia (including Pick's disease)
Normal pressure hydrocephalus
Dementias secondary to metabolic disturbances:
   Thyroid disease
   Vitamin B_{12} deficiency
Dementia with other neurological illness:
   Parkinson's disease
   Huntington's disease
   Wilson's disease
   Multiple sclerosis
Infectious dementias:
   Syphilis
   Creutzfeldt–Jakob disease
Dementia from head trauma
Dementia from brain tumours
Dementia syndrome of depression

Source: Herrmann and van Reekum.[7]

there is no underlying brain lesion, such as a stroke or tumour, which might be causing the symptoms. A single-photon emission computed tomographic (SPECT) scan of the brain provides information on the relative levels of activity in various areas of the brain. The typical finding in Alzheimer's disease is decreased perfusion in the temporal and parietal lobes bilaterally.

Delirium

Individuals who experience an acute disturbance of brain function, generally precipitated by a physical illness or drugs, may develop the syndrome of delirium. This is generally a reversible condition which occurs frequently in older people. Patients with delirium generally display certain behavioural changes such as extreme agitation, at times to the point of violence, or withdrawal and drowsiness to the point of stupor. Delirium is most frequently seen in the general hospital setting in which there are many patients with acute medical illnesses or recent surgery. The diagnostic criteria for delirium are listed in Table 9.5. The classical finding in this disorder is the individual's inability to focus, maintain and shift attention. Patients are generally disorientated and have impaired recent memory. The speech may become rambling and incoherent and patients have reversals of their sleep–wake cycle, generally sleeping excessively during the day while being unable to sleep at night. They sometimes have hallucinations, most commonly visual in nature. Although the condition may fluctuate rapidly, patients may have lucid intervals.

Table 9.5 Diagnostic criteria for delirium

(A) Disturbance of consciousness (i.e. reduced clarity of awareness of the environment) with reduced ability to focus, sustain or shift attention
(B) A change in condition (such as memory deficit, disorientation, language disturbance) or the development of a perceptual disturbance that is not better accounted for by a pre-existing, established or evolving dementia
(C) The disturbance develops over a short period (usually hours to days) and tends to fluctuate during the course of the day
(D) There is evidence from the history physical examination or laboratory findings that the disturbance is caused by the direct physiological consequences of a general medical condition

Adapted from DSM-IV, American Psychiatric Association.[4]

Patients with underlying dementia, or other cognitive problems, are at higher risk for the development of delirium. Although delirium can be seen at any age, it is most common in elderly individuals.

The common causes of delirium are listed in Table 9.6. The most common causes are infection, toxic and metabolic changes, and specific medications.

Patients with delirium need to be investigated to discover the underlying cause of the syndrome. They require baseline laboratory investigations, such as a complete blood count with differential blood chemistry including electrolytes, blood urea nitrogen, creatinine, glucose, calcium, phosphate and liver enzymes, as well as a urinalysis and chest X-ray.

It may be difficult to manage some patients with delirium if they are extremely agitated or violent. The patient may be very confused and frightened and may be paranoid. Patients require gentle reorientation and the staff looking after these patients must speak clearly and slowly and in a direct, supportive fashion. It is important to explain constantly in simple terms exactly what is going on. Patients may be hypervigilant and irritable and, therefore, it is important to place the individual in an optimal environment where he or she is not exposed to excessive noise or stimulation. It is often helpful to involve family and, if possible, for a family member to stay at the bedside as much as possible.

Table 9.6 Common causes of delirium

Category	Examples
Intracranial problems	Strokes, vasculitis, postictal states, meningitis, space-occupying lesions such as tumours and subdural haematomas
Systemic illness	Cardiovascular disease such as myocardial infarction and congestive heart failure, renal or hepatic failure, respiratory insufficiency, anaemia, diabetes, other endocrine disorders
Infection	Generalized sepsis, pneumonia, urinary tract infections, meningitis
Toxic/metabolic	Alcohol, electrolyte problems, acid–base disturbances, hypoxia
Deficiency states	Folate, thiamine, iron deficiency
Trauma	Head injury, surgery, burns
Medications	Analgesics, antihistamines, antiparkinsonian, cardiac, gastrointestinal, psychoactive

Management includes treatment of the underlying disorder as well as maintaining adequate fluid and nutrition. For the acutely agitated, it may be necessary on occasion to use medication to sedate the patient. Physical restraint should only be used as a last resort. Patients who are severely agitated may require constant observation.

The vast majority of patients make a complete recovery from an episode of delirium, although in elderly patients recovery may be slow and it may take weeks to months before the person returns to normal. Many patients will not remember the details of what happened during the delirium and may report that the episode was like a bad dream.

Depression

Depressive disorders and symptoms are frequent in primary-care settings. The prevalence of depressive symptoms in the primary care population has been found to range from 15–25%.[8] The prevalence of major depression among older primary-care patients is 1.8–5.8%.[9] Much higher rates of depression are seen in elderly hospitalized patients and in those residing in long-term care facilities.

It is widely recognized that depression in the elderly is often more difficult to recognize than in younger individuals. Studies suggest that the consequences of unrecognized and untreated depression in older adults may include excessive use of health-care services, increased length of stay during hospitalization, decreased treatment compliance, and increased morbidity and mortality related to underlying medical illness and from suicide.

The clinician should always be vigilant for depressive symptoms in any patient who appears sad or withdrawn, has unexplained physical complaints or is simply failing to thrive. In patients whose pain seems inconsistent with physical findings or appears to be excessive in relation to the underlying physical disorder, depression should be ruled out. The elderly are less likely spontaneously to describe feelings of depression; therefore, the clinician must be more proactive in the detection of these symptoms. Patients who have suffered recent losses are at increased risk of developing depression. In the elderly, these losses may include bereavement, loss of health or loss of role in society. Those living alone are particularly vulnerable and other risk factors include being female, unmarried or widowed and having coexisting physical illness. The rates of completed suicide are particularly high in the elderly, especially white males. Therefore, when depression is suspected, it is important to always ask about suicidal ideation. One study suggested that 70% of those who completed suicide had visited a physician in the month prior to their death.[10] Screening instruments, such as the Depression Rating Scale, can be helpful in detecting the possible presence of depression.[11]

The DSM-IV criteria for depression are listed in Table 9.7 and common medical illnesses and medications associated with depression are listed in Table 9.8. It is particularly important to ask about the presence of the neurovegetative features of depression such as sleep, appetite and energy disturbances. Some disorders such as stroke and Parkinson's disease are strongly associated with the development of depression. In the elderly, it is common to see coexisting depression and dementia. Occasionally, patients can develop the dementia syndrome of depression (pseudodementia) in which a person presents with severe cognitive impairment which diminishes or resolves when the underlying depression is treated. In some patients with certain neurological disorders it may be difficult to recognize depression. Some

patients may have speech difficulty (aphasia) or abnormal prosody (the affective and inflectional colouring of speech), and others may demonstrate pathological crying or amotivational states which are a direct result of underlying neurological disorders.

In patients who have significant depression, it is important to consider the diagnostic possibilities. Patients with severe depression are generally diagnosed as having a major depression, sometimes referred to as clinical depression. However, patients with less severe depression may have an adjustment disorder with depression or dysthymic disorder, which is a chronic, low-grade depression which may last for years. In a patient whose depression appears to be clearly related to a physical illness or a medication, the diagnosis is specified as such, e.g. depression due to stroke. If there is a history of episodes of high mood (hypomania or mania), then a diagnosis of bipolar disorder is made. Patients who have recently become bereaved may simply be suffering from an uncomplicated bereavement. However, it should be noted that if the symptoms of grief become chronic, the possibility of depression must be considered. It is also possible that depressed patients may also be suffering from another non-mood-related psychiatric disorder, e.g. an anxiety disorder, a personality disorder, a somatization disorder, or alcohol or drug abuse or dependency.

Having made a diagnosis, the various management options must be considered. It is most important to consider all factors which may be playing a role in the aetiology of a particular depressive disorder. It is necessary to consider both biological and psychosocial factors. If

Table 9.7 DSM-IV diagnosis of major depression

At least five of the following symptoms have been present nearly every day, for most of the day, during the same 2-week period and represent a change from previous functioning; at least one of the symptoms is either (1) depressed mood or (2) loss of interest or pleasure:

1. Depressed mood, either subjective or reported by others
2. Markedly diminished interest or pleasure
3. Significant change in weight or appetite
4. Insomnia or hypersomnia
5. Psychomotor agitation or retardation
6. Fatigue or loss of energy
7. Feelings of worthlessness or excess of inappropriate guilt
8. Diminished ability to think or concentrate or indecisiveness
9. Recurrent thoughts of death or suicidal ideation

Symptoms cause significant distress or impairment in daily activities, social life or other important areas of functioning

Symptoms are not due to the direct effects of a substance (e.g. drugs of abuse or medication) or a general medical condition

Adapted from DSM-IV, American Psychiatric Association.[4]

Table 9.8 Medical illnesses and medications often associated with depression

Neurological	Collagen–vascular diseases
Stroke	Carcinoma–lymphoma
Parkinson's disease	Viral illness
Hydrocephalus	Hepatitis
Multiple sclerosis	Influenza
Cerebral neoplasms	Mononucleosis
Head injury	Medications
Endocrine	Methyldopa
Hypothyroidism	Propranolol
Hyperthyroidism	Corticosteroids
Cushing's syndrome	L-Dopa
Addison's disease	Cimetidine
	Barbiturates

the patient has an adjustment disorder related to a recent life event, then psychosocial interventions, such as brief psychotherapy, might be indicated. If the patient has a more severe depressive disorder, then generally a combination of antidepressant medication and psychotherapy is indicated. If the presentation is atypical, initial responses to treatment are poor or the diagnosis is unclear, then referral to a psychiatrist may be indicated. Depending on the specific problems and the availability of resources, it might also be beneficial to involve other mental health professionals such as psychologists, occupational therapists and social workers.

Many elderly patients can benefit from psychotherapy, either individual or group therapy. In primary-care settings, even brief supportive psychotherapy, e.g. a 10 min session, may be significantly better than a simple medication visit. It may be important to consider family and other social interventions in some cases. For example, in an elderly person who is very isolated, a referral to a day-care centre may be very important. Education of family members can also be very helpful. The various options for antidepressant medications are discussed later in this chapter. It is important to encourage patients to take their medications regularly, as elderly patients are often non-compliant with treatment. It is also important to be patient and to offer encouragement and reassurance regarding hope for improvement. Some studies suggest that elderly patients may require up to 12 weeks for a full response to antidepressants.

Mania

Some individuals suffer from both episodes of depression and episodes of high, or elevated, mood. When these episodes of high mood are mild, they are referred to as hypomanic episodes and, when severe, they are termed manic episodes. The DSM-IV criteria for a manic episode are listed in Table 9.9. The mood is generally elevated, or expansive, although in some cases it is irritable. The individual often demonstrates grandiose thinking, is very talkative and has reduced need for sleep. Flight of ideas, characterized by thinking that is difficult to follow, with one thought jumping to the next, is often present. The person is often distractible, impulsive and drawn towards pleasurable activities that may be dangerous or illegal. Several medical illnesses and medications are associated with mania, including stroke, multiple sclerosis, hyperthyroidism, corticosteroids, thyroxine, levodopa and amphetamines.

Table 9.9 DSM-IV diagnosis of manic episode

A distinct period of abnormally and persistently elevated, expansive or irritable mood lasting for at least 1 week
During the period of mood disturbance, three (or more) of the following symptoms have persisted (four if the mood is only irritable) and have been present to a significant degree:

1. Inflated self-esteem or grandiosity
2. Decreased need for sleep, e.g. feels rested after only 3 hours of sleep
3. More talkative than usual or pressure to keep talking
4. Flight of ideas or subjective experience that thoughts are racing
5. Distractibility, i.e. attention too easily drawn to unimportant or irrelevant external stimuli
6. Increase in goal-directed activity or psychomotor agitation
7. Excessive involvement in pleasurable activities which have a high potential for painful consequences

Symptoms do not meet criteria for mixed episodes.

Mood disturbance sufficiently severe to cause marked impairment in occupational functioning or in usual social activities or relationships with others, or to necessitate hospitalization to prevent harm to self or others or other are psychotic features

Symptoms are not due to the direct effects of a substance (e.g. drugs of abuse or medication) or a general medical condition

Adapted from DSM-IV, American Psychiatric Association.[4]

Anxiety disorders

The prevalence of anxiety disorders in the elderly is approximately 5%. The most common form of anxiety is phobic disorder. Generalized anxiety disorder (GAD) is also seen frequently and many individuals experience mild symptoms of anxiety which do not meet criteria for a specific diagnosis. GAD is characterized by excessive worry, often about insignificant matters. The anxiety and worry are excessively intense and out of proportion to the situation. Common symptoms include restlessness or feeling on edge, fatigue, difficulty concentrating, irritability, muscle tension and sleep disturbance. Other somatic symptoms include dry mouth, sweating, diarrhoea, urinary frequency, headaches, dizziness, palpitations, tremor and a subjective sense of shortness of breath. Some patients with anxiety disorders develop associated alcohol or tranquillizer abuse or dependence. Panic disorder is characterized by recurrent, unexpected panic attacks. Panic attacks may be associated with particular situations and, therefore, avoidance of those situations is common. Some patients become phobic and avoid crowds as well as situations from which they feel it is difficult to escape. This is called agoraphobia and may result in a severe restriction of activities. These individuals may become housebound and may need companions in order to perform everyday activities.

A phobia is defined as an excessive or persistent fear of a specific situation or of a clearly identifiable object that is out of proportion to the inherent danger. The fear cannot be explained or reasoned away. Some individuals have social phobia in which they are fearful of interactions with other people or performance situations such as public speaking. They often fear that they will act in a way that will be highly embarrassing or humiliating.

Obsessive compulsive disorder is an anxiety disorder in which the manifestations are either obsessions and/or compulsions. Obsessions are thoughts which are defined as recurrent persistent ideas, images or impulses that are experienced as intrusive and inappropriate, and cause marked anxiety or distress. Compulsions are behaviours or mental acts that are repetitive, purposeful and intentional and performed in response to an obsession or to prevent a more dreaded event or situation. The most common compulsions include washing and cleaning, counting, checking and requesting reassurance.

Post-traumatic stress disorder (PTSD) follows exposure to an event which involves death, serious injury or threat to the physical integrity of the person or others and which evokes a response of intense fear, helplessness or horror. This disorder is common in individuals who have been involved in military combat, concentration camps, violent assault or automobile accidents. The individuals experience persisting images of the event, tend to avoid associated stimuli and develop persistent symptoms of increased arousal. They may experience dreams, flashbacks and intense distress when exposed to reminders of the event.

Psychotic disorders

The simplest definition of psychosis is a disorder in which delusions or hallucinations are present. Other definitions have included 'impairment that grossly interferes with the capacity to meet the ordinary demands of life', or gross impairment in reality testing. It is important to note that in the elderly, psychotic symptoms are frequently associated with dementia or delirium and that a number of physical conditions can give rise to psychotic symptoms. Psychotic symptoms can also occur in severe mood disorders such as depression or mania. The most common form of psychosis is the development of paranoid delusions in which a person believes that they are being specifically targeted by others, i.e. people are out to get them in some way. Some individuals are suspicious by nature and perceive the world as a very hostile, selfish, uncaring place. When these individuals make mistakes or experience misfortune, they tend to blame other people. They tend to be extremely sensitive to real or imagined slights or criticisms. When severe, the person may develop delusions with a belief that they are being persecuted, harmed or robbed.

In younger patients, the most common psychotic illness is schizophrenia. This disorder often starts in late adolescence or young adulthood and is characterized by disturbances in thinking, perception, motivation, behaviour and emotions. Many individuals with schizophrenia have significantly impaired functioning. Most patients with schizophrenia develop delusions which often are persecutory in nature. The delusions may be quite bizarre and may include beliefs that one's thoughts are being broadcast from inside one's mind, that thoughts are being inserted into one's mind or that one's thoughts are being controlled. In addition, hallucinations are common, most frequently auditory in nature.

Some individuals may develop a schizophrenia-like illness late in life. Social withdrawal is common, with elaborate or bizarre delusions which are often persecutory. Sensory impairment, particularly diminished hearing, is often associated with this disorder. Other individuals may develop a delusional disorder which is characterized by the presence of a persistent, well-organized delusion. The delusions may be paranoid or may involve jealousy such as concern that one's spouse is unfaithful. With somatic delusions, an individual may believe that he is infested or suffering from a particular physical illness or defect. Other delusional types include erotomania in which the person believes that another person, usually of higher status, is in love with them. A grandiose delusion is a belief of inflated worth, power, knowledge or special relationship to a deity or famous person.

Management

Following the history and examination of the patient, management may include a series of investigations such as blood tests, urine examination, X-rays and neuroimaging techniques. It is extremely important with elderly patients to exclude undiagnosed medical problems which may be contributing to the development of a psychiatric disorder. It is also important to consider the possibility that medications, over-the-counter drugs or alcohol can be contributing to the presentation.

It is very important to involve the family and other caregivers and to provide education with regard to the working diagnosis and management. Various psychosocial interventions, such as the mobilization of community services and referrals to day-care programmes, are often vitally important. Many patients benefit from the involvement of a multidisciplinary team with expertise from a physician (geriatric psychiatrist, geriatrician or a neurologist), nurse, social worker, occupational therapist or psychologist. Sometimes patients require admission to an inpatient unit or day hospital programme and, as noted in the introduction to this chapter, the availability of these services is essential if one is to provide comprehensive care.

Psychotherapy

Many elderly patients can benefit from psychotherapy. Common approaches include supportive therapy, reminiscence or life-review therapy, cognitive therapy and interpersonal therapy. Supportive therapy is particularly helpful for the frail elderly. The therapist takes on an active role in the session, engaging the patient frequently with questions which encourage the expression of feelings. Important components of supportive therapy include ventilation of feelings and realistic reassurance. Reassurance is particularly effective when it arises from a full understanding of both the real issues in a person's life and his or her reactions to them. Reminiscence therapy helps to bolster a person's sense of self by encouraging what is generally considered to be a normal process of ageing, referred to as life review. It is important for older individuals to review and evaluate their lives and to try to develop a meaningful perspective. During the process, some patients may write an autobiography, or make a tape or a video of their lives. It can be most helpful if family members, such as children or grandchildren, are involved in the project. Cognitive therapy has been widely used, particularly for the treatment of depression. It is based on the idea that thoughts produce feelings and that dysfunctional or distorted thoughts can result in a negative, depressive view of the world. Through a process of self-examination and homework, it may be possible to develop insight into this negative pattern of thinking and ultimately to develop a healthier pattern. Finally, interpersonal psychotherapy is based on the theory that interpersonal issues are at the root of many depressions. Therapy focuses on identifying and dealing with issues that arise from interpersonal conflicts, role conflicts and interpersonal losses.

Behaviour management

Some patients benefit from behaviour management strategies which can be particularly helpful in the management of difficult behaviours in cognitively impaired patients. This approach requires attention to cognitive deficits, environmental factors that trigger or maintain the challenging behaviours, and an understanding of staff attitudes, perceptions and expectations. These behaviours must be defined in specific and objective terms. They must then be subjected to an ABC analysis in order to determine the environmental variables that influence them. ABC represents antecedent, behaviour and consequence, each of which must be documented. Following the assessment, an individualized management plan is developed based on the results of the analysis. Behavioural excesses are managed with techniques designed to reduce behaviours, such as extinction, reinforcement of alternative behaviours and time out. When there are behavioural deficits, the approach is to increase appropriate behaviours through gradual reshaping, or retraining, of absent or infrequent behaviours.

Medications

Severe psychiatric disorders, such as those described earlier in this chapter, often require a combined management approach which includes medications to enhance the likelihood of significant improvement. The elderly tend to be more vulnerable to side-effects from medications and a variety of factors can affect drug metabolism in the elderly:

- decreased lean body mass
- increased body fat

- decreased serum albumin
- changes in absorption
- changes in liver function
- decreased kidney function
- changes in drug receptor sensitivity
- changes in amount of neurotransmitters.

It is necessary for the clinician to establish the relative indications and contraindications for medication use in each patient. There should be a specific diagnosis as well as target symptoms which can be used to monitor the effectiveness of treatment. For elderly patients the drugs of choice should, as far as possible, few active metabolites, accumulate in the body to a lesser extent, have a short duration of action and be likely to cause few side-effects. Drugs should be started at very low doses and increased slowly while monitoring for side-effects ('start low, go slow').

Psychotropic medications generally fall into five categories: antidepressants, mood stabilizers, minor tranquillizers, antipsychotics and cholinesterase inhibitors. In primary care, one is most likely to encounter patients on antidepressants or minor tran-

quillizers. A list of the commonly used antidepressant medications can be found in Table 9.10. In general, selective serotonin reuptake inhibitors (SSRIs) are used as first-line agents in the elderly. This group of medications tends to be well tolerated, although they can cause gastrointestinal upset and nervousness on occasion. They are much safer than to the tricyclic antidepressants in the case of overdose.

The most common minor tranquillizers seen in practice are the benzodiazepines. These drugs are primarily used to treat anxiety and insomnia. The favoured benzodiazepines for the elderly are lorazepam, and oxazepam, which have shorter half-lives than diazepam and others in this group. The most common side-effects of benzodiazepines are excessive sedation, confusion and withdrawal reactions. Excessive use of these medications can also lead to falls.

Patients who suffer from bipolar mood disorder are often treated with mood stabilizers such as lithium carbonate, carbamazepine and valproic acid.

Patients suffering from psychotic illnesses or severe agitation or aggression are often treated with antipsychotic medications. A group of newer agents called

Table 9.10 Pharmacological treatment of depression

Class	Drug	Advantage	Disadvantage
TCA	Desipramine Nortriptyline	Well studied, efficacious, low cost, available therapeutic drug monitoring	Anticholinergic effects, orthostatic hypotension, highly toxic in overdose
MAOI	Phenelzine Tranylcypromine	No anticholinergic effects	Orthostatic hypotension, dietary and drug restrictions
SSRI	Fluoxetine Sertraline Paroxetine Fluvoxamine Citalopram	Effective, well tolerated, flat dose response	Potential drug interactions
RIMA	Moclobemide	Well tolerated	Not available in the USA
SNRI	Venlafaxine	Effective	Hypertension with higher doses
NaSSA	Mirtazapine		Not available in Canada; more sedation with lower doses
Other	Trazodone Nefazodone	Useful as a sedative Improves sleep	Sedating, orthostatic hypotension
	Bupropion Amoxapine Maprotiline	Well tolerated, non-sedating	Seizures with high doses Extrapyramidal symptoms Skin rashes, seizures
Psychostimulants	Amphetamine Methylphenidate	Well tolerated, works within days	Not well studied for long-term use

TCA: tricyclic antidepressant; MAOI: monoamine oxidase inhibitor; SSRI: selective serotonin reuptake inhibitor; RIMA: reversible inhibitor of monoamine oxidase; SNRI: serotonin and noradrenaline uptake inhibitor; NaSSA: noradrenaline and specific serotonin antidepressant. Source: Herrmann.[7]

atypical antipsychotic medications, such as olanzapine, risperidone and quetiapine, is preferred in elderly patients. These drugs tend to cause less extrapyramidal side-effects such as parkinsonism and, in addition, patients receiving these medications are less likely to develop tardive dyskinesia than those on the older antipsychotics. The high-potency antipsychotics such as haloperidol frequently cause extrapyramidal side-effects, where as the low-potency antipsychotics, such as chlorpromazine, cause considerable sedation and anticholinergic side-effects.

Finally, several new medications have become available to treat Alzheimer's disease and other dementias. The cholinesterase inhibitors have been found to provide some benefit to individuals with mild to moderate Alzheimer's disease. Two cholinesterase inhibitors, donepezil and rivastigmine, are currently available. Although these medications do not cure the illness, they appear to slow down the rate of progression. There is also some suggestion that these medications may be helpful in treating some of the behavioural disturbances of the dementias. Other agents that might be helpful in the treatment of Alzheimer's disease include vitamin E, selegiline, ginkgo biloba, non-steroidal anti-inflammatory agents and oestrogen replacement in females. It is expected that in the years ahead, numerous agents will become available to modify the progression of the dementias.

References

1 Arie T, Jolley D. Making services work: organization and style of psychogeriatric services. In: Levy R, Post F, eds. The Psychiatry of Late Life. Oxford: Blackwell Scientific Publications, 1982.
2 Shulman K. Regionalization of psychiatric services for the elderly. Can J Psychiatry 1991; 36: 3–8.
3 Rovner BW, German PS, Broadhead J et al. The prevalence and management of dementia and other psychiatric disorders in nursing homes. Int Psychogeriatr, 1990; 13–24.
4 American Psychiatric Association. Diagnostic and Statistical Manual of Mental Disorders. 4th edn. Washington, DC: APA, 1994.
5 Folstein MF, Folstein SW, McHugh PR. 'Mini-mental state'. A practical method of grading the cognitive states of patients for the clinician. J Psychiatric Res 1975: 12: 189–198.
6 Swearer JM, Drachman DA, O'Donnell BF, Mitchell AL. Troublesome and disruptive behaviours in dementia: relationships to diagnosis and disease severity. J Am Geriatr 1988; 36: 784–790.
7 Hermana N, van Reekum R. In: Conn DK et al., eds. Practical Psychiatry in the Long-term Care Facility: A Handbook for Staff. Seattle, WA: Hognefe and Huber, 2001, pp. 42, 166.
8 Katon W, Schulberg H. Epidemiology of depression in primary care. Gen Hosp Psychiatry 1992; 14: 237–247.
9 Hendrie HC, Callahan CM, Levitt EE et al. Prevalence rates of major depressive disorders. The effects of varying diagnostic criteria in older primary care population. Am J Geriatr Psychiatry 1995; 3: 119–131.
10 Conwell Y. Suicide in elderly patients. In: Schneider LS, Lebovitz BD, Friedhoff AJ eds. Diagnosis and Treatment of Depression in Late Life. Washington, DC: American Psychiatric Press,1994.
11 Yesavage K, Brink TL, Lum O et al. Development and validation of a geriatric depression screening scale: a preliminary report. J Psychiatric Res 1983; 17: 37–49.

Further Reading

American Psychiatric Association. Practice guidelines for the treatment of patients with Alzheimer's disease and other dementias of late life. Am J Psychiatry 1997; 154 (5, Suppl).
American Psychiatric Association. Practice guideline for the treatment of patients with delirium. Am J Psychiatry 1999; 156: (5, May Suppl).
Bezchlibnyk-Butler KZ, Jeffries JJ, eds. Clinical Handbook of Psychotropic Drugs 9th edn. Toronto: Hogrefe & Huber, 1999.
Conn DK, Herrmann N, Kaye A et al. Practical Psychiatry in the Long-term Care Facility: A Handbook for Staff. Seattle, WA: Hogrefe & Huber, 2001.
Herrmann N, Lanctôt KL, Naranjo CA. Behavioural disorders in demented elderly patients: Current issues in pharmacotherapy. CNS Drugs 1996; 6: 280–300.
Manley M. The psychiatric interview, history and mental status examination. In: Kaplan MJ, Saddock BJ, eds. Comprehensive Textbook of Psychiatry, Vol. 1. 7th edn. Philadelphia PA: Lippincott, Williams & Wilkins, 2000.
Matthies BK, Kreutzer JS, West DD. The Behaviour Management Handbook: A Practical Approach to Patients with Neurological Disorders, San Antonio, TX: Therapy Skill Builders, 1997.
Schneider LS, Reynolds CF, Lebowitz BD, Friedhoff AJ. Diagnosis and treatment of depression in late life. Results of the NIH Consensus Development Conference, Washington DC: American Psychiatric Press, 1994.
Strub RL, Black FW. The Mental Status Examination in Neurology. Philadelphia, PA: FA Davis, 1977.

10

Spectrum of rheumatic syndromes in the elderly

Lori Albert

'Arthritis' and 'old age' are often linked together. However, the spectrum of rheumatic syndromes affecting the elderly encompasses much more than arthritis. A number of conditions can produce morbidity and disability, such as myositis, polymyalgia rheumatica (PMR) and osteoporosis. While the incidence of some rheumatic diseases, such as systemic lupus erythematosus (SLE), decreases with age, the incidence of others, such as osteoarthritis (OA), increases with age. Some may also have a different clinical expression in the elderly and some, such as PMR, are unique to the older population.

Many of the rheumatic syndromes in the elderly can present to clinicians with a similar and often non-specific clinical picture. For example, SLE, PMR and early rheumatoid arthritis (RA) may all present with aching, stiffness and fatigue, without the specific clinical features that can aid in making a precise diagnosis. The multiple causes of back pain may be difficult to distinguish, and the severity of the underlying condition, such as metastases of an internal malignancy to the spine, may not be immediately obvious. The coexistence of multiple medical problems, particularly neurological ones, may interfere with obtaining a detailed history or carrying out a complete examination, both of which can further complicate making a diagnosis. Therefore, it behooves all those practitioners working with older adults to be mindful of the manifestations of the various rheumatic syndromes. Those individuals with concerning symptoms or new or evolving physical findings should be flagged for further medical evaluation. It is also important to be aware of the potential side-effects and complications that may arise from the treatment of these conditions. A good example of this would be the development of musculoskeletal complications such as osteoporosis and myopathy secondary to corticosteroid therapy for systemic lupus.

Back pain

Back pain is a common and significant source of morbidity in the older adult, as it is in younger individuals. Most patients with low back pain have a mechanical cause for their symptoms. This is defined as pain secondary to overuse of a normal anatomical structure or pain secondary to trauma or deformity of an anatomical structure.[1] Over 50% will have improved at 2 weeks and 90% at 2 months.[2] However, in the elderly patient, especially with new-onset back pain, a number of important medical causes for pain should be considered and ruled out before attributing symptoms to ageing or mechanical back pain.

Many structures in the lumbar spine can give rise to pain: ligaments that interconnect vertebrae, outer fibres of the annulus fibrosus, facet joints, vertebral periosteum, paravertebral musculature and fascia, blood vessels and spinal nerve roots. All parts of the spine also undergo degenerative changes with ageing. These changes may be radiographically evident, but do not necessarily produce pain in and of themselves. However, these age-related changes can become symptomatic if changes are extensive or result in secondary effects on the architecture or biomechanics of the spine (reviewed by Andersson[3]). Changes occur in the disc, with desiccation of the nucleus pulposus and with the development of degeneration and tears in the annulus. Bony excrescences or osteophytes develop from the margins of the vertebral bodies and often occur in conjunction with the loss of disc thickness.

These typically occur in an anterolateral distribution, but those developing posteriorly can contribute to spinal stenosis (see below). Ligamentous hypertrophy as a result of ageing may also contribute to narrowing of the spinal canal.

Autopsy studies have demonstrated the progression of degenerative changes with age, with evidence for significant disc degeneration in most spines by the fourth decade and even earlier.[3] It appears that degeneration is most severe and starts earlier at the L4 and L5 levels than at the L3 level. Degenerative changes can also occur in the facet joints, and appears to be secondary to loss in disc height with increasing stress on the joints.[4] The relationship between ageing and the development of osteoarthritis remains unclear.

Osteoarthritis of the spine with articular degeneration and apophyseal joint sclerosis may be associated with decreased back motion and back pain. Patients may have mild stiffness in the morning. During the day they experience an improvement in their symptoms but have a return of pain at the end of the day after physical activity.

Spondylolisthesis is the forward slippage of one vertebra on to the next as a result of degenerative changes in the spine.[5] This lesion occurs most frequently at the L4–L5 level, and next most commonly at L3–L4, the sites at which degenerative changes are seen. The lesion seems to be more common in women than in men. Spondylolisthesis may cause back pain, typically when the spine is placed in extension (increased displacement) as opposed to flexion (normalization of vertebral body position).

Spinal stenosis[6] occurs when there is narrowing of the spinal canal, nerve root canal or intervertebral foramen as a result of spondylolisthesis, osteophyte formation, ligamentous thickening and disc protrusion. This condition can result from a combination of bony and/or soft-tissue involvement. Normal changes associated with ageing can, if severe and progressive, eventually lead to the clinicopathological diagnosis of lumbar spinal stenosis with central and/or lateral impingement on neural elements.[7] The clinical presentation of stenosis may be back pain, but characteristically there are associated neurological manifestations with pain and/or paraesthesiae radiating into the buttock, thigh or lower leg (Reviewed in Ref. 8). Typically, there is compression of neural elements at the level of the degenerative facet joints, which results in a radiculopathy, most commonly involving the L5

nerve root. These patients will present with leg pain or sciatica, sometimes without back pain. This presentation may be acute and severe if a small disc herniation is superimposed on pre-existing lateral stenosis. Another typical presentation is pseudoclaudication, in which leg pain, paraesthesiae or weakness develops with prolonged standing or walking. Symptoms are relieved by leaning forward and/or resting for a few minutes. Patients often have to sit or lie down to relieve symptoms adequately. In contrast, ischaemic claudication due to arterial insufficiency may present with pain on walking, but is relieved rapidly by standing still and has no postural aggravation. A good distinguishing feature is that those with spinal claudication can ride a bicycle (leaning forward position) while those with ischaemic claudication cannot. In addition, ischaemic claudication is not precipitated by prolonged standing. Acute exacerbations can occur following acute lifting or twisting motions. Often there are few neurological findings on physical examination. There may be limited movement of the lumbar spine and reproduction of symptoms with extension.

Spinal stenosis can lead to emergent situations that require early surgical intervention. Cauda equina syndrome, with compression of the sacral spinal nerve roots, presents with onset of urinary retention or rectal incontinence and associated perianal and/or perineal pain and sensory loss. Myelopathy, manifested by gait disturbances due to weakness and involvement of the posterior columns of the spinal cord with impaired sensory function, may indicate stenosis at the cervical level.

In the setting of spinal stenosis, radiological investigations are required to confirm a clinical diagnosis, and to rule out other potential causes of pain (e.g. tumour metastatic to the spine, osteoporotic fracture or osteomyelitis). Computed tomography (CT) provides the best evaluation of bony tissue. However, magnetic resonance imaging (MRI) is probably the study of choice, as it can identify the soft tissue component of stenosis and gives excellent views of the facet joints. Electromyography (EMG) and nerve conduction studies may have a role in confirming the presence of a nerve root impingement and ruling out other primary neurological disorders which may mimic the symptoms of spinal stenosis.

Another source of back pain seen mainly in the older population is diffuse idiopathic skeletal hyperostosis (DISH). This is a condition of unknown aetiology characterized by the development of non-inflammatory ossification and calcification of paraspinous ligaments.[9] The process is typically most prominent along the lateral side of the anterior longitudinal ligament. This is often associated with excess bone formation at sites where tendons, ligaments or joint capsules insert into bone (entheses). The condition is characterized by spinal immobility and flexion, and moderate pain. However, the radiographic findings are sometimes found incidentally and patients are relatively asymptomatic. If severe, the spinal hyperostosis may contribute to the development of spinal stenosis. Involvement in the neck can lead to dysphagia from impingement on local structures. Peripheral involvement may lead to enthesitis at tendon and ligament insertions, such as medial epicondylitis at the elbow, heel pain and knee pain.

Despite the range of pathological changes contributing to back pain, most of these clinical presentations are managed conservatively. Surgical intervention is reserved for those with intractable pain, or definite and progressive neurological impairment. In general, the goals of management in all of these settings are pain relief and restoration of function. Long-term management then includes muscle strengthening and posture training to correct biomechanical abnormalities and reduce abnormal strain on the spine, thereby lessening the chance of acute strain. This will often alleviate chronic symptoms as well.[10] Older patients often benefit from a supervised programme; this ensures correct performance of exercises to achieve maximal benefit and avoid strain.

Non-narcotic analgesics are preferred for pain relief in most cases. Good relief of pain can often be achieved with the use of acetaminophen used in adequate doses of up to 1 g four times daily. In the absence of liver disease, this is quite a safe approach with minimal side-effects. Many patients benefit from the addition of a non-steroidal anti-inflammatory drug (NSAID).[11] A broad range of NSAIDs is available, with different potencies and risk profiles. The risks of NSAID use are not trivial and include serious gastrointestinal complications such as gastritis, ulcers, perforation and bleeding. This risk increases with prolonged use, and with increasing age and concomitant use of glucocorticoids and anticoagulants. A prior history of ulcer disease or gastrointestinal bleeding also puts patients at higher risk.[12] NSAIDs have other side-effects such as hypertension and interference with hypertension therapy, and increased risk for renal

insufficiency, particularly when combined with medications such as diuretics and certain cardiac drugs. These side-effects arise from NSAID effects on the synthesis of prostaglandins, which are important for many physiological functions, as well as being mediators of pain and inflammation. A new generation of NSAIDs such as celecoxib (Celebrex®) and Rofecoxib (Vioxx®) is more specific and have less impact on the physiological or housekeeping prostaglandin synthesis. Therefore, the risk for the development of significant gastrointestinal complications is reduced with these drugs,[12,13] but they may still put elderly patients at risk for the development of hypertension and renal failure, and should therefore be used cautiously. Pain control is important in the acute episode to allow the patient to increase physical activity and regain confidence. It should be discontinued once the individual resumes normal daily activities. For those with chronic pain, complete relief of pain may not be achieved. However, the goal again should be to support the patient's efforts to be as active as possible.

Narcotic analgesics should be reserved for those with severe pain associated with a herniated disc or severe spinal stenosis. These drugs must be used cautiously in the elderly, because of increased sensitivity to narcotic effects with drowsiness, poor concentration (and thus risk for falling) and impaired clearance of metabolites.

The use of muscle relaxants in those with low back pain to decrease muscle contraction and reduce pain remains controversial.[14] The side-effect of drowsiness suggests that these drugs are probably best avoided in the elderly population.

Tricyclic antidepressants are sometimes used as an adjunct in the management of chronic pain, even in the absence of depression. In the elderly, in particular, side-effects include postural hypotension, dry mouth, cardiac arrhythmias and drowsiness.

Infiltration of facet joints with corticosteroid/local anaesthetic and epidural steroid injections is used by some clinicians, but remains controversial.[15–17] A short course of moderate-dose oral corticosteroid (prednisone 40 mg daily tapering over 1–2 weeks) has also been used. There are limited data to demonstrate the effectiveness of any of these interventions.

The causes of back pain described above increase in frequency in the elderly. However, more ominous medical causes of back pain also increase in frequency in this group. In particular, the incidence of metastatic cancer, infection and osteoporotic fractures increases in the elderly. Red flags on history include constitutional symptoms (fever, sweats, weight loss) and pre-existing malignancy. Other important historical features are a history of trauma, recent infections, risks for osteoporosis and neurological impairment. The clinical examination should be aimed at identifying adenopathy, other organ involvement and a careful neurological assessment. In this age group, it has been recommended that the clinical assessment be accompanied by laboratory tests to rule out significant pathology, including a complete blood count, serum calcium, alkaline phosphatase and back X-rays.[18,19]

Malignancy

Metastatic tumours should be suspected in older patients who present with back pain, especially if the pain is out of proportion to the history or accompanied by night pain, or pain described as more severe at rest.

Bone is a common site of metastasis for carcinomas of the prostate, breast, lung, kidney, bladder and thyroid as well as lymphomas and sarcomas.[20] Metastases of malignancy arising in internal organs to the bone indicates a poor prognosis. This presentation may be associated with systemic symptoms such as fever, night sweats and weight loss. However, this may be the first presentation of widespread disease. Pain is usually severe and unremitting, particularly worsening at night (with recumbency). Pathological fractures may also occur at site of tumour infiltration. If neurological symptoms develop patients should be evaluated promptly for evidence of cord compression. Plain X-rays may show little abnormality. Thus, if the index of suspicion for malignancy is high, further imaging modalities are indicated.

Multiple myeloma is a malignancy of antibody-producing plasma cells in the bone marrow.[21] Bone pain is the most common symptom in myeloma. Pain usually involves the back and ribs. Unlike the pain of metastatic cancer, the pain of myeloma is usually worsened with movement. Severe, persistent pain may indicate the development of a pathological fracture. Bony lesions occur as a result of proliferation of the malignant cells and the activation of bone-resorbing osteoclasts from the production of an activating factor produced by the myeloma cells.

Osteoporotic fractures

Osteoporosis is characterized by low bone mass and microarchitectural deterioration of bone tissue leading to enhanced bone fragility and susceptibility to fractures with lesser degrees of stress than normal bone.[22] Osteoporosis begins to develop in women at the menopause owing to the rapid increase in bone-resorbing osteoclast activity associated with loss of oestrogen. There is also an age-related loss of bone in both men and women that occurs independently of hormonal status. The very elderly are at highest risk of sustaining fractures. Other risks for fracture include previous fracture, risks for falling (such as neurological disease, drug-induced drowsiness and loss of co-ordination) and environmental factors such as loose carpets and uneven surfaces in the home.

Osteoporotic fractures in the spine may occur in the setting of low stress injuries, but may also occur spontaneously. While the latter may be asymptomatic and lead to gradual loss in height, these fractures can be extremely painful. Characteristically, there is abrupt onset of severe back pain but no findings to suggest neurological impairment. X-ray changes may take up to 14–21 days to become apparent. In some cases, radionuclide studies (bone scan) are used to confirm the diagnosis. These fractures can also include the sacrum and pelvic rami.

Pain management is the main issue in caring for these patients. Healing can take up to 4–6 weeks. Simple analgesics such as acetaminophen may be insufficient and narcotic analgesics may be required. Codeine is usually sufficient but its use must be monitored carefully in the elderly. Salmon calcitonin, a naturally occurring hormone, has been demonstrated to have analgesic effects in this setting[23,24] and can be administered subcutaneously or intranasally. The goals of pain management are to allow gradual mobilization to avoid further deconditioning during bed rest.

Once a fracture has occurred, prevention of further fractures is the goal of management. Patients must be evaluated for drug treatment of osteoporosis. This may include calcium and vitamin D and drugs to decrease bone resorption such as bisphosphonates and calcitonin. Patients should also be referred for physiotherapy aimed to improve muscle tone and agility and measures to reduce risks for falling in the home environment.

Referred pain from intra-abdominal organs

Disorders of the vascular genitourinary and gastrointestinal systems can cause pain that is referred to the back. However, it is uncommon to have back pain alone as the only manifestation of visceral disease.[1]

Conditions such as an expanding aortic aneurysm, kidney disease, pancreatitis and peptic ulcer disease should be considered. History should be directed towards identifying organ dysfunction or complications.

Shoulder pain

Shoulder pain is a common complaint in elderly individuals. The shoulder joint may be affected by arthropathies such as RA, crystal disease or generalized OA, although it is uncommon in primary OA. Pain isolated to the shoulder is often extra-articular or soft tissue in origin rather than a true arthritis. The clinical examination is crucial to determining whether this is the problem in an older adult with shoulder pain.

In general, extra-articular problems tend to interfere more with active than passive movements of the shoulder. Specific stressing manoeuvres can also help to isolate the involved structures. However, periarticular conditions that are associated with capsular involvement or capsulitis may demonstrate restriction of passive motion in all directions and it may be difficult to distinguish this problem from a true arthropathy. One should also consider the possibility that shoulder pain is referred in origin, e.g. from the neck or from an intra-abdominal, subphrenic lesion or intrathoracic source such as a Pancoast tumour (lung metastasis with apical involvement). Again, the history and clinical examination will help in sorting out these possibilities; with referred pain, most movements of the shoulder, both passive and active, should be relatively unaffected and testing of rotator cuff function will be painless.

Disorders of the rotator cuff tendons are often grouped under the diagnostic entity of subacromial impingement syndrome (SIS), which describes the compression of the suprahumeral structures against the anteroinferior aspect of the acromion and coracoacromial ligament.[25] The structures most often irritated and inflamed with SIS are the rotator cuff muscles, the long head of the biceps and the subacromial bursa. Impingement leads to oedema, fibrosis and thickening, and ultimately partial or full-thickness tears in the cuff tendons. Inflammation in the bursa may also arise as part of the impingement process and usually coexists with an underlying rotator cuff tendonitis.[26]

In the elderly patient, rotator cuff tendonitis may be the result of thinning and tearing of the cuff tendons.[27] Thus, the elderly patient may present with no history of prior trauma or repetitive activity, but have a gradual history of increasing shoulder discomfort and pain with movement. There may be weakness if a degenerative tear is present. Further limitation of movement occurs if the patient develops a secondary capsulitis. Pain is often felt in the deltoid region or in the humerus. Pain may also be exacerbated by reaching into abduction, elevation or overhead. Many patients experience pain when reaching up behind the back. Night pain is common and may be severe.

The management of these degenerative cuff problems can be difficult.[28] Pain relief is the first goal. This can be done by attempting to reduce inflammation with NSAIDs and physical modalities. Subacromial injection of corticosteroid is often used to achieve this. Physiotherapy also plays an important role, to restore range of motion and to correct abnormal biomechanics in the shoulder. Ultimately, the focus should be on strengthening the rotator cuff muscles to restore their action as stabilizers and depressors (to counterbalance the action of the deltoid muscle) of the humeral head. The rehabilitation of a patient with a torn cuff is usually longer than that of a patient with impingement syndrome without a tear. In general, surgery is usually only considered for those patients with significant loss of function or severe pain that has not responded to conservative measures.

Calcific tendonitis results from chronic deposition of hydroxyapatite or calcium pyrophosphate dihydrate (CPPD) crystals. This may be primary,[29] or occur secondary to previous trauma or metabolic disease such as diabetes mellitus and chronic renal insufficiency. These cases are distinguished by the finding of calcium deposits radiographically. The chronic presentation may be associated with chronic symptoms of pain on movement with a catching sensation probably due to impingement. This is managed in much the same way as the rotator cuff tendonitis. There is also an acute presentation with sudden onset of severe pain and limitation of movement,[26] often in the absence of any previous shoulder symptoms. This presentation usually responds well to injection of corticosteroid.

Bicipital tendonitis often occurs secondary to other rotator cuff pathology. Rupture occasionally occurs owing to chronic impingement and thinning of the tendon. Pain is often felt with shoulder extension and with flexion at the elbow. With a complete rupture, resisted flexion may produce bunching of the biceps muscle belly in the upper arm.

Capsulitis is a condition where painful restriction of shoulder movement occurs originating in the soft tissues.[30] This has also been called frozen shoulder or adhesive capsulitis. In this condition there is restriction of movement in all planes, both active and passive (not just the active limitation of abduction and flexion seen in chronic rotator cuff conditions) and there is a compensatory increase in scapulothoracic motion during flexion and abduction. There are three phases[31] in the development and progression of this condition: mainly painful (3–8 months), then painful and stiff (3–8 months) and eventually less painful but markedly stiff (4–6 months). There is then gradual and spontaneous resolution, with the whole process lasting up to a year, or perhaps more. The condition may be primary, that is of unknown aetiology. It also appears to occur secondary to certain clinical conditions include diabetes mellitus, thyroid disease, pulmonary disorders, cardiac disease including myocardial infarction and surgery, and following cerebrovascular accident.

The goals of treatment are much the same as for the other shoulder disorders described above. Early on, management of pain is important, particularly with a view to maintaining mobility. The use of NSAIDs and local intra-articular steroid injections may improve pain and movement.[32] However, the natural history of resolution of the capsulitis has not been shown to be effectively altered through any specific intervention. Occasionally, manipulation under anaesthesia has been used to speed resolution in the adhesive phase, but this has not consistently been shown to speed recovery or return to full function.[33]

Osteoarthritis

OA is the most common form of arthritis, and occurs, at least radiographically in 70% of persons over the age of 40 years. Joint changes occur as part of ageing, but these may not necessarily be associated with the pathological changes in cartilage and bone seen in OA.[34] The changes in the knee, for example, can be associated with pain. However, the relationship between these changes and the transition to OA (if it occurs at all) remains unclear at present.

The primary site of pathology in OA is the articular cartilage. Normal articular cartilage consists of chondrocytes embedded in an extracellular matrix. The matrix has a high water content and is composed of large proteoglycan aggregates that give cartilage its elasticity and a network of collagen fibres that provides resilience. There are no blood vessels or nerve endings. However, cartilage is a dynamic tissue that continues to be turned over with a balance between degradation and synthesis. With ageing, changes occur in this balanced environment and proteolysis exceeds synthesis.[35] This is largely due to an imbalance between the degradative matrix metalloproteinases and their natural inhibitors, known as tissue inhibitors of matrix metalloproteinases (both of which are produced by chondrocytes). There are also alterations in the matrix water content and changes in the composition of the proteoglycans. This results in a disruption of the organized framework of the matrix, which decreases the tensile strength of the cartilage and makes it stiffer and less deformable. This sets up a situation where the cartilage theoretically does not tolerate mechanical stresses sufficiently, which may result in damage to the tissue. Erosions develop in the cartilage surface, and subsequently vertical clefts develop and deepen. As the disease advances, the cartilage becomes eroded, and leaves denuded, sclerotic and eburnated bone.

There are both systemic and local factors that affect the likelihood that a joint will develop OA.[36] Systemic factors such as age, gender, racial characteristics and genetics may influence the changes that occur in cartilage. Once this vulnerability is in place, local biomechanical factors influence joint breakdown at the macroscopic level. These factors include repetitive joint injury, joint deformity and obesity. Because periarticular muscle acts as a major shock absorber for the joint, loss of muscle strength, bulk and tone in the elderly, as well as age-related degeneration of tendons, may have a significant impact on the progression of disease in a joint, particularly the knee.[37]

OA can be classified as primary (idiopathic) or secondary. Idiopathic OA has a predilection for the distal and proximal interphalangeal (DIP and PIP) joints, zygapophyseal joints of the spine and the hip and knee joints. Secondary OA results from previous joint damage or trauma, prior inflammatory arthritis and certain metabolic or endocrine diseases that lead to accelerated cartilage damage (e.g. diabetes, hyperparathyroidism, acromegaly). The distribution may therefore differ from idiopathic OA.

OA is characterized by pain in the affected joints. Over the course of the day, pain typically worsens with use and is relieved by rest. Morning stiffness may be absent or minimal. However, stiffness after periods of immobility (gelling) are often noted. There may be associated swelling of joints (due to a mild synovitis) as well as cystic changes and bony enlargement. In general, pain from OA gradually worsens over time. Pain may occur with minimal motion or even at rest. Night pain may be seen at this stage. The course may be one of fairly steady progression, although many patients experience exacerbations and remissions in particular joints with an underlying slower progression and gradual loss of mobility and joint function.

Physical examination will reveal pain on passive motion and crepitus, a feeling of crackling as the joint is moved. Joint enlargement may result from synovitis, increased volume of synovial fluid or proliferative changes in cartilage and bone.

Involvement of the fingers is characterized by bony proliferation in the DIP and PIP joints giving rise to bony enlargement called Heberden's and Bouchard's nodes, respectively. This is also termed nodal OA. Patients experience aching and stiffness after use. The base of the thumb or first carpometacarpal (CMC) joint is also typically involved, and exacerbated by twisting and gripping movements. Periodically, these joints can become inflamed, and cystic. This may be part of an erosive picture, or may be due to acute crystal arthropathy involving these small joints. Erosive OA is a distinct syndrome in which Heberden's or Bouchard's nodes are inflamed and erosive changes can be seen on X-ray.

Hip involvement can be characterized by groin pain or pain referred into the buttock, greater trochanter, anterior thigh or even to the knee. Pain and stiffness are usually noted with prolonged standing or walking, but patients also note discomfort getting up from sitting and with the first few steps of walking. The earliest signs of disease are a decrease in internal rotation and abduction.

Involvement of the knee most commonly involves the patellofemoral joint first. This results in pain on descending an incline or stairs. Involvement of medial or lateral compartments can also produce pain after stressful weight bearing, particularly climbing stairs. Flares of OA are commonly seen in the knee following stress and may be associated with increased pain and swelling due to increased synovial fluid. Typical-

ly, this fluid is minimally inflammatory, but can be copious. As noted above, quadriceps weakness may play an important role in the progression of OA of the knee.[37]

OA involving the spine is discussed in the section on back pain.

Unusual patterns of OA, such as involvement of the metacarpophalangeal joints (MCPs), shoulders and ankles, may signify another underlying process, and these patients should be evaluated carefully for other conditions (crystal arthropathy, metabolic disease such as diabetes mellitus, hyperparathyrodism, haemochromatosis, etc.).

There is no known cure or disease-modifying agent in the treatment of OA. Therefore, the goals of management are to control pain and other symptoms and to minimize functional limitation and disability. However, an important caveat is to avoid adverse effects of medications and iatrogenic complications.[38] A management pyramid has been proposed based on the information derived from reviews of randomized clinical trials of different interventions and published guidelines for management. The principle is one of stepped management, with layers of the pyramid being added one to another during the course of managing the individual patient. At the base of the pyramid is weight reduction, exercise and use of assistive devices (canes, orthotics) to improve the biomechanics of affected joints and improve symptoms. The next level involves physical and occupational therapy as well as patient education. Pharmacological interventions can then be added on, starting with acetaminophen and then NSAIDs.[39] Adjuncts to this pyramid that can be introduced at any time include intra-articular corticosteroid injections, hyaluronic acid injections and the use of topical analgesics or capsaicin. Ultimately, surgery may be indicated for intractable pain or disability.

As in the management of back pain, it is preferable to use simple analgesics in the older patient. Acetaminophen has been shown to be comparable to low-dose NSAIDs in patients with knee OA.[40] As noted above, NSAID risks include gastritis, gastric ulceration, acute renal failure, fluid retention and central nervous system (CNS) side-effects in older patients. Therefore, NSAIDs should perhaps be restricted to those in whom non-pharmacological therapy, acetaminophen and intra-articular therapy have been unsuccessful or inadequate.[41] The advent of the more specific Cox-2 inhibitors (Celecoxib, Rofecoxib) and trials demonstrating the protective effective of misoprostal and proton-pump inhibitors in the prevention of NSAID-induced ulcers[42] have increased the use of NSAIDs. Topical therapy with capsaicin has been shown to produce some temporary relief of joint pain.[43,44] These and other 'rubs' are very popular among patients and many are available over the counter. There is evidence that capsaicin and now topical NSAIDs are efficacious for pain relief, but it is not clear that they are significantly better that the cheaper alternatives available over the counter, or even that they are any better than hot or cold packs.

Intra-articular corticosteroid injections are widely used as an adjunct to OA therapy. Controlled studies suggest that injections in the knee are efficacious for only up to 4 weeks. However, in clinical practice many clinicians see much longer lasting responses.[45,46] Intra-articular hyaluronic acid has been shown in some studies to be more effective than placebo injections in patients with knee OA, although there are conflicting data.[47,48] Older patients with moderate to severe pain and functional limitation may be most likely to respond to this treatment[47] and therefore it should be considered to avoid the use of NSAIDs. However, it is expensive and must be paid for by the patient, and many do not want to subject themselves to a series of three to five injections.

Several studies have documented that quadriceps-strengthening exercises are effective in reducing pain and improving function in patients with knee OA,[41,49,50] suggesting that older disabled persons with knee OA can participate in and benefit from aerobic and resistive exercise programmes.

Polymyalgia rheumatica/temporal arteritis

PMR is a rheumatic disease unique to the older population. The diagnosis is rarely made before the age of 50 and 90% of patients are over 60 years old.[51] PMR is an inflammatory condition of unknown aetiology that produces pain and stiffness in the hip and shoulder girdle, as well as the neck and torso, in association with constitutional complaints. Older individuals may present with fever, general decline and non-specific aching. Morning stiffness may be prominent, accentuated by minimal movement. Patients often describe difficulty in dressing without assistance. Pain at night is common. Symptoms have

usually been present for a month or more.[52] Unlike inflammatory myositis, weakness is not a prominent finding, although pain may limit muscle power. Initial presentation with pain and stiffness localized to the shoulders and neck may result in a misdiagnosis as a regional rheumatic problem, such as rotator cuff disease. Conversely, other diseases such as RA and SLE may present early on with a picture suggesting PMR. This is further complicated by the fact that some patients may develop synovitis in the wrists and knees with PMR.[53]

PMR has no clinical feature that is pathognomonic or totally unique from other diagnoses. There is no single diagnostic test that distinguishes it from other inflammatory conditions. Therefore, the diagnosis is a clinical one, based on the constellation of clinical features described above, usually in association with an elevated erythrocyte sedimentation rate.[52] The presence of another specific disease such as RA, polymyositis or chronic infection or malignancy excludes the diagnosis of PMR.

Although there is no diagnostic test, the response to low-dose corticosteroids (15 mg/day or less) is characteristic; patients improve dramatically and rapidly after institution of therapy. The failure to respond to this therapy puts the diagnosis of PMR into question. (see also Chapter 13).

The risks of corticosteroid therapy are legion. Osteoporosis is accelerated with steroid use, especially in the spine, and increases the risk for low-trauma fractures. All patients beginning steroid therapy expected to last beyond 3 months should be started on an osteoporosis prophylaxis regimen of calcium and vitamin D supplementation and potentially other antiresorptive therapy such as bisphosphonates.[54] Avascular necrosis is the death of subchondral bone at hip, knee or shoulder induced by steroid use, and can result in collapse of the affected bone, leading to pain and ultimately joint damage and secondary OA. A non-inflammatory myopathy may develop with proximal muscle weakness. Corticosteroids may increase susceptibility to infection. Steroids may induce abdominal complaints of dyspepsia or bloating. Those on NSAIDs have an even greater risk for gastric ulceration and bleeding. Patients may also develop cataracts, glaucoma, high blood pressure, abnormalities in glucose tolerance and electrolyte abnormalities. Skin becomes fragile and dramatic bruising is often seen. Some patients complain of emotional lability and nightmares.

Ultimately, if the risks for prednisone therapy are too high, patients can be treated symptomatically with NSAIDs or analgesics, as long as monitoring continues to ensure adequate response to treatment. Patients should also be monitored for the development of giant cell arteritis (GCA; see below). PMR in and of itself is not life threatening, but is associated with morbidity and loss of function.

GCA is a common form of vasculitis, or inflammation in the blood vessels, unique to the elderly population and often associated with PMR.[53] The inflammatory process involves the aorta and its proximal branches. The diagnosis rests on a positive biopsy of the temporal artery, but clinical suspicion is needed to direct the biopsy. Patients may present with symptoms of PMR, but the hallmark symptoms that should suggest this potentially serious diagnosis are new-onset headache in the elderly, scalp tenderness, visual changes (double vision, partial or complete blindness in an eye) and jaw or tongue claudication (fatiguing and pain with use, such as chewing meat). Typically patients are unwell, with constitutional complaints, such as fever, weight loss and fatigue, although this is not the rule. Most patients have local symptoms and signs related to arteries, but non-specific presentations are seen in the elderly, such as unexplained fever and non-specific failure to thrive. Onset may be abrupt, but in most instances the symptoms have been present for weeks or months before the diagnosis is established. Headaches are a problem in diagnosis, as many patients develop head pain associated with degenerative changes in the cervical spine. However, all patients with headache should be questioned regarding other symptoms of GCA and should be referred for further evaluation and possible biopsy if there is any concern.

The most serious potential outcome related to this disease is the development of blindness as a result of ischaemia of the optic nerve or tracts secondary to vasculitis of the arteries that supply these structures. Necrosis of the scalp and tongue has also been described.

The treatment of GCA requires the use of high-dose steroids to prevent the development of blindness. Many of these older patients suffer from the side-effects described above because of the high doses that are used.

Rheumatoid arthritis

In contrast to OA, RA typically presents in the childbearing years but may persist into old age. However, a subset of patients may present with new-onset disease at an older age. Approximately 20–30% of cases of RA present after the age of 60 and there is less of a female preponderance than in the younger age group.[55]

Typical seropositive (meaning serum rheumatoid factor-positive) RA is indistinguishable in the elderly from cases with onset at a younger age. Patients present with inflammation in multiple, symmetric, small and large joints, typically involving both hand and foot joints. These patients develop bone erosions on X-ray, as a result of the inflammatory and proliferative synovitis that involves the joints. These patients often develop extra-articular features such as rheumatoid nodules on extensor surfaces. More commonly seen, however, is the pattern of elderly-onset rheumatoid arthritis (EORA) seen in individuals over the age of 60.[56] These patients are rheumatoid factor negative and have less propensity to develop joint erosions. Moderate-sized joints such as shoulders, knees or wrists are involved and fewer joints are involved (typically oligoarticular). Onset may be gradual and early presentations may mimic acute rotator cuff disease in the shoulder, and in some cases may be indistinguishable from PMR. Some patients present with a dramatic onset with multiple joint involvement (polyarticular disease) which is extremely disabling. Constitutional features (fever, weight loss) and most importantly significant morning stiffness (> 1 h) are typically seen. The degree of joint involvement may progress over time.

Extra-articular manifestations, such as nodules, nerve involvement (due to small-vessel vasculitis) and internal organ involvement, are typically absent in EORA patients.[55] These patients do, however, seem to have an increased incidence of secondary Sjögren's syndrome, with the sicca complex of dry eyes and dry mouth. This is the result of autoimmune destruction of tear and saliva glands. Eye symptoms include dryness, gritty or itchy sensation, thick secretions from the eye and sensitivity to light. Oral dryness produces fissuring of lips, difficulty in swallowing dry foods and the development of gingivitis and dental caries.

There is increased mortality and morbidity associated with active, aggressive rheumatoid disease. Large numbers of involved joints, functional limitation and advanced age are all predictors for increased mortality.[57] It is also important to monitor these patients for secondary depression due to changes in lifestyle with limitation in activities of daily living (ADLs) and hobbies, increased dependency on others, social isolation and economic hardship.[58]

Joint damage occurs early, within the first few years of disease, and thus it is important to recognize this disease in its early stages and to refer patients for treatment as soon as possible, as many drugs have the potential to modify the development of joint damage. The armamentarium for treatment of RA has expanded over the last few years. However, almost all have considerable toxicity and require close monitoring for safe use, particularly in the elderly.

In early disease, NSAIDs may be used and often are continued indefinitely. The risks associated with these agents were discussed above. With the availability of the new Cox-2-specific NSAIDs (Celecoxib and Rofecoxib), this therapy is now somewhat safer for use in the elderly.

If patients present with acute and widespread arthritis, with associated constitutional features, low-dose prednisone is often started. Because of the significant potential side-effects of this drug (see above) prednisone is used to bridge the gap until slower acting disease-modifying antirheumatic drugs (DMARDs) are started and become effective (often 6–8 weeks or more). While the response to prednisone therapy is generally good, and it may slow the development of erosions, the potential risks associated with this therapy limit its use. Because RA may be associated with osteoporosis, all patients beginning steroid therapy should receive osteoporosis prophylaxis.

DMARDs are now being started earlier, and the antimalarials (plaquenil), sulfasalazine and methotrexate (or a combination of these drugs) are commonly used.[59,60] The main risks with antimalarials are effects on the eye, with accumulation of drug in the pigmented cells of the retina, resulting in loss of vision. This can be prevented through appropriate dosing and close monitoring by an ophthalmologist. Patients may develop a blue–black discoloration of the skin. Rarely, a neuromuscular syndrome may develop with proximal muscle weakness in the lower extremities. Sulfasalazine may produce gastrointestinal intolerance and, more importantly, decreased blood counts. Methotrexate may also cause gastrointestinal distress and decreased blood counts, and can also be associat-

ed with hepatic toxicity and acute lung disease, with shortness of breath and cough. Intramuscular gold injections are less commonly used these days. The main concerns are bone marrow and kidney toxicity.

Newer therapies include leflunomide (Arava®) and drugs acting against the inflammatory mediator tumour necrosis factor (TNF), which include Etanercept (Enbrel®) and Infliximab (Remicade®).[61] Leflunomide may be associated with alopecia and itching as well as hepatic toxicity. The anti-TNF drugs may be associated with increased risk of infection and malignancy. Long-term experience with these drugs is limited and other side-effects may become apparent over time.

Pharmacological therapy of RA should always be accompanied by patient education regarding the disease and its treatment. Physiotherapy has an important role in preventing joint contractures and restoring function, and includes the prescription of assistive devices, particularly splints, to limit the development of deformities of involved joints.

Systemic lupus erythematosus

SLE is an inflammatory connective tissue disease which is most commonly seen in young women of child-bearing age. However, the disease can have its onset in the elderly. Internal organ involvement (primarily kidney) often dominates the clinical picture and results in more morbidity and mortality than musculoskeletal involvement. Typically, musculoskeletal manifestations include arthralgias and rarely frank arthritis. A classic deforming but non-destructive arthritis, referred to as Jacoud's arthropathy, can result in ulnar deviation of the digits as well as swan-neck deformities in the fingers. It appears that the clinical pattern is different in the elderly, although there is some controversy in this area.[62,63] Many studies suggest a milder disease course in the elderly, with less renal and CNS involvement. Rash and arthritis or arthralgia are the most frequent symptoms in both ealier and late-onset SLE. There is an increase in the frequency of lung involvement (interstitial pneumonitis, serositis), low blood counts (often all cell lines), peripheral neuropathy (with sensory and/or motor dysfunction) and dry eyes/dry mouth complex (sicca) in late-onset disease. Some patients have a tendency to develop blood clots as a result of autoantibodies that interfere with normal blood coagulation and regulatory pathways.

It is also worth noting that certain drugs used in the elderly population for hypertension, cardiac problems or other disorders (e.g. methyldopa, hydralazine, procainamide and isoniazid) can produce an SLE syndrome. This is usually less severe than idiopathic lupus, with fever, arthritis and serositis as the main manifestations.

The time from presentation to diagnosis of SLE is often prolonged in this age group, perhaps because the manifestations may be non-specific early on. The illness may present very much like early RA or PMR. The presence of certain autoantibodies is important in making the diagnosis of SLE. In the elderly, some of these autoantibodies are present but are not specific to the diagnosis of lupus. However, with time, the typical and more specific autoantibodies are usually found.

Treatment of SLE is a complex and depends largely on the severity of the clinical manifestations of disease. NSAIDs and antimalarials are used for those with skin, joint and mild constitutional complaints. The potential side-effects of these drugs have already been discussed in the sections on back pain and rheumatoid arthritis.

Corticosteroid therapy is often required and poses particular risks in the elderly as discussed in the management of PMR. All elderly, patients starting steroid therapy should receive prophylactic therapy for osteoporosis, including calcium supplements, vitamin D supplements and antiresorptive agents such as the bisphosphonates etidronate (Didrocal®), or alendronate (Fosamax®). Patients should also be closely monitored for steroid myopathy, with the development of proximal muscle weakness, and difficulty in arising from a chair or climbing the stairs. Avascular necrosis of the hip appears to be more common in patients being treated with steroids for SLE. Patients may develop severe and persistent aching pain in the groin, buttock or anterior or outer thigh. Patients on steroids should always be closely followed for the development of infection. The usual manifestations may be suppressed by the drug.

Immunosuppressive medications such as azathioprine (Imuran®) or methotrexate may be required to control disease, or to allow prednisone to be discontinued or kept at a lower maintenance dose. With the use of immunosuppressives in the elderly, it is always important to consider whether patients have had any prior exposure to tuberculosis, as reactivation may

occur. The development of bacterial or viral infections is also increased with the use of these drugs. Patients may develop shingles (reactivation of varicella-zoster virus from chickenpox as a young person) with severe pain and blistering lesions in the distribution of one or several dermatomes. Pain can be debilitating and may persists even after lesions have healed (post-herpetic neuralgia). These drugs may also be associated with liver toxicity and bone-marrow suppression, and regular monitoring of blood tests (blood counts, liver enzymes) is required.

For those patients with clotting abnormalities, anticoagulant therapy with coumadin may be required. This puts patients, especially the elderly, at high risk for bleeding complications, especially with minimal trauma. Those also on prednisone may experience excessive bruising owing to the fragility of capillaries associated with prednisone use.

Myositis

Myositis is a disease characterized by acute or chronic inflammation in striated muscle. If there are associated skin findings, this is termed dermatomyositis. Myositis may be idiopathic, associated with an underlying malignancy or be part of another rheumatic disease such as SLE. Inclusion body myositis (IBM) is a distinct form of myositis seen mainly in the elderly population.[64]

The incidence of idiopathic myositis is highest in the fifth and sixth decades of life.[65] Clinically, the disease may present insidiously (over months) or may have a fulminant onset. Fatigue, progressive weakness and sometimes constitutional symptoms may be seen. Muscular weakness is usually proximal and symmetrical, and may be characterized by difficulty in arising from a sitting position, climbing stairs or reaching overhead. Walking becomes increasingly limited and personal care and ADLs may be affected. Although stiffness and aching are not seen as in PMR, some patients will complain of aching in the buttocks, thighs and calves, and some may have tenderness on palpation of major muscle groups.[66] Weakness can also involve the neck and pharyngeal musculature (but there is no involvement of facial or extraocular musculature as in myasthenia gravis), with difficulty in swallowing and risk for aspiration. The heart muscle may also be involved, with rhythm disturbances and even heart failure. Lungs may be involved by an interstitial inflammatory or fibrotic process in some cases, leading to shortness of breath and even respiratory failure.

In those patients with dermatomyositis,[64] the rash may precede the onset of myositis, occur concomitantly or even develop later on. Typically, an erythematous, scaling rash may develop on the bridge of the nose, cheeks, forehead, chest and extensor surfaces, such as elbows, knees and medial malleoli. The classic rash is a violaceous discoloration over the upper eyelid (the heliotrope rash). Other rashes include scaling patches over the MCP and PIP joints, along with erythema and sometimes swelling at the base of the nails. Erythematous rashes may also develop over the back and shoulders (the 'shawl' sign). Photosensitive rashes and itching may also be seen.

IBM is more common in the elderly,[67,68] with a mean age of disease onset of 61 years. It is more common in males than females. This disease typically has an insidious onset, with development over years. Weakness may be asymmetric, and involves distal as well as proximal muscle groups. In the upper extremities wrist and finger flexor muscle groups are involved more commonly than extensors. In the lower extremities knee extensor involvement predominates. Peripheral neuropathy may also be seen, with loss of deep tendon reflexes.

Myositis in the elderly can be associated with an underlying internal malignancy. Data from several studies suggest that this risk is higher for dermatomyositi than for polymyositis, and that the dermatomyositis can precede the development of malignancy by up to 2 years. Therefore, it is reasonable that a search for malignancy is made in older persons with onset of myositis.[69]

The diagnosis of myositis is based on a combination of the clinical picture of weakness, abnormalities in muscle enzyme levels in the blood, EMG studies and usually muscle biopsy.[64]

The mainstay of therapy for myositis is high-dose corticosteroid therapy. This must initially be continued for at least 1 month to control the acute inflammation. There are significant risks associated with this therapy, as noted above in the sections of polymyalgia rheumatica and systemic lupus erythematosus. One of the most significant problems in this group is the development of proximal myopathy secondary to steroids, which may be difficult to distinguish from a flare of myositis or failure of the underlying disease to respond to treatment.

Immunosuppressive therapy such as methotrexate or azathioprine (Imuran®) is often added to achieve and maintain a remission. As noted above (see Systemic lupus erythematosus), complications related to infection are the greatest concern with these drugs, as well as the direct side-effects of bone-marrow suppression and liver toxicity.

Crystal-associated arthritis

Crystal-induced arthropathy can take both acute and chronic forms. However, the acute presentation is usually very dramatic and disabling, and thus the clinical characteristics should be recognized. Acute infectious arthritis should always be considered in the differential diagnosis with this type of presentation, and it should be remembered that infection and crystal arthritis can exist in the same joint.

The two most common crystals causing arthritis are monosodium urate (MSU) (70) and CPPD.[71] In the acute setting, the conditions caused by these crystals are known as gout and pseudogout, respectively.

The classic presentation of crystal arthropathy is a sudden-onset monoarthritis, although polyarticular attacks may occur (and help to distinguish it from infection).[70] The joint may be exquisitely painful, particularly with gout, and is associated with heat, swelling and redness. The redness may extend to the periarticular areas and is sometimes confused with cellulitis. Constitutional symptoms may be present with fever and chills, further confusing the distinction between crystal and infectious aetiologies.

Gout typically has its onset in middle-aged adults. The first MTP joint is often the first joint to be involved, but knees and ankles are seen as well, with the involvement of upper extremity being less common. The frequency may increase in the older age group and becomes more common in women once they become postmenopausal. The features in the older population are somewhat distinct from those in middle-aged adults.[72,73] These include presentation in women, increased association with use of diuretics and polyarticular disease. The polyarticular form may be more indolent and mimic RA. Another feature unique to older individuals is the involvement of DIP joints affected with OA (i.e. Heberden's nodes), which may be mistaken for a flare of OA affecting these joints.

In general, after years of monoarticular attacks, with quiescent intercritical periods, untreated gout may lead to the development of tophaceous deposits within and around joints and in soft tissues (elbows, fingers, ears).

These consist of white chalky material made up of masses of uric acid crystals. The arthritis gradually becomes more destructive, with the development of characteristic erosions in the joints and ultimately destruction.

Pseudogout tends to be associated with onset in older patients.[71] The acute presentation may be less severe than that of gout but can be equally dramatic. Typically, knees and wrists are affected in the acute phase. Acute attacks often occur following trauma, medical illness or surgical procedures. CPPD may be associated with other metabolic diseases such as hypothyroidism, hyperparathyroidism and gout.

CPPD is also associated with a more chronic pattern of arthritis and can result in an accelerated osteoarthritis. However, in this case atypical joints may be involved, such as the second and third MCP joints and wrists. CPPD may also develop with a pseudo-RA pattern, and X-rays and demonstration of crystals become important to avoid using the wrong treatment. Finally, CPPD can lead to a destroyed and deformed joint, such as the neuropathic joint seen in severe diabetes mellitus. Thus, presentations of CPPD can resemble almost any known type of acute or chronic arthritis.[74]

Basic calcium phosphates, which include apatites, have been associated with an idiopathic destructive arthritis of the shoulder (Milwaukee shoulder).[75] Patients present with an inflamed and swollen shoulder with significant loss of function. These crystals can also produce an acute periarthritis, tendonitis or bursitis at any age, which can be exquisitely painful.

Deposition of urate crystals in the joint is related to chronic and sustained hyperuricaemia. The mechanisms responsible for the deposition of CPPD crystals in synovial tissue and articular cartilage are not well understood. However, crystals appear to be able to activate an inflammatory cascade of events with the release of inflammatory mediators and liberation of toxic substances from cells damaged by engulfing crystals.[73] The characteristics of crystals which lead to the dramatic inflammatory response are also poorly understood.

Thus, crystals may produce a broad spectrum of clinical presentations. The correct diagnosis is dependent on the identification of crystals from joint aspirates. Infection should always be ruled out.

The initial goal of treatment is to suppress the acute inflammation. This is achieved through the use of NSAIDs and corticosteroids, either orally or by intra-articular injection. The risk of using NSAIDs in a particular individual must be considered, and if it is felt to be significant steroid therapy may be preferable. Oral steroids are particularly helpful in the setting of a polyarticular attack. Although steroids also have many associated risks, the short duration of the treatment (10–14 days) limits the potential problems. Intra-articular steroids allow systemic therapy to be avoided altogether. Colchicine was used extensively in the past, but toxicity with nausea, vomiting, diarrhoea and risk of bone-marrow suppression have made this an unfavourable choice.

Patients may remain at increased risk for another attack for several weeks after resolution of the acute episode. Small doses of colchicines may have a role here, but patients should be monitored carefully for bone-marrow suppression and myoneuropathy (73).

Treatment should also be considered for the prevention of future attacks. Systemic urate-lowering therapy may be required in those with recurrent episodes of gout or tophaceous deposits. The most effective drug in the older age group is allopurinol. The main concern with this treatment is the risk of an acute hypersensitivity reaction. A rash develops in 3–10% of patients, which may progress to exfoliative dermatitis and even a systemic reaction with internal organ involvement.[76] The drug should be discontinued if any rash develops.

The acute attack of CPPD is managed in the same way as acute gout. However, there is currently no known therapy for the removal or prevention of CPPD crystal deposition in the joints.

Summary

Musculoskeletal problems in older adults can be both diagnostically and therapeutically challenging. Although the spectrum of rheumatic diseases in the sixth decade and beyond can be quite distinct from that in younger individuals, many diseases within the spectrum can have similar clinical features, especially early in the disease course. Management of these conditions is complicated by a remarkable spectrum of toxicities, which are particularly problematic in the elderly. Thus, as discussed in the introduction, all care givers and practitioners working with the elderly should be aware of the presenting features of those diseases that require early investigation and treatment and to ensure that patients are referred appropriately. For those individuals already diagnosed, it is important for all involved in their care to remain vigilant for potential side-effects of therapy. The timely and successful treatment of rheumatic syndromes in older adults can preserve the well-being, longevity and independence of these individuals.

References

1 Borenstein DG. Low back pain. In: Klippel JH, Dieppe PA, eds. Rheumatology 2nd edn. London: Mosby, 1998: 4.3.1–4.3.27.
2 Dixon A StJ. Progress and problems in back pain research. Rheumatol Rehabil 1973; 12: 165–175.
3 Andersson, GBJ. What are the age-related changes in the spine? Baillière's Clin Rheumatol 1998; 12: 161–173.
4 Vernon-Roberts B, Pirie CJ. Degenerative changes in the intervertebral discs and their sequelae. Rheumatol Rehabil 1977; 16: 13–21.
5 Rosenberg NJ. Degenerative spondylolisthesis. J Bone Joint Surg 1975; 57(4): 467–474.
6 Arnoldi CC, Bordsky AE, Cauchoix J et al. Lumbar spinal stenosis and nerve root entrapment syndrome. Definition and classification. Clin Orthop 1976; 115: 4–.
7 Katz JN, Dalgas M, Stucki G et al. Degenerative lumbar spinal stenosis: diagnostic value of the history and physical examination. Arthritis Rheum 1995; 38: 1236–1241.
8 Grobler LJ. Back and Leg Pain in Older adults: presentation, diagnosis and treatment. Clin Geriatr Med 1998; 14: 543–575.
9 Resnick, D, Shaul SR, Robins JM. Diffuse idiopathic skeletal hyperostosis (DISH): Forestier's disease with extraspinal manifestations. Radiology 1975; 114: 513–524.
10 Jackson CP, Brown MD. Is there a role for exercise in the treatment of patients with low back pain? Clin Orthop 1983; 179: 39–45.
11 Berry H, Bloom B, Hamilton EBD, Swinson DR. Naproxen sodium, diflunisal and placebo in the treatment of low back pain. Ann Clin Res 1984; 16: 156–160.
12 Simon LS. Risk factors and current NSAID use (Editorial). J Rheumatol 1999; 26: 1429–1431.
13 Silas S, Clegg DO. Selective Cox-2 inhibition. Bull Rheum Dis 1999; 48(2), 1–4.
14 Johnson EW. The myth of skeletal muscle spasm. Am J Phys Med Rehabil 1989; 68:1.
15 Dilke TFW, Burry HC, Grahame R. Extradural corticosteroid injection management of lumbar nerve root compression. BMJ 1973; ii: 635–637.
16 Jackson RP, Jacobs RR, Montesano PX. Facet joint injection in low back pain: a prospective statistical study. Spine 1988; 13: 966–971.
17 Carette S, Marcoux S, Truchon R et al. A controlled trial of corticosteroid injections into facet joints for chronic low back pain. N Engl J Med 1991; 325: 1002–1007.
18 Bigos S, Bowyer O, Braen G et al. Acute low back problems in adults. Clinical Practice Guideline, Quick Reference Guide No. 14. Rockville, MD: US Department of Health and Human Services, Public Health Service, Agency for Health Care Policy and Research, AHCPR Pub. No. 95–0643. December 1994.
19 Deyo RA, Rainville J, Kent DL. What can the history and physical examination tell us about low back pain? JAMA 1992; 268: 760–765.
20 Engstrom JW, Bradford DS. Back and neck pain. In: Fauci AS, Braumwald E, Isselbacher KJ et al. eds. Harrison's Principles of Internal Medicine. 14th edn. New York: McGraw-Hill, 1998:

73–79.
21 Longo DL. Plasma cell disorders. In: Fauci AS et al. eds. Harrison's Principles of Internal Medicine. 14th edn. New York: McGraw-Hill, 1998: 712–717.
22 Riggs B, Melton LJ. The prevention and treatment of osteoporosis. N Engl J Med 1992; 327: 620–627.
23. Lyritis GP, Paspati I, Karachalios T et al. Pain relief from nasal salmon calcitonin in osteoporotic vertebral crush fractures. A double blind, placebo-controlled clinical study. Acta Orthop Scand 1997; 68 (Suppl 275): 112–114.
24 Lyritis GP, Tsakalakos N, Magiasis B et al. Analgesic effect of salmon calcitonin in osteoporotic vertebral fractures: a double-blind placebo-controlled clinical study. Calcif Tissue Int 1991: 49; 369–372.
25 Calis M, Akgun K, Birtane M et al. Diagnostic values of clinical diagnostic tests in subacromial impingement syndrome. Ann Rheum Dis 2000; 59: 44–47.
26 Dalton SE. The shoulder. In: Klippel JH, Dieppe PA eds. Rheumatology. 2nd edn. London: Mosby, 1998: 4.7.1–4.7.14.
27 Fukuda H, Mikasa M, Yamanaka K. Incomplete thickness rotator cuff tears diagnosed by subacromial bursography. Clin Orthop 1987; 223: 51–58.
28 Wirth MA, Basamania C, Rockwood CA. Nonoperative management of full- thickness tears of the rotator cuff. Orth Clin N Am 1997; 28: 59–67.
29 Uthoff HK, Sarkar K. Calcifying tendonitis. In: Hazleman BL, Dieppe PA, eds. The Shoulder Joint. Bailliere's Clinical Rheumatology. London: Baillière Tindall, 1989: 567–581.
30 Neviaser RJ, Neviaser TJ. The frozen shoulder. Diagnosis and management. Clin Orthop 1987; 223: 59–64.
31 Nash P, Haleman BL. Frozen shoulder. In: Haleman BL, Dieppe PA, eds. The Shoulder Joint. Bailliere's Clinical Rheumatology. London: Baillière Tindall, 1989: 551–566.
32 Steinbrocker O, Arojyros TG. Frozen shoulder: treatment by local injections of depot corticosteroids. Arch Phys Med Rehab 1974; 55: 209–213.
33 Reeves B. The natural history of the frozen shoulder syndrome. Scand J Rheumatol 1976; 4: 193–6.
34 Hamerman D. Lagging and osteoarthritis: basic mechanisms. J Am Geriatr Soc 1993; 41: 760–770.
35 Hamerman D. Biology of the aging joint. Clin Geriatr Med 1998; 14: 417–433.
36 Felson DT, Zhang Y. An update on the epidemiology of knee and hip osteoarthritis with a view to prevention. Arthritis Rheum 1998; 41: 1343–1355.
37 Slemenda C, Brandt KD, Heilman DK et al. Quadriceps weakness and osteoarthritis of the knee. Ann Intern Med 1997; 127: 97–104.
38 Creamer P, Hochberg MC. Osteoarthritis. Lancet 1997; 350: 503–508.
39 Bradley JD, Brandt KD, Katz BP et al. Treatment of knee osteoarthritis: relationship of clinical features of joint inflammation to the response to a nonsteroidal anti-inflammatory drug or pure analgesic. J Rheumatol 1992; 19: 1950–1954.
40 Williams HJ, Ward JR, Egger MJ et al. Comparison of naproxen and acetaminophen in a two-year study of treatment of osteoarthritis of the knee. Arthritis Rheum 1993; 36: 1196–1206.
41 Creamer, P, Flores R, Hochberg MC. Management of osteoarthritis in older adults. Clin Geriatric Med 1998; 14: 435–454.
42 Wolfe MM, Lichtenstein DR, Singh G. Gastrointestinal toxicity of nonsteroidal anti-inflammatory drugs. N Engl J Med 1999; 340: 1888–1899.
43 McCarthy GM, McCarthy DJ. Effects of topical capsaicin in the therapy of painful osteoarthritis of the hands. J Rheumatol 1992; 19: 604–607.

44 Zhang WY, Po ALW. The effectiveness of topically applied cap-saicin: a meta-analysis. Eur J Clin Pharmacol 1994; 46: 517–522.

45 Creamer P. Intra-articular steroids in osteoarthritis: do they work and if so how? Ann Rheum Dis 1997; 56: 634–635.

46 Dieppe PA. Are intra-articular steroid injections useful for the treatment of the osteoarthritis joint? Br J Rheumatol 1991; 30: 199.

47 Lohmander LS, Dalen N, Englund G *et al.* Intra-articular hyaluronan injections in the treatment of osteoarthritis of the knee: a randomized, double blind, placebo controlled trial. Ann Rheum Dis 1996; 55: 424–431.

48 Puhl W, Bernau A, Greiling H *et al.* Intra-articular sodium hyaluronate in osteoarthritis of the knee: a multicenter, double-blind study. Osteoarthritis Cart 1993; 1: 233–241.

49 Ettinger WH, Burns R, Messier SP *et al.* A randomized trial com-paring aerobic exercise and resistance exercise with a health edu-cation program in older adults with knee osteoarthritis. JAMA 1997; 277: 25–31.

50 Fiatarone MA, Marks EC, Ryan ND *et al.* High intensity strength training in nonagenarians: effect on skeletal muscle. JAMA 1990; 263: 3029–3034.

51 Hunder GG, Michet CJ. Giant cell arteritis and polymyalgia rheumatica. Clin Rheum Dis 1985; 11: 471–483.

52 Bengtsson B-A. Polymyalgia rheumatica. In: Klippel JH, ed. Primer on the Rheumatic Diseases. 11th edn. Atlanta, GA: Arthritis Foundation, 1997: 305–306.

53 Hunder GG. Giant cell arteritis and polymyalgia rheumatica. Med Clin North Am 1997; 81: 195–219.

54 American College of Rheumatology Task Force on Osteoporo-sis Guidelines. Recommendations for the prevention and treat-ment of glucocorticoid induced osteoporosis. Arthritis Rheum 1996; 39: 1791–1801.

55 VanSchaardenburg D, Breedveld FC. Elderly-onset rheumatoid arthritis. Semin Arthritis Rheum 1994; 23: 367–378.

56 Terkeltaub R, Esdaile J, Decany F *et al.* A clinical study of older age rheumatoid arthritis with comparison to a younger onset group. J Rheumatol 1983; 10: 418–424.

57 Pincus T, Brooks RH, Callahan LF. Prediction of long-term mor-tality in patients with rheumatoid arthritis according to simple questionnaire and joint count measures. Ann Intern Med 1994; 120: 26–34.

58 Katz PP, Yelin EH. The development of depressive symptoms among women with rheumatoid arthritis. The role of function. Arthritis Rheum 1995; 38: 49–56.

59 O'Dell JR. Triple therapy with methotrexate, sulfasalazine, and hydroxychloroquine in patients with rheumatoid arthritis. Rheum Dis Clin N Am 1998; 24: 465–477.

60 Kelley WN, Harris ED Jr, Ruddy S, Sledge CB eds. Textbook of Rheumatology. 5th edn. Philadelphia, PA: WB Saunders Com., 1997.

61 Jones RE, Moreland LW. Tumor necrosis factor inhibitors for rheumatoid arthritis. Bull Rheum Dis 1999; 48(3), 1–4.

62 Mak SK, Lam EKM, Wong AKM. Clinical profile of patients with late-onset SLE: not a benign subgroup. Lupus 1998; 7: 23–28.

63 Formiga, F, Moga I, Pac M *et al.* Mild presentation of systemic lupus erythematosus in elderly patients assessed by SLEDAI. Lupus 1999; 8: 462–465.

64 Amato AA, Barohn RJ. Idiopathic inflammatory myopathies. Neuro Clin 1997; 15: 615–649.

65 Bohan A, Peter JB, Bowman RL *et al.* Computer-assisted analy-sis of 153 patients with polymyositis and dermatomyositis. Med-icine 1977; 56: 255–586.

66 Mishra N, Kammer GM. Clinical expression of autoimmune dis-eases in older adults. Clin Geriatr Med 1998; 14: 515–542.

67 Sayers ME, Chou SM, Calabrese LH. Inclusion body myositis: analysis of 32 cases. J Rheumatol 1992; 19: 1385–1389.

68 Dalakas MC, Sonies B, Dambrosia J *et al.* Treatment of inclu-sion-body myositis with IVIg: a double-blind, placebo-controlled study. Neurology 1997; 48: 712–716.

69 Sigurgeirsson B, Lindelof B, Edhag O *et al.* Risk of cancer in patients with dermatomyositis or polymyositis: a population based study. N Engl J Med 1992; 326: 363–367.

70 Edwards NL. Gout. Clinical and laboratory features. In: Klippel JH, ed. Primer on the Rheumatic Diseases, 11th edn. Atlanta, GA: Arthritis Foundation, 1997: 234–239.

71 Ryan LM. Calcium pyrophosphate dihydrate crystal deposition. In: Klippel JH, ed. Primer on the Rheumatic Diseases, 11th edn. Atlanta, GA: Arthritis Foundation, 1997: 226–229.

72 TerBorg EJ, Rasher JJ. Gout in the elderly, a separate entity? Ann Rheum Dis 1987; 46: 72–76.

73 Agudelo CA, Wise CM. Crystal-associated arthritis. Clin Geri-atr Med 1998; 14: 495–513.

74 McCarty DJ. Diagnostic mimicry in arthritis: patterns of joint involvement associated with calcium pyrophosphate dihydrate deposits. Bull Rheum Dis 1975: 25; 1438–1440.

75 Dieppe P. Apatites and miscellaneous crystals. In: Klippel JH ed. Primer on the Rheumatic Diseases. 11th edn. Atlanta, GA: Arthritis Foundation, 1997: 222–225.

76 Wallace SL, Singer JZ. Therapy in gout. Rheum Dis Clin North Am 1988; 14: 441–457.

11

Neurological disorders of the elderly

Steven Zylick

This chapter discusses the general neurological changes that occur in the elderly. The discussion focuses on the primary characteristics of structures and functions that change with age and the neurological diseases that these changes may cause. These characteristics include:

- loss of brain size: the loss of brain size parallels other morphological changes in the central nervous system (CNS)
- change in cerebral blood flow: the impact of diminished flow has functional ramifications either acutely or chronically
- changes in the special senses of the elderly, including smell, taste, vision, hearing and balance
- degenerative changes of the spinal column, including central or lateral stenosis and other space-occupying lesions.

Two diseases, Parkinson's disease and multiple sclerosis, will be discussed in more detail. Other common neurological diseases will be discussed in other chapters. These include stroke, headache, infectious diseases, organic brain syndromes, dementia and delirium, and genetic neurodegenerative disorders.

The ageing population and its neurological conditions

The population is slowly shifting to include a larger number of older citizens. With the refinement of life skills, environmental controls and medical services, many people are living longer into the seventh, eighth and ninth decades of life. The knowledge and expectation of living longer lives with an interest in living a quality lifestyle, free of morbid decline or disability, is putting pressure on the development of new insights into well-being and health care.

Many changes are observed as a person ages, many of which are considered to be normal. However, senescence, the manifestation of the ageing process, leads to the decline of cellular functions. This results in a vulnerability to disease, and eventually to death. Many cellular changes and organ diseases associated with ageing have become scientifically understood from the study of older people who required an autopsy after death. This knowledge has then been applied retrospectively to understand the symptoms or behaviours that a person with a particular disease may exhibit. More recently, with the advent of functional magnetic resonance imaging (FMRI), brain activity and patients' symptoms are being correlated more closely with structural changes. This should rapidly expand the understanding of central processing and cellular changes with pathology, much as electromyography (EMG), nerve conduction velocity (NCV) studies and sensory evoked potentials (SEPs) have expanded the functional understanding of the peripheral nervous system (PNS).

The nervous system

Many changes are seen in the nervous system with advancing age. The neurobiological understanding of ageing and its behavioural impact are still poorly understood. The changes most easily seen by others, and complained of by the patient, are changes in sleep patterns, higher brain functions, movements and co-ordination. The gait of the senior patient is affected by biomechanical changes, including loss of muscle tone, degenerative changes to joints and the shortening of ligaments or tendons, and many of these changes

Table 11.1 Chronic diseases of the elderly (age 65–74 years)

Disease	Frequency per 1000 persons
Arthritis	450
Hypertension	350
Hearing impairment	240
Visual impairment	175
Heart conditions	240
Sinusitis	150
Orthopedic impairment	145
Arteriosclerosis	25
Diabetes	90
Varicose veins	75

Source: National Centre for Health Statistics.[1]

may have a neurological basis. Table 11.1 lists the top 10 chronic diseases and their relative frequency per 1000 persons between the ages of 65 and 74 years. Primary neurological disorders, such as hearing and visual impairment, are among the five most common neurological disorders, and hypertension, arteriosclerosis, diabetes and arthritis are frequently the cause of secondary neurological diseases.

Neurological conditions frequently seen by chiropractors

The National Board of Chiropractic Examiners (NBCE) has conducted a job analysis survey of 500 Chiropractors in Canada (1993)[2] and two analyses in the USA (1989 and 2000).[3] Participants were asked to

provide information regarding 115 conditions that they might have seen in the prior year (Table 11.2). The conditions listed were consistent with the International Classification of Disease-9CM codes.

According to the NBCE studies, the most frequently observed neurological disorders presenting to a chiropractor's office were headache, peripheral neuritis or neuralgia, and radiculitis or radiculopathy.[2,3] A comparison of Tables 11.1 and 11.2 indicates that chiropractors may be in an excellent professional position to service many of the ailments of the ageing baby boomer population.

Elderly patients

For the new clinician it may be both interesting and startling to observe the wide variations between patients of the same age, in terms of both structure and function. It is clear that individuals do not age at the same rate, nor do all tissues within a person age at the same rate. Some tissues may undergo rapid changes, possibly due to poor nutrition, blood flow or oxygen, and they may demonstrate accelerated pathology. In addition, cellular tissue may demonstrate programmed obsolescence (senile involution). Cartilage, however, is an exception to this phenomenon. It continues to grow with age, and therefore it does not significantly contribute to the effects of senescence.[4]

In contrast, nerve cells have a very limited capacity to be replaced. Nerve cell division occurs in only a small number of regions, and peripheral nerve axons

Table 11.2 Frequency of neurological conditions presenting to a chiropractor.[2,3]

Neurological Symptom Condition	Average occurrence	
	Canadian Study: NBCE Job Analysis of Chiropractic (1993)	USA Study: NBCE Job Analysis of Chiropractic (2000)
Headaches	Often–routinely (3.76)	Often (3.3)
Peripheral neuritis or neuralgia	Often–routinely (3.10)	Often (2.6)
Amyotrophic lateral sclerosis, multiple sclerosis or Parkinson's	Rarely–sometimes (1.19)	Rarely (0.8)
Tearing or rupture of nerve/plexus	Never–rarely (0.67)	Rarely (1.3)
Stroke or cerebrovascular condition	Never–rarely (0.89)	Rarely (0.7)
Vertebrobasilar artery insufficiency	Never–rarely (0.86)	Rarely (0.5)
Cranial nerve disorder	Rarely–sometimes (1.04)	Rarely (0.8)
Radiculitis or radiculopathy	Sometimes–often (2.54)	Often (2.8)
Loss of equilibrium	Rarely–sometimes (1.88)	Sometimes (1.6)
Brain or spinal cord tumour	Never–rarely (0.44)	Virtually never (0.3)

Table 11.3 Magnetic resonance patterns of age-related changes in 119 subjects (aged 19 months to 80 years)[7]

	Infants to children	Senior's 71–80 years
Intracranial space/whole brain	Increased by 25–27% 26 months to 14 years	Decreased: loss to childhood levels
Grey matter (GM)	Increased by 13% Early to late childhood	Decreased by 13%
White matter (WM)		Slow decline
GM: WM ratio	Decreased exponentially Early childhood to 4th decade	Gradual decline

may regenerate if closely approximated (termed axonal regeneration). Neuronal loss has been estimated at 50 000 neurons per day (from an estimated total of 10 billion neurons), accounting for only a 3% loss throughout life.[5] Many other age-related changes of the nervous system are associated with alterations in cellular structure and neural structure size (dendritic branches). These changes parallel the general reduction in brain weight and size.

Brain size

The brain reaches its maximum mass by the second decade of life, after which it slowly begins to shrink in size. By the age of 80 years, the brain has lost 7% (100 g) of its original size.[5] As brain weight diminishes there is enlargement of the lateral ventricles and a widening of the sulci, representing neuronal loss and replacement gliosis. This cell loss is not consistent in all areas of the CNS. For example, the hippocampus is reported to have a reduction of 27% between the ages of 45 and 95 years, and lumbar anterior horn cells, sensory ganglion cells and Purkinje cells all demonstrate a reduction in size of up to 25%.[6] Conversely, other areas of the brain, such as the vestibular nuclei and inferior olives, do not diminish in size. In addition, magnetic resonance (MR) images of the brain at different ages reflect the varying functional growth and decline over time (Table 11.3).

Neuron count

It is clear that even healthy people experience some loss of brain neurons throughout their lives. Cell death is a normal occurrence during the development of the nervous system. Early in life, cell death is viewed as a 'pruning' of the excessive number of cells initially generated during the proliferation of cellular division of foetal development.[8] This programmed cell death is referred to as apoptosis.

In the adult nervous system there is very little normal cell death. Cell necrosis occurs rapidly in acute neurological disorders and more slowly in chronic diseases (Table 11.4). Chronic neurological diseases are often associated with profuse cell death without obvious signs of cell necrosis. Moreover, there is some evidence that in these chronic disorders the neuronal cell death may involve apoptosis.[8]

In general, the total number of neurons diminishes with age. This is best observed in the larger cells of the nervous system (pyramidal cells of Betz and Purkinje neurons). With age, there is a reduction in the number of neurons in the substantia nigra (dopaminergic cen-

Table 11.4 Examples of nerve cell loss from acute and chronic disorders

Acute disorders (Minutes to hours)	Chronic disorders (Years to decades)
Brain injury as a result of: Trauma Infarction Haemorrhage Infection	Motor neuron disease (aymotrophic lateral sclerosis) Cerebral dementing disease (Alzheimer's, frontotemporal dementia) Degenerative movement disorders (Parkinson's, Huntington's)
Nerve cell loss tends to be more from necrotic processes	Nerve cell death may occur in stepwise decline if disease involves times of acute inflammation–repair (gliosis)–cell loss Nerve cell death may result from apoptosis

Table 11.5 Central nervous system changes with age

Structure	Change
Neuron count	Reduces
Neuron size	Reduces
Cortical mass	Atrophies
Nissl substance	Diminishes
Neurofibrils	Thicken and clump
Amyloid bodies	Accumulate
Lipofuscin pigment	Increases

tre) and locus coeruleus (noradrenergic nucleus). Cell counts of several subcortical nuclei and the cerebral cortex reveal reduced number of neurons with age, which may represent cell loss or shrinkage of neurons.[9]

This reduction in the number of nerve cells continues throughout a person's life and accounts for a loss of approximately 20% of the neurons present at birth. The loss of nerve cells may be higher in persons with certain diseases. In either case, there is a loss of the brain weight and size. These cellular changes include the following (see also Table 11.5):

- Neuronal size and components: The dendritic pattern of neurons appears less branched, there is a loss of dopamine receptors (D_2/D_3-like) in the striatum, and several extrastriatal regions have been associated with both normal ageing and impaired cognitive and motor functions in the elderly.[10]
- Loss of neurotransmitters: Dopamine loss is associated with Parkinson's disease and gamma-aminobutyric acid (GABA) and acetylcholine are associated with Huntington's chorea.
- Cortical mass: The cortical hemispheres undergo atrophic changes. The sulci become broad with reduced size and the gyri and ventricular cavities increase in size.
- Nissl substance: This appears to diminish with age.
- Neurofibrils: These appear to undergo thickening and clumping.
- Amyloid bodies (corpora amylacea): There is an increased number of amyloid bodies. These bodies are most prevalent around the ventricular surface and may represent neuronal degeneration products.
- Lipofuscin pigment: This pigment increases in neurons and glia. Astrocytes are primarily affected, which has a deleterious effect on neuronal function. Oligodendroglia and microglia are not as affected.

- Cerebral blood vessels: Thickening of the arterial wall is seen.
- Cerebrovascular resistance: Increased cerebrovascular resistance will diminish cranial perfusion.
- Reduced level of proteins and enzymes: There is a reduction in the enzymes that produce dopamine and noradrenaline.
- Reduced oxygen utilization: Diminished oxygen utilization may alter cellular metabolic activity with a resulting functional change.
- Circadian rhythms: In humans and animal models, cognitive performance is often impaired when circadian rhythms are disrupted. This includes a general decline in cognitive ability and fragmentation of behavioural rhythms.[11]
- Arachnoid granulations: These structures increase in number and size with age. They tend to become calcified with increasing age.
- Pineal gland: This often develops concretions of calcified material (brain sand) that accumulate with age.

Higher brain functions

Age-related changes may vary between people and these changes may be related to many factors, including genetic make-up, diet, lifestyle and environmental aspects. Some of these age-related changes are normally associated with ageing. However, in some cases, these changes are exaggerated and may become a disease process, such as in the case of dementia. The waning higher brain functions that should not cause any alarm include:

- a decline in the ability to memorize a large body of information
- reduced semantic skills with age; for example, the ability to name objects quickly (some aspects of language are often well maintained in the elderly, such as vocabulary)
- diminished visual–spatial ability: this is the ability to arrange items in a design or three-dimensional design
- a decline in general intelligence in later years
- changes to sleep, mood, appetite, neuroendocrine functions and motor activity (many of these are possibly the result of reduced synthesis and degradation of neurotransmitters or a reduction in receptors).

Memory

FMRI testing allows for the observation of the brain while the patient is actively pursuing a task. In this way, the location in which brain activity is occurring can be mapped. Recent studies have identified the brain sites that are active during common mental tasks. These tests have revealed a difference between older and younger subjects when they are asked to perform memory tasks or rehearsal and recognition tasks. The younger subjects tended to have more brain activity than older subjects in areas of the extrastriate cortex, medial frontal cortex and the right medial temporal lobe, whereas older subjects tended to display increased activity in the insular cortex, right interior temporal lobe and the right frontal gyrus compared with younger subjects.[12] Changing cortical functions may represent a compensation for cell loss (type of central neuroplasticity) but, in the process, some 'normal' memory loss may occur.

Excessive memory loss may become a disease state. Some common disorders of memory include:

• Amnesia: the loss of memory. It may apply to the loss of memory after a trauma or neurological disease (anterograde amnesia), or to the loss of memory prior to these events (retrograde amnesia).
• Dementia: defined as a symptom complex that includes a decline in cognitive and intellectual abilities sufficient to interfere with social and occupational performance in a patient who is alert and awake.[13]
• Delirium: an acute disturbance of mentation often associated with fluctuating levels of consciousness caused by the effects of illness. Delirium may be reversible if the primary disorder is outside the nervous system and is resolved, or it may be chronic if the disease involves the brain. Delirium may be superimposed upon a condition of existing dementia.
• Alzheimer's disease: a global, progressive and fatal encephalopathy, associated with lesions of the hippocampus, temporal and frontal cortex, consisting of neuritic plaques (senile), neurofibrillary tangles and granulovacular degeneration.[14] There is a decline in cognitive and intellectual abilities which interferes with social and occupational life in a patient who is awake and alert. Changes in personality often occur.

These conditions are discussed in more detail in other chapters.

Neuroendocrine functions

Age-related changes or CNS disease may have a significant effect on the endocrine system. The synchronization of gland functions may undergo age-related changes. The loss of endocrine function may lead to endocrine-deficiency diseases, including hypothyroidism, hypogonadism and diabetes.

Endocrine deficiency states may mimic other age-related changes. They may be non-specific and are therefore easy to misdiagnose, or they may be missed altogether. For example, a patient may present with weight gain, dry skin, constipation, high cholesterol levels and fatigue. The question becomes: is the problem just age-related changes or does the patient have hypothyroidism?

The following changes may occur:

• Hypothalamus and pituitary: These may decrease in size with age. Fibrosis, cysts and reduced vascularity may occur. MRI studies have revealed an empty sella in 19% of older patients.[15]
• Prolactin: This may increase with age (hyperprolactinaemia). This is associated with decreased sex steroid production and reduced libido.
• Thyroid hormone: With ageing there is a decrease in thyroid hormone secretion, which appears to be compensated by a decrease in thyroid hormone clearance. Hyperthyroidism is rare in the elderly, but hypothyroidism is often underdiagnosed since it evolves slowly and resembles age-related changes.

> Hypothyroidism may resemble age-related CNS changes, or comorbid disease such as heart disease, arthritis, presbycusis and depression.[15] Symptoms include:
> – dry skin
> – constipation
> – fatigue
> – muscle weakness
> – imbalance (ataxia)

• Growth hormone: The secretion of growth hormone (GH) declines progressively with age and many age-related changes resemble the changes seen in GH deficiency.[12] These include an increased body fat (especially in the visceral/abdominal area), decreased lean body mass, adverse changes in lipoproteins and a reduction in aerobic capacity. The GH decline may also affect the CNS in profound ways, judging from the improved psychological capabilities attributed to GH therapy in GH-deficient patients.[16,17] Benefits reported include improved memory, mental alertness, motivation and work capacity.

The GH decline with age has led to speculation that replacing the GH or stimulating further GH production and release may be beneficial in normally ageing patients.[18–20] This is a controversial subject at present. Some authors argue that there is no benefit for GH therapy above that of exercise and it may contribute to cancer development.[20] Others experts suggest that it has value in minimizing the health consequences of the ageing process, especially in the oldest and most vulnerable sectors of the population who suffer from frailty-associated disorders and cardiovascular disease.[21] The Growth Hormone Research Society[22] has developed consensus guidelines for the diagnosis and treatment of adult GH deficiency, as well as protocols to assist physicians in such areas as definition and diagnosis, testing methods, contraindications and safety concerns, length of therapeutic trials and the pursuit of non-prescription methods to 'normalize' or enhance GH secretion during the ageing process. This last issue is a hot topic in the battlegrounds of nutritional product sales, and many non-medicinal methods to stimulate GH production are flooding the market.

Cerebral blood flow

Blood flow to the brain is reduced as the arterial walls thicken. The reduction may progress slowly over years, producing a general ischaemic state resulting in a loss of CNS nerve cells (reduced cell count). If blood flow is greatly reduced at any time, there is an acute ischaemic episode, which may include syncope, transient ischaemic attack (TIA), reversible ischaemic neurological deficit (RIND) or an ischaemic stroke.

Cerebrovascular perfusion generally declines by 20–28% between the ages of 30 and 70 years.[6] The decline in flow is greatest in the prefrontal cortex, with grey matter affected more than white matter. Perfusion is directly related to cardiac output. Some seniors who are free of cardiovascular disease have cerebral flow and oxygen consumption similar to a 22–year-old person. However, heart disease, anaemia, vascular disease or impaired cerebral autoregulation can cause transient loss of cerebral perfusion accompanied by symptoms of dizziness, lightheadedness and dysequilibrium

(syncope).[23] These symptoms result from reduced oxygen supply to the brain. Moreover, hypoglycaemia is also a frequent cause of these same general symptoms (see Chapter 12; Diabetes and syndrome X).

It is well understood that reduced blood flow is associated with progressive arteriosclerosis, which is a risk for cerebrovascular disease and stroke. Other risk factors include atrial fibrillation, coronary artery disease, hypertension and diabetes.

Autopsy studies reveal that 60–90% of Alzheimer's patients exhibit cerebrovascular disease.[24] An interesting research question being considered at this time is: is it possible that the same risk factors for cerebrovascular disease are also linked to the risk of developing Alzheimer's disease?[24] If this found to be the case, then a clinical approach to Alzheimer's disease might include an emphasis on dietary prevention or medical management of peripheral vascular disease, owing to its effects on CNS blood flow.

Common diseases of altered cerebral blood flow

Syncope

This refers to the transient loss of consciousness resulting from cerebral ischaemia (faint). Prodromal symptoms may include nausea, sweating, giddiness, swaying, vague headache tinnitus or visual dimming ('greying out') which may last from seconds to minutes prior to the loss of consciousness. Loss of postural tone results in a fall to the ground. During the brief unconscious state (coma) the patient usually maintains control of bowel and bladder, pupils are dilated, pulse is slow, blood pressure and respiration reduced and there is facial pallor ('White as a ghost').

With syncope there is risk of a traumatic fall. Usually the fall is more graceful than the fall seen in epilepsy, but in older patients, who may be physically detrained, the fall may be less than graceful and result in an injury. After the fall to the ground, the loss of consciousness and supine positioning normalize cerebral blood flow within 5–10s, and consciousness is regained as vital function and facial colour return. A convulsive syncope may occurs if the unconsciousness is prolonged for more than 20 s. In this case cortical motor neurons may discharge, causing mild, brief clonic jerking of the limbs, face or jaw, resembling a seizure disorder.

The patterned response of reduced cerebral blood flow may occur with many stimuli, which will be briefly noted here:

- Vasovagal or vasodepressor syncope occurs with a sudden fear, emotion or physical injury that initiates a fight or flight response. Excessive vagal nerve stimulation causes peripheral dilatation to shift blood flow quickly to the musculature, reducing cerebral blood flow and causing syncope.
- Micturition syncope (upon urination) occurs as the voiding of the full bladder causes peripheral vasodilatation, especially in the standing posture.
- Exertional syncope occurs with a valsalva manoeuvre that increases the intrathoracic pressure reducing the vascular return to the heart, thus reducing cardiac output. This is a very common cause of syncope or *presyncope* (bouts of light-headedness) resulting from specific activities. For example, physical lifting or exercise during which the patient holds their breath during a lift, rather than exhaling on exertion, is the equivalent of a self-induced valsalva manoeuvre. In the elderly person, breath-holding during exertion is frequently used to compensate for a weak abdominal musculature. Patients with chronic obstructive lung diseases, spells of pertussis (smoker's cough) or patients with laryngitis may cause a self-induced valsalva during a coughing spell.
- Carotid syncope occurs when one or both of the carotid sinuses are massaged, causing reflex cardiac slowing (bradycardia) or a vasodepressor response. Both result in diminished cerebral perfusion. Massage may stimulate carotid sinus hypersensitivity, or the massage may cause carotid compression on one side while the opposite carotid is diseased with arteriosclerotic plaquing.[6] This is a significant cause of falls in the elderly.[25]

In a study of patients aged over 50 years who received only a 5 s massage to the carotid sinus in either the supine or upright position, 1% experienced possible neurological symptoms.[25] In nine of the 1000 patients in this study, transient neurological complications were experienced, including visual disturbances, sensation of 'pins and needles', a sensation of finger numbness in two cases, leg weakness in one case and a sensation of 'being drunk' in another case. In one of 1000 patients mild weakness of the right hand persisted. These symptoms typically resolved within 24 h.[25]

Syncopal episodes due to carotid sinus hypersensitivity may occur with head turning, wearing a tight collar or shaving. They typically occur while the patient is standing and often cause a sudden fall. It is important for a clinician to be aware that therapeutic massage, trigger point pressure, muscle stripping or deep probing during an examination may initiate some of these untoward symptoms.

Many of the premanipulation cervical vertebrobasilar provocation tests require head and neck placement into a position of maximal extension or rotation (George's protocol, Houle's test, Hautant test, etc.). The positioning is thought to determine whether the vessel is patent, or whether it is compromised in one or both vertebral arteries. However, some older patients may have carotid sinus hypersensitivity that may generate false-positive neurological symptoms or signs. If these tests are used, it is prudent to evaluate the patient's history and risk factors for cerebrovascular disease. The neck should then be auscultated for bruits, after which the clinician should test the brachial blood pressure bilaterally prior to provocation testing.

Carotid sinus hypersensitivity

May be stimulated with:

- manual cervical manipulation with rotation or hand positioning on the anterior cervical triangle
- manual muscle therapies: massage, trigger point therapy or deep examination probing
- neck palpation or examination: thyroid, anterior neck musculature, larynx.

May cause:

- transient syncopal episodes
- residual neurological signs (1:1000)
- possible false-positive findings for cervical vertebrobasilar provocation tests.

Significant history and examination:

- history of arteriosclerosis, falling, fainting, light-headed experiences with looking up, rotations or prolonged end-range positioning, neck surgery, masses
- ask about carotid bruit, sounds (whistling/whooshing, pulsing, throat tugging)
- the order of testing may be significant, and should be as follows:
  - (i) auscultate the neck for bruits
  - (ii) test bilateral brachial blood pressure (evaluate for subclavian steal syndrome)
  - (iii) proceed with provocation testing

Orthostatic hypotension

This occurs when pressure-sensitive receptors in the aortic arch and carotid sinus do not signal adequate vasomotor control via centres in the medulla during changes in posture. In these patients, either prolonged standing or arising quickly may cause reduced cerebral blood flow, which in turn may cause syncopal sensations, staggering or falling. This condition differs from vasovagal syncope by not having the systemic autonomic response causing sweating, pallor or nausea.

In the elderly, orthostatic hypotension occurs after prolonged bed rest or illness, or when a sedentary lifestyle contributes to disuse atrophy and poor muscular tone. The use of vasoactive medication and the presence of diabetic neuropathies, Parkinson's disease, hypothyroidism or anaemia contribute to the condition. The elderly are most vulnerable to this type of syncope since the vascular reflexes are progressively impaired with age.[26]

Orthostatic hypotension is strongly indicated with the characteristic history of weakness or fainting with postural changes. On examination, normally the systolic blood pressure will dip slightly upon rising, while diastolic pressure and heart rate rise slightly to compensate. The diagnosis becomes clear if systolic pressure drops by more than 30 mm Hg and diastolic pressure also drops by 15 mmHg upon rising. If the heart rate remains the same, this may indicate autonomic insufficiency, whereas if it increases, this may indicate a failure of the vascular bed to respond to the autonomic system.[27]

Compounding effects

The elderly patient may have many concurrent conditions. Each condition may lead to light-headedness or syncope, and when two or more are present concurrently the effects of ischaemic cerebral blood flow may be seen earlier, last longer and recur more frequently. Thus, the risk factors for syncope are cumulative.

Common cerebrovascular diseases

Aneurysms

These occur as congenital or Berry aneurysms at the branching points of cerebral arteries. The small aneurysms are insignificant and may remain intact for life, but with progressive weakening they can grow to enormous size (2–3 cm diameter).[6] The most common sites of occurrence are the immediate branch points of the circle of Willis. The incidence of aneurysm is 17 in 100 000 and it is more common in women aged 30–50 years. About 40% of ruptured aneurysms cause death and 50% of the survivors rebleed. Symptoms include: very severe acute headache, often frontal, associated nausea, vomiting, photophobia and prostration (extreme exhaustion). After headache begins there may be progressive loss of consciousness or convulsions, hemiparesis, cranial nerve palsies, knuckle rigidity, increased intracranial pressure (papilloedema) and subhyaloid haemorrhage. Differential diagnosis includes migraine and meningitis. Medical treatment is directed towards controlling cerebral oedema, recurrent bleeding and secondary infarction.

Vertebral artery dissecting aneurysm

This is the separation of the tuncia intima from the tunica media with blood entering the separation between the two layers. The separation or aneurysm may progressively tear in a cephalad direction to involve the intracranial portions of the vertebral artery.

Stroke

Stroke is a syndrome characterized by the sudden onset of CNS dysfunction due to cerebrovascular disease (see Table 11.6). It may result from either ischaemia (ischaemic strokes: 80% of cases) or haemorrhage (haemorrhagic strokes: 20% of cases) in brain tissue.

Ischaemic stroke

Factors contributing to ischaemic stroke are listed in Table 11.7. As the blood flow to any part of the cerebral cortex is reduced there will be impairment of brain tissue in the vascular territory of the artery. If the circulation is restored quickly (5–10 min) the ischaemic tissue will recover without permanent damage (reversible ischaemia). With prolonged ischaemia severe permanent damage will occur (irreversible ischaemia).

Reversible ischemia

TIAs are episodes of localized cerebrovascular dysfunction that are completely reversible within 24 h. In most cases they last less than 30 min. Symptoms are specifically localized depending upon whether the anterior–carotid circulation or the posterior–vertebrobasilar circulation is involved.

RIND refers to ischaemic neurological changes that last for more than 24 h with complete or nearly complete recovery.

Table 11.6 Cerebrovascular and vertebrobasilar stroke/ischaemia

Cardiac abnormalities
Cardiac dysrhythmias
Cardiac arrest
Cardiac outflow obstruction (aortic or pulmonary stenosis)
Impaired circulation
Severe muscle wasting
Varicose veins
Prolonged bed rest
Medications: antihypertensives, diuretics, phenothiazines, nitrates
Postsympathectomy operations
Adrenal cortical insufficiency
Orthostatic hypotension (primary)
Reduced brain metabolism
Hypoglycaemia
Anaemia
Hypoxia
Other causes
Hyperventilation
Chronic cough
Lung diseases

Irreversible ischaemia

Stroke-in-progress refers to the slow presentation of an ischaemic stroke over hours or days. The delay in a complete stroke picture may be due to patient compensations (rest, little exertional stress, etc.), vascular shunting or partial healing (partial resolution of the clot).

Complete stroke or cerebral infarction is a permanent neurological injury causing a deficit or death. The affected brain tissue may vary from a small area of necrosis in a non-strategic location of the cortex to a massive lesion with oedema of the cerebral hemispheres. Small lesions may not be detected with routine clinical examinations unless this occur in an important area (e.g. internal capsule). Large lesions will produce deficits that are debilitating or cause death.

Vertebrobasilar stroke/ischaemia is an ischaemic episode occurring in one or both vertebral arteries or the basilar artery.

Pathophysiology of stroke

Ischaemia sets biochemical changes in motion that persist long after the period of ischaemia. These include the release of superoxide radicals, influx of calcium and changes in neurotransmitters, all of which play a role in cell death.

In irreversible brain damage, cells undergo autolysis with a build-up of lactic acid, creatine phosphokinase (CPK) and other products that are released into the blood and cerebrospinal fluid (CSF). The brain becomes soft, demarcations between white and grey matter become vague, and venous haemorrhage develops.

Oedema in the infarcted area is a serious and often life-threatening concern since it contributes to more neurological dysfunction and can lead to herniation of brain tissue and eventually to death. The resolution of oedema within 2 weeks after a severe infarction is an important factor in the patient's recovery and prognosis.

The senses

Smell (olfaction)

Olfactory sense plays a significant role in the perception of foods, odours and air quality. It shares two significant roles with the sense of taste: initiating digestion and having an environmental protective role for sensing noxious substances before ingestion (e.g. spoiled food and poisons).

The olfactory bulb, like other parts of the cerebral cortex, shows evidence of age-related neuron loss. The loss of smell occurs more frequently than that of taste since olfaction has only a single nerve tract (compared with taste which has three nerves) and therefore is more likely to show the effects of nerve cell loss. Four

Table 11.7 Causes and contributory factors of ischaemic stroke

Atherosclerosis	Factors contributing to atherosclerosis include: age (over 40), hypertension, diabetes and smoking
Cardiac emboli	Associated with rheumatic heart valve disease, mural thrombus or mitral valve prolapse
Inflammatory disorders	Such conditions as giant cell arteritis and systemic lupus erythematosus
Lacunar infarction	Result from longstanding hypertension, atherosclerosis or degenerative changes of arterial walls
Migraine	Stroke is a rare complication of migraine headaches
Cardiac disorders	Myocardial infarction, rheumatic heart disease, arrhythmias, endocarditis and mitral valve pro lapse may produce emboli
Haematological disorders	Sickle cell disease and polycythaemia can contribute to cerebral thrombosis

Table 11.8 Common olfactory problems[28]

Peripheral problems affecting smell	Central diseases affecting smell
Viral insult	Multi-infarct dementia
Exposure to toxic fumes	Alzheimer's disease
Head trauma	Parkinson's disease
Calcification of the cribriform plate	Huntingtons' chorea

common odours that become more difficult to identify with age include: coal tar, oil of almonds, oil of peppermint and coffee.[5] The neural structures necessary for smell include the olfactory epithelium, olfactory nerves, olfactory bulb and tract, medial dorsal nucleus of the thalamus, orbitofrontal cortex and the olfactory cortex (to name but a few of the many central connections).

In many elderly patients the loss olfaction results from a multitude of peripheral or central causes. Clinicians generally understand that peripheral problems impact the transduction of stimuli within the nasal mucosa or the peripheral olfactory fibres to the mucosa, identified as a difficulty in the threshold of smell. Conversely, lesions affecting central olfactory networks are identified as the inability to identify specific odours or to compare odours. This simple peripheral–central view has recently been questioned (28). Some experts believe that the olfactory pathways are simply selectively vulnerable to destruction by various disease processes. An interesting theory is that environmental agents that are related to the aetiology of the disease may pass into the CNS through the highly active transport systems of the olfactory receptors. Common olfactory problems are listed in Table 11.8.[28]

Do human pheromones exist?

Volatile pheromones are significant triggers for reproductive behaviour in many animal species. The physiology of pheromome perception requires a vomernasal organ and an accessory olfactory system. The belief that humans lacked a vomernasal organ has been recently questioned and has fuelled the search for human pheromones.[29] They have not been identified to date, but commercial researchers continue to search.

Taste (gustation)

Food intake declines in the elderly and they frequently report having a poor appetite. The changes in the sense of taste may account for part of the poor appetite. Taste involves the perception of sweet, sour, bitter and salt. Poor appetite may also result from a reduced sensory-specific satiety (decreased pleasantness of food as it is consumed)[30] (Table 11.9).

Neural circuits that mediate taste include the cranial nerves VII, IX and X, the solitary nucleus in the brainstem, the ventroposteromedial nucleus of the thalamus and the insularopercular cortex.[31] Since three different nerves convey taste information to the brain, it is rare for patients to have a complete loss of taste (ageusia).

From childhood to the age of 80 years there may be as much as a 70% reduction in the number of taste buds as a result of the progressive degeneration of taste papillae. This loss of taste is exacerbated by a concurrent loss of saliva flow and reduced amylase content (the enzyme that hydrolyses starch). Age-related impairment of taste sensation has an insidious effect on the health of the person. The clinical impact ranges from reduced eating pleasure, to reduced perception of bitter and saltiness, to a slowing of the protective reflexes associated with the accidental ingestion of substances.

There has been considerable research into the development of the swallowing mechanism, from the time when swallowing develops *in utero* to the senior years. Normal ageing does not by itself appear to impair swallowing, in spite of reduced oropharyngeal muscular tension, speed of responses, taste sensitivity and smell, but the duration of swallowing and oesophageal motility do slow with age.[32] Oropharyngeal dysphagia (difficult symptomatic swallowing) should be viewed as a specific result of pathological disease and not as a sign of normal ageing.

Smoking has been reported to reduce the taste of food, making flavoursome foods taste flat, while simple tongue brushing can increase taste sensation in the geriatric patient.[33] Other suggestions for patients with diminished taste include the enhancement of food flavours using herbs, spices or monosodium glutamate (MSG),[34] provided the patient does not experience any MSG side-effects such as headache.

Table 11.9 Taste changes with age and side effects

Reduced pleasure in eating	Loss of interest in food
	Weight loss
	Anorexia
	Malnutrition
	Unbalanced food habits contributing to chronic disease
Reduced sense of sweetness and saltiness	Often leads to excessive consumption of refined foods
	Overuse of added sugar and salt
Dietary focus on softer foods leads to reduced mastication (chewing)	Osteopenia of the mandible
Diminished taste with reduced taste reflex reactions	Slower reflex rejection of accidental ingestion of drugs, household cleaners, etc.
	Poorer co-ordination of deglutition (swallowing), (e.g. of pills or poorly chewed food, may contribute to choking, aspiration or regurgitation

Nutritional utilization

Good nutrition is essential for the maintenance of body systems, especially the CNS. Malnutrition presenting as undernutrition or obesity presents a health liability that may contribute to chronic fatigue, disease, poor quality of life and lowered resistance to infections.

The prevalence of protein-energy malnutrition has been estimated by Mion et al.[35] as occurring in 15% of community-dwelling seniors, 5–12% of homebound seniors, 20% to 65% of hospitalized patients and 5–85% of institutionalized seniors.[35] In protein-energy malnutrition there is depletion of lean body mass and adipose tissue, weight loss and diminishing gastrointestinal functions, resulting in the poor distribution and reduced perfusion of a nutrient-deficient state. Reduced glucose and other essential nutrients may affect brain functions.

Alcohol stimulates the hypothalamic–pituitary–adrenal (HPA) axis, stimulating the secretion of stress hormones (glucocorticoids), with resulting premature and/or exaggerated ageing.[36] The older person may also be more susceptible to the effects of alcohol, that is less tolerant of it effects, and suffer more adverse consequences, including falls, fracture, subdural haematoma, anaemia, gastritis, liver disease, pancreatitis, alcoholic amnesic syndrome and dementia.

Many amino acids and vitamins are precursors for neurotransmitters. Their deficiencies and role in dementias are considered important, but their specific effects in the prevention or treatment of dementias, especially Alzheimer's disease, are uncertain.[37] The control of blood pressure and other nutritional factors may have a more direct role for multi-infarct dementia. Table 11.10 lists the significant nutrients for neurotransmitter production. Deficiencies may lead to an acceleration of age-related changes or may enhance other disease processes.

Vitamin E, ginkgo biloba and other nutrients are being researched as possible modulators of the development or progress of dementia. Deficiencies in three significant vitamins, folate (folic acid), vitamin B_{12} and vitamin B_6, are frequently associated with neurological disease of the young and pregnant patients, and also proving to be significant for the elderly.

Table 10 Essential requirements for central nervous system neurotransmitters[37]

Amino acids	Vitamins
Tyrosine	Vitamin A
Tryptophan	Vitamin B_6
Threonine	Vitamin B_{12}
Histidine	Thiamin
Choline	Niacin
	Riboflavin
	Vitamin C
	Vitamin D
	Vitamin E
	Folic acid

Folate [recommended dietary allowance (RDA) 200 μg in men, 150 μg in women)]

Folate deficiency anaemia resulting from deficiency or a drug deficiency is most frequently seen in the elderly.[38] Low folate levels are associated with increased plasma homocysteine levels (a risk factor for coronary heart disease) and peripheral neuropathy, and may be important for the regulation of mood or preventing depression.[39] Marginal deficiencies have been detected in patients with depressive disorders; therefore, supplementation in patients receiving antidepressant therapy may aid the treatment outcome.

Sources of folate include green leafy vegetables, orange juice, grain products and fortified cereals, with the highest concentrations in spinach, liver and yeast extract. It is lost from food during cooking, leached out with boiling and is otherwise degraded with light, heat and air.

Vitamin B_{12} (RDA 2 μg in elderly men, 1.6 μg in elderly women)

Vitamin B_{12} deficiency is commonly associated with peripheral neuropathy, as well as dementia and cognitive impairment. It is reported to be present in up to 15% of the elderly because of a loss of intrinsic factor, which aids its absorption, and malabsorption of food cobalamine.[40] Malabsorption may result from achlorhydria, gastric atrophy, bacterial overgrowth and stomach infection with Helicobacter pylori. Grains and cereals are often fortified with vitamin B_{12}. Intramuscular injections are routinely used when patients present with signs of anaemia or malnourishment.

Vitamin B_6 (RDA 2 mg in men, 1.6 mg in women)

Vitamin B_6 is a cofactor in the production of several essential neurotransmitters. Deficiency is associated with peripheral neuropathy and convulsions. In one study, the prevalence of vitamin B_6 deficiency was found to be over 23% among elderly men and women.[41] Diminished levels have been associated with reduced lymphocyte proliferation, impaired interleukin-2 production and high homocysteine.[42]

Vision

Visual acuity

In a population-based study, the rate of visual impairment in 80-year-old people was 15–30 times that in 40–50 year olds.[42] It is estimated 13% of people aged over 85 years are blind, and 50% of blind Americans are over the age of 65 years.[41]

The visual system undergoes significant losses beginning in the mid-forties and almost 90% of people require visual aids by the sixth decade.[41] These

Table 11.11 Structural changes in the visual system affecting vision[6]

Changes	Effects
Loss of retro-orbital fat pad	Results in recession of eyes
Loss of elastic tissue of brow and upper lid	Leads to ptosis
	Reduced upper visual field
Loss of elastic tissue of lower lid	Leads to lower lid sagging with tearing eyes (poor siphoning of tears via the punctum)
Reduced tear production	Causes dry eyes
Cornea becomes more spherical	Development of astigmatism
Thinning of cornea and conjunctiva with loss of endothelium	Leads to corneal oedema and hazing
Anterior chamber of eye becomes shallower	May contribute to an acute angle closure glaucoma (during dilation)
Iris fibrous structure changes leading to small, fixed pupils	Impairs light transmission
Aqueous humour develops yellow autofluorescent pigmentation	Contributes to blue–green confusion
Lens develops opacities	Reduces light transmission
Loss of flexibility of lens	Loss of accommodation for near vision (presbyopia)
Central cells of lens lose cellular identity	Central lens becomes crystalline and micro-opacities develop
Outer lens continues to grow with new cells on the surface of the lens	Contributes to increased intraocular pressure
Ciliary muscle weakens	Reduced speed of accommodation

changes result from changes to the neurological and non-neurological structures of the eye. The neurological structures include the retina and optic nerve, which change in the sixth decade, whereas the non-neurological structures (muscles, shape of eye ball, cornea) begin to change earlier, between the ages of 35–45[43](Table 11.11).

Age effects on visual processing

Visual–spatial abilities such as drawing a three-dimensional figure or arranging blocks, are impaired in older patients. There is some evidence that age-related reorganization of cortical activation occurs.[44] In one study, subjects were shown visual patterns while undergoing positron emission tomography (PET) to study where the blood flow was enhanced during the visual process. Young subjects tended to activate the occipitotemporal pathway, whereas older subjects activated occipital and frontal regions. Other aspects of the visual system will impact on the processing speed in the elderly, as summarized in Table 11.12.

Cataracts

With age, the lens of the eye becomes harder, thicker, less flexible and more yellow. The yellow causes blue–green wavelengths to be absorbed, resulting in more difficulty with colour discrimination, and more illumination is required in order to read.[46]

The exact reasons for the development of a cataract are not completely understood. It is thought that the lens may become overhydrated, with the nuclear proteins clustering together to form densities (opacifications). The changes may be initiated or promoted by photo-oxidative damage.[47] Other causes of cataracts have been identified. These include: blunt trauma, electrical shock, ionizing radiation, large osmotic shifts of fluid balance, diabetes mellitus and many drugs (e.g. long-term use of corticosteroids).

Table 11.12 Visual changes with age[45]

Visual speed of procession	Reading speed is slower
Light sensitivity	Significant loss of twilight and darkness vision
Dynamic vision	Watching moving objects becomes difficult and slower
Near vision	Difficulty with small print
Speed of searching	Difficulty in finding an object quickly in a complex view

Clinically, patients with cataracts gradually find that their visual acuity declines, and they experience more difficulty in bright light due to glare. The increased myopia allows them to read without glasses, or they may require new glasses, and spoke-shaped opacities may be seen upon examination of the eye. Non-surgical management of cataracts includes eyeglass correction. Cataract surgery may involve the use of intraocular lens implants with reported visual acuity improvements to 20/40 or better.[48]

The lens has high concentrations of glutathione and ascorbic acid (antioxidants) which decrease with age.[47] Poor nutrition and deficiencies of trace minerals have caused cataracts in animals, but the association with diet and the value of supplementation remain uncertain.

Presbyopia

Clinically, the most frequent visual problem in the elderly is the inability to focus on items too close to the eye (presbyopia). This causes them to read printed text at arms' length from the eye. The presbyopic changes have been shown to occur most rapidly in the fourth decade. In one large sample of 3645 patient reports, presbyopic additions during the ages 40–50 years were approximately 0.25 dioptres per 2 years. After the age of 50 years, the change increased more slowly at a rate of 0.25 dioptres in 8 years.[49]

The clinical approach to this visual acuity difficulty is with a prescription for corrective lenses. Other simple suggestions for coping with presbyopia include:

- bright light for reading
- hand magnifiers
- avoiding glare
- yellow lenses for night driving
- tinted or ultraviolet lenses to reduce daytime glare
- Large-print computer screens or texts.

Glaucoma

Glaucoma is increased intraocular pressure that is too high for the health of the optic nerve. If pressure is prolonged nerve atrophy and visual loss will occur. Therefore, early detection and treatment are essential to limit the visual loss. Glaucoma is the second most common cause of blindness in the older population. Unfortunately, the prevalence of glaucoma increases with age and nearly half of the patients diagnosed are not aware of symptoms.[50]

Certain patients are more susceptible to glaucoma. The risk factors include: high intraocular pressure, black race (1 in 10 elderly blacks versus 1 in 50 elderly whites), old age, family history, myopia, high hyperopia (extreme farsightedness), diabetes and vascular disease.[50] There are two types of glaucoma: acute angle-closure glaucoma and open-angle glaucoma.

Acute angle-closure glaucoma only occurs in 0.1% of patients over the age of 40 years, and most frequently between the age of 50 and 70 years in patients who are highly hyperopic.[50] In this condition the iris makes excessive contact with the lateral margins of the cornea and the anterior chamber is narrow. The rapid rise in intraorbital pressure leads to severe unilateral eye pain (less than 5% are bilateral) with an oedematous cornea and blurred vision with halos or rainbows around lights. This condition may be misdiagnosed as acute sinus pain, migraine or cluster headache. It requires immediate ophthalmological referral.

Open-angle glaucoma accounts for 70% of glaucoma cases. It has no mechanical obstruction at the anterior chamber angle (cornea–iris angle) and the intraocular pressure may or may not be elevated above the norm (21 mmHg).[15] The condition is painless without a feeling of pressure, even when the intraocular pressure is increased, because it has developed very slowly. Visual field loss occurs in the peripheral vision and paracentral visual fields. Examination may reveal variation in the thickness of the disc rim, notches, cupping or splinter haemorrhages.

The ophthalmoscopic examination is often difficult in the older patient because of smaller pupil size. It is always comforting to the primary contact clinician to know that the patient has had a recent ophthalmological examination, where the specialized tests of tonometry (intraocular pressure test), gonioscopy (examination of the anterior chamber) and a dilated fundus (examination of the retina) are used. Periodic ophthalmological examination is recommended for patients with high risk (positive family history, black race, severe myopia or diabetes of at least 5 years' duration).[51]

The initial glaucoma treatment focuses upon the reduction of intraocular pressure with medications. Many of these medications are applied as drops to the eye, which drain to the nasopharynx and may have systemic side-effects. The clinician should be aware of these effects since they may present confusing symptoms for other concurrent conditions.

The clinician should consult the Compendium of Pharmaceutical Supply Co. (CPS) for specific concerns any one medication type.
This list is offered since patients may not realize that a few eye drops may have systemic effects.

Bradycardia
Depression
Exacerbation of COPD/asthma
Impotence
Dry mouth
Fatigue
Hypertension
Cardiac dysrhythmias
Lethargy
Anorexia
Paraesthesia
Blood dyscrasias

Some surgical therapies are available (laser, direct surgery) which attempt to open the cornea–iris angle or create a hole to the posterior chamber to prevent the anterior chamber from developing increased pressure.

Retinal detachment occurs in 1:10 000 people, and most frequently in patients over 50 years. It is a tear or hole in the retina and may occur after cataract surgery, after trauma or in patients with myopia.[51] The separation occurs between the neural layer and the pigmented layer. The tear allows liquified vitreous to enter the subretinal space. Symptoms include prodromal light flashes in 50% of cases, progressing to a visual field defect, perception of a curve in a straight line or loss of central vision if the macula is detached. The earliest sign is elevation of the retinal area so that it is out of focus, arteries and veins in the separate area appear almost black, and the separated area may have wrinkles.[51]

Surgical management include: laser coagulation when subretinal fluid has not accumulated, scleral buckling when subretinal fluid is present; in more complex cases direct surgery is necessary (transplanar vitrectomy).

Diabetic retinopathy (or maculopathy) is most frequently seen in patients with poor diabetic control over 50 years of age and after 10–15 years of type II diabetes mellitus (15). Early signs include microaneurysms, retinal haemorrhage (dot or blot), cotton-wool spots and venous beading. There is also a risk for developing retinopathy or maculopathy. Loss of vision is usually due to macular oedema, which reduces the retinal neural activity in the affected areas, although visual loss may also occur in a retina free of abnormalities.[52]

Early treatment of diabetic retinopathy is effective, but is dependent upon early detection and initiation of treatment in the presymptomatic stage. Therefore, regular screening of patients is advocated. Recent screening techniques involve digital camera photographic evaluation of the retina, which appears to be more specific and sensitive than hand-held ophthalmoscopy.[53]

Giant cell arteritis is a granulomatous inflammatory disease of the arteries of the external carotid system causing a thrombosis within the most affected artery.[6] Inflammation and occlusion of one or both ophthalmic arteries will result in visual loss or blindness (25% of patients). Patients may have other symptoms, including weight loss, malaise, headache, jaw claudication and muscle weakness. Treatment of choice is with a high dosage of anti-inflammatories (steroids). Patients suspected of having this condition require immediate ophthalmological referral.

Retinal vascular occlusions occur most frequently in patients aged over 60 years with associated systemic conditions including diabetes, systemic hypertension, arteriosclerosis and blood dyscrasias.[6] Retinal vein occlusions (branch or central veins) present with a loss of central vision (macular oedema) or visual field defects, and an ophthalmological view of haemorrhage, retinal oedema and cotton-wool spots.

Retinal artery occlusion presents with white oedematous infarction of the retina with sudden, severe painless loss of vision. Blockage of a retinal branch artery causes a field defect, whereas a central artery occlusion affects the whole retina. Thromboembolic phenomena such as cholesterol emboli from carotid arteries, platelet–fibrin emboli from arteriosclerotic plaques or calcific emboli from cardiac valves are often the cause.[15] Embolic diseases of the brain (stroke, transient ischaemic attack) or the heart (angina, myocardial infarction) are often associated.

The sudden onset of visual loss usually draws the patient to a hospital for evaluation, but senior patients may instead choose bed rest, as some patients erroneously assume that they will be fine in the morning. Immediate treatment is necessary to ensure the preservation of visual acuity, but even with treatment the prognosis is often poor.[6]

Hearing

In terms of function, hearing appears to exhibit more variation than other biological systems. It peaks at the age of 10 years, as opposed to 25 years as is the case for most other physiological functions. Noticeable changes may be seen in the third or fourth decade, followed by the loss of high-pitched sounds (14–20 kHz) in the senior years.[6] The decline in the higher frequencies may be detected with audiometric testing. The reduction in hearing may be 40–50 dB for frequencies higher than 1000 Hz.

The tones of normal speech frequency are only slightly affected, but the loss of speech perception is often profound. This may result from a decline in central procession. The reaction times for hearing are slower, with poorer sound localization, which suggests changes to central perception processing.

The age-related changes of central auditory neural circuits in the inferior colliculus have revealed a reduction in GABA neurons, GABA concentrations, receptors and glutamic decarboxylase activity.[54] These changes may represent central changes of auditory sensitivity, cell loss or progressive deafferentation. The hearing reduction occurs with non-neurological factors as well as changes in the cochlea and auditory pathway.

The auditory reflexes become slower, with atrophy occurring within the auditor pathways which may contribute to confusion in sound localization and communication within a group or with extraneous noise. Biaural performance (listening with both ears) is often degraded in the elderly as a result of poor temporal coding in addition to audiometric sensitivity.[55] This would account for more difficulty in speech recognition with competing noise.

Structural changes in the auditory system affecting hearing are shown in Table 11.13.

Presbycusis (age-related hearing loss) occurs in nearly all people in their senior years for a number of reasons. Most cases result from cochlear hair cell degeneration and are well managed with the fitting of a hearing aid for sound amplification. Severe hearing loss is generally due to cochlear disease or other disease of the auditory pathways. These may require lip-reading training, assistive listening devices or, in some cases, cochlear implants.

The impact of presbycusis may seriously impact the patient's social communications and contribute to

Table 11.13 Structural changes in the auditory system affecting hearing: age-related hearing loss (presbycusis)

Non-neurological	Effects
Pinna size increases, with decreased flexibility	
Loss of elasticity of external auditory meatus, becoming narrower	Reduced sound conduction
Reduced, drier cerumen often accumulating	Reduced sound conduction
More rigid or thickened (although more translucent) tympanic membrane	
Stiffening of ear ossicles with ligament and articulation degeneration	Reduced sound conduction
Atrophy of inner ear muscles: tensor and levator veli palatini, salpingopharyngeal muscles	Loss of middle ear equalization or drainage
Stiffening of basilar and Reisner's membrane	Reduced sound-wave transduction
Atrophy of the blood vessels (stria vascularis)	Reduced flow to inner ear
	Reduced endolymph formation
Neurological	
Loss of hair cells and supporting cells of the organ of Corti	Reduced sound transduction
Loss of ganglion cells and auditory nerve fibre	Reduced sound transmission
	May be associated with extraneous sound generation (tinnitus)
Loss of neurons of temporal gyrus or parietal association areas	Reduced sound perception

social isolation from family and friends, introversion, depression and possibly dementia. An early referral for an audiogram will initiate an accurate diagnosis and treatment alternatives for the older person with hearing problems

Hearing aids are an unfortunate reality. Many patients feel that they do not have as bad a problem as others would have them think. Many patients with significant hearing loss choose not to wear them and may even deny that they need them.

Vestibular function

Dizziness is another common complaint in geriatric medicine. In chiropractic practices, as reported in the Canadian NBCE Job Analysis Study (1993),[2] the complaint is seen as frequently as one or two cases per month.

The vestibular system is concerned with balance, postural reflexes and eye motions. The labyrinth is made up of two otolith organs, the utricle and the sacculus, together with the ampullae located in the three semicircular canals. The otoliths function to convey information on static head positioning and linear acceleration motion. The semicircular canals convey more information on rotational acceleration of the head. These organs project to brainstem oculomotor nuclei via the vestibular portion of cranial nerve VIII, then to the thalamus, cerebellum and sensory cortex.

Disruption to the vestibular system results in the perception of dizziness, vertigo, nausea, unsteadiness and nystagmus. Disease of the labyrinth gives rise to peripheral symptoms which involve more severe intermittent vertigo, nystagmus and often hearing symptoms (loss or tinnitus). Disease of the brainstem gives rise to more constant central symptoms of less severe vertigo, nystagmus and, rarely, hearing loss. Only the common peripheral diseases will be briefly described in this chapter, and the central aetiologies are listed in Table 11.14.

Unilateral vestibular hypofunction (UVH) is a common vestibular dysfunction in the senior population.[56] The effect arises from a disturbed vestibulospinal reflex inducing various degrees of postural sway, dysequilibrium or falls depending upon the person's ability to compensate with visual and proprioceptive cueing.

Benign positional vertigo (BPV) is the sensation of vertigo only when the head is turned in a specific manner or when the head is in a certain position. The patient will describe vertigo sensations when they lie

Table 11.14 Diseases of the elderly commonly presenting with vertigo or ataxia

Acute conditions	Chronic conditions
Drug intoxications	Multiple sclerosis
Wernicke's encephalopathy	Alcoholic cerebellar
Vertebrobasilar ischaemia or	degeneration
infarction	Posterior fossa tumours
Cerebral Haemorrhage	Friedreich's ataxia
Inflammatory disorders	
(Viral or bacterial)	

down, turning in bed, shoulder-checking while driving, or an odd combination of neck motions. The patient learns to avoid these offending positions.

This condition is the most common cause of peripheral vertigo, with a mean age of occurrence of 54 years (range 11–84 years)[57] and, in one study, the incidence was 107 cases per 100 000 per year.[58] BPV accounts for 30% of vertigo complaints. No cause is usually identified, but it commonly occurs after head trauma, such as in patients with whiplash-associated disorders (WAD)[59] or after a recent infection of the vestibular structure causing debris (otolith crystals) to fall into the posterior semicircular canal.[60]

The syndrome is characterized by brief episodes (seconds to minutes) of severe vertigo, which may be accompanied by nausea and vomiting, with specific head positioning. Lying on the side with the affected ear down is often the most irritating position. Hearing loss is not common. The Nylon–Baran test or Halpike manoeuvre is used to duplicate the patient's symptoms. Medical therapy is directed towards the suppression of the symptoms by various drugs. Other treatment options include specific exercises that attempt to fatigue the stimulus, or the repositioning of the otolith or debris with the modified Epley manoeuvre or the Semont manoeuvre.[61] In some patients the episodic vertigo may resolve within a few months, whereas in others it is recurrent (see Chapter 14).

Cervical vertigo refers to a syndrome characterized by vertiginous feelings or a woozy feeling, tinnitus and diminished neck mobility. These symptoms are usually triggered by neck motion. Dysfunctional joint positioning and injury to cervical vertebral structures (myofascial structures, nerves and blood vessels) are important causes of the impairment to cervical proprioceptive input to the brainstem.

The differentiation between vestibular vertigo and cervical vertigo can be established with the pivot-chair test.[62] The seated patient experiences symptoms of body rotation while the head is held stabilized. Treatment of the cervicothoracic spine is aimed at reducing joint dysfunction and vertebral neuromuscular–proprioceptive integrity with spinal manipulation, physical therapy and exercise. The upper cervical spine appears to be the most significant focus of therapy, owing to the large range of motion, importance of the neck-righting reflexes and the path of the vertebral artery in this area.

Ménière's disease is characterized by repeated episodes of vertigo (minutes to days) associated with tinnitus and progressive hearing loss. Hearing loss progresses with each episode of vertigo. These symptoms are unilateral in 90% of cases, and may last for 4–8 h. Men are affected more than women, between 20 and 50 years of age.[6] There an increased volume of labyrinthine endolymph, but the exact aetiology is often unknown.

At the time of the first acute attack the patient may have noticed the slow onset of tinnitus, hearing loss and a sensation of fullness in the ear. Caloric testing (cold or warm irrigation of the outer ear to observe nystagmus) usually reveals impaired vestibular function.

Acute attacks involve vertigo, nausea and vomiting, which may occur at intervals of weeks to years. Tinnitus is often only a minor annoyance and may not be mentioned initially.

In more severe attacks the autonomic symptoms intensify (pallor, sweating, and increased nausea) and are associated with vertigo, nausea, vomiting and tinnitus. At times the onset of the recurrent attacks is preceded by an aura (fullness in the ear, increased tinnitus or further hearing loss). Some attacks may start only with a sudden sense of vertigo. Nystagmus is present only during the acute attack of vertigo, and is absent between bouts. The episodes of vertigo diminish as hearing loss progresses. Therapies include medications similar to those for benign positional vertigo and a variety of surgical procedures for the removal of endolymph. Spinal manipulation and traction have been used where there is mechanical and osteoarthritic irritation localized to the cervical vertebrae, resulting in autonomic otovestibular disorder.

Central vestibular and cerebellar disorders

Many conditions can cause disequilibrium at the brainstem level by affecting the tracts or nuclei involved with the integration of visual, labyrinthine or proprioceptive functions. Table 11.14 lists the more common acute and chronic conditions that affect the elderly.

Balance

In Canada each year 30% of all persons over the age of 65 and 50% of all persons over the age of 80 years fall. In one province of Canada, Ontario, 23 7000 persons aged 65 and over seek hospital care for falling each year. They are hospitalized for an average stay of 17 days, more than two-thirds will fall for a second time within 6 months, and the risk of death from the fall may be between 15 and 50%.[63] (see also Chapter 14).

These statistics emphasize the importance of balance evaluation and treatment for the elderly patient. The chiropractor is one of the best suited professionals to evaluate the elderly for this function, since chiropractors tend to see their patients more frequently than other health practitioners, they are skilled in the assessment of the three component systems subserving balance, and they have the hands-on skills to treat patients in the office with low-technology, cost-effective procedures.

The ability to maintain body position over a base of support is static balance[64] (station), whereas the ability to move in a weight-bearing posture without falling is dynamic balance (gait).[56]

Static balance

Static balance, also referred to as steadiness, is the ability to control postural sway in stationary standing and is easily measured as a change in the centre of pressure (force) under the feet (base of support). In quiet standing the amplitude and frequency of postural sway are greater in the older person[65] and greater in women than in men.[66] Sway is increased if the eyes are closed, during an attention-demanding activity (e.g. arithmetic problem) or during a physical activity (maximum grip strength)[67] and the recovery from perturbations is slower. Thus, postural balance and stability require more conscious awareness in elderly than in young persons as a result of diminished feedback and neuromuscular integration.

Postural sway and the evaluation of postural balance are significant for the older patient because of the correlation with the risk of falling.[68] Two simple tests of static balance are described in Table 11.15.

Table 11.15 Clinical tests of static balance[64]

Rhomberg	Stand with feet together (small base of support) Eyes open: visual cueing Eyes closed: labyrinthine and proprioception problems will be magnified
One-leg stance ('stork' stand)	Stand on one leg (10 s) Many seniors have difficulty with this test. It may be clinically important just to note the difference between right and left

Dynamic balance

Dynamic balance, also referred to as dynamic stability, is the ability to react to perturbations of stability using internal and external cues. With body movements the centre of gravity for the body moves over the base of support during motor activities (such as gait, reaching, pushing and pulling). Dynamic balance is also required during the transition from one posture to another (i.e. sitting to standing, lying to sitting, etc.). During transitions the centre of gravity must be controlled during the shift from one base of support to another.

In a study comparing balance on a moving platform, comprising 53 subjects aged 17–89 years), ageing was associated with reduced head stabilization and a stronger coupling between head motion and hip motion.[69] With ageing the centre of pressure does not approach the edges of the base of support. The older patients appear not to lean too far to one side or the other, and they maintain more stiffness within their axial skeleton. There are many tests in the literature to help to assess dynamic stability, and two simple functional tests are described in Table 11.16.

Table 11.16 Clinical test of dynamic stability

Functional reach test[70]	The functional reach is the maximum distance a person can reach forward beyond the length of their arm while standing still
Get up and go[63,70]	The patient is asked to stand up from a seat, walk 3 m, turn around and sit down

Symmetry

Symmetry is described as the equal distribution of weight among the weight-bearing pressure points of one's body.[68] The location of pressure points and the number of pressure points may vary with a person's posture, but will always relate to the balance of body mass over the gravitational pull. Examples include the buttocks in stable sitting, the feet in a standing posture, or the knees and hands in the quadruped position.

Patient symmetry is evaluated during a postural examination of the body and with the specific orthopaedic evaluation of the musculoskeletal system. During a physical examination, the contour, size and range of motion are compared from one side to the other in search of structural imbalance.

The spinal cord and the ageing spinal column

Osteoarthritis

Osteoarthritis (OA) is a common chronic disease of the elderly that often results in significant physical disability. It affects approximately 80% of adults over the age of 65, and women more than men.[71] It is classified as primary when no clear underlying aetiology is present and secondary when a mechanical, infective or metabolic cause can be identified. There are many secondary causes of OA, such as the diseases frequently found in the elderly, including infection, gout, rheumatoid arthritis, Paget's disease and metabolic bone disorders. These will not be discussed in this chapter but are significant in their own way because they cause secondary neurological disease.

OA is often described as 'wear and tear' changes to the joints, where the effects of the wearing out are faster than the reparative phases. As it develops, cartilage that normally covers bone, reducing the friction or absorbing shock, begins to crack and wear away, eventually exposing the body surfaces to each other at the joints. The joint capsule, ligaments, tendons and muscles begin to change in texture and suppleness, contributing to joint stiffness. Eventually the joints begin to form osteophytic spurs, abnormal thicknesses or fluid-filled pockets (cysts). During this progressive degenerative process, joint pain due to inflammation may be experienced periodically or chronically.

Degenerative disc disease

This is the progressive thinning, dehydration and altered biomechanics associated with repetitive injury or ageing. Over time, the central portion of the disc (nucleus) begins to tear through the rings of the fibrous layers of the disc (annulus), resulting in disc derangement, disc bulge, disc protrusion or herniation. New bone growth (osteophytic spurring) occurs around the disc in areas where the outer annular fibres are stressed most by a pulling-away or are fractioned at their attachment from the bone. The following conditions may occur:

- spondylosis: a general term for the degenerative changes resulting from OA affecting the vertebrae, intervertebral disc, surrounding ligaments and connective tissue, sometimes with pain or paraesthesia radiating down the an extremity if nerve roots are compressed (intervertebral encroachment radiculitis)
- arthrosis, arthropathy: disease of a joint
- spondylarthrosis: combined degeneration of both vertebrae and joint arthritis
- Stenosis: narrowing of a duct or canal. With regard to the vertebrae it may refer to central stenosis where the central vertebral canal is compromised, or lateral stenosis (IVF stenosis) where the intervertebral foramens is compromised.

The general features of degenerative spinal disease involving the disc, bone or joint may include:

- hypertrophied facet
- osteophytic processes from margins of vertebrae or joints
- disc flattening
- disc bulges
- subluxation of facet joints.
- degenerative spondylosisthesis (e.g. L5 over S1)
- lateral recess encroachment
- hypertrophy or buckling of ligamentum flavum
- ossification of posterior longitudinal ligament.

In this chapter only a few of the common neurological conditions are discussed as they result from the increasing size of the vertebrae and/or decreasing size of canal (central stenosis) or intervertebral foramen (lateral stenosis). Stenosis of the canal may result from changes to the vertebral unit from a number of changes listed above. The cardinal symptoms of lumbar spinal stenosis is neurogenic claudication (claudiospinalis), the symptoms of cervical stenosis may be cervical myelopathy, radiculopathy or both within the cervical spine,[72] and the cardinal symptom of lateral stenosis (IVF) is radiculopathy.

Cervical spondylitic myelopathy (CSM) is spinal cord compression that results from cervical degenerative disease changes (spondylosis deformans). Degenerative disc disease (spondylosis) and degenerative joint disease (arthrosis) are common findings among the elderly. The changes progressively narrow the spinal canal and possibly the IVF, causing progressive pressure to the spinal cord (myelopathy), nerve roots (radiculopathy) or both (myeloradiculopathy).[62] The most commonly affected levels of the cervical spine, in order of frequency, are C5–C6, C6–C7 and C4–C5.[73]

With the diminishing cervical canal the spinal cord may be compressed anteriorly with posterior osteophytic spurs, by calcifications of the posterior longitudinal ligament or from posterior disc bulges. It may be compressed posteriorly or posterolaterally by the buckling of the ligamentum flavum, zyagophyseal osteophytic spurring or by the lamina if the canal is congenitally small. The pressures on the spinal cord may be compounded by each other as well as by the biomechanical motions of the spine (Figure 11.1).

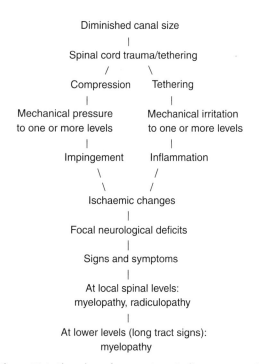

Diminished canal size
|
Spinal cord trauma/tethering
/   \
Compression   Tethering
| |
Mechanical pressure   Mechanical irritation
to one or more levels   to one or more levels
| |
Impingement   Inflammation
\   /
\   /
Ischaemic changes
|
Focal neurological deficits
|
Signs and symptoms
|
At local spinal levels:
myelopathy, radiculopathy
|
At lower levels (long tract signs):
myelopathy

Figure 11.1 Flow chart of progressive spinal/root compression.

The clinical findings of CSM include the following:

- The patient may have a chronic history of radiculopathy.
- The patient may spontaneously develop symptoms after a seemingly trivial minor injury.
- Symptoms may include reduced dexterity, clumsiness, arm pain, unsteady gait with long-tract signs of spasticity, hyperreflexia and extensor plantar response.
- Motor abnormalities are most predominant, such as weakness and atrophy of upper extremities and progressive loss of dexterity.
- Lhermitte's sign with flexion or extension of neck is an important indicator of spinal compression. (Lhermitte's sign is the provocation of numbness, burning, coldness, tingling and electric shock sensation with neck flexion.)
- A neurological level of involvement is identified with reflex changes or sensory changes. For example, when the biceps reflex is diminished or absent and the triceps reflex hyperreflexic, this would indicate that the involved level is C5–C6.
- Radiographic signs in the cervical spinal canal: 10–11 mm indicates absolute stenosis (61), less than 12 mm indicates a high risk (74).
- Patients with congenital spinal stenosis usually have long-tract signs early in the condition.
- Sphincter disturbances may occur but are not an outstanding feature.
- Pain is not a dominant complaint.
- The stenotic canal usually measures less than 1.2 cm on X-ray
- Congenital narrowing of a canal may involve many segments and narrowing may be associated with blocked vertebrae.
- Computed tomographic (CT) myelography, tomography or MRI may be used to provide further detail.

Concurrent arm and leg pain in the elderly

Many elderly patients present with a number of complaints that may camouflage an important diagnosis such as CSM. When confronted with a complex patient history, the clinician is advised to focus the history-taking along the time line in order to identify an accurate temporal pattern of the details (chronology of symptoms). This will help to weed out insignificant symptoms. All the while, the clinician must search for symptoms that may represent a focal neurological finding. These may or may not be associated with injury.

The clinician who is seeing an elderly patient for the first time who complains of a specific upper arm weakness and paraesthesia must be cautioned not to make a quick diagnosis of radiculitis without considering the possibility of concurrent cervical stenosis. The clinician should establish the significance of any hobbling, leg limping or weakness, and ask specific questions about bowel and bladder functions (frequency or excessive dribbling), observing excessive underclothes staining for either, prior to any provocative cervical examinations involving extreme flexion or extension positioning.

> A small cervical spinal canal (12–13 mm) in a patient who has concurrent arm, neck and leg symptoms demands further evaluation.

Indications for surgical referral would include progressive impairment without remission. The best surgical results are observed in patients who have symptoms of less than 6 months' duration, mild cord changes and few sensory changes and should be considered at an early stage of the disease.[72]

Conservative care is used for patients who are a poor surgical risk. Education and counselling are helpful to identify positions of exacerbation, such as extreme flexion or extension. Supportive care may also involve a cervical collar to restrict mobility or to avoid reinjury. Physical therapy can relieve pain and medications are used to control inflammation. Reflex-based manual techniques and soft-tissue therapies may offer symptom relief.

Other causes of myelopathy

There are many other causes of myelopathy. These include herniated central discs, tumours, spinal cord trauma, ankylosing spondylitis, Paget's disease, rheumatoid disease (atlantoaxial dislocation), spinal cord tumours,[6] multiple sclerosis, amyotrophic lateral sclerosis and metastatic tumours.[75] The effects of radiation therapy for tumours around the spine, causing delayed spinal cord necrosis and myelopathy, may occur months or years after the therapy.[74]

Caudal equina claudication (neurogenic intermittent claudication)

Neurogenic intermittent claudication is a spinal canal mass lesion occurring below the T10, and is characterized by lower limb paraesthesia or pain, bowel or bladder dysfunction brought on by walking or standing and relieved by rest in a lumbar flexion position.[76,77]

In the younger patient an acute caudal equina syndrome may be seen with an acute disc prolapse of L2/L3, causing bilateral multiple root compression requiring emergency surgery. This is not the clinical picture in the elderly patient. The elderly patient may have had a long history of periodic low back pain associated with aggravating positions, or pain may be only a minor complaint, while other patients present with weakness as a predominant complaint. There may be nerve root symptoms of one nerve root (monoradicular), less commonly involving several roots or even the complete caudal equina. When pain is present it is distinctly paraesthetic in quality, described as numbness, coldness or burning in the lumbosacral or sciatic distribution. The mechanism may be a combination of mechanical compression and vascular ischaemia of one or more roots of the caudal equina.

Clinical findings

- Physical examination may be unrevealing in 50% of cases.
- Varying degrees of other lumbar and sacral root signs occur.
- Muscle wasting may be very obvious when lumbar roots are affected.
- Exercise in some postures may worsen neurological signs (e.g. lumbar extension).
- X-ray may reveal spinal canal narrowing, severe spondylosis or secondary conditions, such as ankylosing spondylitis, Paget's disease, fluorosis or achondroplasia.
- CT and MRI are more helpful than X-ray.
- Central stenosis is often associated with IVF stenosis; therefore, there is often a combined caudal equina compression and lateral entrapment.

Differential diagnosis
Primary tumours of the caudal equina

The most common tumours are ependymomas and neurofibromas. In general, the primary symptoms may present as low back pain and/or sciatica with a sudden or gradual onset. Pain may be worse with lying down and at night. Other symptoms develop after the onset of pain; these may be years later and include paraesthesia, leg weakness, bowel dysfunction and less frequently bladder or sexual dysfunction. On examination there are no characteristic features. The straight leg raise (SLR) test is often abnormal. Root compression signs may be absent or widespread. Less commonly patients may have painless weakness of the legs, sphincter disturbance, caudal equina syndrome or spinal subarachnoid haemorrhage.

Malignant diseases of the caudal equina, nerve roots or spinal nerves

In the elderly, secondary diseases of vertebral metastasis usually result from breast or prostate, primary bone tumours or multiple myeloma. All may result in signs and symptoms similar to other compression neuropathies in various ways. They may appear with clinical features that resemble compression of nerve roots in IVF, compression of the conus medularis of caudal equina, collapse of a vertebra (compression fracture with minimal trauma) or with invasion of spinal nerves outside the IVF or the lumbosacral plexus.

Three clinical pictures of caudal equina lesions in the adult

Patten[73] delineates three simple clinical presentations of a caudal equina lesion based upon the location of the lesion: lateral one, central–internal and central–external lesions.

Lateral caudal equina syndrome occurs from a space-occupying lesion developing lateral to the caudal equina, or in a high location it may affect the base of the spinal cord (T12–L2). The syndrome most frequently results from a neurofibroma, causing L4 radicular symptoms (thigh pain, quadriceps weakness and areflexia as well as tibialis anterior weakness).

A central–internal lesion (conus lesion) occurs from a space-occupying lesion developing centrally within the conus medularis or filum terminale. The syndrome may result from an ependymoma, possibly resulting in only back pain (maybe for years) until the mass is large enough to compromise the roots. Root lesions may occur from S5 to S4 and progressively up to the lumbar roots. Symptoms of genito-urinary pain, bladder or sexual dysfunction will precede lumbar radiculopathy (leg pain, loss of ankle strength and reflex, etc.).

A central–external lesion occurs from a mass lesion outside the caudal equina. The syndrome may result from primary bone tumours (cordomas,

Paget's) or metastatic disease (prostatic) resulting in unusual radiculopathies (L2 or L3 root pain) or radiculopathies that do not resolve with conservative care.

Radiculitis and radiculopathy

Radiculitis is the inflammation of the root of a spinal nerve, whereas radiculopathy refers to a disease process of the nerve roots. The radiculopathies can involve only sensory symptoms or purely motor symptoms, but most often involve both. If both are involved, then the signs of pain radiating into a limb (dermatomal) and weakness (myotomal) of specific muscles with reduced reflex

Table 11.17 Spinal nerve root examination[78]

Root	Level	Muscle test	Sensory
C5	C4–C5	Deltoid (C5/C6) Shoulder abduction	Lateral shoulder
C6	C5–C6	Biceps (C5/C6) Extensor carpi radialis longus and brevis Wrist extension	Thumb/first finger
C7	C6–C7	Triceps (C7/C8) Flexor carpi radialis Wrist flexion	Middle finger
C8	C7–T1	Flexor carpi ulnaris (C7/C8/T1) Flexor digiti superficialis Flexor digiti profundus Finger flexion	Medial forearm
T1	T1–T2	Abductor digiti minimi (C8/T1) Dorsal interossei (finger abduction) Palmar interossei (finger adduction) Finger abduction and adduction	Medial Arm
L4	L4–L5	Tibialis anterior (L3/L4/L5) Foot inversion Quadriceps (L2/L3/L4)	Medial leg/foot
L5	L5–S1	Extensor hallucis longus (L5/S1) Toe extension	Lateral leg/dorsal foot
S1	S1–S2	Gastrocnemius (S1) Soleus (S2) Peroneus longus and brevis (S1) Foot eversion	Lateral leg/foot Sole

testing are useful for the identification of the involved vertebral level. However, if only the motor (anterior) root or only the sensory (dorsal) root is involved, the classical radicular findings become a little more confusing for the undergraduate. The clinical picture may become even more blurred if the older patient presents in a detrained habit, with disuse atrophies, or with excess adipose tissue that hides atrophies. Finally, the typical clinical picture of a patient presenting with radiculopathy would also include residual effects of past radiculopathies, diminished reflexes (especially the Achilles reflex), and possibly the effects of past surgery, current medications or other chronic disease, all of which present a clinical challenge for even the most experienced clinician.

The clinical findings for primary root lesions are summarized in Table 11.18.

Superficial sensory changes may occur in the corresponding dermatome, but because of dermatomal overlap, the sensory changes may be minimal or difficult to interpret. The perception of the patient's paraesthesia in a dermatome (with normal testing) may be interpreted as an early root sign.

Prior to muscle testing it is wise to inspect involved joints for arthritic changes and, when testing the frail patient, to apply force equal and opposite to the patient's effort, ensuring that the patient is told to apply force slowly. Many older patients have a swift initial impulse of force with poor recruitment or endurance. Excessive ballistic overloading may cause delayed-onset muscle soreness.

Nerve root irritation is generally considered to be a precursor phase or final resolving phase of a root inflammation (radiculitis). It may have a mechanical aetiology, such as intervertebral pressure or repetitive root trauma (tethering). Alternatively, it may have a chemical aetiology, such as the presence of local inflammatory products from discs or facets.

The most frequently aetiology seen in a chiropractic practice is vertebral joint dysfunction (vertebral subluxation). The early signs of radiculopathy are often thought to represent the neuropathophysiological component of the vertebral subluxation on the spinal roots. The effects on the root are the precursors of radiculopathy and by definition are not associated with the 'hard signs' of radiculopathy.

The signs of nerve root irritation (early signs of radiculitis) are valuable to assist the clinician in identifying the clinical picture, and are as follows.

Sensation

- Sensory changes with the primary modalities (light touch, vibration, hot and cold) may not be helpful since the root irritation may be of sufficient intensity to block sensory afferent impulses completely.
- Paraspinal hyperesthesia (see below) may seen at the involved vertebral level.

Muscular

- Motor changes with muscle testing will reveal 5/5 testing (unremarkable).
- The clinician should observe for atrophy. Oblique lighting is often helpful. Muscle atrophy is commonly seen in the supraspinatus and infraspinatus as a flattening of the muscle with an obvious bony look to the spine of the scapula. The triceps may also appear flabby. The speed of the wave of percussion after the muscle is struck with a reflex hammer should be observed, then compared with the opposite muscle.
- The muscles are palpated for mild loss of tone. Peripheral muscles any be difficult to compare as a result of the patient's handedness.

Autonomic

- The autonomic changes are not consistent signs and are difficult to interpret, but may at times prove helpful. One should observe for autonomic changes such as autonomic instability:
  (i) Pilomotor effect: when this is present, it may be seen when the patient undresses. Cold air falling upon the skin produces a pilomotor effect (goose pimples) in the affected dermatome.
  (ii) vasomotor effect: when this is present, poor circulation may be observed or felt as cooler to the touch.

Supersensitivity

- Tender motor points[79–81] may be palpated as myalgic spots or increased sensitivity of muscles undergoing partial denervation. The motor point is the most excitable point of a muscle, usually located in the central belly of the muscle. It is the area of greatest concentration of nerve endings. The muscle is palpated for tenderness with firm pressure at the area of the motor point. Excessive sensitivity may represent partial denervation hypersensitivity.

- Motor-point tenderness may be measured with a pressure algometer or graded from the reactions to examination (similar to grading trigger points):
  grade 0: no tenderness with firm pressure
  grade 1: some tenderness, not unpleasant
  grade 2: some tenderness, unpleasant
  grade 3: acute tenderness, patient reacts vigorously (jumps)
  Pressure that elicits tenderness of grade 2 or 3 may induce autonomic signs, pilomotor effects in the dermatome or sweating in the axillae or hands.

Hyperaesthesia syndrome

(Dorsal ramus compression) is a syndrome that may occur at any vertebral level, but is more common in the low back. The most common cause is a twisting, lifting action of the body. The syndrome includes one symptom and three signs, namely:

- clearly defined area of hyperesthesia adjacent to the spinal cord
- localized paravertebral tender spot (associated with area of hyperesthesia)
- dull ache in the involved area (the only symptom)
- limitation of movement of the trunk by pain.

The most common cause is a lifting or twisting action that initially causes a sharp pain lasting for only a few seconds. A pain-free interval of minutes to up to 2h may occur, after which a dull ache may begin.

On examination there is a minor limitation in the gross ranges of motion due to pain. The scratch test (with the patient prone, an open safety pin is drawn down the spine 5 cm from the midline) may indicate the involved areas where the pin feels sharper. The patient may feel that the clinician is pressing harder in a specific area, it may feel 'sharper', it may 'tickle', feel 'hot' or 'hurt'. The skin-rolling test (rolling a small flap of skin along the spine between the fingers) will illicit similar results, but the scratch test will stimulate the pain fibres more specifically. Skin rolling may be done as a second test since it involves other pressure receptors. Skin rolling may also indicate for subcutaneous adhesions that may result from myofascial pain or injury (trigger points, scar tissue, fibromyalgia, etc.). A tender spot within the deep paraspinal musculature will be found, possibly due to local hypertonus of dorsally innervated segmental muscles.

The aetiology for this syndrome is not known. One possible cause is the impingement of the dorsal ramus as it passes through the posterior musculature, or as it passes under the retroarticular ligaments. The symptoms in this case would be the result of a denervation supersensitivity, similar to nostalgia paraesthetica in the thoracic spine.

Therapy may involve local pulsed therapeutic ultrasound (inflammation reduction), the Nimo technique, muscle stripping and vertebral adjustment of segments (reduction of tonus). Prognosis is excellent unless chronic neuropathic change occurs leading to denervation atrophy of a small group of paraspinal muscle fibres.

This syndrome as it appears in the medical literature is a very good partial description of a vertebral subluxation complex (VSC). The theoretical aetiology of dorsal ramus compression distal to the IVF would therefore classify it as a peripheral neuropathy. Central to the VSC model is a central excitatory state of the spinal cord (facilitated segment) with reflex-based ramifications: somato-somato reflexes, somato-visceral reflexes, and so on.

Peripheral neuropathy

Peripheral neuropathy (PN) is a category of neuropathic diseases that involve the PNS, all neural structures outside the brain and spinal cord. The olfactory bulbs and optic nerves remain part of the CNS. The cardinal features include the impairment of one or more peripheral nerves, usually resulting in sensory disturbance, loss of reflex and flaccid distal muscle weakness, and sometimes affecting cranial or autonomic nerves.[6]

There are many causes of PN, with the pathology involving the degeneration of the nerve fibre through wallerian degeneration, axonal degeneration or segmental degeneration. In developed countries the most common causes are related to diabetes mellitus, alcoholism, chronic lung disease, neoplasm, renal disease, thyroid disease, medications, vitamin B_{12} deficiency and an increasing number of acquired immunodeficiency syndrome (AIDS)-related polyneuropathies.[82] About half of the diabetics over the age of 60 have some peripheral neuropathy. In general, approximately 20% of the elderly have some form of peripheral neuropathy.[83]

Double crush ('multiple crush') is the concept that the existence of two sites of simultaneous compression, or a second (later) site of compression, placed either proximal or distal to the first (earlier) site of compression, will result in significantly poorer neural function than will a single site of compression. The constraint on axoplasmic flow could also be a metabolic neuropathy, thus supporting the high association between diabetes and carpal tunnel syndrome.[84]

Peripheral neuropathies have been classified in different ways, according to their various clinical characteristics (see Table 11.18).

Peripheral neuropathy is common in the elderly, resulting in reduced poor distal proprioception and strength that hinder balance, causing 50% of patients to fall each year.[84]

The clinician can help patients with peripheral neuropathy to prevent falls by teaching them and their families about peripheral nerve dysfunction and its effects on balance. Helpful strategies include advising patients to substitute vision for the lost somatosensory function, the correct use of a cane, the importance of proper shoes and orthotics, and suggestions to perform exercises for balance and upper extremity strengthening.

> In elderly patients, loss of heel reflexes, decreased vibratory sense (improving proximally), impaired position sense of the toe and inability to maintain unipedal stance for 10 s (in three tries) suggest the possibility of peripheral neuropathy, and these patients are at greater risk for falling.[84]

Selected peripheral neuropathies

Diabetic neuropathy

This involves different possible patterns of nerve injury:

- diabetic polyneuropathy
- diabetic mononeuropathy (femoral neuropathy is the most common)
- diabetic amyotrophy (characterized by proximal lower extremity weakness and atrophy
- diabetic vascular mononeuritis multiplex
- thoracolumbar polyradiculoneuropathy
- autonomic neuropathy
- sensorimotor polyneuropathy: the most common pattern which may be associated with peripheral nerve entrapment syndromes such as carpal tunnel syndrome.

Alcoholic neuropathy

This involves ethanol toxicity with nutritional and vitamin B_1 (thiamine) deficiency. It is an axonal motor and sensory neuropathy with insidious onset. Demographic trends reveal the elderly comprise a fast-growing segment of the population and alcohol-related problems are anticipated to increase.[85] In addition to liver disease, dementia, confusion, peripheral neuropathy, insomnia, late-onset seizure disorder, incontinence, diarrhoea, myopathy, depression, fractures and adverse reactions to medications may be anticipated.

Herpes zoster

This viral infection of the cervical nerve root is less common than in the thoracic nerve roots, but if present will occur in any dermatome (C2 and C3 most frequently) or the trigeminal distribution. In the ageing patient, herpes zoster is a frequent cause of diminished quality of life. The skin lesions often appear as immunity declines

Table 11.18 Peripheral neuropathies classified by different characteristics

Rate of onset of the condition	Acute (< 1 week)
	Subacute (< 1 month)
	Chronic (> 2 months)
Aetiology	Idiopathic (no known cause)
	Toxic (external poison or metabolic waste)
	Hereditary (genetic cause)
	Secondary to disease
Pathology	Axonal degeneration
	Segmental demyelination
	Mixed
Type of nerve fibres	Motor, sensory, autonomic, mixed
Size of nerve fibre involved	Small, large, mixed
Distribution of changes in the body	Proximal, distal, diffuse
Pattern of nerves affected	Mononeuropathy (one peripheral nerve affected)
	Mononeuritis multiplex (two or more peripheral nerves affected in a similar way, often by a systemic disease, (e.g. diabetes)
	Symmetrical (affecting bilateral structures)
	Polyneuropathy (affecting several nerves)
	Polyradiculoneuropathy (affecting several nerve roots)

with age but rarely pose a significant threat, except when ocular structures (trigeminal distribution) are involved. Early identification and the initiation of treatment within 48–72 h of disease onset offer the greatest chance of minimizing neurological sequelae.[86]

Pain may precede the lesion, persist after acute eruptions or continue long afterwards (post-herpetic neuralgia or PHN). While the pain in younger patients is transient and bearable, the elderly often have more prolonged and more intense pain.

Although a wide range of therapies is available, most are not effective. Traditional analgesics offer little benefit for the treatment of PHN. The best results for pain relief have come from capsaicin and tricyclic antidepressants. Other therapies that have been tried include: anticonvulsants, transcutaneous electrical nerve stimulation (TNENS) and nerve blocks.[97]

Multiple sclerosis

Multiple sclerosis (MS) is characterized by focal deterioration of the CNS myelin. It may occur in various areas, and clinically may manifest as impaired motor, sensory, cerebellar, visual or other system dysfunctions. Typically, the disease follows a relapsing and remitting course with progressive neurological impairment as the plaques grow. The specific signs and symptoms will vary from patient to patient and even from attack to attack within one patient.[88]

The onset of MS is rare in childhood (0.3–0.4%), with approximately 60% of MS cases beginning between ages 20 and 40 years. The other cases of MS begin in the fifth or sixth decade.[89] Initial signs of motor deficits in one or more extremities occur in 50% of patients. These may be associated with the sensation of numbness or tingling in the extremity, or a band-like sensation around the trunk. In 25% of patients, monocular blindness may be the initial sign. Other signs may include unsteadiness of gait due to cerebellum and cerebellar tract lesions, brainstem lesions or deficits due to ocular mobility causing nystagmus, vertigo or, if the patient has spinal cord lesions, tingling or electric shock-like sensations down the back and into the sides with passive neck flexion (Lhermitte's sign).[88,90]

In general, lower extremities are affected earlier and more frequently than the upper extremities. Symptoms may consist of spasticity, flexor spasms or hyperreflexia. Two-thirds of patients show problems with sphincter control. Over 65% of patients complain of fatigue. With longstanding progression of the disease, there may be euphoria, denial of the illness and depression. Some factors are known occasionally to precipitate a relapse, such as infections, trauma, lumbar puncture, emotional illness and even pregnancy.

The aetiology of MS is not completely understood. There is support for genetic causes,[98] primarily because it is more prevalent in monozygotic twins with MS than in dizygotic twins,[92] but only about 15% of MS cases have a familial pattern.[93] Environmental triggers, immune system deficiencies and infectious diseases are also suspected.[90] Viral illnesses (mumps, measles, rubella) occurring late in childhood have been associated with increased risk for developing MS.[94]

The geographical distribution reveals a high-risk prevalence for the northern latitudes.[89,95]

Table 11.19 Classification of multiple sclerosis (MS) according to Rose[97]

Definite MS	Probable MS
Patient has a relapsing and remitting course with at least two bouts separated by no less than 1 month	Patient has a history of relapsing and remitting symptoms with clinical evidence of only one lesion.
Patient has a slow or stepwise progressive course extending over at least 6 months	
There are documented neurological signs resulting from more than one site of white matter central nervous system pathology (focal defects)	There is only a single bout of symptoms with signs of multi-focal white matter disease followed by variable symptoms and signs
These symptoms begin between 10 and 50 years of age	
CSF shows protein components from myelin and there is evidence of white matter lesions on CT or MRI scans	CSF shows basic protein components of myelin and there is evidence of white matter lesions on either CT or MRI scans
There is no better neurological explanation for the symptoms	There is no better neurological explanation for the symptoms

CSF: Cerebrospinal fluid; CT: Computed tomographic; MRI: Magnetic resonance imaging.

- 1 in 100 000 equatorial regions
- 6–14 in 100 000 southern USA and Europe
- 30–80 in 100 000 Canada and northern USA.

The diagnosis of MS is usually one of exclusion. If the patient has an acute onset of focal neurological symptoms (e.g. visual deficit, hemiparesis), the clinical evaluations are focused first to rule out ischaemic states, migraine variants or small mass lesions. The challenge is then to identify a recurring pattern. The patient who experiences an insidious development of less significant signs or signs that are attributed to another disorder (e.g. depression) is likely to have a delay in establishing a definitive diagnosis. One should beware of the patient who infrequently visits doctors ('haven't seen a doctor since they cut the umbilical cord!') or the patient who does not consistently see the same practitioner (e.g. uses only walk-in clinics or hospital emergency departments for health care).

In years past, the appearance of new neurological signs or aggravation of current signs had been used as a clinical indication of MS (bath water test).[96] However, this test is not advocated at this time since it has been correlated with prolonged debilitation after testing.

A classification described by Rose[97] describes criteria for the clinical identification of MS characteristics based upon three levels of confidence (Table 11.19). The history of the disease is unpredictable, remissions occur in at least 20% of the MS patients and an exacerbating remitting course is the most frequent form.

Pathology

The MS lesions consist of scattered multiple delineated areas of demyelination found anywhere in the CNS white matter. The most predominant areas affected are the periventricular areas, spinal cord, brainstem, optic nerves and optic chiasm. MS does not involve the peripheral myelin. Nerve cells undergo demyelination, although the axons are relatively preserved.

Laboratory tests

Some laboratory tests may be helpful in the diagnosis of MS, although the diagnosis is usually made on a clinical basis. Tests of CSF may show an increase in mononuclear pleiocytosis in CSF protein and elevated immunoglobulin G (IgG). CT and MRI scans are helpful in localizing lesions.

The differential diagnosis may include spinal cord lesions such as tumours, myelopathy and spinocere-bellar degeneration. The most difficult differentiation is between MS and lupus erythematosus.

Treatment

No specific treatment is established at this time. Some treatments claiming results include:

- Low-fat diets.
- Hyperbaric oxygenation.
- Adrenocorticotropic hormone (ACTH) may be beneficial during the acute phase.
- Corticosteroids may encourage the rate of recovery during a bout of MS.
- β-Interferon may diminish the number of exacerbations.
- Spinal cord stimulation (SCS): Dorsal column stimulation to relieve intractable pain with electrodes implanted in the spinal cord has given some patients relief and the ability to regain voluntary control over arms, legs and sphincters.[98] Some authors have reported up to 50% success for chronic pain and 80% for acute pain.[99] These methods have been criticized for their temporary effects and poor patient compliance (18% after 1 year) (100). In approximately 50% of paraplegic or hemiplegic patients SCS caused a decrease in reflex activity (spasticity).[101]
- Physical therapies: Symptomatic treatment is individualized for the patient and may require occupational or physical therapy to rehabilitate motor power, ataxia, impaired sensation or intention tremor, and to prevent excessive spasticity, contracture and compensatory patterns. Common problems addressed with physical therapy include decubitus ulcerations, bowel and bladder problems, sexual dysfunction, gait and spasticity control.
- TENS for pain modification.
- Ultrasonic stimulation of lymphatics was used in patients where spastic paraparesis was the predominant clinical feature.[102] The response was an 80% subjective improvement, but only a 19% objective change, such as a rise in the B-lymphocytes and a fall in the T-lymphocytes.[103]
- Electrical stimulation: Paraplegic patients receiving stimulation to the knee extensors/flexors, or hemiplegic patients receiving stimulation to the ankle flexor/extensors demonstrated a decreased reflex activity (spasticity) which lasted for more than 30 min.[101]
- Interferential therapy: Bowel and bladder dysfunctions are particularly disabling for the MS patient's

lifestyle and work life. Objective improvements have been seen with interferential therapy applied on the lumbosacral spinal marrow for treating urinary frequency, urgency or incontinence.[104]

- Aquatic exercise programmes for gait, conducted in a cool swimming pool, help to maintain fitness (mobility, aerobic capacity and body mass) without the risk of trauma or falls. The cool water also prevents body overheating, which may occur with the same exercise intensity in an exercise programme on dry land.
- Kegel exercises: To eliminate or improve simple urinary stress incontinence a series of exercise to promote the strength of the pelvic-floor musculature may be taught to the patient. The patient begins by intermittently stopping and starting the flow of urine without breath-holding. The exercise should focus on the genitourinary muscles without abdominal or gluteal muscle contraction. The exercise should be performed several times per day. With progressive control the hold-time of the exercise may be built up to 10–15 s of maximum contraction.
- Elevator exercise: This is a slight modification of the Kegel exercise. The patient is asked to contract the pelvic muscles at progressively higher tension and hold them for 5 s first at 25% of strength ('first floor'), then 50% of strength (second floor), then at 75% of strength (third floor) and then at maximum strength (top floor). The procedure is reversed while the tension is slowly released through the successive floors. Patients may be more motivated if told that the pelvic–floor muscles play a role in sexual activities).

Respiratory muscle training

An exercise training programme for improving respiratory muscle strength and ventilatory capacity is indicated for the patient who has poor exercise/endurance tolerance, poor coughing strength or an impairment of the force of speech. A 1 week programme using inspiratory or expiratory resistive loads improved maximum static inspiration (PImax) by 31%, expiratory pressures (PEmax) by 31% and voluntary ventilation by 21%.[105]

Parkinson's disease

Movement disorders are common among the elderly. The most common neurological movement disorder is Parkinson's disease (PD).[106] Paralysis agitans: PD is alternatively called 'paralysis' refers to the loss of motion and 'agitans' to the tremor. The usual onset is between the ages of 40 and 70 years, with the most frequent onset occurring in the sixth decade, and only very rarely does it occur as early as the third decade.[107] It is present throughout the world, with a higher prevalence in men.[108] Since the diagnosis is based on the clinical presentation, the prevalence rate varies widely from 10 to 405 per 1000, and this rate increases with age.[109] In North America, 1% of patients over the age of 65 years are affected by this disease (approximately 1 million people).

Parkinson's classification

The disease is classified as:

- primary (idiopathic)
- secondary (acquired)
- heredodegenerative
- multiple system degeneration (Parkinson's plus).

Primary idiopathic PD occurs with the unknown loss of the pigmented cells that produce dopamine in the substantia nigra of the midbrain.[110] It is confirmed at autopsy by the presence of Lewy bodies in the same area.

Acquired PD can result from infections, medications, toxins, vascular disease, tumours, normal pressure hydrocephalus, hepatocerebral degeneration, hypothyroidism and parathyroid abnormalities.[110]

Heredodegenerative disorders are a group of rare disorders that account for less than 1% of cases of PD. They include Huntington's disease, Wilson's disease and spinocerebellar degeneration.[110]

The group classified as multiple system degeneration (Parkinson's plus) offers the greatest diagnostic challenge since there is much overlap with other diseases. Often patients who do not respond to standard parkinsonian therapy, or who deviate from known clinical patterns, are considered in this category. Diseases may include progressive supranuclear palsy, Shy–Drager syndrome and the parkinsonism–dementia–amyotrophic lateral sclerosis complex.[110]

Differential diagnosis

Some disease conditions are known to resemble PD, such as encephalitis and iatrogenic effects of medications (phenothiazines) (Table 11.20). Drug-induced Parkinson's symptoms are confirmed by withdrawing the drug to observe for the resolution of symptoms.

Table 11.20 Conditions that may resemble Parkinson's disease

Disease or pathology resembling Parkinson's disease	Characteristic sign
Senile tremor (essential tremor)	A fine, quick tremor that is more obvious during intentional movements
Progressive supranuclear palsy	Dystonic postures of head and neck, mild dementia, with impairment of vertical gaze, (defective conjugate gaze)
Lacunar infarcts (Binswangers disease)	Unilateral or bilateral corticospinal tract signs hyperactive facial reflexes, hypertension and atherosclerosis of small blood vessels and multiple strokes
Infections, e.g. human immunodeficiency virus, tuberculosis	May cause extrapyramidal signs
Repeated trauma (multiple concussions)	Dementia pugulistica refers to cognitive changes seen in boxers years after trauma.[111] Dementia, Parkinson's, pyramidal and cerebellar signs
Normal pressure hydrocephalus	An acquired condition leading to changes in mentation, gait disturbance and urinary incontinence
Tumours	May cause a mass effect with pressure on the nigrostriatal tract

Several studies have examined the association between environmental factors and PD. Exposure to pesticides or wood pulp has been implicated, as well as activities such as vegetable farming, rural living and drinking well-water.[112] However, no specific environmental toxins have been identified as the primary cause of PD.

Parkinson-like symptoms have rarely occurred after head injury, lacunar infarcts and vertebrobasilar ischaemia.

Pathophysiology

PD is a degenerative disease of the CNS primarily affecting the substantia nigra. There is a consistent loss of melanin-containing cells in the substantia nigra, locus coeruleus and the dorsal nucleus of the vagus nerve. There is also a decreased concentration of the neurotransmitter dopamine. Tyrosine hydroxylase, a significant enzyme for dopamine, also diminishes.[113] The failure of dopamine to control the basal ganglia results in rhythmic and synchronous bursts of impulses within the cortex–basal ganglia thalamus–cortex loop, which is seen in the pyramidal tract as a tremor.

The exact aetiology of PD is not understood. Some toxins that are known to cause PD include carbon monoxide, ethanol, methanol, manganese and a synthetic heroin derivative (MPTP, 1-methyl-4-phenol-1,2,3,6-tetrahydropyridine), which offers a valuable research tool.[114]

Diagnosis and clinical features

The early identification of the PD patient has been a research priority. Many studies have tried to identify patients in the preclinical phase with the hope of improving care. To date, no indicators have been found before the parkinsonian signs are seen and often the diagnosis may take 5 years or more to confirm (without autopsy).[107]

The diagnosis of PD is based on the patient's history and physical examination. Patients often relate a history spanning many years where they may recall subtle signs of incoordination or slowness of motions. This period may represent a preclinical phase.[115] Early symptoms are difficult to identify and are often ignored. Some of the first complaints may be stiffness and soreness of the axial girdle musculature[116] or unexplained tiredness or fatiguability.[117] The slowness of motions, diminished spontaneous motions and changes in the face and body may be thought to be changes of normal ageing, and therefore initially ignored.

It is during this phase that patients may become frustrated by the subtle decline in their functional state. They may consult numerous doctors in search of answers: 'What is it', 'Why me', 'What's going to happen now?' and so on. For many patients, being a diagnosed is both a blessing and fear. On the one hand, they feel blessed with a great relief from the anxiety and frustration of months or years of uncertainty. On the other hand, a new fear develops as they come to understand the disease, realize their future path and begin to cope with its meaning (see also Chapter 23).

Signs of Parkinson's disease

Bradykinesia

This may be seen in the gait as a failure to swing one or both arms, while the difficulty in moving the feet results in a shuffling gait. Writing becomes slower and smaller (micrographia). There is a lack of facial tone, expression or emotion (hypomimia), with drooling and infrequent blinking, at a rate of 5–10/min (normal 15–20/min).

Tremors

An action tremor may be present in a patient's hands many years before the classic alternating 'pill-rolling' tremor (4–6 Hz) and, if unilateral, it strongly suggests the diagnosis of PD. Complete relaxation may abolish the tremor and intentional motions may diminish the tremor for a short time. An action tremor may occur at a higher frequency.

Cog-wheel rigidity

The altered muscle tone causes muscular rigidity. The rigidity is interrupted by the superimposed tremor and gives rise to the ratchet or cog-wheel sensation when a joint is passively moved. Cog-wheel rigidity may be more evident if the patient is asked to perform two tasks at the same time. For example, opening and closing one hand rapidly will reveal more rigidity in other prominent muscles of the trunk or another limb.

Glabella tap sign (Myerson's sign)

Repeated tapping of the bridge of the nose will result in a failure to inhibit the reflex eye-blinking.

Tendon jerks

These usually remain normal (plantar flexion), a negative Babinski sign. The plantar responses are down-going.

Posture

The patient's posture becomes progressively more flexed as the condition advances, reflecting a loss of postural reflexes and postural instability. The poor balance and the risk of a fall are hazardous to the patient.

The PD patient has less postural sway during standing compared with normal patients. It is thought that the increased musculoskeletal stiffness may be an adaptation to compensate for postural instability by avoiding overbalancing.[118] The stiff posture would limit the movement of the centre of body mass.

Loss of righting reflexes

PD patients have reduced righting reflexes. These are important for maintaining balance during gait and maintaining stability in stationary positions (standing and sitting). During gait there is a forward tilting with increased walking speed, the arms do not swing freely and the stride length is shortened (festination of gait). At times the loss of balance may cause the patient to fall backwards (retropulsion).

Autonomic changes

Postural hypotension, salivation and urinary urgency may occur in 25% of patients.

Higher brain functions

Depression is common and dementia may occur late in the disease as a result of cerebral atrophy.

Axial rigidity during locomotion

Stiffness of the body is seen that is comparable to the rigidity of the limbs. With systematic manipulation of walking speed on a treadmill, the co-ordination deficits and rigidity in trunk movement may be revealed. A recent study suggests that the signs of axial stiffness and reduced co-ordination of trunk movement are a sensitive early measure for PD diagnosis.[119]

Freezing

This is a delay and difficulty in beginning a motor function, such as initiating walking.[120] It may occur more frequently on turning or in narrow spaces. The patient may complain that freezing has contributed to falling or that it is embarrassing in public.

Reduced reaction time

The difficulty in initiating movements also results in poorer reaction times during transitions (laying to sitting, sitting to standing, etc.) or with repetitive motions such as simple pronation/supination motions of the arms.[121] The reaction times may vary from arm to arm, as well as at different times of the day. In patients who have been diagnosed and are receiving medication, reaction times may vary according to their medication schedule: poor before the medication the best 30–40 min after the ingestion of medication. This helps the patient to plan events, such as shopping, with little risk of freezing during the outing.

Movement time

The time taken to perform simple acts is increased. This has been used as an outcome measure for the study of motor control and performance deficits in patients.[122,123] This sign is a result of the bradykinesia and reduced reaction time.

Sequential acts

Many daily activities are composed of a series of movements needed to achieve a goal. For example, walking requires a series of inherent and learned motor patterns that coordinate many actions, such as the leg and arm movement, spinal movement, pelvis weight shifts, and many muscular stabilization functions of the pelvis and shoulder girdles. The PD patient has a great deal of difficulty with movement sequences that are performed automatically.[124]

Simultaneous acts

Other daily activities may include the performance of two motor tasks at one time; for example, walking while pulling a trolley, standing up while holding a plate or walking while reaching to grasp an object. PD patients have difficulty in executing these simultaneous motor activities.[125] It is thought that the mechanisms for these motor deficits may be a result of disordered motor planning or the inability to produce the strength and timing needed for the motor act.

Festination gait

The involuntary tendency to take short, small, accelerating steps during walking may be seen in some Parkinson's patients. The gait is usually slow with decreased stride length, decreased cadence and an increased time spent in the double-support phase. The increased cadence is considered to be a result of poor control of stride length.[126]

Cognitive changes

Fisk and Doble[127] provided a recent review of the cognitive changes in PD patients. Dementia and mood changes represent two generalized behavioural deficits. Memory impairments and conceptual ability represent two special cognitive deficits.

- Dementia: The features of dementia include impairment of memory as well as slowed information processing, and mood and personality disturbances. The phrase subcortical dementia is often used

by clinicians to distinguish it from the dementia of Alzheimer's disease.[127]
- Mood changes: Social withdrawal and isolation may occur if the patient has a poor perception of their functional ability, embarrassment or concurrent disease. Depression is common in PD patients.[128] The physical signs of depression are difficult to differentiate from the usual facies of the PD patient.
- Memory: PD patients may develop dementia, but they have the capacity to learn new information.[129] They are able to learn to use cues to aid their memory, such as lists, notes and electronic schedules. This is significant for maintaining an independent lifestyle for as long as possible.
- Conceptual ability: Neuropsychological testing has revealed that patients often show inflexibility or perseverant behaviours,[129] which could be misinterpreted as a stubborn or uncooperative attitude.

Assessment tools for diagnosis and management

Three tools that may be helpful for the evaluation of PD and its progression are Hoehn and Yahr's Staging[130] (Table 11.21), Schwab and England's Activities of Daily Living (ADLs) assessment (Table 11.22) and the Unified Parkinson's Disease Rating Scale (UPDRS) (Table 11.23). The differential diagnosis of PD is summarized in Table 11.24.

Treatment

PD is one of the few neurodegenerative diseases in which the symptoms can be improved with medication. The improvements in motor strength, co-ordination, skills and ambulation have a dramatic influence on the patient's lifestyle. Medical treatment is directed towards reducing cholinergic activity within the basal ganglia and increasing dopamine activity.[106] It is directed towards the balancing of dopamine and acetylcholine, but does not affect the pathological process. Drugs commonly used for the treatment of PD are listed in Table 11.25.

Selegiline

This drug is a monoamine oxidase (MAO) B inhibitor. The two enzymes MAO A and B play a significant role in the breakdown of dopamine. This drug increases dopamine levels and may have a neuroprotective effect in the early stages of the disease.

Table 11.21 Staging of Parkinson's disease: Hoehn and Yahr scale[130]

Stage 1 Unilateral features of Parkinson's disease (tremor, rigidity or bradykinesia)	(a) Signs and symptoms on one side only (b) Symptoms mild (c) Symptoms inconvenient but not disabling (d) Usually presents with tremor of one limb (e) Friends have noticed changes in posture, locomotion and facial expression
Stage 2 Bilateral features of stage 1 with possible speech, posture and gait abnormalities	(a) Symptoms are bilateral (b) Minimal disability (c) Posture and gait affected
Stage 3 Worsened bilateral features with balance difficulties, but independent living	(a) Significant slowing of body movements (b) Early impairment of equilibrium on walking or standing (c) Generalized dysfunction that is moderately severe
Stage 4 Unable to live independently	(a) Severe symptoms (b) Can still walk to a limited extent (c) Rigidity and bradykinesia (d) No longer able to live alone (e) Tremor may be less than at earlier stages
Stage 5 Requires wheelchair and is unable to get out of bed	(a) Cachectic stage (b) Invalidism complete (c) Cannot stand or walk (d) Requires constant nursing care

This scale was developed in the 1960s to describe the severity of Parkinson's disease. The scale reflects progressive severity of the condition, but is not a linear indicator of the disease.
This rating system has been largely supplanted by the Unified Parkinson's Disease Rating Scale, which is much more detailed and complex.

Table 11.22 Schwab and England's Activities of Daily Living[131]

Percent of daily activities	Description
100%	Completely independent. Able to do all chores without slowness, difficulty or impairment
90%	Completely independent. Able to do all chores with some slowness, difficulty or impairment. May take twice as long
80%	Independent in most chores. Takes twice as long. Conscious of difficulty and slowness
70%	Not completely independent. More difficulty with chores. Some chores may take three or four times as long. May take a large part of the day to do chores
60%	Some dependency. Can do most chores, but very slowly and with great effort. Makes errors. Some chores impossible
50%	More dependent. Helps with half of chores. Difficulty with everything
40%	Very dependent. Can assist with all chores but can do few alone
30%	With effort, occasionally does a few chores alone or begins alone. Much help needed
20%	Can do nothing alone. Can provide slight help with some chores. Severe invalid
10%	Totally dependent, helpless
0%	Vegetative functions such as swallowing, bladder and bowel function are not functioning. Bed-ridden

This assessment evaluates the effect on the Parkinson's disease patient's daily living. The rating can be assigned by the rater or by the patient.

Table 11.23 Unified Parkinson's Disease Rating Scale (UPDRS)

The UPDRS is a rating tool used to follow the longitudinal course of Parkinson's disease. It is made up of an assessment of mentation, behaviour and mood, the activities of daily living and motor assessments.

Each section is evaluated by interview. Some sections require multiple grades to be assigned to each extremity. A maximum score of 199 points is possible (i.e. total disability); a score of 0 indicates no variations from the norm (i.e. no disability).

(1) *Mentation, behaviour, mood*
  (a) Intellectual Impairment
    0 None
    1 Mild (consistent forgetfulness with partial recollection of events, with no other difficulties)
    2 Moderate memory loss with disorientation and moderate difficulty handling complex problems
    3 Severe memory loss with disorientation regarding time and often place, severe impairment with problems
    4 Severe memory loss with orientation only to person, unable to make judgements or solve problems
  (b) Thought disorder
    0 None
    1 Vivid dreaming
    2 'Benign' hallucinations with insight retained
    3 Occasional to frequent hallucinations or delusions without insight, could interfere with daily activities
    4 Persistent hallucinations, delusions or florid psychosis
  (c) Depression
    0 Not present
    1 Periods of sadness or guilt greater than normal, never sustained for more than a few days or a week
    2 Sustained depression for >1 week
    3 Vegetative symptoms (insomnia, anorexia, abulia, weight loss)
    4 Vegetative symptoms with suicidal thoughts
  (d) Motivation/initiative
    0 Normal
    1 Less assertive, more passive
    2 Loss of initiative or disinterest in elective activities
    3 Loss of initiative or disinterest in day-to-day (routine) activities
    4 Withdrawn, complete loss of motivation

(2) *Activities of daily living*
  (a) Speech
    0 Normal
    1 Mildly affected, no difficulty being understood
    2 Moderately affected, may be asked to repeat
    3 Severely affected, frequently asked to repeat
    4 Unintelligible most of the time
  (b) Salivation
    0 Normal
    1 Slight but noticeable increase, may have night-time drooling
    2 Moderately excessive saliva, may have minimal drooling
    3 Marked drooling
  (c) Swallowing
    0 Normal
    1 Rare choking
    2 Occasional choking
    3 Requires soft food
    4 Requires nasogastic or gastric tube
  (d) Handwriting
    0 Normal
    1 Slightly small or slow
    2 All words small but legible
    3 Severely affected, not all words legible
    4 Majority illegible
  (e) Cutting food/handling utensils
    0 Normal
    1 Somewhat slow and clumsy but no help needed
    2 Can cut most foods, some help needed
    3 Food must be cut, but can feed self
    4 Needs to be fed
  (f) Dressing
    0 Normal
    1 Somewhat slow, no help needed
    2 Occasional help with buttons or arms in sleeves
    3 Considerable help required but can do something alone
    4 Helpless
  (g) Hygiene
    0 Normal
    1 Somewhat slow but no help needed
    2 Needs help with shower or bath, or very slow in hygienic care
    3 Requires assistance for washing, brushing teeth and going to the toilet
    4 Helpless
  (h) Turning in bed/adjusting bed clothes
    0 Normal
    1 Somewhat slow, no help needed
    2 Can turn alone or adjust sheets, but with great difficulty
    3 Can initiate, but not turn or adjust alone
    4 Helpless
  (i) Falling: unrelated to freezing
    0 None   (Continued)

1 Rare falls
2 Occasional, less than one per day
3 Average of one per day
4 More than one per day
(j) Freezing when walking
0 Normal
1 Rare, may have starting hesitation
2 Occasional falls from freezing
3 Frequent freezing, occasional falls
4 Frequent falls from freezing
(k) Walking
0 Normal
1 Mild difficulty, may drag legs or decrease arm
  swing
2 Moderate difficulty, requires no assistance
3 Severe disturbance, requires assistance
4 Cannot walk at all, even with assistance
(l) Tremor
0 Absent
1 Slight and infrequent, not bothersome to patient
2 Moderate, bothersome to patient
3 Severe, interfere with many activities
4 Marked, interferes with many activities
(m) Sensory complaints related to parkinsonism
0 None
1 Occasionally has numbness, tingling and mild
  aching
2 Frequent, but not distressing
3 Frequent painful sensation
4 Excruciating pain

(3) *Motor examination*
(a) Speech
0 Normal
1 Slight loss of expression, diction and volume
2 Monotone, slurred but understandable, moderately
  impaired
3 Marked impairment, difficult to understand
4 Unintelligible
(b) Facial expression
0 Normal
1 Slight hypomimia, could be poker face
2 Slight but definite abnormal diminution in
  expression
3 Moderate hypomymia, lips parted some of the time
4 Masked or fixed face, lips parted 6 mm (1/4 inch)
  or more, with complete loss of expression
(c) Tremor at rest
Face
0 Absent
1 Slight, infrequent
2 Mild, present most of the time
3 Moderate, present most of the time
4 Marked, present most of the time

0 Absent
1 Slight, infrequent
2 mild, present most of the time
3 Moderate, present most of the time
4 Marked, present most of the time
LUE
0 Absent
1 Slight, infrequent
2 Mild, present most of the time
3 Moderate, present most of the time
4 Marked, present most of the time
RLE
0 Absent
1 Slight, infrequent
2 Mild, present most of the time
3 Moderate, present most of the time
4 Marked, present most of the time
LLE
0 Absent
1 Slight, infrequent
2 Mild, present most of the time
3 Moderate, present most of the time
4 Marked, present most of the time
(d) Action or postural tremor
RUE
0 Absent
1 Slight, present with action
2 Moderate, present with action
3 Moderate, present with action and posture holding
4 Marked, interferes with feeding
LUE
0 Absent
1 Slight, present with action
2 Moderate, present with action
3 Moderate, present with action and posture holding
4 Marked, interferes with feeding
(e) Rigidity
Neck
0 Absent
1 Slight or only with activation
2 Mild or moderate
3 Marked, full range of motion
4 Severe
RUE
0 Absent
1 Slight or only with activation
2 Mild or moderate
3 Marked, full range of motion
4 Severe
LUE
0 Absent
1 Slight or only with activation
2 Mild or moderate

3 Marked, full range of motion

4 Severe

RLE

0 Absent

1 Slight or only with activation

2 Mild or moderate

3 Marked, full range of motion

4 Severe

LLE

0 Absent

1 Slight or only with activation

2 Mild or moderate

3 Marked, full range of motion

4 Severe

(f) Finger taps

Right

0 normal

1 Mild slowing and/or reduction in amplitude

2 Moderately impaired, definite and early fatiguing, may have occasional arrests

3 Severely impaired, frequent hesitations and arrests

4 Can barely perform

Left

0 Normal

1 Mild slowing and/or reduction in amplitude

2 Moderately impaired, definite and early fatiguing, may have occasional arrests

3 Severely impaired, frequent hesitations and arrests

4 Can barely perform

(g) Hand movements (open and close hands in rapid succession)

Right

0 Normal

1 Mild slowing and/or reduction in amplitude

2 Moderate impaired, definite and early fatiguing, may have occasional arrests

3 Severely impaired, frequent hesitations and arrests

4 Can barely perform

Left

0 Normal

1 Mild slowing and/or reduction in amplitude

2 Moderately impaired, definite and early fatiguing, may have occasional arrests

3 Severely impaired, frequent hesitations and arrests

4 Can barely perform

(h) Rapid alternating movements (pronate and supinate hands)

Right

0 Normal

1 Mild slowing and/or reduction in amplitude

2 Moderate impaired, definite and early fatiguing, may have occasional arrests

3 Severely impaired, frequent hesitations and arrests

4 Can barely perform

Left

0 Normal

1 Mild slowing and/or reduction in amplitude

2 Moderately impaired, definite and early fatiguing, may have occasional arrests

3 Severely impaired, frequent hesitations and arrests

4 Can barely perform

(i) Leg agility (tap heel on ground, amplitude should be 7.5 cm)

Right

0 Normal

1 Mild slowing and/or reduction in amplitude

2 Moderately impaired, definite and early fatiguing, may have occasional arrests

3 Severely impaired, frequent hesitations and arrests

4 Can barely perform

Left

0 Normal

1 Mild slowing and/or reduction in amplitude

2 Moderately impaired, definite and early fatiguing, may have occasional arrests

3 Severely impaired, frequent hesitations and arrests

4 Can barely perform

(j) Arising from chair (patient arises with arms folded across chest)

0 Normal

1 Slow, may need more than one attempt

2 Pushes self up from arms or seat

3 Tends to fall back, may need multiple tries but can arise without assistance

4 Unable to arise without help

(k) Posture

0 Normal erect

1 Slightly stooped, could be normal for older person

2 Definitely abnormal, moderately stooped, may lean to one side

3 Severely stooped with kyphosis

4 Marked flexion with extreme abnormality of posture

(l) Gait

0 Normal

1 Walks slowly, may shuffle with short steps, no festination or propulsion

2 Walks with difficulty, little or no assistance, some festination, short steps or propulsion

3 Severe disturbance, frequent assistance

4 Cannot walk

(m) Postural stability (retropulsion test)

0 Normal

1 Recovers unaided

2 Would fall if not caught

3 Falls spontaneously   (Continued)

4 Unable to stand
(n) Body bradykinesia/hypokinesia
   0 None
   1 Minimal slowness, could be normal, deliberate character
   2 Mild slowness and poverty of movement, definitely abnormal, or decreased amplitude of movement
   3 moderate slowness, poverty or small amplitude
   4 Marked slowness, poverty or amplitude

RUE: right upper extremity: LUE: left upper extremity; RLE: right lower extremity; LLE: left lower extremity.

Table 11.24 Differential diagnosis in Parkinson's disease[108,112,132]

Disease	Description
Essential tremor (familial tremor) (107)	Postural tremor mainly of the upper extremities, most obvious with arms outstretched (as in the finger-to-nose test)
	Tremor is 12–14 Hz. It may involve the head, arm or voice. Tremor may worsen with stress, whereas alcohol may temporarily diminish it
Huntington's disease (133)	Degenerative congenital (autosomal-dominant) condition displaying chorea, personality changes and dementia
Wilson's disease (133)	Congenital (autosomal-recessive) disorder of copper metabolism resulting in tremor ('wing-beating'), dysarthria, rigidity, bradykinesia, dystonia and psychiatric disturbance

Dopamine

Levodopa is the most potent anti-PD medication used today.[134] Exogenous dopa (e.g. levodopa, or levodopa plus a decarboxylase inhibitor which helps to prevent breakdown in the liver) is often prescribed. There may be peripheral side-effects (hypotension, nausea and vomiting) as well as central ones (confusion and depression dyskinetic movements).

One controversy currently being investigated is the concern that levodopa is a neurotoxin that adds to oxidative stress and cell death, possibly contributing to the progression of the disease.[135]

Table 11.25 Common drugs and surgical procedures used for Parkinson's disease

Drugs
  Selegiline
  Levodopa
  Dopamine agonists:
    Bromocriptine
    Pergolide
    Pramipexole
    Ropilirole
  Anticholinergics and amantadine
  Catechol-*O*-methyltransferace inhibitors as an adjunct to levodopa (tolcapone)
Surgery
  Stereotactic surgery
  Human foetal and medullary transplantation
  Deep brain stimulation

Dopamine agonists

These drugs directly stimulate dopamine receptors. An example is bromocriptine,[136] which is used when levodopa responsiveness is lost and may provide some neuroprotection in younger patients. Other agonists are available and are used in complex regimens to reduce the periods of immobility (freezing). Side-effects may include hypotension and confusion.

Anticholinergic drugs

These drugs function by restoring the balance between dopamine and acetylcholine neurotransmitters in the basal ganglia. An example is benzhexol.[136] They have effects that are useful in controlling tremor, but little effect on the rigidity and slow movements associated with PD. Side-effects may include confusion, visual blurring, urinary retention and dry mouth.

Amantidine

This is an antiviral drug that helps to reduce rigidity. The mechanism of action is not completely understood, but its effect is to increase dopamine release, block reuptake of dopamine and stimulate dopamine receptors.

COMT inhibitors as an adjunct to levodopa (tolcapone)

Catechol-*O*-methyltransferase (COMT) is one of the primary enzymes for the metabolism of levodopa, dopamine, adrenaline, noradrenaline and their metabolites.[137] COMT inhibitors make more levodopa available by preventing or slowing its metabolism, thereby increasing levodopa availability to the brain with less variation in plasma levels.[137] It decreases the off-time in patients with a fluctuating response to levodopa (On–off phenomenon). In this way, it improves the patients' activities of daily living. The most common side-effect is an acute dyskinesia after initiation of the drug, and after continued use some patients may develop severe diarrhoea or increased liver transaminase.

Stereotactic surgery

Surgical techniques were developed in Sweden by Dr Lars Leksell in the 1950s but were discontinued in the 1960s when levodopa was introduced. Unfortunately, the response to levodopa tends to wear off, and in later stages of the disease may itself produce dyskinesias.[138]

Pallidotomy is a surgical procedure to remove over-active dopaminergic neurons in a portion of the basal ganglia and globus pallidus, to reduce the tremors and dyskinesias of PD.[138]

Human foetal and medullary transplantation

This surgical technique involves the transplantation of tissue capable of synthesizing and releasing dopamine to the striatum of the PD patient. The procedure is experimental and has raised many ethical concerns.

Deep brain stimulation

The use of bilateral deep brain stimulation of the thalamus, subthalamic nuclei or globus pallidus is a new experimental technique for patients who are responsive to levo-dopa but suffer from wild on–off fluctuations in motor function.[139,140] This new technique is used in carefully selected patients to control unwanted symptoms and to improve the quality of life with the PD.

Psychiatric counselling

Depression, psychosis, confusion, agitation, hallucinations and delusions may all occur in PD patients. These may respond to modifications in the medications, including decreasing levo-dopa or dopamine agonists or discontinuing anticholinergics, amantidine or selegiline.[135] Medical supervision is necessary and at times counselling should be advocated. The psychiatric complications may be very debilitating for the patient's well-being, for their family and in social interactions.

The frequency of depression varies widely, occurring in between 18 and 70% of PD patients.[140] The variation results from the speed of the disease process, the advancing age of the patient and other predisposing factors. Counselling and treatment (antidepressant therapy) are helpful.

The patient's family is very important. They may provide not only significant levels of care and support, but also information. The family may be the first to identify early signs of depression or behavioural changes. Counselling should be considered for family members to help them to understand the disease, to advise them on their role as a loving support crew, but also on the need to apply 'tough love' to motivate the PD patient if necessary, to consider respite care, and to consider or cope with transitions to institutional care if necessary.

The chiropractor must not assume that the patient is receiving adequate attention from other health professionals. Patients may have been misdiagnosed or left in the dark without their questions answered, received in adequate follow-up, missed specialist appointments, or may have other concurrent conditions that have been identified (e.g. depression, suicidal tendencies, malnutrition or alcoholism).

Chiropractic, rehabilitation and physical therapies

The patient with PD is advised to kept as active as possible and to avoid any unnecessary bed rest which may increase flexion contractures, poor balance and unwanted muscle atrophy. Motor disabilities may lead to myofascial pain, falls, social isolation and lifestyle changes. The patient often seeks chiropractic care for their movement conditions.

Chiropractic care is aimed at improving spinal mobility, adjusting vertebral joint subluxation, treating spinal pain syndromes and providing health-care counselling or referrals. Physical therapies and rehabilitation may focus on improving musculoskeletal function (strength, flexibility, range of motion), and prescribing programmes for endurance, balance and co-ordination, gait, relaxation, diet and rejuvenation therapies (spa, massage). Supportive chiropractic care of the PD patient may be helpful to promote the postural correction, spinal mobility and gait. General physical exercise will not modify the progression of the disease, but exercise may decrease the rate of physical decline from disuse atrophy. This may increase the survival rate of the PD patients.[141]

Heavy weight training and prolonged hard exercise should be avoided. The training effects may cause prolonged periods of exhaustion and possibly reduce the duration of drug effects.[142] Moderate exercise should be advised to maintain cardiovascular capacity, basic strength, flexibility and agility. Patients should be encouraged to maintain an active lifestyle on a daily basis.

Postural flexibility exercises are helpful to attempt to diminish the anterior flexion deformity. Lying supine on a small pillow placed under the mid-thoracic kyphosis while breathing deeply may aid in kinesthetic awareness and elongation of the thoracic curvature. Deep respiratory excursion exercises may improve thoracic expansion and preserve lung volume. Flexibility exercises for the calf, hip flexor, pectoralis and cervical musculature may help the patient to feel less stiff.

Aerobic exercise twice per week has been shown to improve estimated maximum oxygen consumption and heart rate.[143] Exercise programmes may be recommended at least three or four times per week (20 min per session), but the preference is to maintain a daily schedule of activity that is within the capacity of the individual. A daily programme will encourage continuity as it becomes a part of the patient's lifestyle. In addition, the benefits of improving mood, energy level and sleep may be realized daily.

Exercise programmes may be divided into two smaller sessions (10 min each) in one day if the patient does not have the endurance to exercise for 20 min at one time. The type of exercise prescribed should parallel the patient's functional skills and the stage of PD (Hoehn and Yahr Scale; Table 11.21):

- younger or stage 1 patients may have very few limitations (swimming, bicycle riding, jogging);
- older or stage 2 and 3 patients, may avoid aggressive activities in favour of stable exercises (pool fitness, exercise bike, 'mall walking', i.e. walking in shopping malls where the climate is controlled and the floor is smooth);
- more disabled or stage 4 and 5 patients, who may not be able to walk well or may confined to a wheelchair, should be encouraged to follow a seated exercise programme.

Improvements in gait
The gait of 10 patients with idiopathic PD was studied before and after a single osteopathic manipulation.[144] In comparison to a separate group of 10 PD patients who received a sham manipulation, the manipulation group displayed statistically significant improvements in their gait. Observed changes included improved stride length, cadence and maximum velocities of upper and lower extremities after treatment. This study sheds light on the possible impact of joint manipulation upon kinesthetic awareness and motor functions in these patients. Further studies are needed to identify the duration of these effects.

Improvements in physical measures
Rehabilitation therapies for improving strength, range of motion and relaxation, and initiating movements with basic gymnastic programming have demonstrated improvements.[145] Improved motor coordination, strength and gait were realized with supervised or unsupervised programmes or by increasing general activities such as climbing stairs, catching a ball or hitting a punch-bag.[134,145,146]

Improvements in activities of daily living
In a study that used a home exercise programme, improvements were seen in the patient's ability to tend to their personal care (self-care), feeding and mobility.[147]

Supportive physical activity care
Comella et al. evaluated disability in PD patients after 1 month of intensive physical rehabilitation.[148] There were significant improvements in the ADLs (Table 11.22) and in the UPDRS (Table 11.23). The improvements returned to baseline 6 months after patients returned to a sedentary lifestyle. This indicates that patients need continued encouragement and the guidance of a long-term maintenance programme for physical activity.

Walkers
At stage 3 balance difficulties become a significant concern with a risk of falling. A fall could be fatal, it may initiate many secondary health issues or it could further the deterioration of the PD. During this stage, canes, walking frames or wheelchairs may be useful periodically, especially when the patient is fatigued.

Two-, three- and four-wheeled walking frames are available. They have been shown to improve mobility and prevent falls when balance becomes difficult.[149]

Prognosis of Parkinson's disease

Patients with PD live with a chronic degenerative disease that usually progresses slowly. For an individual patient it is difficult to attempt to estimate the rate of progression from stage to stage, but a rough guideline is 2.5 years between stages.[150] Medication appears to be successful for 4–6 years, then medication-related side-effects and poor balance become problematic between 5 and 10 years. With dopamine-replacement therapy the life expectancy of patients with PD is approximately equal to that of people without PD.[150]

Of all the symptoms of PD patients report that in the first decade with the disease the most problematic symptom is tremor, then 12–14 years after diagnosis, imbalance becomes the main complaint.[151]

Reference:

1 National Center for Health Statistics, Current estimates from the National Health Interview Survey, USA, 1994

2 National Board of Chiropractic Examiners. Job Analysis of Chiropractic. A project report, survey analysis, and summary of the practice of chiropractic within the United States. Greeley, CO: NBCE, 2000.

3 National Board of Chiropractic Examiners. Job Analysis of Chiropractic. A project report, survey analysis, and summary of the practice of chiropractic within Canada. Greeley, CO: NBCE, 1993.

4 Aihie Sayer A, Osmond C, Briggs R, Cooper C. Do all the systems age together? Gerontology 1999; 45(2): 83–86.

5 Kenney RA. Physiology of Aging. 2nd edn. Chicago, IL: Year Book Medical Publishing, 1989: 94.

6 Adams RA, Victor M, Ropper AH. Principles of Neurology. 6th edn. New York: McGraw-Hill, 1997.

7 Courchesne E, Chisum HJ, Townsend J et al. Normal brain development and aging: quantitative analysis at in vivo MR imaging in healthy volunteers. Radiology 2000; 216: 672–682.

8 Honig LS, Rosenberg RN. Apoptosis and neurologic disease. Am J Med 2000; 108: 317–330.

9 Krandel ER, Schwartz JH, Jessell TM. Principles of Neural Science. 3rd edn. Norwalk, CT: Appleton & Lange, 1991: 976.

10 Kaasinen V, Vilkman H, Hietala J et al. Age-related dopamine D2/D3 receptor loss in extrastriatal regions of the human brain. Neurobiol Aging 2000; 21: 683–688.

11 Antoniadis EA, Ko CH, Ralph MR, McDonald RJ. Circadian rhythms, aging and memory. Behav Brain Res 2000; 114: 221–233.

12 Cummings DE, Merriam GR. Age-related changes in growth hormone secretion: should the somatopause be treated? Semin Reprod Endocrinol 1999; 17: 311–325.

13 American Psychiatric Association Diagnostic and Statistical Manual of Mental Disorders (DSM-IV). 4th edn. Washington, DC: APA, 1994.

14 Rogers AM, Simon DG. A preliminary study of dietary aluminum intake and risk of Alzheimer's disease. Age Aging 1999; 28: 205–209.

15 Gallo JJ, Busby-Whitehead J, Silliman RA, Murphy JB. Reichl's care of the elderly. Clinical Aspects of Aging. 5th edn. New York: Lippincott, Williams & Wilkins, 1999.

16 Nynerg F. Growth hormone in the brain: characteristics of brain targets for the hormone and their function. Front Neuroendocrinol 2000; 21: 330–348.

17 Ho KK, Hoffman DM. Aging and growth hormone. Horm Res 1993; 40: 80–86.

18 Veldhuis JD, Iranmanwsh A, Weltman A. Elements in the pathophysiology of diminished growth hormone secretion in aging humans. Endocrine 1977; 7: 41–48.

19 Lamerts SW. The somatopause: to treat or not to treat? Horm Res 2000; 53 (Suppl 3): 42–43.

20 Corpas E, Harman SM, Blackman MR. Human growth hormone and aging. Endocr Rev 1993; 14: 20–39.

21 Johannsson G, Svensson J, Bengtsson BA. Growth hormone and aging. Growth Horm IGF Res 2000; 10 (Suppl B): S25–S30.

22 Hartman ML. The Growth Hormone Research Society consensus guidelines for the diagnosis and treatment of adult GH deficiency. Growth Horm IGF Res 1998; 8 (Suppl A): 25–29.

23 Mehagnoul-Schipper DJ, Vloet LC, Colier WN et al. Cerebral oxygenation declines in healthy elderly subjects in response to assuming the upright position. Stroke 2000; 31: 1615–1620.

24 Kalaria RN. The role of cerebral ischemia in Alzheimer's disease. Neurobiol Aging 2000; 21: 321–330.

25 Richardson D, Bexton R, Shaw F et al. Complications of carotid sinus massage – a prospective series of older patients. Age Aging 2000; 29: 413–417.

26 Lipsitz LA. Orthostatic hypotension in the elderly. N Engl J Med 1989; 321: 952–957.

27 Caplan L, Kelly JJ. Consultation in Neurology. Toronto: BC Decker, 1988.

28 Doty RL. Influence of age and age-related diseases on olfactory function. Ann NY Acad Sci 1989; 561: 76–86.

29 Bartoshuk LM, Beauchamp GK. Chemical senses. Ann Rev Psych 1994; 45: 419–449

30 Rolls BJ. Do chemosensory changes influence food intake in the elderly? Physiol Behav 1999; 66: 193–197.

31 Frank ME, Hettinger TP, Mott AE. The sense of taste: neurobiology, aging and medication effects. Crit Rev Oral Biol Med 1992; 3: 371–393.

32 Sonies BC. Oropharyngeal dysphagia in the elderly. Clin Geriatr Med 1992; 8: 569–577.

33 Winkler S, Garg AK, Mekayarajjananonth T et al. Depressive taste and smell in geriatric patients. J Am Dent Assoc 1999; 130: 1759–1765.

34 Schiffman SS. Intensification of sensory properties of foods for the elderly. J Nutr 2000; 130(4S Suppl): 927S–930S.

35 Mion LC, McDowell JA, Heaney LK. Nutritional assessment of the elderly in the ambulatory care setting. Nurse Pract Forum 1994; 5: 46–51.

36 Lister RG, Eckardt MJ, Weingartner H. Ethanol intoxication and memory: recent developments and new directions. In: Galanter M, ed. Recent Developments in Alcoholism. New York: Plenum, 1987: 111–126.

37 Beattie BL, Louie VY. Nutrition and aging. In: Gallo JJ, Busby-Whitehead J, Sillman RA et al., eds. Reichel's Care of the Elderly. 5th edn. New York: Lippincott, Williams & Wilkins, 1999: 225–240.

38 McNulty H. Folate requirements for health in different population groups. Br. J Biomed Sci 1995; 52: 110–119.

39 Alpert JE, Fava M. Nutrition and depression: the role of folate. Nutr Rev 1997; 55: 145–149.

40 Carmel R. Cobalamin, the stomach and aging. Am J Clin Nutr 1997; 66: 750–759.

41 Cruz JA, Moreiras-Varelo O, Van Staveren WA et al. Intake of vitamin and minerals. Euronut SENECA investigators. Eur J Clin Nutr 1991; 45(Suppl 3): 121–138.

42 Tielsch JM, Sommer A, Witt K, Katz J. Blindness and visual impairments in the urban population: the Baltimore Eye Survey. Arch Ophthalmol 1990; 108: 286–290.

43 Gallo JJ, Fulmer T, Paveza GJ, Reichel W. Handbook of Geriatric Assessment, 3rd edn. Gaithersburg, MD: Aspen, 2000: 229–231.

44 Levine BK, Beason-Held LL, Purpura KP et al. Age-related differences in visual perception: a PET study. Neurobiol Aging 2000; 21: 577–584.

45 Myelin SN, Ribaya-Mercado JD, Russell RM et al. Vitamin B_6 deficiency impairs interleukin 2 production and lymphocyte production in elderly adults. Am J Clin Nutr 1991; 53: 1275–1280.

46 Carter WJ. Effect of normal aging on skeletal muscle. In: Maloney FP, Means KM, eds. Physical Medicine and Rehabilitation: Rehabilitation and the Aging Population, Vol. 4. Philadelphia, PA: Hanley & Belfus, 1990: 1–7.

47 Head KA. Natural therapies for occular disorders, part two: cataracts and glaucoma. Altern Med Rev 2001; 6: 141–166.

48 Brenner MH, Curbow B., Javitt JC et al. Vision changes and quality of life in the elderly. Arch Ophthalmol 1993; 111: 680–685.

49 Blystone PA. Relationship between age and presbyopic addition using a sample of 3,645 examinations from a single private practice. J. Am Optom Assoc 1999; 70: 505–508.

50 American Acadamy of Ophthalmology Practice Pattern Committee. Primary Open-angle Glaucoma. San Francisco, CA: American Acadamy of Ophthalmology, 1996.

51 La Heij EC, Hendrikse F. Retinal detachments and retinal surgery. Ned Tijdschr Geneeskd 1999; 143: 781–185.

52 Greenstein VC, Holopigian K, Hood DC et al. The nature and extent of retinal dysfunction associated with diabetic macular edema. Invest Opthalmol Vis Sci 2000; 41: 3643–3654.

53 Garvican L, Clowes J, Gillow T. Preservation of sight on diabetes: developing a national risk reduction programme. Diabet Med 2000; 17: 627–634.

54 Caspary DM, Milbrandt JC, Helfert RH. Central auditory aging: GABA changes in the inferior colliculus. Exp Gerontol 1995; 30: 349–360.

55 Grose JH. Binaural performance and aging. J Am Acad Audiol 1996; 7: 168–174.

56 Norre ME, Forrez G, Beckers A. Vestibular dysfunction causing instability in aged patients. Acta Otolaryngol 1987; 104: 50–55.

57 Baloh RW, Honrubia V, Jacobson K. Benign positional vertigo: clinical and oculographic features in 240 cases. Neurology 1987; 37: 371–378.

58 Froehling DA, Silverstein MD, Mohr DN et al. Benign positional vertigo: incidence and prognosis in a population-based study on Olmsted County, Minnesota. Mayo Clin Proc 1991; 66: 596–601.

59 Oostenderp RAB, VanEupen AAJM, VanErp JMM, Elvers HWH. Dizziness following whiplash injury: a neuro-otological study in manual therapy practice and therapeutic implications. J Manipulative Physiol Ther 1999; 7: 123–130.

60 Barker RA, Barasi S. Neuroscience at a Glance. Oxford: Blackwell Science, 1999.

61 Souza T. Differential Diagnosis for the Chiropractor. Protocols and Algorithms. Gaithersburg, MD: Aspen, 1997.

62 Conley T, Schoenman K, Pudik T. Cervical spondylotic myelopathy. Top Clin Chiropractic 1995; 2(3): 48–53.

63 Institute for Clinical Evaluative Sciences. Get up and go! Identifying risk factors and preventing falls in elderly patients. Inform Newslett 1998; Sept 4(4): 1–4.

64 Duncan PW, Studenski S, Chandler J, Prescott B. Functional reach: predictive validity in a sample of elderly male veterans. J Geront Med Sci 1992; 47: M94.

65 Brockhurst JC, Robertson D, James-Groom P. Clinical correlates of sway in old age: sensory modalities. Age Aging 1982; 11: 1–10.

66 Overstall PW, Exton-Smith AN, Imms FJ, Johnson AL. Falls in the elderly related to postural imbalance. BMJ 1977; i: 261–264.

67 Stelmach GE, Zelaznik HN, Lowe D. The influence of aging and attentional demands on recovery from postural instability. Aging 1990; 2: 155–161.

68 Nichols DS. Balance retraining after stroke using force platform biofeedback. Phys Ther 1997; 77: 553–558.

69 Nardone A, Grasso M, Taratola J et al. Postural coordination in elderly subjects on a periodically moving platform. Arch Phys Med Rehabil 2000; 81: 1217–1223.

70 Duncan PW, Weiner DK, Chandler J, Studenski S. Functional reach: a new clinical measure of balance. J Geront Med Sci 1990; 45: M192–M197.

71 Spirdso WW. Physical Dimensions of Aging. Windsor, Ontario: Human Kinetics, 1995.

72 Richter M, Kluger P, Puhl W. Diagnosis and therapy of spinal stenosis in the elderly. Z Prtho Ihre Grenzgeb 1999; 137: 474–481.

73 Bland JH. Disorders of the Cervical Spine. Toronto, WB Saunders Co., 1994.

74 Sasaki T, Kadoya S, Lizuka H. Roentgenological study of the sagittal diameter of the cervical spinal canal in normal adult Japanese. Neurol Med Chir (Tokyo) 1998; 38: 83–88.

75 Young WF. Cervical spondylotic myelopathy: a common cause of spinal cord dysfunction in older persons. Am Fam Physician 2000; 62: 1064–1070, 1073.

76 Patten J. Neurological Differential Diagnosis. 2nd edn. New York: Springer, 1995.

77 Finneson BE. Low Back Pain. Toronto: JB Lippincott Co., 1973.

78 Glick TH. Neurological Skills. Examination and Diagnosis. Boston, MA: Blackwell Scientific, 1993.

79 Gunn CC. 'Prespondylosis' and some pain syndromes following denervation supersensitivity. Spine 1980; 5: 185–195.

80 Gunn CC. Tenderness at motor points. J Bone Joint Surg 1976; 58-A: 815–825.

81 Gunn CC, Milbrandt WE. Utilizing trigger points. Osteopathic Physician 1977; 44: 29–52.

82 Richardson JK, Ashton-Miller JA. Peripheral neuropathy: an often-overlooked cause of falls in the elderly. Postgrad Med 1996; 99: 161–172.

83 Richardson JK, Ashton-Miller JA, Lee SG, Jacobs K. Moderate peripheral neuropathy impairs weight transfer and unipedal balance in the elderly. Arch Phys Med Rehabil 1996; 77: 1152–1156.

84 Dellon AL, Mackinnon SE. Chronic nerve compression model for the double crush hypothesis. Ann Plast Surg 1991; 26: 259–264.

85 Fink A, Hays RD, Moore AA, Beck JC. Alcohol-related problems in older persons. Determinants, consequences, and screening. Arch Intern Med 1996; 156: 1150–1156.

86 Landow K. Acute and chronic herpes zoster. An ancient scourge yields to timely therapy. Postgrad Med 2000; 107: 107–108, 113–114, 117–118.

87 Schmader K. Herpes zoster in the elderly: issues related to geriatrics. Clin Infect Dis 1999; 28: 736–739.

88 Adams RD, Victor M, Ropper AH. Principles of Neurology. 6th edn. New York: McGraw-Hill, 1997.

89 Polliack ML, Barak Y, Achiron A. Late-onset multiple sclerosis. J Am Geriatr Soc 2001; 49: 168–171.

90 Compston A. Multiple sclerosis. In: Brain's Diseases of the Nervous System, Walton J, ed. Oxford: Oxford University Press, 1993: 366–382.

91 Compstom DAS. The dissemination of multiple sclerosis. The Langdon-Brown Lecture 1989. J R Coll Physicians Lond 1990; 24: 207–218.

92 Ebers GC, Bulman DE, Sadovnick AD. A population-based study of multiple sclerosis in twins. N Engl J Med 1986; 315: 1638–1644.

93 Ebers GC. Genetic factors in multiple sclerosis. Neurol Clin 1983; 1: 645–654.

94 Dean G. On the risk of multiple sclerosis according to age at immigration. In: Field EJ, Bell TM, Carnegie PR, eds. Multiple Sclerosis Progress in Research. Amsterdam: North-Holland, 1986: 197–207.

95 Kurtzke JF, Gudmundsson KR, Bergmann S. Multiple sclerosis in Iceland: evidence of a post war epidemic. Neurology 1982; 32: 143–150.

96 Berger JR, Shweremata WA. Persistent neurological deficit precipitated by hot bath test in multiple sclerosis. JAMA 1983; 249: 1751–1753.

97 Rose AS, Ellison GW, Myers LW, Tourtellotte WW. Criteria for the clinical diagnosis of multiple sclerosis. Neurology 1976; 26: 20–22.

98 Cook AW. Electrical stimulation in multiple sclerosis. Hosp Pract 1976; 11(4): 51–58.

99 Ray CD. Electrical stimulation: new methods for therapy and rehabilitation. Scand J Rehabil Med 1978; 10: 65–74.

100 Bates JA. Therapeutic electrical stimulation. The transistorized placebo? Electroencephalogr Clin Neurophysiol 1978; 34(Suppl): 329–334.

101 Vodovnik L, Rebersek S, Stefanovska A et al. Electrical stimulation for control of paralysis and therapy of abnormal movements. Scand J Rehabil Med 1988; 17(Suppl): 91–97.

102 Orlowska E, Pakszys W, Kotowicz J et al. Attempt at treating multiple sclerosis by means of ultrasound stimulation of the lymphatic system. Neurol Neurochir Pol 1978; 12: 587–593.

103 Orlowska E, Gornas P. Effects of ultrasound stimulation of the lymphatic system on changes in the subpopulations of peripheral blood lymphocytes in multiple sclerosis. Neurol Neurochir Pol 1980; 14: 283–288.

104 Van Poppel H, Ketelaer P, Van Weerd A. Interferential therapy for detrusor hyperreflexia in multiple sclerosis. Urology 1985; 25: 607–612.

105 Olgiati R, Girr A, Hugi L, Haegi V. Respiratory muscle training in multiple sclerosis: a pilot study. Schweiz Arch Neurol Psychiatr 1989; 140: 46–50.

106 Marsden CD. Parkinson's disease. J Neurol Neurosurg Psychiatry 1994; 57: 672–668.

107 Adams RD, Victor M, Roper AH. Principles of Neurology. 6th edn. New York: McGraw-Hill, 1997.

108 Martilla RJ, Rinne UK. Epidemiology of Parkinson's disease in Finland. Acta Neurol Scand 1979; 53: 82–102.

109 DeRijk MC, Breteler MM, Graveland GA. Prevalence of Parkinson's disease in the elderly: the Rotterdam study. Neurology 1995; 45: 2144–2146.

110 Stacy M, Jankovic J. Differential diagnosis of Parkinson's disease and other parkinsonism plus syndromes. Neurol Clin 1992; 10: 341–355.

111 Margante L, Rocca WA, DiRosa AE. Prevalence of Parkinson disease and other types of parkinsonism: a door-to-door survey in three Sicilian municipalities. Neurology 1992; 42: 1901–1907.

112 Martilla RJ, Rinne UK. Epidemiological approaches to the etiology of Parkinson's disease. Acta Neurol Scand 1989; 126: 13–18.

113 McGeer P et al. Aging, Alzheimer's disease and the cholinergic system of the basal forebrain. Neurology 1984; 34: 741.

114 Tanner CM, Ben-Shlomo Y. Epidemiology of Parkinson's disease. Adv Neurol 1999; 80: 153–159.

115 Korman K, James JA. Medical management of Parkinson's disease in the elderly. Top Geriatr Rehabil 1993; 8: 1–13.

116 Swash M, Schwartz MS. Neurology: A Concise Clinical Text. Toronto: Baillière Tindall, 1989.

117 Stern G, Lees A. Parkinson's disease: The Facts. Oxford: Oxford University Press, 1991.

118 Dietz V, Berger W, Horstmann GA. Posture in Parkinson's disease: impairment of reflexes and programming. Ann Neurol 1988; 24: 660–669.

119 Van Emmerik RE, Wagenaar RC, Winogrodzka A, Wolters EC. Identification of axial rigidity during locomotion in Parkinson's disease. Arch Phys Med Rehabil 1999; 80: 186–191.

120 Carr JH, Sheppard RB. Neurological Rehabilitation: Optimizing Motor Performance. Oxford: Butterworth Heinemann, 1999.

121 Evarts EV, Teravainen H, Calne DB. Reaction time in Parkinson's disease. Brain 1981; 104: 167–186.

122 Berardelli A, Dick JPR, Rothwell JC et al. Scaling of the size of the first agonist EMG burst during rapid wrist movements in patients with Parkinson's disease. J Neuro Neurosurg Psych 1986; 49: 1273–1279.

123 Benecke R, Rothwell JC, Dick JPR et al. Performance of simultaneous movements in patients with Parkinson's disease. Brain 1986; 109: 739–757.

124 Benecke R, Rothwell JC, Dick JPR et al. Disturbance of sequential movements in patents with Parkinson's disease. Brain 1987; 110: 361–379.

125 Schwab RS, Chafetz ME, Walker S. Control of two simultaneous voluntary motor acts in normal and Parkinsonism. Arch Neurol Psych 1954; 72: 591–598.

126 Wall JC, Turnbull GI. The kinematics of gait. In: Turnbull GI, ed. Physical therapy management of Parkinson's disease. New York: Churchill Livingstone, 1992: 49–67.

127 Fisk JD, Doble SE. Cognitive deficits. In: Turnbull GI, ed. Physical therapy management of Parkinson's Disease. New York: Churchill Livingstone, 1992: 69–89.

128 Mayeux R, Stern Y, Rosen J. Depression, intellectual impairment and Parkinson's disease. Neurology 1981; 31: 645–650.

129 Lees AJ, Smith E. Cognitive deficits in the early stages of Parkinson's disease. Brain 1983; 106: 257–270.

130 Hoehn MM, Yahr MD. Parkinsonism: onset, progression and mortality. Neurology 1967; 17: 427–442.

131 Gillingham FJ, Donaldson MC, eds. Third Symposium of Parkinson's Disease. Edinburgh: Livingstone, 1969: 152–157.

132 Heilman KM, Watson RT, Greer M. Handbook for Differential Diagnosis of Neurological Signs and Symptoms. New York: Appleton-Century-Crofts, 1977.

133 Gibb WRG. Neuropathology of movement disorders. J. Neurol Neurosurg Psych 1989; June(Suppl.): 55–67.

134 Palmer S, Mortimer JA, Webster DD et al. Exercise therapy for Parkinson's disease. Arch Phys Med Rehabil 1986; 67: 741–745.

135 Klein RB, Knoefel JE. Neurologic problems in the elderly. In: Gallo J, Busby-Whitehead J, Rabins PV et al., eds Reichel's Care of the elderly: Clinical Aspects of Aging. 5 edn. New York: Lippincott Williams & Wilkins, 1999: 260–274.

136 Olanow CW. Medication in Parkinson's disease. Neurology 1998; 50(3 Suppl 3): S1–S7.

137 Nissens E, Touminen R, Perhoniemi V, Kaakkola S. Catechol-O-methyltransferase activity in human and rat small intestine. Life Sci 1988; 42: 2609–2614.

138 Fine J. Pallidotomy relieves symptoms of Parkinson's disease. N Engl J Med 2000; 342: 1708–1714.

139 Ghika J, Villemure JG, Fankhauser H *et al.* Efficiency and safety of bilateral contemporaneous pallidal stimulation (deep brain stimulation) in levodopa-responsive patients with Parkinson's disease with severe motor fluctuations: a 2-year follow-up review. J Neurosurg 1998; 89: 713–718.

140 Waters CH. Managing the late complications of Parkinson's disease. Neurology 1997; 49: S49–S57.

141 Kuroda K, Tatara K, Takatorige T *et al.* Effect of physical exercise on mortality in patients with Parkinson's disease. Acta Neurol Scand 1992; 86: 55–59.

142 Fertl E, Doppelbauer A, Auff E. Physical activity and sports in patients suffering from Parkinson's disease in comparison with healthy seniors. J Neural Transm 1993; 5: 157–161.

143 Bridgewater KL, Sharpe MH. Aerobic exercise and early Parkinson's disease. J Neurol Rehabil 1996; 10: 233–241.

144 Wells MR, Giantinoto S, D'Agate D *et. al.* Standard osteopathic manipulative treatment acutely improves gait performance in patients with Parkinson's disease. J Am Osteopath Assoc 1999; 99(2): 92–98.

145 Bilowit DS. Establishing physical objectives in the rehabilitation of patients with Parkinson's disease (gymnasium activities). Phys Ther Rev 1956; 36: 176–178.

146 Szkely BC, Kosanovich NN, Sheppard W. Adjunctive treatment for Parkinson's disease: physical therapy and comprehensive group therapy. Rehabil Lit 1982; 43: 72–76.

147 Hurwitz A. The benefit of a home exercise regimen for ambulatory Parkinson's disease patients. J Neurosurg Nurs 1989; 21: 180–184.

148 Comella CL, Stebbins GT, Brown-Toms BA, Goetz C. Physical therapy and Parkinson's disease: a controlled trial. Neurology 1994; 44: 376–338.

149 Mahoney J, Euhardy R, Carnes M. A comparison of a two-wheeled and a three-wheeled walker in a geriatric population. J Am Geriatr Soc 1992; 40: 735–736.

150 Hoehn MM. The natural history of Parkinson's disease in the pre-levodopa and post-levodopa eras. In: Cedarbaum JM, Gancher ST, eds. Neurological Clinics. Philadelphia, PA: WB Saunders & Co., 1992: 331.

151 Wendall CM, Hauser RA, Nagaria MH *et al.* Chief complaints of patients with Parkinson's disease. Neurology 1999; 52(Suppl 2): A90.

Further reading

Afifi, AK, Bergman RA. Basic Neuroscience; A Structural and functional approach 2nd edn. Baltimore: Urban & Schwarzenberg, 1986

Ajmani RS, Metter EJ, Jaykumar R *et al.* Hemodynamic changes during aging associated with cerebral blood flow and impaired cognitive function. Neurobiol Aging 2000; 21: 257–269.

Barker RA, Dunnett SB. Neural Repair, Transplantation and Rehabilitation. East Sussex: Psychology Press, 1999.

Bartoshuk LM, Beauchamp GK. Chemical senses. Annu Rev Psychol 1994; 45: 419–449.

Bushnell TG, Cobo-Castro T. Complex regional pain syndrome: becoming more or less complex? Man Ther 1999; 4: 221–228.

Calne DB, Eisler T. The pathogenesis and medical treatment of extrapyramidal diseases. Med Clin North Am 1979; 63: 715–727.

Canadian Task Force on the Periodic Health Examination. Periodic health examination, 1995 update: 3. Screening for visual problems among the elderly. Can Med Assoc J 2995; 152: 1211– 1222.

Glover JR. In Burger AA, Tobis JS. Approaches to the Validation of Manipulation Therapy. Springfield, Ill: Charles C Thomas, 1977: Chapter 9.

Kaplan LR, Kelly JJ. Consultation in Neurology. Toronto: BC Decker, 1988.

Kosnik W, Winslow L, Kline D *et al.* Visual changes in daily life throughout adulthood. J Geront Psych Sci 1988; 43: 63–70.

Kraft GH, Freal JE, Coryell JK. Disability, disease duration, and rehabilitation service needs in multiple sclerosis: patient perspectives. Arch Phys Med Rehabil 1986; 67: 164–168.

McLeod JG, Lance JW. Introductory Neurology. 2nd edn. London: Blackwell Scientific Publications, 1989.

Morgante L, Rocca WA, DiRosa AE. Prevalence of Parkinson's disease and other types of parkinsonism: a door-to-door survey in three Sicilian municipalities. Neurology 1992; 42: 1901–1907.

Morley JE, Silver AJ. Nutritional issues in nursing homes care. Ann Intern Med 1995; 123: 850–859.

Perkin DG, Rose FC, Blackwood W, Shawdon HH. Atlas of Clinical Neurology. Philadelphia, PA: JB Lippincott, 1986.

Prinz PN, Bailey SL, Woods DL. Sleep impairments in healthy seniors: roles of stress, cortisol, and interleukin-1 beta. Chronobiol Int 200; 17(3): 391–404.

Rampling R, Symond P. Radiation myelopathy. Curr Opin Neurol 1998; 11: 627–632.

Terrett AGJ. Vertebrobasilar Stroke Following Manipulation. West Des Moines, IA: National Chiropractic Mutual Insurance Co., 1996.

Weisberg L, Strub RL, Garcia CA. Essentials of Clinical Neurology. Gaithersburg, MD: Aspen, 1989.

Wells MR, Giantinoto S, D'Sgate D *et. al.* Standard osteopathic manipulative treatment acutely improves gait performance in patients with Parkinson's disease. J Am Osteopath Assoc 1999; 99: 92–98.

12

Diabetes and syndrome X

Brian J Gleberzon

Diabetes is thought to affect 1 out of every 15 people in affluent countries such as Canada and the USA.[1] The USA is thought to have over 16 million people with diabetes, half of whom are thought to be undiagnosed,[2–4] with an additional 30–40 million who have impaired glucose function.[5] There are two types of diabetes, type I and type II. In the past, type I was often referred to as juvenile-onset diabetes or insulin-dependent diabetes mellitus (IDDM) and type II as non-insulin-dependent diabetes mellitus (NIDDM).[1] Table 12.1 compares type I and type II diabetes. Type II diabetes accounts for over 80% of all diagnosed cases of diabetes and is thought to affect 1 in 5 people over the age of 65 years.[3,5]

In the USA, the health-care costs associated with type II diabetes quadrupled during the 1990s and exceeded $100 billion in 1995, or 15% of the total annual health-care expenditure.[3,4,6] This exceeds the health-care costs of both cancer and heart disease.[3] This also represents 28% of the national (Medicare) health-care budget for elderly Americans.[7] Diabetes is the fourth leading cause of death in the USA, accounting for 180 000 deaths each year, predominant due to coronary heart disease.[8] In one inner-city hospital in the USA, 20% of all 950 beds were occupied by patients with diabetes, with treatment primarily directed towards microvascular and macrovascular complications.[4,7]

In the USA, elderly patients with diabetes average 3.7 visits per year to a physician specifically for care of their diabetes. About 30% of diabetics between 65 and 74 years are of age hospitalized each year, a rate one-third higher than the same group without diabetes.[5]

Elderly diabetic patients are of particular concern to health-care providers because research suggests that poor glycaemic control may interact synergistically with other age-related pathologies, such as dementia, which may in turn accelerate diabetic complications.[5,8] It is for this reason that chiropractors and other providers of complementary and alternative medicine (CAM) must possess a thorough understanding of the aetiology, pathomechanics and accepted interdisciplinary management guidelines for diabetes.

The definition of diabetes has recently been modified by the American Diabetic Association.[2,4,5] Several criteria may be used independently to establish the diagnosis of diabetes. These are: (i) a 75 g oral glucose tolerance test with a 2 h value of 200 mg/dl or more, (ii) a random glucose tolerance test with a 2 h value of 200 mg/dl or more with typical symptoms of diabetes, and (iii) a fasting plasma glucose of 126 mg/dl or more on one or more than one occasion.[2] Normal fasting levels of blood glucose are 80–90 mg/dl and should be less than 115 mg/dl.[1,9] While diabetes may be suspected in patients with characteristic clinical signs and symptoms, confirmation requires blood tests to be performed. A CAM practitioner must therefore refer patients suspected of having diabetes to a med-

Table 12.1 Comparison of type I and type II diabetes

Feature	Type I	Type II
Age of onset	< 40 years old	> 40 years old
Prevalence	20%	80%
Symptoms	Classic	Variable
Weight	Lean	Often over weight
Family history	Uncommon	Very common
Ketosis	Present	Often absent
Endogenous insulin	Decrease	Variable
HLA-related	Positive	Uncertain
Islet cell pathology	Positive	Positive
Islet cell antibodies	Positive	Positive
Insulin treatment	Essential for survival	Variable
Neurovascular complications	Present	Present

ical practitioner for confirmation. The Expert Committee on the Diagnosis and Classification of Diabetes recommends a routine test of all individuals at the age of 45 years and at least every 3 years thereafter.[2]

To understand both types of diabetes, it is useful to describe them using the three 'Ds' of an epidemiological approach: distribution, dynamics and determinants. Preventive strategies and current therapeutic approaches used to manage both types of diabetes will also be discussed.

Distribution of diabetes

The prevalence of diabetes increases with age in all populations.[1,5] In affluent, urbanized countries, diabetes is thought to affect at least 6% of the population, with estimates as high as 10%.[10] Of those affected, 80% present with type II diabetes, with symptoms typically becoming apparent after the age of 40 years. In Native American populations, the incidence of diabetes exceeds 30%.[11]

There is a considerable racial predilection with regard to the prevalence of type II diabetes.[5] The incidence of type II diabetes has been increasing steadily since the 1960s among minority groups.[3,5] Among those over the age of 65 years, the prevalence of diabetes in the USA in Hispanics, blacks and Caucasians is 33%, 25% and 17%, respectively.[1,6]

The prevalence of diabetes increases with age in all populations. Not only do elderly Hispanics and African-Americans demonstrate a prevalence of diabetes that exceeds 20%, but an additional 25% are afflicted by impaired glucose tolerance.[5] Diabetes shows little gender preference, although it is slightly more frequent among women with advancing age.[5]

Dynamics of diabetes

Understanding the pathophysiology of diabetes is the most effective way to explain its signs, symptoms and pathological sequelae. Classic signs and symptoms of diabetes include:

- polyuria
- polyphagia
- polyuria
- ketonuria
- rapid weight loss.

Although diabetes is often described in terms of an endocrine disorder (which is appropriate considering that diabetes is the most common of the endocrine disorders), it can also be discussed as a neurological and/or nutritional condition. The normal changes associated with insulin and pancreatic function have been described in Chapter 5, Normal ageing. It is important to note that, although insulin resistance in older patients and in older patients with diabetes, including non-obese elderly patients, is well documented, insulin action and glucose tolerance can be preserved, even among the very old.[5] This is because the development of diabetes is not only determined by genetic factors, but also affected by extrinsic factors including diet, medications, level of activity, chronic illness and stress.[1,5]

Diabetes is essentially a disorder of insulin function. Insulin, produced by the endocrine component and β-cells of the pancreas, facilitates the uptake and utilization of glucose, amino acids and fatty acids by cells and tissues, promoting the synthesis of glycogen, proteins and lipids.[9] Insulin can therefore be classified as an anabolic hormone. The absence of the anabolic effect of insulin accounts for the pathomechanics of diabetes.

In the presence of excess carbohydrates, insulin promotes the synthesis and storage of glycogen in the liver and muscles.[9] This is achieved because insulin increases the permeability of cells to glucose, particularly in target tissues of muscle and adipose cells. This physiological effect is absent in most neurons of the brain, because brain cells are normally permeable to glucose without hormonal intermediates.[9]

Excess carbohydrates that cannot be stored as glycogen are converted, under the influence of insulin, into fats, mainly as triglycerides, which are stored in adipose tissue.[9] This is achieved by the dual effects of insulin inhibiting hormone-sensitive lipase while promoting glucose uptake into fat cells. This is an important feature of the physiological effects of insulin because, even though diabetes is often discussed in terms of 'blood sugar', it is the abnormalities of fat metabolism that account for the clinical features of acidosis and arteriosclerosis that result in the death of diabetic patients.[9,12]

Insulin also has the direct effect of promoting amino acid uptake into cells for protein synthesis.[9] This occurs because insulin increases amino acid permeability into cells, and insulin stimulates messenger RNA (mRNA) translation activity, resulting in increased protein synthesis by ribosomes.[9] Insulin also increases DNA transcription into RNA, while concomitantly inhibiting protein catabolism. Lastly, insulin inhibits gluconeo-genesis by the liver.[9]

In the absence of insulin and its physiological effects, there is a derangement in the glucostatic function of the liver. Initially, there is an increase in serum levels of glucose. The lack of insulin promotes hepatic catab-olism of glycogen, proteins and, most importantly, triglycerides.[9] The hydrolysis of stored triglycerides results in the release of large quantities of fatty acids and glycerol into circulating blood. Moreover, the lack of insulin stimulates the liver to convert stored fatty acids into phospholipids and cholesterol, which are released into the bloodstream as lipoproteins.[9] This process also results in the production of ketone bod-ies, which can result in ketosis. Ketosis can subse-quently cause severe acidosis and coma, leading to death.[9]

The change in serum glucose results in osmotic changes by causing fluid to leave cellular structures and enter the bloodstream.[9] This results in both intracel-lular dehydration and extracellular dehydration because of an increase in urination (osmotic diuresis).[9] Polyuria is one of the characteristic clinical manifes-tations of diabetes. Diabetic patients, because they experience dehydration, are often continually thirsty (polydipsia).[1,9] However, because thirst perception is decreased in the elderly, the recognition by clinicians of volume depletion must rely on atypical presenta-tions such as orthostasis, unsteadiness and confusion.[5]

Because biochemical nutrients cannot enter cellu-lar structures and thus remain in the bloodstream, they can be considered technically 'out of the body' and are eventually excreted. This leads to another classic sign of diabetes: polyphagia. The person is continual-ly hungry, even though they have a seemingly adequate diet. This has been described as 'starvation in the midst of plenty'.[12] The constituent metabolites fail to enter cellular structures, structures that require glucose, pro-tein and fatty acids to function and survive. In order to increase the bioavailability of glucose, proteins and fatty acids, the diabetic patient will catabolize other biochemical structures, thus liberating the required biochemical sources of energy.

As described previously, catabolism of lipids, which results in ketosis, leads to a lowering of the pH of serum.[9] The physiological response to this metabolic acidosis is to stimulate characteristic rapid and deep breathing patterns called Kussmal breathing.[9] More-over, the increased circulation of cholesterol leads to an increased risk of the development of artheroscle-rotic plaquing of arterial walls, particularly those arter-ies which are narrow and tortuous in their design.[9] Such arteries include those of the heart (coronary arteries), retina and kidney. The net effect of lipid mobilization and arterial plaquing, therefore, is dam-age to cardiac tissue, glomerosclerosis of kidney tissue and visual impairment (often blindness). It has been estimated that one-third of persons with diabetes develop kidney problems, and diabetic retinopathy is the most frequent cause of new blindness among adults aged 20–74: in patients who have had type II diabetes for longer than 20 years, nearly 60% have some degree of retinopathy.[10,13]

Diabetes is the leading cause of blindness in adults, the most frequent cause of end-stage renal disease, a leading cause of lower limb amputation and an important risk factor for atherosclerotic vascular dis-ease.[3] Diabetic atherosclerosis is a leading cause of impotence, and is a leading contributory factor to neu-rovascular damage in the legs and feet.[10] Because dia-betic patients often experience diminished sensory perception, they are often unaware of sores or infec-tions in their lower limbs. This often leads to gangrene and subsequent amputation:[10] 50% of non-traumat-ic amputations in the USA occur in diabetic patients.[10,13]

Microvascular disease also affects neurological functions. A common development is peripheral sen-sory polyneuropathy, the hallmarks of which include paraesthesias, numbness, and tingling and burning sensations in a glove-and-stocking distribution.[13] Other forms of neuropathy include cranial mononeuropathy, typically of cranial nerves III and VII, peripheral mononeuropathies, autonomic neu-ropathy and diabetic neuropathic cachexia.[13] Clinical features of diabetic autonomic neuropathy include postural dizziness, gustatory sweating and pupillary abnormalities.[13]

Catabolism of proteins can detrimentally affect immune function. Immunoglobulins are a rich source of amino acids, and seem to be vulnerable to degradation.[12] Moreover, the catabolism of proteins contributes to the wasting away of diabetic patients.[12]

It is important for a clinician to be aware that many of the dramatic symptoms attributed to other organ systems are aggravated by the development of diabetes. These include urinary incontinence (Chapter 18), weight loss and weakness mistakenly attributed to malignancy.[5] Samos and Roos describe other specific syndromes associated with diabetes in older patients. One of the most common conditions, seen in up to 10% of diabetic patients, is a painful shoulder peri-arthrosis, with moderate to severe limitation of motion of the glenohumeral joint.[5] Some other neuropathic syndromes, although less common, are more dramatic, but often resolve spontaneously.[5] This includes diabetic amyotrophy, which consists of asymmetric weakness of muscle groups, pain and wasting of the pelvic and thigh muscles with minimal change in sensory abilities. This typically occurs in men. Spontaneous resolution often occurs within a year of onset. Diabetic neuropathic cachexia is a similar syndrome, presenting in older diabetic patients with peripheral painful neuropathy, dramatic weight loss and depression. Fortunately, this condition typically abates within 1 year of its onset, with a good recovery and prognosis.[5]

For reasons not entirely understood, older diabetic patients present with an increased frequency of depression, anxiety and forgetfulness.[5,8] A study released in 2000 reported that diabetes is associated with lower levels of cognitive function and greater cognitive decline among older women.[8] Moreover, a combination of low basal metabolic heat production, decreased muscle mass, decreased shivering, diminished peripheral blood flow, high surface to body mass ratio and impaired autonomic nervous system function contribute to an increased susceptibility to hypothermia.[5] Older diabetic patients also fail to mount a fever in response to an infection, thereby delaying the diagnosis of serious infections such as malignant otitis externa, polymicrobial necrotizing fascitis and tuberculosis, which is very common in nursing homes.[5]

Determinants of diabetes

Several different pathways could account for diabetes. Diabetes could be the result of the loss or destruction of the insulin-producing β-cells. Alternatively, insulin may be produced in adequate amounts, but it may be destroyed after leaving the pancreas, before affecting peripheral target cells. Another explanation could be that insulin is produced in adequate amounts and reaches its target tissue safely, but the end organ may be resistant to the physiological effects of insulin.

Type I diabetes

It is now considered unequivocal that type I diabetes is the result of the selective destruction of the β-cells in the pancreatic islets of Langerhans.[14] The current concept is that, among certain susceptible individuals, there is an autoimmune response mediated by T-lymphocytes (T-cells) that reacts specifically to one or more β-cell proteins (autoantigens).[14] There are several lines of evidence to support the concept that type I diabetes is a T-cell-mediated autoimmune disease.[14]

First, bone-marrow cells from type I diabetic subjects transferred type I diabetes into human leucocyte antigen (HLA)-compatible siblings who received bone-marrow transplantation for the treatment of various types of leukaemia.[14] Secondly, type I diabetes occurs after pancreatic transplantation.[14] This may indicate that normal islet cells can be targeted by the autoimmune response which is usually activated in response to transplantation.[14] Thirdly, many diabetic patients exhibit signs and symptoms of other autoimmune disorders.[14] Lastly, immunosuppressive agents have been demonstrated to slow the progression of islet cell damage in patients with type I diabetes.[15]

The question remains: what initiates the autoimmune response to islet cell proteins? As early as 1980, researchers predicted that certain individuals with particular HLA alleles were susceptible to particular mutagens (possibly chemical, but more likely to be viral) that trigger an autoimmune response to either islet cells or insulin, such as HLA-DR3 or DR4.[1,14,16]

Studies in animal models have revealed that certain environmental factors may promote, while others may protect against the development of diabetes.[14] In essence, the development of diabetes is influenced by the net effect of genetic and environmental factors on immunological responses.

This concept posits that T-cells specific for islet β-cell molecules normally exist, but are constrained by immunoregulatory (self-tolerant) mechanisms. Diabetes results when one or another immunoregulatory mechanism fails, allowing islet cell autoreactive T-cells to become activated, expand clonally, and result in a cascade of immune and inflammatory processes in the islets (insulitis), culminating in β-cell destruction.[14]

During the late 1990s, a great deal of attention was paid to the theoretical link between cow's milk and the development of type I diabetes in children.[17–22] The theory posits that early consumption of cow's milk may expose the immune system to a foreign protein possessing immunological cross-reactivity with an antigen present in pancreatic β-cells.[17] Although some studies support this theory,[17,19] most researchers have refuted it.[22]

Combining all available evidence can produce a unified theory, which includes genetic, viral and autoimmunological factors. In this unified theory, a viral agent infects a host. In those individuals with particular HLA allelic combinations, there is either the development of T-cells that target self-antigens (often called 'forbidden clones', which are thought to be selected against during embryological development) or a failing of the autoregulatory mechanism that promotes self-tolerance by T-cells to self-antigens that exist naturally. In any event, the T-cells target, attack and destroy the person's self-antigens on the pancreatic islet cells. The destruction of self-tissue further stimulates the production of more self-destructive T-cells, exacerbating the process. The self-antibodies eventually destroy the host tissues and organs.

Type II diabetes

Type II diabetes is characterized by three main metabolic disorders: insulin resistance, decreased pancreatic β-cell function and elevated hepatic glucose synthesis.[3–5,23] Of these proposed mechanisms, insulin resistance by peripheral tissues appears to be the most important.[5,23] Insulin resistance results in a 60–80% reduction in glucose uptake in skeletal muscle, and resistance worsens with the progression of diabetes.[3,5,23] Insulin resistance appears to be related to obesity.[3,5,23] This association between diabetes and obesity was demonstrated in a study that found that obesity at 25 years of age strongly predicted the development of diabetes in middle age.[24]

There is a strong genetic and environmental causative role in the development of type II diabetes. Genetic factors may be classified into two types: (i) primary diabetogenes, which result in the development of diabetes (analogous to oncogenes which predispose a person to various cancers) and (ii) secondary or diabetes-related genes, such as those that predispose a person to obesity.[6] Indeed, obesity seems to play a permissive role in the development of type II diabetes, with 60–80% of diabetic patients classified as clinically obese.[4,6]

Type II diabetes clearly has a genetic basis. Concordant rates for type II diabetes approach 100%.[6] However, the mode of inheritance of type II diabetes remains uncertain. What is known is that diabetes does not appear to follow simple mendelian models, but is instead a result of a polygenetic effect.[6] Because the mode of inheritance is so complex, type II diabetes has been described as a 'geneticist's nightmare',[6] and because there are subtypes of type II diabetes, multiple genetic theories are necessary to account for the different genetic patterns. Clearly, type II diabetes is a genetically heterogeneous entity.[6,25]

An intriguing theory, called the 'thrifty gene hypothesis', was developed to explain the development of type II diabetes among Native American, such as the Pima of Arizona. This hypothesis was first proposed by James Neel, a geneticist at the University of Michigan, in the 1960s, and the theory has stood up to scrutiny reasonably well over the past 40 years.[25]

The striking prevalence of type II diabetes in many Native American groups created suspicions that there might be a predisposition to the disease, which was manifested with a reservation-style life.[11,25] Neel opined that it was possible that these groups might possess a particular genotype that conferred relative advantage to survivability in a traditional hunter–gatherer lifestyle that would be disadvantageous in a different lifestyle. In essence, a change to a Western dietary pattern would compromise a complex homoeostatic mechanism.[25]

Imagine an environment that has times of relative food availability, countered by times of famine. Such an environment would certainly exist in Arizona, with a short growing season and sparse rain. In such an environment, it would be relatively beneficial to develop a 'quick insulin trigger', which allowed the immediate and complete anabolism of any consumed food, especially in times of sparse food availability.

However, in a different environment, in which food was continually available and its acquisition required minimal effort (such as on a reservation), a quick insulin trigger would be unnecessary, but still activated. Food would continue to be anabolized quickly as a guard against future hard times, a future that never materialized. (Consider the similarities to sickle cell anaemia: the heterozygous form of sickle cell anaemia confers greater survivability in environments in which malaria is endemic, but can be fatal in other environments, such as high altitudes.) Under such conditions, the quick insulin trigger, which would be constantly active, may result in either pancreatic fatigue or peripheral resistance.[25]

Syndrome X

The confluence of three diseases, namely type II diabetes, hypertension and obesity, has led many to describe a new syndrome, Syndrome X.[8,25–28] This condition is sometimes referred to as metabolic syndrome X. Metabolic syndrome X should not be confused with cardiac or microvascular syndrome X, which is characterized by angina, ischaemia-like electrocardiograms, normal coronary angiograms and no evidence of coronary spasm, even though both conditions are further characterized by insulin resistance and endothelial dysfunction.[28–30]

Epidemiological evidence acquired during the 1980s and 1990s has revealed that insulin resistance and the compensatory hyperinsulinemia are common to, and result in, not only type II diabetes, but also ischaemic vascular diseases, hypertension, obesity, lipid alteration and coagulative disturbances.[26–28,32]

The conditions comprising metabolic syndrome X all seem to have a general common cause, which some colloquially call 'civilization syndromes' or 'altered lifestyle syndromes'.[25] In essence, a lifestyle associated with living in industrialized societies results in an increased risk for the development of syndrome X. According to Neel, this is not surprising considering the reliance on highly refined carbohydrates and high-fat content in the diet, coupled with a sedentary lifestyle.[25] Lastly, Neel cited recent calculations indicating that our hunter–gatherer and agrarian predecessors required 3000 kcal/day, whereas a high-technology lifestyle requires only 2000 kcal/day or less.[25]

Diabetes prevention, predisposing factors and treatment

Diabetes clearly has a strong genetic link, and the manifestation of diabetic symptoms is provoked by the lifestyle endemic to industrial societies. So what is a chiropractor, or other CAM provider, to do? In those patients with type I diabetes, insulin is the standard method used to control the progression of diabetic symptoms; however, non-pharmacological approaches are as important to the successful management of diabetes as pharmacological interventions, especially for type II diabetes.

Because the neurovascular complications associated with diabetes contribute to high rates of both morbidity and mortality in older patients, a CAM practitioner can play an important role in the management of diabetes by being aware of the early signs and symptoms of diabetes, as well as being cognizant of the predisposing risk factors for its development:[3]

- minority ethnicity
- older age
- obesity
- high waist-to-hip ratio
- low birthweight
- family history of diabetes
- history of gestational diabetes
- physical inactivity
- certain medications (corticosteroids, β-blockers, thiazide, diuretics, diazoxide, cyclosporine and niacin).

Early detection, coupled with aggressive comanagement by a patient's health-care team, can significantly diminish the devastating complications of diabetes. This team should include the CAM provider, a nutritionist, a podiatrist if required and certainly an endocrinologist.

Traditionally, poor glycaemic control has been tolerated and even thought to be acceptable in the elderly with confirmed diabetes.[5] However, the current tendency among endocrinologists is for tighter control among all persons with diabetes, even in cases of mild diabetes.[5] The basis for this newer approach is that the pathophysiological consequences of hyperglycaemia, in concert with other changes associated with the normal ageing process and other coexisting pathologies, may accelerate the onset and course of clinical complications. Many authors report that retinopathy, macroangiopathy, neuropathy and nephropathy develop more rapidly in those older patients with poor glycaemic control.[5] Poor glycaemic control is an important predictor of coronary heart disease in elderly women.[5] Of particular relevance to health-care providers who perform cervical adjustments is that older patients with type II diabetes are at greater risk for cerebrovascular accidents than are younger persons with type I diabetes.[5] Moreover, a stroke that occurs in an older diabetic patient is associated with higher mortality and morbidity, and poor glycaemic control is thought to contribute to increased stroke severity and prolonged recovery.[5]

There are two primary goals of treatment for the older diabetic patient. These are (i) prevention of acute symptoms and acute complications (such as coma and hypoglycaemia) and (ii) prevention of chronic complications. Retrospective studies suggest that good blood glucose control reduces the likelihood and severity of stroke, heart disease, visual impairments, nephropathy and even cognitive dysfunction.[5] There is an inclination, therefore, to achieve euglycaemia (normal blood glucose levels) regardless of advancing age.[5] Additional physiological benefits include a decline in nocturia, polyuria and hypovolaemia, fewer infections, better wound healing, a slower progression of retinopathy, cataract development, neuropathy and nephropathy, and better control of dyslipidaemia, which in turn leads to a lower risk of cardiovascular disease.[5]

Dietary management

The goal of treatment is to alleviate symptoms and arrest pathological deterioration by normalizing fasting and postprandial blood glucose levels.[1,5,13] The primary method to achieve this result diabetes education, dietary changes, exercise and weight loss.[4,8,13,23,33] A practitioner can recommend that patients consume more frequent yet smaller meals to minimize insulin stress, but patients must be encouraged to be vigilant towards any changes in routine that may precipitate hypoglycaemia (unexpected exercise, missed meals) if a hypoglycaemic agent is being used.[23]

Weight reduction is the major goal of dietary therapy, primarily by means of caloric restriction, which is thought to enhance insulin sensitivity in peripheral cells.[4,23] Reduction of both total and saturated fat content and replacement with complex carbohydrates to 50–55% of dietary calories is consistently recommended to lower the risk of atherosclerotic disease.[4,23] Low-protein diets are often recommended for those patients with nephropathy and evidence of diabetic glomerosclerosis.[23] High-fibre diets are also thought to be beneficial for lipid control.[23,34] A 2000 study by Chandalia et al. reported that high intake of dietary fibre had a positive effect on patients with Type II diabetes.[34] Specifically, the researchers found that dietary fibre, particularly of the soluble type, above the levels recommended by the American Diabetic Association, improved glycaemic control, decreased hyperinsulinaemia and lowered plasma lipid concentration in patients with type II diabetes.[34] The absence of weight loss in the group of patients consuming a high-fibre diet indicated that the improvement was not simply the result of caloric restriction.[35]

Chandalia et al. noted with regret that, despite the evidence of benefit, dietary fibre intake by persons with diabetes did not increase significantly during the 1990s.[34,35] This was attributed to both a lack of patient education and a limited awareness by physicians as to the benefits of dietary treatment to manage diabetes successfully.[35]

Exercise

Exercise is a non-pharmacological treatment for many clinical conditions, including atherosclerosis, sleep disorders, depression and diabetes.[36] For the diabetic patient, exercise seems to enhance insulin sensitivity, perhaps by selectively reducing abdominal obesity.[4,13,23] Exercise has also been shown to enhance glucose uptake and non-oxidative glucose disposal, and to improve lipid balance.[23] The only precautions to be taken prior to recommending an exercise programme for diabetic patients are to ensure the patient does not have advanced coronary artery disease or suffer from severely impaired visual or proprioceptive disorders and, for those patients with peripheral neuropathies, to monitor any foot trauma carefully.[5,23] Because loss of muscle mass contributes to insulin resistance, a clinician should pay preferential attention to resistance exercises in severely sacropenic patients.[5,36]

Physical activity exerts a pronounced effect on insulin sensitivity, which in turn potentially lowers blood glucose and lipid levels. Exercise training may also improve other physiological and metabolic abnormalities associated with type II diabetes, such as lowering body fat, reducing blood pressure and normalizing dyslipoproteinaemia.[37]

Pharmacological approaches

It would be remiss not to discuss the pharmacological agents commonly used in the management of diabetes, even though the administration of such agents is beyond the scope of practice for CAM providers. For no other reason, it is important for drug-free practitioners to be aware of the most commonly prescribed medications that patients may be taking, since CAM practitioners can play an important role in patient management by being cognizant of the possibility of iatrogenic drug reactions (see Chapter 22).

Sulfonylurases

Sulfonylurases and related agents have been used to treat type II diabetes since the 1940s. Since the primary effect of these drugs is to increase insulin secretion, the major indicator for their use is hypoglycaemia.[4,5,23] To be effective, however, sulfonylurases require functional pancreatic β-cells. Notable side-effects include hypoglycaemia, weight gain and hyperinsulinaemia.[13] Second-generation sulfonylurases, which include glipizide (Glucotrol) and glyburide (DiaBeta or Micronase), cause fewer interactions and present a more favourable safety profile.[5,38]

Insulin

Insulin is indicated for type II diabetic patients for (i) initial stabilization of patients with severe hyperglycaemia, (ii) established patients with hyperglycaemic crisis, and (iii) patients in whom oral hypoglycaemic agents have failed.[4,13] Lispro (Humalog), a brand of recombinant human insulin, is often recommended.[13] Practitioners should be aware that insulin therapy may result in weight gain in obese type II diabetic patients, and increases the risk of hypoglycaemia.[4,23] In older patients with type II diabetes, especially those with atherosclerotic cardiovascular disease, insulin regimens may avoid hypoglycaemia and hyperinsulinaemia, factors that are associated with an increased risk of cardiovascular events.[23] No specific insulin-dosing regimen has been identified as being preferentially beneficial for the elderly diabetic patient.[5] Although insulin therapy is always a stressful approach, insulin injections for older patients are particularly problematic and complex. This is because older patients may have visual impairments that complicate both the drawing and injection of the drug, impaired manual dexterity, decreased sensation in the hands, limited access to injection sites (perhaps because of restricted ranges of motion) and problems monitoring blood levels.[5] Both physical and cognitive impairments may further impede insulin use, and hypoglycaemia is associated with severe psychomotor deficits.[5]

Metformin

A second-generation biguanide, metformin, is often recommended for those patients who are both obese and display signs of insulin resistance.[4,23,38] The pharmacological action of metformin is to decrease both hepatic gluconeogenesis and peripheral insulin resistance.[4,5] Moreover, metformin does not cause weight gain and it improves the lipid profile by causing a decline in the very low-density lipoprotein triglycerides, total cholesterol and very low-density cholesterol levels, while increasing the high-density lipoprotein cholesterol levels.[4,5] However, side-effects include abdominal discomfort, anorexia, diarrhoea and, more importantly, lactic acidosis.[5]

Thiazolidenediones

For patients with insulin resistance, thiazolidenediones may be used. These drugs (also known as Troglitazone or Rezulin) have as their effect a decrease in peripheral insulin resistance, and a reduction in fatty acids by sensitizing hepatic and peripheral tissue to insulin[4,13] The major concern of these drugs is their risk of hepatotoxicity, a clinical circumstance identifiable by both allopathic and CAM practitioners.[4]

Combination therapy

On occasion, a medical practitioner may choose a combination therapy to correct most pathophysiological defects found in type II diabetic patients.[4,23,38] For example, metformin and insulin may be recommended for obese patients, whereas the practice of adding metformin to sulfonylurea is used to optimize glycaemic control and delay the need for exogenous insulin.[13]

Botanical medicines

Many CAM practitioners, particularly naturopaths and homoeopaths, preferentially use botanical medicines to achieve powerful clinical results for a wide range of clinical conditions, including diabetes. There is mounting evidence for the benefits of ginseng, cat's claw (for general improvement in diabetic symptoms), aloe vera (for wound healing), and capsicum and evening primrose (for the treatment of diabetic neuropathy).[39]

Cultural engineering

Neel, the proponent of the thrifty gene hypothesis to explain type II diabetes, has suggested a strategy to manage diabetes and other metabolic syndrome X diseases associated with the lifestyle of an industrial world: cultural engineering.[25] Neel advocates a return to, wherever feasible, a paleolithic lifestyle, which Eaton *et al.* term a 'paleolithic prescription'.[40] Specifically, this shift would involve a diet comprised of a high dietary fibre content, a decline in refined carbohydrate and sodium consumption, less saturated fat in the diet and a much higher level of physical activity.[25,40] Neel opines that cultural engineering, analogous to genetic engineering which has as its goal the effort to improve the genome, has as its goal the conscious development of an environment (in the broadest sense) in which the human genome can find its optimal expression.[25] In the case of persons living in industrial societies, the optimal expression of the human genome may require a shift towards a cultural lifestyle that emulates a healthy approach to diet and physical activity.

Chiropractic adjustments

A review of the chiropractic literature describing chiropractic care and diabetes demonstrates a true paucity of articles. The articles that are available regrettably tend to be based only on anecdotes and are poorly referenced.

The quintessential chiropractic–diabetic anecdote is the story involving Joseph Clay Thompson, contemporary and student of BJ Palmer. According to the story, young Clay developed diabetes mellitus as the result of a severe blow to the head while unloading lumber from a truck.[41] The company physician gave Clay only 7–10 days to live after he failed to respond to the traditional medical treatments available at that time. On the suggestion of his father, Clay presented to a chiropractor, Dr James Dick, who had helped the senior Thompson years earlier. Dr Dick adjusted Clay for 16 consecutive days, after which time the patient demonstrated no signs or symptoms of diabetes. This episode in Clay's life led him to enrol at Palmer College at the age of 37.[41] Eventually, Thompson became head of research at Palmer College and developed the Thompson terminal point technique, which is among the most widely used Name techniques today.

The three articles that specifically discuss diabetes and chiropractic recount one case each of the successful resolution of a patient's diabetes while under chiropractic care.[42–44] Two articles emphasize the importance of chromium,[42,44] and two articles discuss the concept that chiropractic adjustments enable the patient's body to restore homoeostasis, which ultimately leads to a reduction in the patient's diabetic profile.[43,44] One author emphasized that he was not treating the patient's diabetes, but was restoring the patient's homoeostasis by chiropractic adjustments, particularly to the mid and lower thoracic segments.[43] Another of the authors stated that the key correction was to the fifth cervical vertebra, with 'its known involvement with blood sugar metabolism' (sic).[44] Unfortunately, this latter statement was not

referenced, and the author is unaware of the source of this assertion. Also, and somewhat perplexingly, the chiropractor did not indicate that the C5 segment was among those that he identified as being subluxated during the patient's physical examination.[44]

In an article exploring psychoneuroimmunology, Morgan reports that several studies suggest that behavioural modification directed at stress management may contribute significantly to the treatment of type I diabetes.[45] This may be explained by the association between elevated T-cell activity in response to grief experiences among diabetic patients.[45]

New frontiers or brave new worlds?

Transplantation of either entire pancreatic organs or islet cells has met with tremendous success since the early 1990.[7,46–53] Xenotransplantation, using neonatal porcine pancreas, has been found to normalize glucose levels in test mice.[48,49] Techniques that specifically transplant islet β-cells into diabetic subjects have been used successfully for over 10 years.[7,47] Immunoisolation techniques, such as islet cell microencapsulation, are often used in order to avoid tissue rejection by the host recipient.[52] Still other techniques use human cells that have been genetically engineered to produce insulin.[51]

In May 2000, Shapiro et al. revealed the results of a study that some consider a giant step towards the development of a cure for diabetes.[54] The team of researchers transplanted islet cells into patients with type I diabetes, and provided the patients with a new steroid-free immunosuppressive regimen. All five of the patients who received the transplanted islet cells demonstrated an immediate and sustained independence from insulin, once sufficient islet mass was transplanted, and have currently remained off insulin, with a median follow-up of 6.2 months.[54] This is in stark contrast to the only 12.4% of diabetic patients who have received transplanted cells who become insulin independent beyond 1 week, and the only 8.25% who achieve insulin independence beyond 1 year.[54] There were no episodes of acute rejection, complications have been minor and there were no elevations in lipid profiles.[54]

A much more controversial avenue of experimental research involves the transplantation of human foetal pancreatic tissue.[53] The use of human foetal tissue for the treatment of such diseases as Parkinson's and diabetes may circumvent the recipient's immunological response, but such procedures involve a deeper dilemma of biomedical ethics which may defy a solution. Is it appropriate in the twenty-first century to harvest tissue from one human to provide spare parts for another, despite a noble purpose? If the use of foetal tissue is approved, will this result in a nefarious underworld trade in aborted foetuses for transplantation? Will parents be allowed to procreate for the express purpose of cannibalizing tissues from an unborn child to a living sibling, or even a parent?

References

1 Abrams W, Beers M, Berkow R. The Merck Manual of Geriatrics. 2nd edn. Whitehouse Station NJ: Merck & Co., 1995: 997–1021.

2 Expert Committee on the Diagnosis and Classification of Diabetes Mellitus. Report of the Expert Committee on the Diagnosis and Classification of Diabetes Mellitus. Diabetes Care 1997; 20: 1–15.

3 Goldberg R. Prevention of type 2 diabetes. Med Clin North Am 1998; 82: 805–817.

4 Mahler R, Adler M. Type 2 diabetes mellitus: update on diagnosis, pathophysiology, and treatment. J Clin Endocrinol Metab 1999; 84: 1165–1170.

5 Samos LF, Roos B. Diabetes mellitus in older patients. Med Clin North Am 1998; 82: 791–802.

6 Sacks D, McDonald J. The pathogenesis of type II diabetes mellitus. Am J Clin Pathol 1996; 105: 149–156.

7 Ratner RE. Type 2 diabetes mellitus: the grand review. Diabet Med 1998; 15(Suppl 4): S4–S7.

8 Gregg EW, Yaffe K, Cauley JA et al. Is diabetes associated with cognitive impairment and cognitive decline in older women? Arch of Intern Med 2000; 160: 174–180.

9 Guyton AC, Hall JE. Textbook of Medical Physiology. 9th edn. Toronto: WB Saunders, 1997: 971–983.

10 Butler RN, Rubenstein AH, Gracia AMG, Zweig SC. Type 2 diabetes: causes, complications, and new screening recommendations. Geriatrics 1998; 53(3): 47–54.

11 Bennett PH. Type 2 diabetes among the Pima Indians of Arizona: an epidemic attributable to environmental change? Nutr Rev 1999; 57(5 Pt 2): S51–S54.

12 Ganong WF. Review of Medical Physiology. A Lange Medical Book. 18th edn. Stamford, CT: Appleton & Lange, 1997: 315–323.

13 Dagogo-Jack S, Santiago JV. Pathophysiology of type 2 diabetes and modes of action of therapeutic interventions. Arch Intern Med 1997; 157: 1802–1817.

14 Rabinovich A, Skyler JS. Prevention of type 1 diabetes. Med Clin North Am 1998; 82; 739–752.

15 El Mansour A, Martignat L, Maugendre S et al. Cyclosporin depresses pancreatic islet expression of antigens for islet cell autoantibodies in non obese diabetic mice. J Autoimmun 1996; 9: 29–39.

16 Verge CF, Eisenbarth GS. Strategies for preventing type 1 diabetes mellitus. West J Med 1996; 164: 249–255.

17 Cavallo MG, Fava D, Monetini L et al. Cell-mediated immune response to beta casein in recent-onset insulin-dependent diabetes: implications for disease pathogenesis. Lancet 1996; 348: 926–928.

18 Ellis TM, Atkinson MA. Early infant diets and insulin-dependent diabetes. Lancet 1996; 347: 1464–1465.

19 Timberlake A, Wagner W. Cow's milk: friend or foe? Today's Chiropractic 1994; 23(2): 22–24.

20 Scott FW, Kolb H. Cow's milk and insulin-dependent diabetes mellitus. Lancet 1996; 348: 613.

21 Schatz DA, Maclaren NK. Cow's milk and insulin-dependent diabetes mellitus. Innocent until proven guilty. JAMA 1996; 276: 647–648.

22 Norris JM, Beaty B, Klingensmith G et al. Lack of association between early exposure to cow's milk protein and beta-cell autoimmunity. JAMA 1996; 276: 609–614.

23 Feinglos MN, Bethel MA. Treatment of type 2 diabetes mellitus. Med Clin North Am 1998; 82: 757–786.

24 Brancati FL, Wang NY, Mead LA et al. Body weight patterns from 20 to 49 years of age and subsequent risk of diabetes mellitus: the Johns Hopkins precursors. 1999; 159: 957–963.

25 Neel JV. The 'thrifty genotype' in 1998. Nutr Rev 1999; 57(5): S2–S9.

26 Okapcova J, Hrnciar J, Kurray P et al. Insulin resistance and the coronary syndrome. Vnitr Lek 1999; 45: 3–10.

27 Pogatsa G. From type 2 diabetes to metabolic X syndrome. Orv Hetil 1999;140: 635–640.

28 Granberry MC, Fonseca VA. Insulin resistance syndrome: options for treatment. South Med J 1999; 92: 2–15.

29 Chen JW, Lin SJ, Ting CT. Syndrome X: pathophysiology and clinical management. Chin Med J 1997; 60: 177–183.

30 Buus NH, Bottcher M, Bottker HE et al. Reduced vasodilator capacity in syndrome X related to structure and function of resistance arteries. Am J Cardiol 1999; 83: 149–154.

31 Goodfellow J, Owens D, Henderson A. Cardiovascular syndrome X, endothelial dysfunction and insulin resistance. Diabetes Res Clin Pract 1996; 31(Suppl): S163-S171.

32 Wannamettee SG, Shaper AG, Durrington PN, Perry IJ. Hypertension, serum insulin, obesity and the metabolic syndrome. J Hum Hypertens 1998; 12: 735–741.

33 Lipkin E. New strategies for the treatment of type 2 diabetes. J Am Diabet Assoc 1999; 99: 329–334.

34 Chandalia M, Abhimanyu G, Lutjohann D et al. Beneficial effects of high dietary fiber intake in patients with type 2 diabetes mellitus. N Engl J Med 2000; 342: 1392–1398.

35 Rendell M. Dietary treatment of diabetes mellitus (Editorial). N Engl J Med 2000; 342: 1440–1441.

36 Gleberzon BJ, Annis R. The necessity of strength training for the older patient. J Can Chiropractic Assoc 2000; 4(2).

37 Wallberg-Henriksson H, Rincon J, Zierath JR. Exercise in the management of non-insulin-dependent diabetes mellitus. Sports Med 1998; 25(1): 25–35.

38 Butler RN, Rubenstein AH, Gracia AMG, Zweig SC. Type 2 diabetes: treatment goals and pharmaceutical therapies. Geriatrics 1998; 53(4): 42–49.

39 Boon H, Smith M. The Botanical Pharmacy. The Pharmacology of 47 Common Herbs. Kingston: Quarry Press, 1999.

40 Eaton SB, Eaton SB III, Konner MJ. Paleolithic nutrition revisited: a twelve-year retrospective on its nature and implications. Eur J Clin Nutr 1997; 51: 207–216.

41 Noyman B. The Thompson technique: a low-force, high-velocity approach. Today's Chiropractic 1996; 25(2): 68–73.

42 Evans GW. Diabetes and aging: the chromium connection. Today's Chiropractic 1994; 23(2): 40–42.

43. Inselman PS. Even diabetics need good nutrition. Am Chiropractor 1998; 20(6): 14–16.

44 Kfoury PW. Chiropractic and holistic management of type II diabetes mellitus. Digest Chiropractic Econ 1995; 37(4): 39–42.

45 Morgan L. Psychoneuroimmunology, the placebo effect and chiropractic. J Manip Physiol Ther 1998; 21: 484–491.

46 Berger A. Transplanted pancreatic stem cells can reverse diabetes in mice. BMJ 2000; 320: 736.

47 Weir GC, Bonner-Weir S. Islet transplantation as a treatment for diabetes. J Am Optom Assoc 1998; 69: 727–732.

48 Yoon KH, Quickel RR, Tatarkiewicz K *et al*. Differentiation and expansion of beta cell mass in porcine neonatal pancreatic cell clusters transplanted into nude mice. Cell Transplant 1999; 8: 673–689.

49 Rayat GR, Rajotte RV, Korbutt GS. Potential application of neonatal porcine islets as treatment for type 1 diabetes: a review. Ann N Y Acad Sci 1999; 875: 175–188.

50 Contreras JL, Eckhoff DE, Cartner S *et al*. Long-term functional islet mass and metabolic function after xenoislet transplantation in primates. Transplantation 2000; 69: 195–201.

51 Falqui L, Martinenghi S, Severini GM *et al*. Reversal of diabetes in mice by implantation of human fibroblasts genetically engineered to release mature human insulin. Hum Gene Ther 1999; 10: 1753–1762.

52 Lanza RP, Jackson R, Sullivan A *et al*. Xenotransplantation of cells using biodegradable microcapsules. Transplantation 1999; 67: 1105–1111.

53 Brooks-Worrell BM, Peterson KP, Peterson CM *et al*. Reactivation of type I diabetes in patients receiving human fetal pancreatic tissue transplants without immunosuppression. Transplantation 2000; 69: 166–172.

54 Shapiro J, Lakay JRT, Ryan E *et al*. Presented at the Transplant 2000 Conference, 1st Joint Meeting, American Society of Transplant Surgeons and American Society of Transplantation, May 13–17, 2000. Chicago, IL.

13

Immobility and muscular disorders

Brian J Gleberzon

The old adage 'use it or lose it' is nowhere more appropriate than when discussing the care of older patients. There is often a vicious cycle of pain, dysfunction and disuse atrophy associated with many clinical conditions that preferentially affect older patients. Many clinical conditions that present with pain as a primary symptom are discussed throughout this text. This chapter will focus on two muscular disorders that result in significant immobility: fibromyalgia (FM) and polymyalgia rheumatica (PMR). Issues of bed rest and pain management will also be reviewed.

Fibromyalgia

FM is a form of non-articular rheumatism.[1] For a diagnosis of FM, there must be chronic diffuse musculoskeletal aching lasting for 3 months, accompanied by soft-tissue tender points.[1–3] Axial skeletal pain (pain of the cervical spine, anterior chest, or thoracic or lumbar region) must be present.[2,3] The American College of Rheumatology (ACR) has established diagnostic criteria for FM.[4] These are:

- diffuse musculoskeletal pain of at least 3 months' duration
- stiffness that is worse in the morning
- tenderness to digital palpation of at least 11 of 18 specific points (Table 13.1)

The ACR defines pain as widespread when the pain is reported in all of the following areas: Pain in the left side of the body, pain in the right side of the body, pain above the waist, pain below the waist and axial skeletal pain.[4]

FM is commonly associated with stiffness, general fatigue, paraesthesias, headaches, dysmenorrhoea and a swollen feeling of the tissues.[2,5] Irritable bowel syndrome, and especially Crohn's disease, is very common in patients with FM.[6] One of the most distinctive features of FM is non-restorative sleep.[1,2,5]

In 90% of cases, FM presents in women.[1,2] Caucasian women between the ages of 40 and 60 years are the most likely persons to present with FM.[1] Although its exact prevalence is unknown, it has been estimated that 3–6 million individuals in the USA have FM.[1] FM accounts for 2% of all visits to family medical physicians, 10% of general internal medicine referrals and 20% of referrals to rheumatologists, making it the third or fourth most common reason for rheumatological referral.[1,7] One article reports that the average person with FM has waited for 10 years before being correctly diagnosed, has seen 12 doctors and has tried between 12 and 15 medications.[8]

Table 13.1 Diagnosis of fibromyalgia through palpation of 18 sites*[3]

1. Occiput	At the suboccipital muscle insertion
2. Low cervical	At the anterior aspects of the intertransverse spaces of C5–C7
3. Trapezius	At the midpoint of the upper border
4. Supraspinatus	Above the spine of the scapula near the medial border
5. Second rib	Upper lateral aspect of the second costrochondral junction
6. Lateral epicondyle	2 cm distal to the epicondyles
7. Gluteal	In the upper outer quadrant of the buttocks in the anterior fold of muscle
8. Greater trochanter	Posterior to the trochanteric prominence
9. Knee	At the medial fat pad proximal to the joint line

* Pain can be elicited on the left or right side, or both.

For most patients, symptoms appear to begin gradually and unexpectedly in adulthood; however, for some patients, the onset of FM can be attributed to trauma (especially whiplash), acute sprain, muscle spasm, nerve root irritation or lumbosacral sprain, viral infection, overactivity or surgery.[1,2] Some patients have reported a preceding episode of emotional or physical stress.[1] Other self-reported conditions that accompany FM include bursitis, chondromalacia, vertigo, constipation, diarrhoea, temporomandibular joint dysfunction, sinus and thyroid problems, allergies, bruxism and sciatica.[1]

There is often a familial association with FM, with 12% of patients reporting symptomatic children and 25% symptomatic parents.[1]

Because the symptoms are fairly vague, FM is often a diagnosis of exclusion. That is, FM is suspected when no other cause can be identified, and it remains an aggregate of identified symptoms and signs not (as yet) attributable to any specific aetiology.[1,2] Although the aetiopathogenesis of fibromyalgia is still enigmatic, there is no shortage of proposed theoretical models. Common aetiological theories are sleep disturbances, lack of exercise, microtrauma, chemical imbalance, emotional stress, psychological disturbances, autonomic dysfunction, genetic predispositions, viral causes, immunological, neurohormonal and neurotransmitter aberrations, nutritional deficiencies, toxic habits, and muscle strength deficits and deconditioning.[1–3,5] Some authors suggest that FM is related to mechanical dysfunctions and myofascial pain syndromes,[2] while one study linked fibromyalgia to post-traumatic stress disorder.[9]

There is an abundance of clinical evidence that FM is related to a disturbance of sleep. Smythe and Moldofsky report a profound disturbance in stage 4 sleep due to intrusions in alpha-rhythms during normal non-rapid eye movement (REM) sleep.[1,5] A recent study conducted at the University of Toronto Centre for Sleep and Chronobiology revealed that patients with FM have diurnal impairments in speed of performance on complex cognitive tasks, which accompanied light stage 1 sleep.[10] The patients in this study also reported diffuse pain and non-restorative sleep symptoms of sleepiness, fatigue and negative mood.[10]

Patients who engage in regular aerobic exercise appear to be relatively protected from developing FM.[1] Although patients with FM tend to be sedentary and rank below the average level of physical activity, it is not clear whether this results in FM or vice versa.[1]

Various chemical and hormone imbalances have been theorized to result in FM. These include deficiencies of somatomedin C, tryptophan and serotonin.[1] Other possible biochemical agents involved in FM include endorphins, prostaglandin E_2, noradrenaline and substance P.[1] Bell et al. proposed that FM is the result of an 'environmental chemical intolerance' (CI) mechanism.[11] The authors claim that severe CI is a characteristic in 20–47% of persons with chronic fatigue syndrome and/or FM. The authors posit that chemical, biological and/or psychological stimuli can initiate and elicit sensitization via the olfactory system to the limbic, mesolimbic and hypothalamic pathways.[11]

Some researchers maintain that FM is caused by dysfunction of the neuroendocrine axes[12] or elevated activity of corticotropin-releasing hormone (CRH) of the hypophysis.[13] Others argue that the most widely accepted model for the pathogenesis of FM invokes a central nervous system mechanism, such as nociception and allodynia, rather than any pathology of the muscles.[14]

One of the more interesting explanations for FM is presented by Winfield.[15] He compared the stress-laden life of today's world with that of our prehistoric forebears. In both cases, humans rely on neuroendocrine systems and pain-regulatory mechanisms that protect us during times of stress. However, he proposed that these protective mechanisms are maladaptive in psychologically and physiologically vulnerable persons who experience chronic stress. Winfield opined that persons with FM become vulnerable because of long-lasting psychological and neuropsychological effects of negative experiences from childhood. Now ill-equipped with cognitive, emotional and behavioural skills as adults, they display maladaptive coping strategies, demonstrating low self-efficacy and negative mood when confronted with the inevitable chronic stressors of modern life. Winfield concludes that these individuals do not have a discrete disease in and of itself, but are simply the most ill in a continuum of distress, chronic pain and painful tender points in the general population.[15]

Winfield is not the only author to question whether FM is a separate and distinct disorder. Some argue that FM is a type of chronic fatigue syndrome, chronic pain syndrome or myofascial pain syndrome, while others consider each to be a separate clinical entity. Because of the similarities in clinical presentation, it is imperative that a clinician be able to perform a differential diagnosis between FM and those conditions that it most resembles. Physicians who are unaware of these different conditions may label a patient with chronic pain as neurotic or a malingering.[16]

Differential diagnosis

Because there are no characteristic laboratory or radiographic findings for FM, the differential diagnosis of FM from other, similar conditions requires a great deal of skill on the part of the clinician.[1] FM does not cause articular swelling, damage or degeneration, nor are changes in laboratory findings such as sedimentation rate, uric acid or rheumatoid factor of any diagnostic value.[3] In particular, a clinician must be able to differentiate between FM and myofascial pain syndrome (MPS) (Table 13.2).

A key element in the differential diagnosis between FM and MPS is the determination of the presence of trigger points or tender points.[3] According to Schneider, tender points are defined as discrete areas of soft tissue that are painful to about 4 kg of palpatory pressure, whereas trigger points are defined as hyperirritable spots located within a taut band of skeletal muscle that are painful to compression and give rise to characteristic referred pain and autonomic phenomena.[3] Trigger points are often described as 'knots' or 'nodules' that are elicited in taut muscular bands described as 'ropy'.[3]

The most distinctive difference between tender points and trigger points is the difference between the cause and effect of a clinical condition.[3] The tender points characteristic of FM are the effect, not the cause, of the condition; or, rather, the syndrome classified as FM is characterized by a certain number of tender points in distinctive locations. Alternatively, trigger points are the causative agents of MPS.[3]

Treatment

Conventional treatment of FM has used a multipronged approach including psychotherapy, patient education, stretches, cardiovascular exercises, nutritional supplements, postural training exercises, manipulation to restore proper biomechanics, acupuncture, cognitive behavioural therapy or electromyographic biofeedback training, lifestyle changes to reduce stress and strategies to normalize sleep patterns.[1-3]

Current medical management consists of low doses of antidepressants, such as amitriptyline or cyclobenzaprine .[1-3] These drugs are thought to normalize sleep disorders. However, amitriptyline was found to be effective in only 30% of patients and cyclobenzaprine in only 39% of cases.[1]

In one study, oral malate and magnesium at doses of 1200–2400 mg and 300–600 mg, respectively, were shown to reduce tender-point pain by 41% after 4 weeks and 67% after 8 weeks.[1] Botanical medicines thought to be of benefit for general 'rheumatism' are

Table 13.2 Differential diagnosis of fibromyalgia and myofascial pain syndrome[1,3]

Feature or symptom	Fibromyalgia	Myofascial pain syndrome
Pain pattern	Bilateral and widespread	Regional: specific pain pattern
Female: male ratio	10–20:1	1:1–2
Onset	Variable: trauma (?)	Trauma/overuse
History presentation	Chronic, widespread pain, morning fatigue and stiffness, pain with no known cause	History of acute or chronic muscle strain or injury
Soft-tissue findings	Tender points	Trigger points
Sleep disorders	Common, strong correlation	May be secondary to pain
Morning fatigue	Present, debilitating	Absent
Palpable changes	None	Nodular and ropy
Associated symptoms	Many	Few
Skin-roll tenderness	Common	Uncommon
Jump response	Seldom	Frequent
Muscle metabolism	Impaired systemically (?)	Impaired locally
Treatment approach	Treatment is systemic. Low-dose antidepressants, aerobic exercise psychotherapy, self-help modalities and manual therapies (manipulation)	Treatment is regional. Ischaemic compression, spray and stretch, needle injections, manipulations secondary to joint dysfunction
Prognosis	Seldom cured	Usually good

cat's claw and burdock, whereas German chamomile, hops, lemon balm and passion flower are all thought to improve sleep patterns.[17] A commonly used homoeopathic medicine is *Rhus toxicodendron*.[1]

Exercise, especially low-impact aerobic exercise, is thought to be a key component of FM treatment, especially for older patients.[1,18] Brisk walking, swimming and cycling may all improve symptoms of FM by improving strength, posture, general fitness and flexibility, relieving stress, improving blood flow to muscles and contributing to a general improvement in well-being.[1,19]

A study by Berman *et al.* reported that real acupuncture was more effective than sham acupuncture for improving symptoms of FM.[20] This led the authors to suggest that further high-quality double-blind randomized trials be conducted to establish the effectiveness of acupuncture for FM.[20]

Blunt *et al.* conducted a randomized control crossover trial to demonstrate the effectiveness of chiropractic management for FM.[2] The study used pain levels, cervical and lumbar ranges of motion, strength, flexibility, tender points, myalgic scores and perceived functional abilities as outcome measures.[2]

The investigators' rationale for chiropractic care in the management of FM was the inhibition of pain, relaxation of paraspinal muscles, breaking of articular adhesions and increased range of motion.[2] Chiropractic management included spray and stretch techniques, soft-tissue therapies, patient education and spinal manipulative therapy. The results revealed improvement in patients' cervical and lumbar ranges of motion, straight leg raising and reported pain levels.[2]

Previous studies examining the effectiveness of manipulation for patients with FM revealed that 37–45% of patients reported moderate to great improvement.[1]

Many studies describe a interdisciplinary approach for the effective management of FM, typically using medical, psychological and physical therapies.[21–23] A study by Singh *et al.* revealed that mind–body interventions including patient education, meditation techniques and movement therapy (qigong) appeared to provide effective adjunctive therapy for patients with FM.[23]

Relaxation methods provided a moderate to great level of improvement in FM symptoms in 66% of patients, followed by rest (47%), narcotics (46%) and

chiropractic care (46%).[1,3] Physical modalities such as heat, massage, mechanical supports, interferential current and transcutaneous electrical nerve stimulation (TENS) provided relief in 37% of patients.[1] Exercise was reported to provide relief in 32% of patients.[1] Chiropractic care provided no relief in only 16% of patients, compared with the 45% of cases in which medications provided no relief of symptoms.[1]

It seems evident, therefore, that effective treatment of FM is best accomplished with a team effort. Pharmacological support to improve sleep patterns should be augmented with exercise, rest and relaxation techniques, nutritional supplements, psychotherapy, self-help groups, patient education and chiropractic care.

Polymyalgia rheumatica

PMR is characterized by pain and stiffness of the proximal joints of the shoulder and pelvic girdle.[24] The onset of symptoms is typically abrupt and insidious.[24] Although muscle strength is unaffected in PMR, mild to moderate muscle weakness may be revealed on physical examination owing to the natural reluctance of the patient to exert maximum force with a stiff, sore joint.[24] The erythrocyte sedimentation rate (ESR) is typically elevated in patients with PMR to 40 mm/h or more, although ESR is normal in 13% of cases.[24] C-reactive protein, fibrinogen and α-2-globulins are usually increased.[25] Temporal arteritis presents in 15% of patients with PMR and 50% of patients with temporal arteritis have symptoms of PMR.[18,25]

PMR occurs most commonly in women and almost exclusively in persons over the age of 50 years.[18,24] The prevalence of PMR has been estimated at 0.5% in the USA.[18,24]

Despite general agreement on the clinical features and symptoms of PMR, there is no standard test with which to make a definitive diagnosis. This is especially problematic because PMR has a long list of differential diagnoses. These include FM, polymyositis, systemic lupus erythematosus, Parkinson's disease, hypothyroidism, neoplasms and rheumatoid arthritis (RA).[18,24] The most difficult condition to distinguish from PMR is RA. Both PMR and RA share similar clinical profiles, and patients who develop RA after the age of 60 are more likely to present with PMR-like symptoms such as abrupt onset, involvement of large joints and absence of rheumatoid factor.[24] Further confounding the definitive diagnosis of PMR is the fact that PMR often presents with atypical features such as peripheral synovitis, muscle weakness, carpel tunnel syndrome, asymmetric pain, onset before the age of 50 and a normal ESR.[24] Although typically involving the proximal joints, pain and stiffness of the extremities occur in between 50 and 83% of patients in clinical trials.[24,26]

Unlike most other clinical conditions, the positive response of patients to low-dose corticosteroids is considered to be pathognomonic of PMR. If the patient fails to demonstrate rapid improvement in symptoms within 1 or 2 days to a 10–20 mg/day dose of corticosteroids, the clinician must question the original diagnosis.[18,24]

Temporal arteritis, also known as giant cell arteritis, commonly copresents in patients with PMR, and vice versa.[25] As in PMR, 50% of patients with temporal arteritis present with constitutional signs including low-grade fever, night sweats, anorexia, weight loss, malaise, fatigue and depression.[25] Temporal arteritis typically involves the cranial branches of the carotid artery, but can also affect other large and medium-sized arteries.[18]

Headache is the most common symptom of temporal arteritis, seen in two-thirds of patients.[18] The headaches are often described as boring or lancing in nature[25] Other clinical findings are scalp tenderness, scalp artery tenderness and pain with chewing (jaw claudication).[25] Visual impairments are common and are the most worrisome feature of temporal arteritis.[18,25] Impaired visual acuity, transient blurring of vision, diplopia, ptosis, amaurosis fugax or scintillating scotomata often occur, with visual loss occurring in 10–20% of patients.[25] Diagnosis is confirmed by temporal artery biopsy.

A delay in the diagnosis of temporal arteritis may lead to catastrophic results, such as stroke and blindness.[25] Temporal arteritis can also result in myocardial infarction, ischaemia of the limbs and bowel, dementia and stroke.[25]

Treatment of temporal arteritis is high-dose corticosteroid therapy, with the initial dose of oral prednisone being 40 mg/day.[25] As in the case of PMR, dramatic improvements in constitutional symptoms usually occur within 2 days of commencing treatment.[25] The initial dosage level continues for 2 weeks, with a total duration of therapy of 3 years or more, as is the case with PMR.[18,25] However, prolonged corticosteroid use is not without its risks, and the side-effects of chronic steroid administration can be fatal, especially in older patients.[25] These include infection, difficulties in controlling diabetes and hypertension, cognitive changes and, most importantly, development of osteoporotic fractures.[25]

Pain and bed rest

A common fallacy about ageing is that pain is a normal consequence of growing old. The literature is inconsistent with respect to the incidence of reported pain with age. Although one study reported a three-fold increase in persistent pain between the ages of 18 and 80 years, another larger study indicated that there is an age-related decrease in pain in all anatomical the sites other than joints.[27]

Osteoarthritis is by far the most common pain-producing disorder in older patients.[27] Painful syndromes of neurogenic origin, such as trigeminal and postherpetic neuralgia, occur frequently among older persons.[27] Although the neural elements responsible for pain perception do not appear to decline with age, there is evidence to suggest that there are alterations in the neural pathways involved in nociception; this may account for the apparent decline in reported pain.[27] Alternatively, the lower prevalence of pain may be due to either a reticence to report pain or a degree of stoicism.[27]

Chronic pain may have a major impact on a person's quality of life, and may result in changes in affect or mood, such as depression.[27] The depression, in turn, may exacerbate the condition responsible for the pain (such as immobility-induced osteoporosis) or it may enhance the perception of the pain.[27]

As detailed in Chapter 6, the location, character, intensity and quality of the pain must be ascertained during the patient interview, as this may enable the clinician to diagnose the aetiology of the pain.

Principles of pain management

Treatment of pain should be directed primarily at the underlying cause, if it can be identified. This is especially true if the pain is neoplastic in origin. The psychological and affective impairments associated with the pain should be managed concurrently, which may require referral to a mental health specialist. If non-pharmacological approaches are ineffective, the patient should be referred to his or her medical doctor for the prescription of appropriate medications.[27] Wherever possible, medications should be given orally, and constant pain requires regular administration of analgesics to maintain a constant state of analgesia. As discussed in Chapter 22, Iatrogenic drug reactions, the use of opioids, non-steroidal anti-inflammatory drugs (NSAIDs) and other medications is not without risk, particularly in the older patient. For example, in the USA, NSAIDs are thought to cause between 8000 and 16 000 deaths and more than 100 000 hospitalizations annually.[28]

Bed rest

Pain, which can be caused by clinical conditions as diverse as osteoarthritis, cancer and myofascial pain syndromes, or acute occupational or recreational injuries, may result in a patient either seeking or being prescribed bed rest. The problem, however, is that within 48 h of complete bed rest, muscle mass and metabolic efficiency (as measured by maximum oxygen uptake) decline by 1% per day.[18] Within 1–2 days of best rest for an older patient, even ordinary activities may require a marked increase in cardiac output to meet the demands of deconditioned muscles. Typically, 2 days of recovery are required for every single day of bed rest.[18]

Finally, bed rest for extended periods may result in pressure sores, stasis pneumonia, pulmonary embolism, urinary tract infections, and muscle atrophy and deconditioning.[18]

References

1 St Clair S. Diagnosis and treatment of fibromyalgia syndrome. J Neuromusculoskeletal Syst 1994; 2(3): 101–111.
2 Blunt K, Rajwani M, Guerriero R. The effectiveness of chiropractic management of fibromyalgia: a pilot study. J Manipulative Physiol Ther 1997; 20: 389–399.
3 Schneider M. Tender points/fibromyalgia vs. trigger points/myofascial pain syndromes: a need for clarity in terminology and differential diagnosis. J Manipulative Physiol Ther 1995; 18: 398–406.
4 Wolfe F, Smythe HA, Yunus MB et al. The American College of Rheumatology 1990 criteria for the classification of fibromyalgia. Report of the Multi-center Criteria Committee. Arthritis Rheum 1990; 33: 160–172.
5 Ghayoumi A. Multiple disciplinary approach to fibromyalgia. J Chiropractic 1994; 31(11): 83–86.
6 Buskila D, Odes LR, Neumann L, Odes HS. Fibromyalgia in inflammatory bowel disease. J Rheumatol 1999; 26: 1167–1171.
7 Wallace DJ. The fibromyalgia syndrome. Ann Med 1997; 29: 9–21.
8 Goldberg P. Fibromyalgia: understanding its causes and resolution. Part I of II. Today's Chiropractic 1998; 27(5): 20–27.
9 Amir M, Kaplan Z, Neumann L et al. . Posttraumatic stress disorder, tenderness and fibromyalgia. J Psychosom Res 1997; 42: 607–613.
10 Cote KA, Moldofsky H. Sleep, daytime symptoms, and cognitive performance in patients with fibromyalgia. J Rheumatol 1997; 24: 2014–2023.
11 Bell IR, Baldwin CM, Schwartz GE. Illness from low levels of environmental chemicals: relevance to chronic fatigue syndrome and fibromyalgia. Am J Med 1998; 105(3A): 74S-82S.
12 Crofford LJ. Neuroendocrine abnormalities in fibromyalgia and related disorders. Am J Med Sci 1998; 315: 359–366.
13 Neeck G, Riedel W. Hormonal pertubations in fibromyalgia syndrome. Ann NY Acad Sci 1999; 876: 325–338.
14 Russell IJ. Neurochemical pathogenesis of fibromyalgia. Z Rheumatol 1998; 57 (Suppl 2): 63–66.
15 Winfield JB. Pain in fibromyalgia. Rheum Dis Clin North Am 1998; 25: 55–79.
16 Bennett RM. Emerging concepts in the neurobiology of chronic pain: evidence of abnormal sensory processing in fibromyalgia. Mayo Clin Proc 1999; 74: 385–398.
17 Boon H, Smith M. The Botanical Pharmacy. The Pharmacology of 47 Common Herbs. Kingston: Quarry Press, 1999.
18 Lonergan E. Geriatrics. A Lange Clinical Manual. 1st edn. Stamford, CT: Appleton & Lange, 1996.
19 Gleberzon BJ, Annis RA. The necessity of strength training for the older patient. J Can Chiropractic Assoc 2000; 4(4).
20 Berman BM, Ezzo J, Hadhazy V, Swyers JP. Is acupuncture effective in the treatment of fibromyalgia? J Fam Pract 1999; 48: 213–218.
21 Turk DC, Okifuji A, Sinclair JD, Starz TW. Interdisciplinary treatment of fibromyalgia syndrome: clinical and statistical significance. Arthritis Care Res 1998; 11: 186–195.
22 Keel PJ, Bodoky C, Gerhard U, Muller W. Comparison of integrated group therapy and group relaxation training for fibromyalgia. Clin J Pain 1998; 14: 232–238.
23 Singh BB, Berman BM, Hadhazy VA, Creamer P. A pilot study of cognitive behavioral therapy in fibromyalgia. Alternative Ther-Health Med 1998; 4(2): 67–70.
24 Brooks RC, McGee SR. Diagnostic dilemmas in polymyalgia rheumatica. Arch Intern Med 1997; 157: 162–168.
25 Dwolatzky T, Sonnerblick M, Nesher G. Giant cell arteritis and polymyalgia rheumatica: clues to early diagnosis. Geriatrics 1997; 52(6): 38–40, 43–44.
26 Salvarani C, Cantini F, Macchioni P et al. Distal Musculoskeletal manifestations in polymyalgia rheumatica: a prospective followup study. Arthritis Rheum 1998; 42: 1561–1562.
27 Abrams W, Beers M, Berkow R. The Merck Manual of Geriatrics. 2nd edn. Whitehouse Station: Merck & Co., 1995.
28 Cohen J. Avoiding drug reactions. Effective low-dose drug therapies for older patients. Geriatrics 2000; 55(2): 54–64.

14

Instability: falls, fractures and disorders of gait and proprioception

Brian J Gleberzon

Instability is a serious problem in older patients. Not only can it seriously diminish their activities of daily living and hamper their social interactions, but it is also a major contributing factor to the risk of falls and fracture. Instability can be caused by many different factors, which may be categorized as either intrinsic or extrinsic. Intrinsic causes of instability include disturbances of gait, deterioration of those mechanisms responsible for proprioception and balance (cerebellar, labyrinthine and visual systems), diminished neck righting reflexes, adverse drug reactions, acute illnesses (such as fever), peripheral neuropathies, foot problems, dementia, decline in muscle strength and diminished baroreceptor control.[1–5] In a recent article, Morgenthal[4] listed the major intrinsic risk factors for falls. These were: poor vision, cardiovascular disease, lower extremity dysfunction, disorders of gait and balance, bladder dysfunction, cognitive impairments, neurological disorders and medication use. Other specific intrinsic medical conditions that may lead to an increased risk of falling include nocturia and Parkinson's disease (PD). PD has been reported to increase the risk of falling 10-fold.[2] Disorders that negatively affect sensory input, such as diabetic neuropathy or vitamin B_{12} deficiency, may also contribute to instability.[2] Extrinsic causes of instability are those related to environmental hazards, such as slippery floors, inadequate lighting, lack of handrails or bathroom grab-bars, and uneven outdoor walkways and pavements. Some authorities have concluded that environmental hazards may interact critically with individual behaviours and intrinsic health risks to increase the likelihood of falling.[6]

Intrinsic risk factors for falling are often cumulative. For example, among the most important intrinsic risk factors are hip weakness, balance impairment and taking prescription medications (particularly four or more).[7] Patients with none of these risk factors have a 12% chance of sustaining a fall in a 1 year period. Those persons with all three have a risk factor approaching 100%.[7]

Instability may manifest as vertigo, dizziness or disequilibrium. These conditions may be the result of pathologies to the vestibular apparatus or they may be the consequence of adverse drug reactions. From a clinical perspective, the most serious sequella of instability is the patient falling and suffering a fracture.

Falls and fractures

Falls and subsequent fractures are a leading cause of morbidity and mortality among the elderly. Death due to a fall is the sixth leading cause of death in older patients[2] and the leading cause of death due to injury.[3] Seventy five per cent of persons who die from a fall are over the age of 65.[2,4] The death rate from falls rises exponentially with increasing age for both genders in all racial groups.[2,3]

About one-third of community-dwelling elderly people fall once a year.[2,3,8] This rate rises to 50% in those over the age of 80.[7] The fall rate is even higher in nursing homes.[8] Homes and nursing-care facilities are the most common locations where fatal falls occur, with an estimated annual incidence of 1500 falls per 1000 persons.[9,10] Five per cent of falls in the elderly result in a fracture and one-fifth of these are hip fractures.[1,7]

The estimated lifetime risk of hip fracture occurrence is about 14% in postmenopausal women and 6% in men.[9] The incidence of hip fractures predominates in women over men by a factor of four to one.[11] In North America, falls account for 250000 hip fractures each year.[2,7] Demographic projections indicate that, by the year 2050, about 650000 hip fractures will occur annually, about half of them occurring in those aged 85 years and older.[2,12] One in three women and one in six men who live to the age of 90 will sustain a hip fracture.[2] In the year following a hip fracture, mortality rates for these patients increase by 15%.[2]

In the USA, falls accounted for 14000 deaths and 22 million visits to hospitals and physicians' offices in 1996.[10] The death rate directly attributable to falls increases with age and the death rate from falling is consistently higher in men until the age of 75,[10] despite the fact that falls occur more frequently in women of this age.[2] After the age of 75, the frequency of death-related falls is similar in both genders.[2]

Not only does the rate of falling increase with age, but the injury rate is highest among the old old (persons 85 years and older).[7] Among the elderly who fall, the risk of hospitalization is 10 times greater and the risk of dying eight times greater than in children who fall.[7] Among older persons, falls also account for 90% of wrist, forearm and pelvic fractures.[2] Even in the absence of fracture, a fall results in serious injury in 25% of all cases.[13] Looking at falls and fractures from another perspective, one study reported that 96% of all fractures were the result of a fall and 85% of the fractures involving a fall occurred at the patient's home.[14]

It is estimated that half of all older persons limit their activities in some way to avoid the risk of falling, which imposes strict limitations on the ability of these individuals to pursue a higher quality of life.[13,15] Even if not fatal, falls result in an inordinate amount of pain, social isolation, immobility, loss of self-confidence, health-care costs and premature nursing-home placement.[3]

A prospective study reviewed the profile of a homogeneous group comprising 832 urban older persons who had sustained a hip fracture from a fall.[16] All were community dwelling, cognitively intact and previously ambulatory. Most fractures occurred in patient's the home, particularly in patients who were older, less healthy and poor ambulators. More than 75% of the fractures resulted from a fall while the patient was either standing or walking. In this study, most falls occurred during the daytime.[16]

The economic impact of trauma in older patients is a matter of growing concern to public-health practitioners and providers.[17] A study conducted in 1996 reported that older persons incurring one or more injurious falls resulted in increased annual hospital costs of $11 042, nursing-care costs of $5325 and total health-care costs of $19 440.[17] Incurring two or more injurious falls increased costs substantially. These findings led the researchers to conclude that 'health care costs of falls are pervasive and substantial, and they increase with fall frequency and severity'.[17] In the USA, the overall economic burden of caring for older patients who fall and sustain an injury is estimated at $12.4 billion.[7] Discharge from hospital often leads to placement in a nursing home, with falls listed as the reason for 40% of admissions to these facilities.[3,7]

The health-care burden directly attributed to falls and fractures is not isolated to the USA. For example, the World Health Organization (WHO) has estimated that 1.7 million hip fractures occurred world-wide in 1990 and some experts have predicted the global number of hip fractures to exceed 6.25 million by 2050.[18,19] These predictions are also based on studies conducted in Australia,[20,21] Spain,[22] Germany,[23] Japan,[24] Norway,[25] Sweden,[26] France[27] and Finland.[28]

The study conducted in Finland reported some very disturbing findings.[28] The investigators reported increases in fall-induced injuries of 284% between 1970 and 1995, with an increase in death rates of 80%. The researchers concluded that, for reasons unknown, the number of fall-induced injuries had increased at a rate that cannot by explained simply be demographic changes.

Many falls are the direct result of adverse side-effects to certain prescription medications. The determination of whether or not the use of various prescription medications is the direct cause of falls and fractures has been the subject of at least 50 epidemiological studies.[8] In particular, patients prescribed psychotrophic drugs or antidepressants are at an increased risk of falling.[7,8,29,30] Other medications associated with dizziness and increased rates of falling include neuroleptics, hypnotics and sedatives, and a combination of drugs with hypotensive effects.[28–31] Some studies have found associations between non-steroidal anti-inflammatory drugs (NSAIDs) and an increased risk of falling.[8] Improving drug regimens is probably one of the most important and effective means of reducing falling risk in older persons, especially among the frail elderly.[31] Other adverse and iatrogenic drug reactions are discussed in Chapter 23.

The importance of 'safety-proofing' a patient's home for injury prevention, as well as the benefits of hip protectors, will be discussed at the end of this chapter.

History assessment and physical examination

If a patient presents subsequent to a fall, or is otherwise judged to be at risk for falling, it is imperative that a practitioner conduct a thorough history and physical examination. If a patient has sustained a fall, the practitioner must determine whether immediate referral to a hospital is warranted.

If the practitioner judges that the patient has not sustained a fracture or other serious injury, the doctor can then ask the 'SPLAT' questions:[2,3,15]

- Symptoms associated with the fall (vertigo, disequilibrium, nausea, headache)
- Prior falls
- Location of the fall
- Activity at time of fall
- Time of day the fall occurred.

These questions are designed to determine the conditions under which the fall occurred.

Physical examination should include a postural and gait assessment, noting any significant structural abnormalities in the lower limb (especially of the feet) or any pathognomonic gait patterns (such as the shuffling gait pattern of PD). Blood pressure, should be measured supine, sitting and standing. The patient's pulse should be recorded. General muscle strength of the major gait and postural muscles (gastrocnemius, hamstrings, quadriceps, psoas) should be assessed. According to McCarthy,[5] peripheral neuropathy is one of the least recognized causes of falls. The clinical hallmarks of peripheral neuropathy are the loss of the distal lower extremity sensation and motor function that gradually improves proximally.[5]

Several instruments are available to assess the balance of older patients.[32] These include the Berg Balance Scale, the Clinical Test of Sensory Interaction and Balance (CTSIB), the Functional Reach Test, the Tinetti Balance Test of the Performance-Oriented Assessment of Mobility Problems and the Physical Performance Test.[32]

The Berg Balance Scale is one of the more commonly used tests to assess balance.[32] Although the test requires about 15 min to administer, very little equipment is involved. Several different components of balance are assessed during the 14 items of the test:[32–34]

1. Patient asked to go from a seated position to a standing position, with no support.
2. Patient asked to stand unsupported for 2 min.
3. Patient asked to sit unsupported with feet on the floor for 2 min.
4. Patient asked to go from a standing position to a seated position.
5. Patient asked to move from a chair to a bed and back again.
6. Patient asked to stand unsupported with eyes closed.
7. Patient asked to stand unsupported with feet together.
8. Patient asked to reach forward as far as they can while standing unsupported.
9. Patient asked to pick up an object from the floor while standing unsupported.
10. Patient asked to look over their left and right shoulders while standing unsupported.
11. Patient asked to turn around 360 degrees while standing unsupported.
12. Patient asked to place each foot alternately on a stool (each foot four times).
13. Patient asked to walk heel-to-toe (tandem).
14. Patient asked to stand on one leg.

The Berg Balance Scale has consistently demonstrated high reliability and validity.[32]

A useful test is the 'get up and go test'.[3,7,32] To administer this test, the patient is asked to arise from a standard arm chair, walk 3 m across the room, turn around and walk back to the chair and sit down.[3,7] A practitioner can also record the amount of time a patient requires to perform this test (called the timed get up and go test).[32]

If a patient reports vertigo, other specific tests should be performed. Specific tests include the Dix–Hallpike manoeuvre in cases of suspected benign paroxysmal positional vertigo and the sitting rotatory chair test to differentiate between cervicogenic and vestibular vertigo (see below).

Disorders of gait

Walking is best thought of as controlled falling. The centre of mass the body travels outside the body's base of support during 80% of the stride cycle, and maximum toe clearance during forward propulsion is 2 cm above the ground.[35] In order to propel oneself, co-ordinated actions of the foot, lower limb, pelvis, torso, trunk and head must all be involved. The spine is vital for proper gait kinematics, since it attenuates horizontal acceleration of the trunk to provide a stable platform for the head.[35]

Gait, balance, the ability to negotiate stairs and other mobility tasks decline with age.[4] For example, it has been estimated that 2 million Americans have difficulties with such essential mobility tasks as the ability to stand independently or the ability to stand from a seated position.[4] In older patients, these difficulties may be the result of adverse drug reactions, inactivity (immobility) with a concomitant loss of muscle strength and joint flexibility, a loss of proprioceptive and balance mechanisms, various disease processes (such as PD) or injury.[2,13]

An individual's gait invariably changes with age. Significant gait disturbances occur in more than 15% of older persons and up to 25% of them require a walking aid.[2] Older men tend to have a wide-based gait, whereas older women adopt a narrow-based, waddling gait.[2] In general, older persons often walk slowly, with a reduction in stride length, force of push-off, toe clearance, arm swing, and hip and knee rotation.[2,3,13] An extrapyramidal pattern emerges, resulting in a stance of general flexion with increased muscle tone, poverty of motion and bradykinesia.[3] There is also an increase in postural sway. Both feet tend to remain on the ground for a longer period during the gait cycle. In older persons, there is a decline in the variability of muscle activity patterns and an increase in head horizontal acceleration.[35] This type of gait pattern is often referred to as senile gait.

A study by Lee and Kerrigan sought to identify kinetic differences between elderly 'fallers' and 'non-fallers'.[36] Their study revealed that, among those patients who tend to fall, there was a significantly greater peak torque in hip flexion, hip adduction, knee extension, knee varum, ankle dorsiflexion and ankle eversion.[36] Ankle dorsiflexion was significantly decreased in the fall group.[36]

Another study conducted at the Sunnybrook Health Science Center (University of Toronto) sought to determine predictors of the likelihood of future falls among ambulatory older adults.[37] Based on his findings, the investigator concluded that such observed changes in gait as decreased stride length and speed and prolonged double support (standing on both feet) time may be stabilizing adaptations related to the fear of falling, whereas stride-to-stride variability in the control of gait is an independent predictor of falling. Stride-to-stride variability may therefore be a useful measure to identify individuals at a high risk of falling.[37] The study concluded that, contrary to common expectations, a wider stance does not necessarily increase stability, but instead seems to reflect an increased likelihood of experiencing a fall.[37]

The fear associated with falling was identified as a risk factor for sustaining a fall during a study by Luukinen et al.[38] This group identified other risk factors for falling such as abnormal heel–shin test, reduced knee extension strength, reduced grip strength, poor distant visual acuity, low supine pulse rate, inability to carry a 5 kg load 100 m, not engaging in heavy outdoor work and no habitual exercise.[38] The importance of exercise, including strength training, is discussed further in Chapter 28.

Other physiological changes associated with an increased risk of falls

Many concomitant age-related physiological changes that occur in older patients predispose them to a fall. An important contributory factor to postural control and balance is provided by the activity of the mechanoreceptors of the facet (zygapophyseal) joints of the cervical spine.[3] Impairment of the mechanoreceptors from such structural changes as cervical spondylosis can result in a feeling of unsteadiness during movements, especially movements involving head rotation.[3] Changes to the visual system may result in a decrease in accommodation, visual acuity, adaptation to darkness, peripheral vision acuity, glare tolerance and contrast sensitivity, all of which contribute to an increased risk of falling.[2,39]

Incontinence may indirectly lead to an increase in falling risk. The patient may, in an effort to diminish incontinent episodes, purposefully restrict fluid intake; this could lead to dehydration and postural hypotension. Alternatively, nocturia may increase the risk of falling simply because the patient is travelling to the bathroom more often, especially at night and often in the dark, potentially tripping over hazards such as furniture, loose carpets or even family pets.

Types of vertigo

Dizziness is an all-encompassing term employed by patients and may include true vertigo (sense of motion), disequilibrium (sense of lacking co-ordination with erect posture or during purposeful movements) or imbalance. Fifty to sixty per cent of older patients living at home and 80–90% of patients in outpatient clinics report episodes of dizziness.[13] By the age of 80, one in three persons will have suffered a fall, resulting in significant morbidity: vestibular symptoms precede these falls in more than half of the patients.[13]

Balance and orientation information is received from the vestibular, visual and somatosensory receptors and is correlated, integrated and co-ordinated in the cerebellum and vestibular nuclei.[1] Perception, adaptation and modulation of received information occur in the frontal cortex and the thalamus.[1]

Vertigo is the cardinal sign of vestibular disease, although it may be the result of pathology or dysfunction of the labyrinth, vestibular nerve, vestibular component of the eighth cranial nerve, vestibular nuclei, cervical afferent nerves, cerebellum or other supratentorial structures.[1,40,41] Vertigo may be experienced as either a sensation of spinning (subjective vertigo) or that the world is spinning about one's self (objective vertigo).[40] A vertiginous patient will often describe symptoms that include unsteadiness, giddiness, lightheadedness and disequilibrium.[40] However, it is imperative to differentiate true vertigo from simple lightheadedness, dizziness or tinnitus.[15] Accompanying symptoms of true vertigo include nausea, vomiting, staggering and nystagmus.[15] Vertebrobasilar insufficiency may present with similar symptoms to vertigo. However, unlike vertigo, vertebrobasilar insufficiency also presents with numbness, diplopia, drop attacks, dysphagia, dysarthria and ataxia, and is not fatiguable or habituable with repeated provocative head positioning.[15,40] Lastly, tinnitus, defined as a ringing in the ears for which there is no outside source, accompanies specific vertiginous conditions such as Ménière's syndrome.[1]

Vertigo may result from either central or peripheral causes. Central causes include arteriovenous malformation, cerebral haemorrhage, brainstem vascular disease, tumours and demyelinating diseases such as

multiple sclerosis.[40] Vertigo of peripheral origin includes conditions affecting the vestibular system (such as Ménière's syndrome) or proprioceptive sense organs of the cervical spine (such as cervical vertigo or Barre–Lieou syndrome). The most common cause of peripheral vertigo is believed to be benign paroxysmal positional vertigo (BPPV).[1,40] Moreover, certain pharmaceuticals exhibit vestibulotoxic effects. These include salicylates, barbituates, tranquillizers, antihistamines, arsenic, mercury and lead.[40]

Central vertigo may be differentiated from peripheral vertigo by observing the patient's nystagmus and the direction in which the patient tends to fall.[15] In cases of peripheral vertigo, nystagmus is accentuated by looking towards the unaffected ear and is improved by visual fixation.[15] The nystagmus itself is a jerk nystagmus with a fast phase contralateral to the side of damage.[1] The patient tends to fall away from the side of the fast component of the nystagmus.[15]

Conversely, in cases of central vertigo, the patient's nystagmus is accentuated by looking towards the side of the lesion and is not improved by visual fixation. The patient tends to fall towards the fast component of the nystagmus.[15] There is a course jerk nystagmus with the fast component ipsilateral to the side of lesion.[1]

Vertigo of cerebellar origin is often associated with incoordination and intention tremor, nystagmus and ataxic stance; the patient tends to fall to the affected side if he or she walks around.[1] Infarction of the portion of the cerebellum supplied by the posterior inferior cerebellar artery can lead to an intense vertigo which is virtually indistinguishable from vertigo of a labyrinthine origin.[1] However, symptoms indicative of this type of medullary syndrome may include nausea, vomiting, ipsilateral Horner's syndrome, loss of pain and temperature sensation, difficulty swallowing, hoarseness and intractable hiccups.[1]

Other medical tests used to differentiate between the different causes of vertigo include electronystagmography (ENG), audiograms and duplex Doppler scans.[1]

Benign paroxysmal positional vertigo

The most common cause of peripheral vertigo in the general population is BPPV, and it is also the most common cause of vertigo in older adults.[1] This condition is a clinical syndrome characterized by recurrent, brief episodes of vertigo and rotary nystagmus which is precipitated by specific positions of the head related to the effects of gravity.[31] BPPV accounts for 17–30% of all cases of vertigo presenting to vestibular clinics.[40] BPPV is most commonly seen in individuals over the age of 40 years, with the highest age distribution between 50 and 70 years.[40] It is more prevalent in women. BPPV is considered to be self-limiting, but may last for several months.[15]

Most cases (over 50%) of BPPV are idiopathic, although some cases have followed incidences of head trauma, infection or surgery.[40] Owing the presence of nystagmus and the intensification of symptoms by changes in head position, many investigators suspect that the posterior semicircular canals are involved in BPPV. Other possible pathophysiological explanations for BPPV include cupulolithiasis (the 'heavy cupula' theory) and canalithiasis, free-floating endolymphatic densities in the posterior semicircular canal.[40] However, there is currently no definitive theory to explain the pathophysiology of BPPV and its aetiology remains enigmatic.

The diagnosis of BPPV is confirmed if there is an acute onset of vertigo and nystagmus by provocative positioning of the head with the affected ear placed downwards. The vertigo and nystagmus have a brief latent onset period (between 1 and 30 s) and the vertigo and nystagmus are of limited duration (15–30 s). Characteristic rotary nystagmus is elicited by a head-hanging position and is reversed on upright sitting. A distinguishing test is the fatiguability of vertigo by the Dix–Hallpike (or Nylen-Barany) manoeuvre with repeated positioning.[1,40,42]

The Dix–Hallpike is both a diagnostic and a therapeutic manoeuvre for BPPV. The patient is seated on an examination table. The doctor then rapidly guides the patient into a supine head-hanging position. That is, the patient's head would be hanging over the end of the examination table, with the neck in 30–45° of extension and 30–45° of rotation.[1,40] This procedure provokes a rapid rotary nystagmus and an episode of vertigo. The side of rotation that results in the nystagmus and vertigo indicates the involved ear; the lowermost ear is thought to be the one involved.[40] For example, if a left cervical anterior rotary position was observed to produce symptoms of BPPV, the clinician would diagnosis that the left ear was the site of pathology. Clearly, it is vital for the practitioner to explain fully the details of the manoeuvre to the patient before starting the test.

After confirming the diagnosis of BPPV and determining the side of ear involvement, the practitioner can use the Epley's canalith repositioning procedure for therapeutic benefits.[43] After the Dix–Hallpike procedure, the patient is allowed to sit upright for approximately 10 min. This is thought to allow endolymphatic particles to settle into gravity-dependent positions of the posterior semicircular canals. The patient is then repositioned in the Dix–Hallpike position. The patient is directed to gaze downwards towards the affected ear with the eyes open. An episode of nystagmus and vertigo is likely to be precipitated, and the patient must be reassured. The patient is then rotated 180° into a lateral recumbent position. This results in the opposite ear pointing towards the floor. This final position is held for 2–3 min and the patient is assisted to a seated position.[43]

The procedure is thought to reposition the particles into the utricle of the inner ear. Nystagmus should be absent when the patient is returned to the upright position. The patient is then instructed to maintain an upright position for the next 48 h.[43] It is imperative that the patient maintains this position, and does not look upwards or downwards or lie in a horizontal position. After 48 h, it is theorized that the particles will not re-enter the posterior semicircular canals and the patient can resume normal activities.[43]

Treatment with vestibular suppressant medications is of limited usefulness, except during episodes of exacerbation. Patients usually respond well to vestibular exercises, and in most cases spontaneous resolution occurs within 1 year.[15]

Epley reported success rates of 90% using this manoeuvre.[43] However, due to the provocative nature of the procedure, a practitioner must exercise caution when contemplating its use on older patients.

Cervical or cervicogenic vertigo

Cervical vertigo is the second most commonly diagnosed cause of vertigo.[41] There are three probable pathophysiological mechanisms of cervical vertigo: (i) vascular compression or stenosis of the vertebral artery, (ii) altered proprioception input (abnormal neck reflex), and (iii) vasomotor changes caused by irritation to the cervical sympathetic chain.[41,44]

Diagnostic criteria of cervical vertigo include: dizziness, episodes of recurrent balance instability, tinnitus and, less commonly, hearing loss. Patients may also report neck pain, restricted ranges of cervical motion, headaches and earaches.[41] Cervical vertigo may result from injuries sustained following a motor vehicle accident.[44]

Fitz-Ritson proposed a model to explain cervicogenic vertigo.[44] In his model, the C2 dorsal root ganglia convey sensory information from the joints and muscles of the neck to brainstem nuclei. These same nuclei are also connected to the ocular muscles. This model may explain the interrelatedness of cervicogenic vertigo and nystagmus.[44]

The key procedure used to assess cervicogenic vertigo was first described by Fitz-Ritson.[44] For this procedure, sometimes referred to as the sitting rotary chair test, the patient is seated in a chair that can rotate. The doctor stands behind the patient. For the first part of the test, the patient is instructed to shake their head from side to side as far and as quickly as possible. If this results in vertiginous symptoms, the vertigo may either originate from the labyrinthine compartments or it may be cervicogenic, stemming from the muscles and joints of the neck.

For the second part of the test, the patient is asked to rotate their entire body from side to side to acquaint themselves with this motion. The doctor then holds the patient's head steady with slight cephalad traction. The patient is instructed to close their eyes and to continue rotating on the chair from side to side. This action essentially negates the involvement of labyrinthine elements and involves only cervical elements. The doctor should be prepared for the onset of patient symptoms.[44]

If no symptoms are observed with the head held steady, the practitioner can conclude that the vertigo is of labyrinthine origin, whereas cervicogenic vertigo would be diagnosed if symptoms occurred during both procedures.[44] In cases of cervicogenic vertigo, deep palpation will usually elicit suboccipital tenderness, and joint restrictions (or subluxations) are often detected in the C1–C3 levels.[1] Vertigo may be provoked during either motion palpation or cervical joint play.[1]

A recent study sought to determine the therapeutic results in a group of patients with cervical vertigo using conservative active and passive modalities.[41] Passive treatment included spinal manipulative therapy to specific cervical and thoracic segments, soft-tissue techniques, electrotherapy (interferential current) and labyrinth-sedation drugs. Active treatment included biofeedback and exercise. The treatment periods lasted for between 15 and 77 days (mean 41 days). Sixty per cent of the 15 patients in the study reported a complete remission of their vertigo, with another three patients (20%) reporting consistent improvement. The

authors concluded that very favourable results were achieved in cases of cervical vertigo using active and passive treatment protocols that included spinal manipulative therapy.[39] Other authors have also suggested a plan of management for cervicogenic vertigo that includes spinal manipulative therapy and soft-tissue therapy.[1,45]

Ménière's syndrome

The cause of Ménière's syndrome is unknown.[13] It is characterized by a classic constellation of four symptoms: dizziness characterized as episodic spinning or whirling vertigo, (ii) fluctuating, low-frequency sensorineural hearing loss, (iii) tinnitus, and (iv) a sensation of fullness in the ear (13, 46). Typically, attacks are not triggered by positions or other events.[1] Episodes of vertigo may last for 1 or 2 h,[15,46] during which the patient will usually prefer to lie on their unaffected side, with the affected ear up.[1] Because symptoms may or may not develop concurrently, a careful history and complete physical examination are necessary for an accurate diagnosis.[46] If Ménière's is present but untreated for 10 years or more, hearing loss may increase as the vertiginous episodes gradually subside.[46]

Management of Ménière's syndrome includes sodium restriction and the avoidance of caffeine, alcohol and nicotine.[15] Sedatives, antiemetics, antihistamine, antidepressants and vestibular suppressants are often prescribed.[15,46] Many vestibular suppressants have anticholinergic effects, which in the elderly may cause mental confusion and urinary incontinence.[13] Surgery, including cochlear implantation, may be necessary in severe, unresponsive cases.[46,47] Conservative management includes the treatment of secondary neuromusculoskeletal manifestations.[1]

Chiropractic care and peripheral vertigo

Douglas suggested that spinal manipulative therapy and soft-tissue therapy are appropriate treatments for peripheral vertigo, including Ménière's disease.[1] It was the author's opinion that manual therapies would stimulate proprioceptors in the cervical spine, which could either normalize input to the vestibular nuclei by restoring more normal joint and muscle function, or aid in the neurological adaptation process.[1]

In a more recent article, Kessinger and Boneva described a case study of a 75-year-old woman with a longstanding history of vertigo, tinnitus and hearing loss who responded favourably to upper cervical specific chiropractic care.[48] The authors reported that this patient experienced an alleviation of her symptoms, that structural and functional improvements were evident through radiographic examination, and that audiological function improved. It is interesting to note that, over the course of 3.5 months and 29 office visits, the patient received only three upper cervical specific adjustments.[48]

Vertebrobasilar insufficiency

In the elderly, vertebrobasilar insufficiency (VBI) is an important cause of vertigo and disequilibrium.[13] VBI often results from arteriosclerosis with insufficient collateral circulation. It may also be the result of compression of vertebral arteries by cervical spondyloses, postural hypotension or a subclavian steal syndrome.[13] The differential diagnoses of VBI and BPPV have been described previously.

Postural or orthostatic hypotension

Orthostatic hypotension occurs in 15–22% of community-dwelling seniors and is defined as a drop in systolic blood pressure of 20 mmHg or more when the patient stands from a seated position.[2] Orthostatic hypotension is characterized by vertigo, lightheadedness and syncope, which is the sudden transient loss of consciousness characterized by unresponsiveness and loss of postural control.[2]

Various physiological changes may predispose an older person to syncope or orthostatic hypotension. Diminished baroreflex sensitivity, reduced cardiac output and reduced pulmonary function can all reduce cerebral oxygen flow by as much as 40%.[2] Certain medications, autonomic insufficiency syndromes, cardiovascular disease, dehydration and multiple cerebral infarcts may all cause orthostatic hypotension. Syncope can also occur after eating a large meal, urination, defecation, coughing or even swallowing.[2]

Other causes of instability

Other possible causes of vertigo or dizziness in older patients include acute vestibular neuritis, cranial trauma, eighth cranial nerve vascular compression, acoustic neuroma and multiple sclerosis.[1]

Botanical medicines and instability

Several animal studies have demonstrated the clinical effectiveness of gingko for vestibular disorders.[49] In vestibular neurectomized cats, gingko was found to improve posture, locomotor balance and spontaneous neck muscle activity. One clinical trial of patients with recent onset of idiopathic vertigo found that gingko decreased the intensity, frequency and duration of vertiginous symptoms compared with a placebo.[49] Gingko has also been reported to be effective in cases of 'chronic cerebral insufficiency'.[41] With improvement in: memory loss, difficulty concentrating, confusion, fatigue, physical strength, headache, depressive moods, anxiety, dizziness and tinnitus.[49] Gingko has also been reported to be of benefit to patients with dementia and depression.[49]

Preventive strategies: treating instability, the importance of home assessments and community-based programmes

McCarthy suggested that five domains should be addressed in the patient who exhibits peripheral neuropathy and balance instability:[5] education, physical training, footwear assessment, eye examinations and support during walking.[5] The use of a supportive device is especially important for the unstable person when walking in unfamiliar or poorly lit places, or while walking on irregular, soft terrains. If the use of a cane is recommended, McCarthy advised that the cane should be planted in the ground opposite the lower extremity that is contralateral to the cane hand (for example, if the cane is in the left hand, it is swung forward and placed in the ground at the same time as the right leg and foot).[5] Moreover, in order to gain the most benefit from a cane, the patient should be able to bear 20–25% of his or her body weight on the cane (this can be checked using a bathroom scale).[5] It is important that the clinician emphasize to the patient that the use of a cane does not imply that the patient is frail, and that its use may potentially prevent the tragic consequences of a fall.

Education and therapy aimed at reducing potential risk factors of falling among older patients have been shown to reduce the risk of falls by 7–12%.[7] A field practitioner may consider suggesting to an older patient (or their carer) that an at-home inspection be conducted to identify and remove potential risk factors for falling.

A study in Australia sought to determine the cost-effectiveness of a home assessment programme aimed at reducing hazards in older persons' homes.[13] Cost-effectiveness was estimated by determining the cost of the programme related to the cost per fall prevented and the cost per injury prevented.[20] Over a 1 year period, the investigators determined the cost of the programme to be $172 per person. The associated cost per fall prevented was estimated at $1721 per person and the cost per injury prevented at $17 298. The investigative team concluded that injury-prevention programmes aimed at 'safety-proofing' a patient's home are substantially cost-effective in terms of both health-care savings and enhanced quality of life for the patient.[20]

Another study conducted in Miami, USA, however, found that home assessments may not have the large potential benefit that was previously thought, but did conclude that the usefulness of grab-bars should be evaluated further.[50]

Norton et al. concluded from a study conducted in Australia that strategies aimed at preventing falls and fractures among the old old and among institutionalized individuals should focus primarily on modification of intrinsic (health) factors, while the modification of extrinsic factors has the greatest potential for prevention among the younger, community-dwelling seniors.[14]

Killinger, Hawk, Azad and their team at Palmer College of Chiropractic have emphasized the importance of community-based programmes targeted at older patients.[51,52] Such programmes have as their goals health education, health promotion and prevention strategies.[51,52] Community-based programmes can provide information on issues of importance to older patients such as osteoporosis, osteoarthritis, diet and nutrition, exercise and how to safety-proof a person's home.[51,52] The importance of this approach is addressed in greater detail by Killinger in Chapter 30. Moreover, from a pedagogical perspective, Mootz and Haldeman recently concluded that 'for health professional students to understand the natural history of health-related events over time and to achieve the goal of collaborative practice, curricula must be community oriented'.[53] Such programmes may enable students to develop important clinical skills that they might not otherwise have had an opportunity to develop during their internship.

The Harstad injury-prevention study is a prospective evaluation of the introduction of a community-based environmental hazard-prevention programme.[54,55] This study has been in progress for 8 years. The first 3 years were allocated to establishing baseline data.

Interventions and data collection have been ongoing for the past 5 years. A reduction in falls resulting in fracture were reported during the second year of the study.[54] However, Gillespie et al. of the Cochrane Review commented that, because the investigation was neither controlled nor randomized, its optimistic conclusions may be a reflection of examiner bias and confounding factors.[55]

A community-based educational outreach programme was designed at the Canadian Memorial Chiropractic College (CMCC) in 1999.[56] In recognition of the International Year of the Older Patient, the Ministry of Health of Ontario, Senior's Secretariat, accepted applications for outreach programme initiatives. The proposal submitted by Gleberzon of CMCC was accepted and the project was cofunded by the Ontario Chiropractic Association. An excellent resource guide, 'Creating a Community Health Forum' by Dr Irwin Goldzweig of Meharry Medical College, was consulted and used in designing the programme.[57]

Student interns were recruited and trained as the programme's presenters. A focus group was conducted with older members of the community and a content-expert facilitator, in order to identify those areas of greatest concern to older persons, and to determine the best manner in which the information should be presented. The use of focus groups to obtain the opinions, feelings and perception of older persons has been advocated by experts in gerontological research.[58] The focus group revealed that issues of concern were osteoporosis, osteoarthritis and injury prevention. The programme was advertised on a senior community-bulletin internet website. Activity co-ordinators from different prospective sites contacted the outreach programme supervisor (Gleberzon) and presentations were scheduled at mutually convenient times.[56]

Twenty different presentations at 12 different sites were conducted between September 1999 and March 2000. Outcome measures (surveys) indicated that the programme was well received by the target audience. Each person in attendance was given a handout with a checklist of recommendations to safety-proof their homes:[56]

- Replace 60 watt bulbs with 100 watt bulbs.
- Ensure all walkways and stairs are in good repair.
- Ensure there is a clear pathway from the bed to the bathroom. This may involve removing or relocating ottomans, low tables, benches, or even family pets.

- Remove any loose area or throw rugs, especially if they are on slippery surfaces such as hardwood floors.
- Place grab-bars in bathroom by toilets and bathtubs.

In addition, each presentation site was given two posters, entitled 'Chiropractic Care of the Older Patient', and 'Osteoarthritis, Osteoporosis and Preventative Strategies for the Older Person' (Figures 14.1, 14.2).

Interns reported that the community-based outreach programme was a wonderful experience. They felt that their appreciation of the special needs and concerns of older patients was enhanced. The interns also reported that their public-speaking skills were improved, and that these skills would be useful for other presentations that they may conduct once they were in private practice.[56]

Community-based programmes can help to develop important interdisciplinary and social-support networks. According to Healthy People 2000, 'social support networks are of critical importance in promoting the health and independence of older adults'.[59]

One might argue that an academic institution such as a chiropractic college has an obligation to provide outreach presentations as a community service. Programmes such as the one described here are also viewed favourably by both the community and the profession at large. As Goldzweig summed up '… good medicine means going beyond the walls of the operating room, the emergency room and the examination room. It means going to the people before they end up in any of these "rooms" and helping them to change their lives in a way that will foster their health, their well-being and their happiness'.[57] The author strongly encourages any individual or organization to consider implementing a similar outreach programme for the older people in their communities.

The Cochrane Review recently assessed the effectiveness of different programmes designed to reduce the incidence of falls in community-dwelling, institutionalized or hospitalized elderly people.[55] The Review assessed 18 trials and one preplanned meta-analysis. These trials targeted either intrinsic or environmental risk factors, using such interventions as exercise programmes designed to improve strength or balance, educational programmes, medication optimalization programmes, and environmental hazard modification in homes or institutions. The reviewer

concluded that health-care providers contemplating fall-prevention programmes should consider interventions that target both intrinsic and extrinsic (environmental) risk factors of individual patients.[55] The reviewers also concluded that 'at present, exercise programs alone appear of uncertain effectiveness in the prevention of falls'.[55]

Hip protectors

Since the 1970s, several studies have investigated the potential use of hip protectors for the prevention of hip fractures subsequent to a fall.[60] This approach stems out of other research that indicates that falls usually occur while the patient is walking or standing, and that the fracture occurs on the side that impacts the ground. Several different kinds of padded hip protectors have been developed, most of which consist of plastic shields or foam pads that are kept in place by specially designed underwear pockets into which the device is inserted.[60]

The Cochrane Review has recently assessed the effectiveness of hip protectors in reducing the incidence of hip fractures in elderly persons following a fall.[60] The researchers reviewed six randomized trials involving 1752 participants. All six studies involved older persons living in either nursing homes or residential care centres, three in the Scandinavian countries, one in Japan, one in the UK and one in Australia. (An additional 11 studies were found by the researchers but they were not included in their review as these studies were still ongoing.) The reviewers concluded that hip protectors appear to reduce the risk of hip fracture subsequent to a fall within selected populations at high risk (e.g. patients living in long-term care facilities).[60]

In one study reviewed, the occurrence of hip fracture was 16/660 (2.4%) in those persons allocated to wear hip protectors compared with an incidence of 63/951 (6.6%) in those persons not allocated to wear protectors.[60] However, the reviewers noted that hip protectors offer a very visible reminder to their wearers and their care givers. Thus, the reduction in the incidence of hip fracture may be attributed to changes in the behaviour of either the wearer or care givers (or both), rather than to the protectors themselves.[60] Lastly, the reviewers commented that their conclusion were based on five trials of low to moderate quality.[60]

The reviewers also concluded that no significant adverse effects of the hip protectors were reported, but compliance, particularly in the long term, was poor.[60] The only reported adverse effect associated with the use of hip protectors was skin irritation. Several strategies to increase wearer compliance include offering a larger selection of hip-protector colours, using different fabrics for the underwear pockets (cotton instead of Nylon), and the use of button flies on underwear instead of Velcro (some men reported that they did not like the 'ripping' sound of the Velcro).[61]

Summary

Although there are several risk factors that an older person may have that can lead to a fall and fracture, many of these risks can be minimized or avoided. The adage that the best treatment is often prevention is nowhere more important than in the case of fall and fracture prevention. Chiropractors can facilitate many of these preventive strategies by suggesting that their patients 'safety-proof' their homes, engage in exercise, be mindful of iatrogenic drug reactions and, if they have known intrinsic risk factors (such as advanced osteoporosis) or live in a high-risk residence (such as a nursing home), consider wearing hip protectors. Finally, many causes of instability, such as gait disorders, vertigo and certain peripheral neuropathies, can be successfully managed by chiropractic care.

References

1 Douglas F. The dizzy patient: strategic approach to history, examination, diagnosis, and treatment. Chiropractic Technique 1993; 5(1): 5–16.

2 Abrams W, Beers M, Berkow R. The Merck Manual of Geriatrics. 2nd edn. Whitehouse Station: Merck & Co., 1995.

3 Bowers L. Clinical assessment of geriatric patients: unique challenges. Top Clin Chiropractic 1996; 3(2): 10–22.

4 Morgenthal AP. The geriatric examination: neuromusculoskeletal system and mental status examination. Top Clin Chiropractic 2000; 7(3): 50–57.

5 McCarthy KA. Peripheral neuropathy in the aging patient: common causes, assessment and risks. Top Clin Chiropractic 1999; 6(4): 56–61.

6 Connell BR, Wolk SL. Environmental and behavioral circumstances associated with falls at home among elderly individuals. Arch Phys Med Rehabil 1997; 78: 179–186.

7 Tibbitts M. Patients who fall: how to predict and prevent injuries. Geriatrics 1996; 51(9): 24–31.

8 Cumming RG. Epidemiology of medication-related falls and fractures in the elderly. Drugs Aging 1998; 12: 43–53.

9 Lauritzen JB. Hip fractures. Epidemiology, risk factors, falls, energy absorption, hip protectors, and prevention. Dan Med Bull 1997; 44: 155–168.

10 Hoskin AF. Fatal falls: trends and characteristics. Stat Bull Metrop Insur Co 1998; 79(2): 10–15.

11 Parker MJ, Pryor GA. Hip Fracture Management. Oxford: Blackwell Scientific Publications, 1993.

12 Brody JA. Prospects for an aging population. Nature 1985; 315: 463–466.

13 Lonergan E. Geriatrics. A Lange Clinical Manual. 1st edn. Stamford, CT: Appleton and Lange, 1996.

14 Norton R, Campbell AJ, Lee-Joe T, Butler M. Circumstances of falls resulting in hip fractures among older people. J Am Geriatr Soc 1997; 45: 1108–1112.

15 Ferri F, Fretwell M, Watchel T. Practical Guide to the Care of the Elderly Patient. 2nd edn. St Louis, MO: Mosby-Year Book, 1997.

16 Aharonoff G, Dennis M, Elshinaway A et al. Circumstances of falls causing hip fractures in the elderly. Clin Orthop 1998; 348: 10–14.

17 Rizzo J, Friedkin R, Williams C et al. Health care utilization and costs in a Medicare population by fall status. Med Care 1998; 36: 11174–11188.

18 Smith RD, Widiatmoko D. The cost-effectiveness of home assessment and modification to reduce falls in the elderly. Aust N Z J Public Health 1998; 22: 436-440.

19 WHO Study Group. Assessment of fracture risk and its application to screening for postmenopausal osteoporosis. WHO Technical Report Series No. 843. Geneva: World Health Organization, 1994.

20 Melton LJ III. Hip fractures: a worldwide problem today and tomorrow. Bone 1993; 14(Suppl 1): S1–8.

21 Hill K, Schwarz J, Flicker L, Carroll S. Falls among healthy, community-dwelling, older women: a prospective study of frequency, circumstances, consequences and prediction accuracy. Aust N Z J Public Health 1999; 23: 41–48.

22 Padilla Ruiz F, Bueno Cavanillas A, Peinado Alonso C et al. Frequency, characteristics and consequences of falls in a cohort of institutionalized elderly patients. Aten Primaria 1998; 21: 437–442, 445.

23 Von Rentein-Kruse W, Micol W, Oster P, Schlierf G. Prescription drugs, dizziness and accidental falls in hospital patients over 75 years of age. Z Gerontol Geriatr 1998; 31: 286–289.

24 Aoyagi K, Ross PD, Davis JW et al. Falls among community-dwelling elderly in Japan. J Bone Miner Res 1998; 13: 1468–1474.

25 Bergland A, Petterson AM, Laake K. Falls reported among elderly Norwegians living at home. Physiother Res Int 1998; 3: 164–174.

26 Johansson B. Fall injuries among elderly persons living at home. Scand J Caring Sci 1998; 12: 67–72.

27 Pepersack T. Falls in elderly persons: evaluation of risk and prevention. Rev Med Brux 1997; 18: 227–230.

28 Kannus P, Parkkari J, Koskinen S et al. Fall-induced injuries and death among older adults. JAMA 1999; 281: 1895–1899.

29 Leipzig RM, Cumming RG, Tinetti ME. Drugs and falls in older people: a systematic review of meta-analysis: I. Psychotropic drugs. J Am Geriatr Soc 1999; 471: 30–39.

30 Thapa PB, Gideon P, Cost TW et al. Antidepressants and the risk of falls among nursing home residents. N Engl J Med 1998; 339: 875–882.

31 Monane M, Avorn J. Medications and falls. Causation, correlation and prevention. Clin Geriatr Med 1996; 12: 847–858.

32 Whitney S, Poole J, Cass S. A review of balance instruments for older patients. Am J Occup Ther 1998; 52: 666–671.

33 Berg KO, Maki BE, Williams JI et al. Clinical and Laboratory measures of postural balance in an elderly population. Arch Phys Med Rehabil 1992; 73: 1073–1080.

34 Berg KO, Wood-Dauphinee SL, Williams JI, Gayton D. Measuring balance in the elderly. Preliminary development of an instrument. Physiother Can 1989; 41: 304–311.

35 Frank J. Geriatric gait instability. Presented at the CMCC 5th Annual Conference of Advancements in Chiropractic: A Comprehensive Approach to the Geriatric Patient, Oct. 30, 1999.

36 Lee LW, Kerrigan DC. Identification of kinetic differences between fallers and nonfallers in the elderly. Am J Phys Med Rehabil 1999; 78: 242–246.

37 Maki BE. Gait changes in older adults: predictors of falls or indicators of fear. J Am Geriatr Soc 1997; 45: 313–320.

38 Luukinen H, Koski K, Laippala P, Kivela SL. Factors predicting fractures during falling impacts among home-dwelling older adults. J Am Geriatr Soc 1997; 45(11): 1302–1309.

39 Ivers RQ, Cummings RG, Mitchell P, Attebo K. Visual impairment and falls in older adults: the Blue Mountain Eye Study. J Am Geriatr Soc 1998; 46: 58–64.

40 Van der Velde GM. Benign paroxysmal positional vertigo. Part I: Background and clinical presentation. J Can Chiropractic Assoc 1999; 43(1): 31–39.

41 Bracher ES, Almeida CI, Almeida RR et al. A combined approach for the treatment of cervical vertigo. J Manipulative Physiol Ther 2000; 23: 96–100.

42 Baloh RW, Jacobson KM. Neurology. Neurol Clin 1996; 14: 85–101.

43 Van der Velde GM. Benign paroxysmal positional vertigo. Part II: A qualitative review of non-pharmacological, conservative treatments and a case report presenting Epley's 'canalith repositioning procedure', a non-invasive bedside manoeuvre for treating BPPV. J Can Chiropractic Assoc 1999; 43(1): 41–49.

44 Fitz-Ritson D. Assessment of Cervicogenic vertigo. J Manipulative Physiol Ther 1991; 14: 193–198.

45 Fitz-Ritzon D. The chiropractic management and rehabilitation of cervical trauma. J Manipulative Physiol Ther 1990; 12: 17–26.

46 Knox GW, McPherson A. Meniere's disease: differential diagnosis and treatment. Am Fam Physician 1997; 55: 1185–1190.

47 Adair RA, Kerr AG. Streptomycin perfusion of the labyrinth in the treatment of Meniere's disease: a modified technique. Clin Otolaryngol 1999; 24: 55-–57.

48 Kessinger RC, Boneva DV. Vertigo, tinnitus, and hearing loss in the geriatric patient. J Manipulative Physiol Ther 2000; 23: 352–362.

49 Boon H, Smith M. The Botanical Pharmacy. The Pharmacology of 47 Common Herbs. Kingston: Quarry Press, 1999.

50 Sattin RW, Rodriguez JG, DeVito CA, Wingo PA. Home environmental hazards and the risk of fall injury events among community-dwelling older persons. Study to Assess Falls Among the Elderly (SAFE) group. J Am Geriatr Soc 1998; 46: 669–676.

51 Hawk C, Killinger L, Zapotocky B, Azad A. Chiropractic training in care of the geriatric patient: an assessment. J Neuromusculoskeletal Syst 1997; 5: 15–25.

52 Killinger L, Azad A, Zapotocky B, Morschhauser E. Development of a model curriculum in chiropractic geriatric education: process and content. J Neuromusculoskeletal Syst 1998; 6: 146–153.

53 Mootz RD, Haldeman S. The evolving role of chiropractic within mainsteam health care. Top Clin Chiropractic 1995; 2(2): 11–21.

54 Ytterstad B. The Harstad injury prevention study: a community-based prevention of fall fractures in the elderly evaluated by means of a hospital based injury recording system in Norway. J Epidemiol Community Health 1996; 50: 551–558.

55 Gillespie LD, Gillespie WJ, Cumming R et al. Interventions for preventing falls in the elderly (Cochrane Review). In: The Cochrane Library, Issue 4. Oxford: Update Software, 2000

56 Gleberzon BJ. Developing a community-based educational program for older persons. J Can Chiropractic Assoc 2001; 45(1), 18–24..

57 Goldzweig IA. Creating a Community Health Forum. Health Promotion for the Ethnic Minority Elderly. A manual produced with the support of the US Administration on Aging, the American Association of Retired Persons, the National Eldercare Institute on Health Promotion, and the Meharry Consortium Geriatric Education Center. Meharry Medical Center, 1996.

58 Gray-Vickrey P. Gerontological research: use and application of focus group. J Gerontol Nurs 1993; 19(5): 21–27.

59 Healthy People 2000: National Health Promotion and Disease Prevention Objectives. Washington, DC: US Department of Health and Human Services, 1990.

60 Parker MJ, Gillespie LD, Gillespie WJ. Hip protectors for preventing hip fractures in the elderly (Cochrane Review). In: The Cochrane Library, Issue 4. Oxford: Update Software, 2000.

61 Clarke BS, King RO. Compliance with the use of PROHIP® hip protectors in a long term care setting. Presented at the Canadian Association of Gerontology Conference and 29th Annual Scientific and Educational Meeting, Edmonton, Alberta, Oct. 26–28, 2000.

15

The ageing heart

Sherryn N Levinoff Roth

You are only as old as your arteries

Thomas Sydenham (1624–1689)

Age is the most important risk factor with respect to cardiovascular disease. Men and women aged 65 years or older in the USA and Canada (1999 data)[1,2] comprise 12.7% and 12.4%, respectively, of the total population and this population accounts for more than 50% of the total visits to physicians' offices and 20% of Canadian health-care dollars spent.[3,4] Ageing causes major changes in physiology and anatomy. These changes lead to disease processes, the most common being coronary heart disease (CHD) and hypertension with all their sequelae. Patients with cardiovascular disease (CVD) can decompensate with any unexpected changes or stresses in life or with illness in another system. Treatment of the elderly for non-cardiac illness using medication or other modalities may impact on the cardiovascular system and precipitate cardiac events.

The following changes occur in the heart and blood vessels as people age.

The arteries stiffen. The middle layer of the blood-vessel wall (the media) between the vessel lining (endothelium) and the outer muscle layer thickens and becomes less able to stretch and relax with systole and diastole. More collagen is deposited in the media and between the muscle fibres. The elastic fibres become frayed and less effective. These changes in the arteries increase wall tension in the left ventricle and force the heart to work harder to accomplish the same work.

Diastolic filling becomes a most important factor in the function of the elderly ventricle. According to Starling's law, within physiological limits, a larger diastolic volume in the ventricle results in a greater force of contraction and ultimately a greater cardiac output.[5] Therefore, to maintain adequate cardiac reserve, the ventricle must be well filled. The contribution to diastolic filling from atrial contraction becomes an increasingly important factor in maintaining diastolic filling in a stiff heart, with the atrial contraction contributing more than 50% of the filling in the elderly but only 20–30% in a younger population.[6,7] Consequently, changes in heart rhythm which alter the ability of the atrium to contract and/or adequately fill the ventricle, such as atrial fibrillation where there is no effective atrial contraction, will reduce the cardiac output, and may precipitate congestive heart failure (CHF), myocardial infarction (MI) or cardiogenic shock.

With ageing, often in association with coronary artery disease (CAD), the myocardium becomes less able to relax and allow the blood to enter the left ventricle. This inability of the heart to relax is termed diastolic dysfunction.[8,9] Diastolic dysfunction is distinctly different from systolic dysfunction, i.e. reduced contractility due to depressed function of the left ventricle, often associated with heart damage due to MI or myocarditis from a virus, toxin, etc. If a heart with diastolic dysfunction develops a rapid heart rate associated with anaemia, fever or hyperthyroidism, there may not be enough time between beats for the ventricle to fill adequately and cardiac output will fall.

Vasoreceptor and neurohormonal activity changes with age, often with resultant hypertension, left ventricular hypertrophy (LVH) and cardiac enlargement: (i) serum catecholamines, adrenaline and nor-adrenaline levels increase with ageing, downregulating the receptors and making the response to stress less effective and adaptive;[10–12] (ii) The renin–angiotensin system (RAS) is a feedback loop mediated by the kidney which can cause vasoconstriction and other negative effects (Figure 15.1). Even though renin levels may fall with ageing, the RAS may be activated by the presence of atherosclerosis in the renal arteries, leading to hypertension, stiffer vessels and higher renin levels. Isovolumic relaxation time (the time between the end of ventricular systole and when the mitral and tricuspid valves open, allowing blood to enter and fill the ventricles in diastole) prolongs. This leaves less filling time between heartbeats, compromising cardiac output and potentially leading to congestive heart failure;[13,14] and (iii) Nitric oxide, which relaxes arterial wall smooth muscle and prevents atherogenesis in healthy blood-vessel walls, falls with ageing, leading to inappropriate vasoconstriction.[15]

As the heart enlarges, the wall tension increases and the shape of the heart changes, becoming more globular, enlarging the annulus or the support structures of the mitral and tricuspid valves. The mitral and tricuspid valves begin to leak, causing added stress on the ventricles to maintain adequate forward flow. A vicious cycle occurs with progressive failure of the heart to supply adequate oxygen to the body.[16] With exercise, the heart size normally increases. In the elderly the size may dilate to the point where it is not an advantage according to Starling's law and cardiac output may begin to decrease with exercise, causing symptoms of fatigue and shortness of breath.

The maximum heart rate reached with exercise decreases with increasing age, as does the maximal oxygen consumption by the heart. In general, skeletal muscle mass is also reduced with ageing and therefore exercise tolerance in the elderly is reduced.[17]

This chapter will deal with the most common cardiac problems that occur in the elderly heart and many of the available treatments.

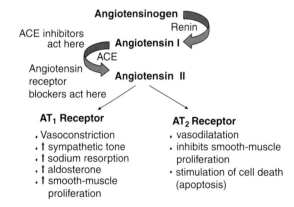

Figure 15.1 Renin–angiotensin–aldosterone system.

Ischaemic heart disease

Good advertising increased the awareness of the most serious risk factors causing ischaemic heart disease, i.e. smoking, diabetes mellitus, hypertension, elevated serum cholesterol, strong family history, physical inactivity and obesity. According to the Framingham data, however, age alone is an even more important risk factor for development of CVD than multiple risk factors in a younger patient. The relative risk of developing CVD in a 38-year-old woman with elevated low-density lipoprotein (LDL) cholesterol, low high-density lipoprotein (HDL) cholesterol and elevated blood pressure, who also smokes, is 4 (one point for each risk factor), while that of a 60-year-old woman with *no* risk factors is 8 (point count for age ≥ 60).[1] Older Canadians are more likely to have at least one of the three major modifiable risk factors (smoking, hypertension, elevated cholesterol) for CVD than those who are younger. In the 18–34 age group, 48% of the population has one or more of these major risk factors, compared with 85% in the 65–74 age group.[18]

Type II diabetes mellitus is a very strong risk factor for CVD that affects a large segment of the elderly population. The annual incidence is 8.6 cases per 1000 for Canadians aged 65 years or greater with an estimated prevalence of 8.9–16.6% of the 65 years or greater population.[19] To mitigate the effect on the heart, the American Diabetes Association has decided that all diabetics should be treated as if they have CVD, even though there are no apparent signs or symptoms of heart disease. They should be started on cholesterol-lowering 3-hydroxy-3-methylglutaryl-coenzyme A (HMG-CoA) reductase ('statin') medication regardless of the lipid levels.[20]

There is a misconception about the incidence of coronary disease in women. The general public and many health professionals including physicians answered incorrectly when asked whether heart disease was less or more prevalent in women than breast cancer: the reality is that the incidence of heart disease is 10 times more prevalent in woman than breast cancer.[21] Women have a similar incidence to men of coronary disease, with the following differences: (i) the onset is delayed by approximately 10 years compared with men, i.e. the incidence starts to increase approximately at the time of menopause (50–55 years), and equals or surpasses the incidence of that in men by the age of 75 years (Figure 15.2); (ii) women often have

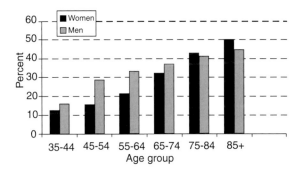

Figure 15.2 Percentage of total deaths due to cardiovascular diseases by age group and gender, Canada, 1997. Source: Statistics Canada, 1999 (22); courtesy of Heart & Stroke Foundation of Canada.

atypical symptoms and are more likely to present with angina rather than MI; (iii) when women do have MI, they have an increased mortality and complication rate compared with men.[23,24]

Ischaemic heart disease is a term that applies to a full spectrum of pathological syndromes. This ranges from early plaque formation in the walls of the arteries causing no symptoms, through partially blocked arteries that do not significantly obstruct blood flow (less than 50% obstruction); through tightly blocked arteries that limit blood flow downstream, to totally occluded vessels. In general, when an artery occludes

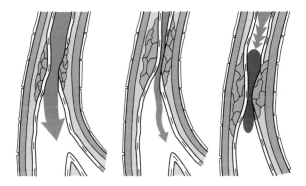

Figure 15.3 Occluding thrombus. Fibrous cap disruption exposes lipid-rich core to platelets and fibrinogen, forming thrombus. Adapted from an International Thrombosis Education Initiative, American College of Cardiology, courtesy of Dr MJ Davies, University of London.

totally and suddenly, there is myocardial damage. Major stenosis (greater than 70% narrowed) is likely to be associated with angina pectoris, i.e. anterior retrosternal chest pain, left or bilateral arm pain and/or shortness of breath on exertion. Lesions less than 50% stenosed do not usually cause symptoms. If the artery lining (endothelium), erodes and the plaque ruptures, exposing the lipid-rich core to the blood, platelets aggregate, fibrin forms and ultimately an occlusive thrombus forms, blocking blood flow and causing MI or actual damage to the heart muscle[25] (Figure 15.3). Very often there is some warning that an MI is about to occur. The patient experiences pain at rest lasting for less than 20 min when the thrombus forms but it spontaneously recedes without causing damage. This is unstable angina or an intermediate or acute coronary syndrome.

MI occurs with increasing frequency in advanced age, and the incidence of complications and death with an MI also increases with age.[26] Increasing age is the most important long-term adverse prognostic factor after an infarction. Nearly 50% of patients who die after hospitalization for acute MI are aged >75 years.[27] According to the first Global Utilization of Streptokinase (SK) and tPA (tissue plasminogen activator) for Occluded coronary arteries (GUSTO I) trial, the duration of hospital stay increased by 10-fold, as did the 30 day mortality between patients under 65 years compared with those greater than 85 years. Both thrombolytic agents are associated with higher rates of stroke in older patients. Because the incidence of haemorrhagic stroke with SK is slightly lower than that with tPA, SK is advocated for patients over the age of 75 years.[28]

Plaque rupture and formation of an obstructing thrombus, often associated with a partially obstructive plaque, can trigger MI or unstable angina. Initial treatment can be either medical or invasive management. Regardless of the choice of acute event management, all patients should be encouraged to participate in risk-modification measures to prevent further episodes.

Medical management

The cornerstone for medical treatment of patients with coronary artery disease is antiplatelet medication, i.e. medication that will prevent platelet aggregation. Acetylsalicylic acid (ASA) is the most common medication used, usually enteric coated, to protect the patient from gastrointestinal upset. Chewable ASA given as soon as possible after the onset of symptoms of MI has been shown to reduce mortality by 25%.[29] The positive results seem to relate just as much to the elderly (>65 years) as to the younger patients.

In ASA-allergic or ASA-intolerant patients, ticlodipine or clopidigrel can be used. New oral 2B/3A platelet receptor inhibitors are being studied to block all pathways for platelet aggregation, but to date these drugs have not been shown to improve outcomes consistently in patients with angina or an intermediate coronary syndrome.[30,31]

Patients presenting to the emergency room with electrocardiographic (ECG) changes indicative of MI are assessed for treatment with thrombolytic therapy. Thrombolytic drugs such as tPA or SK lyse the clot in approximately 1 h in 80% or more of cases. The sooner the drug is given, the earlier circulation is restored and the smaller the area of damage.[28] In some areas, paramedics are instructed to administer the thrombolytic in the ambulance to save valuable time. Unfortunately, elderly patients often delay calling for help and thus present to the hospital long after cell damage has begun.

All patients who have an acute coronary syndrome or MI should be anticoagulated with heparin.[32] Low molecular weight heparin given subcutaneously has been used successfully;[33] this has a more predictable effect, ensuring that the patient becomes anticoagulated promptly without excessive dosage, and leads to a reduced occurrence of unstable angina.

Unless blood pressure is extremely low, all patients with CAD should be prescribed an angiotensin-converting enzyme (ACE) inhibitor drug in increasing doses as tolerated to reduce mortality and the chances of a subsequent coronary event. In the Heart Outcomes Prevention Evaluation (HOPE) trial, using ramipril as the ACE inhibitor, more than half of the patients were at least 65 years old; many were also diabetic and hypertensive. The overall relative risk of events (death from cardiovascular causes, MI or stroke) was reduced to 0.78 (17.8% reduced to 14%) with treatment on ramipril. The elderly benefited even more than the younger patients did.[34]

β-Adrenergic-blocking medication has been shown to reduce mortality and morbidity with the first and subsequent infarcts, reduce the infarct size and reduce 1 year mortality.[35] β-Blockers can be given intravenously initially on presentation in the emergency room and thereafter orally. This is particularly important to the elderly who have the highest mortality with infarction.[27]

Invasive management

Invasive management refers to treatment with coronary angiography to define the anatomy of the coronary arteries followed by either (i) direct percutaneous coronary angioplasty (PTCA, balloon dilatation of a partially or totally occluded artery), with or without stenting, or (ii) coronary artery bypass grafting (CABG). Aggressive invasive management of CAD in the elderly is practised to a lesser or greater degree depending on the country. Direct angioplasty on presentation to the emergency room with an MI has been shown to be effective, salvages more myocardium and causes fewer problems such as bleeding than the thrombolytic drugs.[36] In the USA, patients tend to undergo coronary angiograms much earlier and more frequently in the course of investigation and treatment than in Canada or most European countries.[37] Caution should be exercised in that complication rates for procedures and surgery are higher in the elderly than in younger population, but there may be an ultimate improved outcome with aggressive management.[38] When medical management fails or is clearly inappropriate, it is reasonable to consider more aggressive management.

CABG surgery was introduced in 1968. Three very large American and European trials have shown that patients who have had CABG have less angina and, in specific subgroups with multivessel CAD, may live longer than patients who are treated with medical therapy alone.[29–41] Medical therapy, however, has improved significantly since these studies. The Bypass Angioplasty Revascularization Investigation (BARI) trial compared the results of randomized study of angioplasty (without stenting) and CABG in patients with multivessel disease: 5 year survival rates, rehospitalization and revascularization rates, and MI rates were not statistically different in any group including the elderly except for diabetics. Diabetics had an 80.6% 5-year survival when treated with CABG, but only 65.5% survival when treated with PTCA.[42] Studies are ongoing to determine whether the use of stents has modified the recommendation that CABG be the preferred treatment for diabetics. In a large trial of acute MI in an population aged 65 years or greater including approximately 22% diabetics, thrombolytic therapy was compared with primary angioplasty; the mortality in both groups was significantly better than a third group that received no reperfusion strategy, but the primary angioplasty group had an improved mortality at 30 days after the MI.[43]

Elderly patients are now commonly undergoing CABG when indicated for relief of symptoms, and longevity is also improved. Mortality in octogenerians having CABG is 8% and morbidity includes a 7% incidence of stroke compared with 1% in a patient group aged less than 70 years. Older patients spend more time in the intensive care unit (ICU) postoperatively.[44,45] This becomes a problem in that precious ICU beds become blocked and limited resources are used less effectively. Once bypassed, most elderly patients return to a better quality of life than preoperatively but it often takes months until they achieve the level that a younger patient would have achieved in weeks.

Arrhythmias and heart block

The incidence and complexity of arrhythmias increase with advancing age. This may be related to the increased incidence of associated CAD and hypertensive heart disease as well as the increased left ventricular wall thickness (LVH), and calcification in the mitral and aortic annular tissue. Elderly patients without anatomical heart disease can also experience arrhythmias. This may be related to altered electrical or nerve impulse formation and conduction system deterioration which occurs with ageing. Using 24 h ambulatory electrocardiographic monitoring, it has been shown that more than 75% of patients over the age of 70 without identified cardiac disease will have some ventricular extrasystoles, and 10–20% will have frequent ventricular couplets and frank ventricular tachycardia.[46] Ambulatory monitoring is essential: these arrhythmias must be correlated with symptoms before contemplation of treatment. The Cardiac Arrhythmia Suppression Trial (CAST) showed that antiarrhythmic medications given post-MI that cause no symptoms can lead to an increased mortality.[47]

When significant arrhythmias occur in the elderly either fast or slow, they are less well tolerated than in a younger population. The elderly heart depends on an appropriate length of time for diastolic filling. If the heart rate increases without a change from sinus rhythm, diastolic filling time decreases and the atria do not have time to empty completely into the ventricle, causing blood to back up in the lungs, liver, pleural space and legs. Tachycardia can be caused by common problems such as an acute febrile illness, e.g. hyperthyroidism or profound anaemia. The back-up becomes even more pronounced if the rhythmic change is associated with the loss of atrial contraction and its contribution to ventricular filling, precipitating pulmonary oedema and/or circulatory collapse.

If the heart rate slows below a critical rate, haemodynamic collapse occurs with poor perfusion of the brain, kidney and other vital organs. This may cause a stroke, a fainting spell, an MI or CHF.

The most common arrhythmia in the elderly is atrial fibrillation, present in almost 10% of the population 65 years of age or older. The incidence increases steadily with advancing years.[48] This arrhythmia is part of a larger syndrome called sick sinus syndrome in which the sinus node loses control as the pacemaker of the heart. The heart rate may be either very slow but sinus, or atrial fibrillation and very fast or very slow. Atrial fibrillation may be paroxysmal initially, lasting for only minutes to hours, often waking patients suddenly from their sleep at night with symptoms of palpitations and shortness of breath. The co-ordinated atrial contraction is lost. The rapid heart rate and the loss of atrial contraction may cause markedly reduced diastolic filling time and life-threatening illness.

Some of the many medications used to slow the heart rate in atrial fibrillation include digoxin, β-blockers, amiodarone, and some calcium-channel blockers such as diltiazem. In addition to ensuring that the heart rate is controlled, it is most important that patients over the age of 65 years who develop atrial fibrillation are anticoagulated with oral warfarin. The annual incidence of embolic stroke increases with age: 7.3% in patients 60–69 years of age, 20% in patients 70–79 years of age and 30.8% per year in patients 80–89 years of age.[49,50] By using low-level anticoagulation with warfarin, the incidence of embolic stroke and death decreases dramatically to near-normal levels for an age-matched population without atrial fibrillation.[51,52] Aspirin does not significantly affect the incidence of embolic stroke in atrial fibrillation.[53] Bleeding may occur as a result of anticoagulation, but the results of a haemorrhage are rarely as damaging and permanent as a stroke.

Once the heart rate slows, the patient usually stabilizes. For best cardiac output and cardiac efficiency, sinus rhythm should be maintained. If patients do not spontaneously revert to sinus rhythm, they should be anticoagulated for a minimum of 3 weeks and then cardioverted with a trial of antiarrhythmic medication or, if necessary, a carefully timed, low-level, direct current shock. Amiodarone has been shown to be the most effective drug to convert and maintain sinus rhythm.[54] Sometimes the sinus node continues to control the heart beat, but the rate slows to less than 50 beats/min. This may be spontaneous or may be caused by the very medication that is being used to prevent recurrence of atrial fibrillation. A pacemaker, with a lead either in the ventricle alone (single chamber) or in both the atrium and ventricle (dual-chamber pacing), will maintain adequate heart rate (Figure 15.4a, b).

Some patients may not revert to sinus rhythm by any method used. If the ventricular rate is well controlled, atrial fibrillation is often well tolerated and compatible with a reasonably active lifestyle. Occasionally, despite maximal medication and an attempt at cardioversion, patients continue to fibrillate rapidly. Percutaneous transvenous ablation of the atrioventricular (AV) node (causing complete heart block with no impulses reaching the ventricle) in conjunction with a permanent ventricular pacemaker can be very effective in resolving the problem.

With increasing age, there is an increased incidence of complete heart block, i.e. total loss of conduction of the atrial impulse through the AV node to the ventricles. The atria and the ventricles beat at different rates without any relationship to each other. The intrinsic ventricular rate is usually 35–40 beats/min.

Permanent pacing is indicated in this situation in order to return to a normal lifestyle. There is still controversy over whether there is an advantage in dual-over single-chamber pacing. Despite the expected physiological advantage, according to a recent Canadian trial, there is only a trend towards but not a significant advantage in quality of life or mortality with dual- versus single-chamber pacing.[55] Since a simple demand ventricular pacemaker that senses intrinsic ventricular beats costs approximately one-fifth of a dual-chamber pacemaker, more than 70% of the pacemakers implanted in Canada at this time are single-lead pacemakers to the ventricle only.

Approximately 250 000 pacemakers are implanted in North America annually; 16 000 were implanted in Canada in 1999.[56] The use of pacemaker implants steadily increases with age among men and women, and is highest in the 85-plus age group.[57] They are implanted transvenously in the upper chest under local anaesthesia, often as an outpatient procedure (Figure 15.4a, b). Lithium batteries power pacemakers; they are very reliable and often last for 10–12 years or more. The circuitry is very sophisticated: the device will sense an intrinsic electrical depolarization, i.e. if the patient has a spontaneous heart beat, the pacemaker detects this and does not fire; the pacemaker can be set to vary its rate according to activity by sensing skeletal muscle or respiratory action so that when the patient is walking quickly the paced rate will speed up, and when the patient is sitting watching televi-

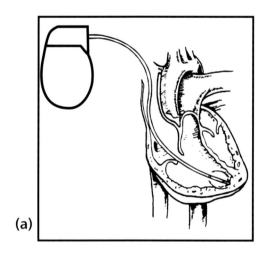

(a)

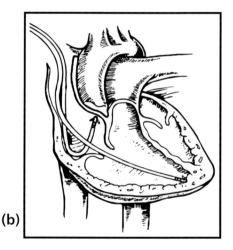

(b)

Figure 15.4 Pacemakers. (a) Single-chamber system: the pacing lead is implanted in the atrium or ventrical, depending on the chamber to be paced and sensed; (b) Dual-chamber systems have two leads; one implanted in both the atrium and the ventricle. Courtesy of Medtronic Inc.

sion or resting it will slow down; the device will track arrhythmias such as atrial fibrillation, and switch modes from dual- to single-chamber pacing if required. The device can be programmed to slow its rate during sleeping hours and perform many other useful functions. All programming is done by computer-generated signals to the device from the skin surface. Proximity to a magnetic field or sensing repetitive electrical stimulation, such as with arc welding or tuning a car, will inhibit the device, causing it temporarily to cease pacing; therefore it is imperative that patients with pacemakers are not treated with cautery or an electrical muscle-stimulating treatment such as transcutaneous electrical nerve stimulation (TENS), which is likely to turn off their pacemaker. A magnet over the pacemaker device eliminates the sensing circuitry if an electrical field environment is essential. A magnet should only be applied in controlled situations with the patient on a cardiac monitor to avoid causing cardiac arrest by a pacer spike falling in the wrong part of the cardiac cycle.

Hypertension

Hypertension or high blood pressure is defined as a systolic blood pressure (SBP) ≥ 140 mmHg or diastolic blood pressure (DBP) ≥ 90. Hypertension is a major risk factor for CAD, stroke, kidney failure, CHF and peripheral vascular disease.[58] Both SBP and DBP increase with age in the Western industrialized world. SBP continues to rise until 70–80 years of age, but DBP levels off at approximately 50–60 years. People with the highest blood pressures in their younger years will have the greatest increases with ageing. African-Americans have a higher incidence of hypertension than Caucasians after the age of 30. The risk of cardiovascular morbidity and mortality relates to both SBP and DBP, and increases with rising blood pressures. The risk with each increment in blood pressure becomes more significant the older the patient subset.[59] There are two comprehensive reports relating to the detection and management of hypertension: the sixth Joint National Committee on Prevention, Detection, Evaluation, and Treatment of High Blood Pressure (JNC-6) and the 1999 World Health Organization/International Society of Hypertension (WHO/ISH) Hypertension Guidelines.[60,61]

Hypertension in the elderly is undertreated and for many years was significantly underestimated as a major risk factor for cardiovascular events in this group. Studies such as the Systolic Hypertension in the Elderly (SHEP) trial and the Swedish Trial in Old Patients with Hypertension (STOP-Hypertension) have shown the benefits of appropriate blood-pressure treatment in the elderly.[62,63] In the SHEP trial, patients 60 years of age and older with SBP 160–219 mmHg and DBP < 90 mmHg. were treated with a low-dose diuretic, ± a β-blocker ± methyldopa ± hydralazine, in that order, in the treatment arm versus placebo. The treated cohort showed a 33% reduction in all stroke, a 50% reduction in the incidence of CHF and a 27% reduction in cardiovascular events. In the STOP-Hypertension trial, people aged 70–84 years with SBP between 180 and 230 mmHg or DBP between 105 and 120 mmHg were treated with one of three different β-blockers or a potassium-sparing diuretic versus placebo. Total cardiovascular events were reduced by 33% and stroke by about 35% in the treatment arm. There was also a trend towards a reduced incidence of MI.

The elderly, those aged 65 years or older make up approximately 12% of the population of Western countries and consume more than 20% of health-care funds.[64] According to the SHEP trial data, 8% of those aged 60–69 years, 11% of those aged 70–79 and 22% of those aged 80 or greater had isolated systolic hypertension. The problem is more prevalent in African-Americans (71.8%), Hispanic Caucasians (52.9%) and Mexican-Americans (54.9%) in patients 65–74 years of age. Men have a slightly higher prevalence than women (56.4% versus 52.5%). SBP is responsible for more CVD, cardiovascular accidents and CHF, but DBP elevation is more related to CVD in younger patients.[65] It is therefore important to focus on this single risk factor, i.e. systolic hypertension, which, if well treated, would significantly reduce health-care costs.

All health-care personnel who deal with the elderly should have an accurate means of checking blood pressure: the cuff should be inflated to 250mm Hg and deflated slowly to avoid missing the true SBP. Blood pressure should be taken as the average of at least two readings in the sitting position after the patient has rested for no less than 15 min. Blood pressure should be taken in both arms since there may be subclavian artery narrowing giving a falsely low reading in one arm. 'White coat syndrome', fear of medical personnel in labcoats, can elevate SBP; 24 h ambulatory blood-pressure monitoring should be done to confirm hypertension.

If blood pressure is elevated, it should be a priority for treatment. A curable cause for the hypertension is rarely found in the elderly (less than 0.5% of hypertensive patients). Occasionally, when the arteries become thickened and do not compress well with the blood-pressure cuff, there will be pseudoelevation of the blood pressure.[65] When treated, these elderly patients will often complain of dizziness when they stand (orthostatic hypotension), which may worsen after diuretics or other antihypertensive medication are started for the elevated sitting blood pressure. A standing blood-pressure determination should be obtained in patients complaining of dizziness who are also on medication.

Hypertension can be defined and classified according to Table 15.1. A patient's risk and prognosis can be stratified according to blood pressure, risk factors and target organ damage as listed. Evidence for target organ damage includes: LVH (thickening of the heart muscle) as identified on an ECG, echocardiogram or, less accurately, by radiogram; proteinuria and/or slight elevation of plasma creatinine concentration; ultrasound or radiological evidence of atherosclerotic plaque (carotid, iliac and femoral arteries, or aorta); and generalized or focal narrowing of the retinal arteries (by funduscopy).

Appropriate treatment of the hypertension will prevent and may reverse target organ damage. All randomized trials to date have shown clear evidence of a lower incidence of major cardiovascular events after high blood pressure was treated with antihypertensive drugs. There is no evidence yet that the main benefit of treating hypertension is due to a particular drug property rather than to lowering blood pressure per se.[60] The Veterans Administration Cooperative Study on Antihypertensive Agents demonstrated that treating to a target blood pressure using diuretics, a non-selective adrenergic blocker and a vasodilator sequentially with follow-up of 3.3 years led to a major reduction in stroke and CHF. In patients older than 60 years, there was a significant decrease in cardiovascular events, from 62.8% to 28.9%.[67] Many other studies were done, including a meta-analysis of five large trials showing that, with treatment, stroke was reduced by 34%, CHD by 19% and vascular deaths by 23%, all of which were highly significant.[68] Aggressive management of mild to moderate hypertension is now advised in diabetics, since they are at very high risk for the early development of target organ damage.[69]

Accordingly, treatment is decided based on risk according to a flow chart (Figure 15.5). Lifestyle modifications should be encouraged in all patients. These modifications include cessation of smoking, weight reduction, moderation of alcohol consumption, reduction of salt intake and increased physical activity. Less well-known modifications are increased potassium intake (often found in fruits and vegetables), increased calcium intake, reduction in caffeine, relaxation and biofeedback. The loss of 4.5 kg in weight has been shown to reduce SBP by 4 mmHg. Fast-food diets are very high in salt content; reduction of salt intake

Table 15.1 Stratifying risk and quantifying prognosis (adapted with permision from1999 WHO/ISH Hypertension Practice Guidelines[61])

Other risk factors & and disease history	Blood pressure (mmHg)		
	Grade 1 (mild hypertension) SBP 140–159 or DBP 90–99	Grade 2 (moderate hypertension) SBP 160–179 or DBP 100–109	Grade 3 (severe hypertension) SBP ≥ 180 or DBP ≥ 110
I. No other risk factors	Low risk	Medium risk	High risk
II. 1–2 risk factors*	Medium risk	Medium risk	Very high risk
III. ≥ 3 risk factors, TOD† or diabetes	High risk	High risk	Very high risk
IV. Associated clinical conditions: coronary, renal, vascular, retinal, cerebrovascular disease	Very high risk	Very high risk	Very high risk

*Risk factors: level of systolic and diastolic blood pressure (SBP and DBP), men > 55 years, women > 65 years, smoking, cholesterol > 6.5 mmol/l (250 mg/dl), diabetes, family history of premature cardiovascular disease.
†Target organ damage: left ventricular hypertrophy by electrocardiography, echocardiography or X-ray; proteinuria, ultrasound or X-ray evidence of athosclerotic plaque; generalized or focal narrowing of retinal arteries.

has been shown to reduce blood pressure gradually over periods of several weeks to a few years.[59,70–72]

Health-care personnel should review the elderly patient's medications since some medications cause fluid and salt retention, aggravating the hypertension. In particular, many elderly patients are taking non-steroidal anti-inflammatory drugs (NSAIDs) for their various aches and pains. Non-pharmacological therapy with intermittent acetaminophen is preferred for the hypertensive patient.[73]

If, after the appropriate interval of treatment by lifestyle modification, blood pressure is still elevated above 140/90, drug treatment should begin. The lowest dose of medication should be used initially to avoid adverse effects. Often two medications prescribed in combination at lower dose are more effective and tolerated better than a single drug at higher strength. For better compliance, dosing once or at most twice per day is advised. Diuretics, β-blockers, ACE inhibitors and calcium-channel blockers are the first-line therapy, with angiotensin receptor-blocking agents, direct vasodilators and β-blockers as second-line therapy.[74]

Current medications are much improved over those available in the 1980s; they are more effective at lowering blood pressure with fewer side-effects, and it is only the rare patient whose blood pressure cannot be successfully treated. Often the problem is a lack of compliance, with the elderly patient forgetting or refusing to take the medication. They may also confuse the dose regimen.[75,76]

Sometimes the patient is embarrassed to talk about side-effects. Diuretics, a cornerstone in blood-pressure management, are often avoided by the elderly since the increased urine output may cause incontinence or accidents. β-blockers may slow the heart rate and cause fatigue, impotence, dizziness or syncope. The elderly often have coexisting vascular disease, and dropping the blood pressure beyond a critical point can precipitate strokes or transient ischaemic attacks, angina or MI, deteriorating renal function and leg claudication.[77]

Congestive heart failure

CHF is a clinical diagnosis that occurs when the heart is unable either to supply an output sufficient for the body and its organs, or to pump out the venous return, which causes fluid to back up in the lungs, legs, liver and abdomen.

The incidence of CHF increases with increased age. It affects 1.9% of the population and is the most common diagnosis in the Western world for patients over the age of 65 years. It is responsible for a very high per-

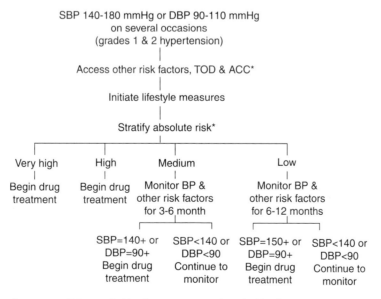

Figure 15.5 Initiation of treatment. SBP: systolic blood pressure; DBP: diastolic blood pressure; TOD: target organ damage; ACC: associated clinical conditions (cardiovascular and renal disease); BP: blood pressure. *See Table 15.1. Adapted with permission from1999 WHO/ISH Hypertension Practice Guidelines.[61]

centage of health-care expenditure (estimated at $20 billion/year). As the mean age of the population increases, the rate of diagnosis of CHF is reaching epidemic proportions (affecting approximately 5 million Americans), with more than 400 000 new cases being diagnosed annually in the USA.[78,79] CHF is mainly a diagnosis of the elderly: 80% of admissions occur in patients aged 65 years or older, with more than 50% of those admissions in patients 75 years or older.[80]

The causes of CHF in the elderly are numerous but often relate to the previously described syndromes, i.e. CAD with ischaemia and infarction, chronic hypertension, degenerating heart valves and arrhythmias. The patient's description of the onset of symptoms and a background knowledge of the patient's past medical problems are critical in determining the aetiology. For example, if the onset of shortness of breath is sudden and preceded by left-sided chest pain, MI or an acute coronary syndrome is the likely cause, whereas if the symptoms have been present in a milder form with progressive deterioration for a month and the patient has a history of chronic hypertension, a hypertensive cardiomyopathy would be the more likely cause.

CHF can be due to left ventricular systolic or diastolic dysfunction. Systolic and diastolic dysfunction are best distinguished by non-invasive techniques such as echocardiography with Doppler studies:

- systolic dysfunction: with recurrent MI or chronic pressure overload such as with longstanding hypertension or a stenosed aortic valve, the heart may dilate and myocardial contractility diminishes with a reduced amount ejected per beat;
- diastolic dysfunction: this less understood entity is very prevalent in the elderly. Diastole was thought to be a passive process wherein the heart muscle merely relaxes and the blood flow into the ventricle. It is known now that this is an active process and energy is required during diastole.[81] The thicker and less distensible the ventricle, the less likely it will be able to relax effectively. CHF caused by diastolic dysfunction is a difficult and often frustrating problem to treat, especially when systolic function appears to be normal.

The common symptoms reported by patients with CHF include shortness of breath on exertion or at rest, inability to lie flat, fatigue, weakness, weight loss and swelling of the legs or abdomen. The physical findings may include crepitations (crackles) in the lower lungs, unexplained wheezing, elevated jugular venous pressures, ascites (fluid in the abdomen), enlarged tender liver and swollen lower extremities. A chest X-ray may show an enlarged cardiac silhouette, dilated upper lobe vessels, interstitial oedema with Kerley B lines (looking like short horizontal lines 1–3 cm in length in the lower lobes peripherally stacked one above the other), pleural effusions, pulmonary oedema (fluid within the alveolar sacs) with a 'butterfly pattern' infiltrate seen radiating out from the hilar areas, fluid in the interlobar fissures and dilated pulmonary arteries.

Long-term treatment is often not effective in the elderly and there is a 50% readmission rate to hospital for CHF within 3 months of the initial admission. Simply educating patients to restrict fluid intake and salt content in the diet is very helpful.[82] Patients should weigh themselves daily each morning on arising. Excessive weight gain indicates accumulation of fluid. Diuretics are used to reduce the congestion. Digoxin's effect is limited but may be of some help in dilated hearts or with tachycardia control. It has been shown to reduce the number of hospitalized days in CHF patients.[83] Vasodilators, especially ACE inhibitors, are often helpful in controlling heart failure by reducing enhanced neurohumoral activation, lowering blood pressure, reducing the work of the heart and, specifically, ACE inhibitors are effective in reducing mortality and morbidity.[84–88]

Recent studies have shown that β-blockers are effective in reducing mortality and morbidity in patients with moderate to severe systolic dysfunction.[89–95] Other drugs such as dobutamine and phosphodiesterase inhibitors, which are positive inotropes and increase contractility, are avoided on a chronic basis since they are associated with an increased early mortality.[96–97]

Many new innovative treatments for CHF patients with severe systolic dysfunction have been developed, with promising results. Sleep apnoea has been linked to heart failure and treatment with continuous positive-pressure breathing machines has been shown to improve heart function in selected cases.[99,100] A new types of pacemaker which paces both right and left ventricles simultaneously, causing resynchronization, has been shown to improve cardiac output and quality of life.[101] Automatic implantable cardiac defibrillators reduce the very high incidence of sudden death associated with extremely poor left ventricular function.[102–104] Left ventricular assist devices are currently in use as a bridge to heart transplantation, with fully implantable permanent models in testing.

Heart-failure clinics have evolved since the mid-1990s. These specialized clinics carefully monitor patients who have recently been started on treatment for CHF, sometimes by using telemetry home monitoring. The clinic personnel continue to educate patients about salt and fluid retention, medication compliance, and early reporting of excessive weight gain and new or worsening symptoms. In this manner, quality of life improves and readmission rates can be reduced in the elderly from 47% to less than 25%.[105–108]

Valvular heart disease

A murmur heard when listening to the heart of an elderly patient does not necessarily signify significant valvular disease. Most echo-Doppler studies on the elderly will show some thickening of the aortic and mitral valve leaflets, minor leaking of the mitral, tricuspid, aortic and pulmonary valves, but no significant haemodynamic abnormalities.

Aortic stenosis (narrowing of the aortic valve opening with a pressure gradient across the valve) is a common debilitating valvular lesion in the elderly. It may be caused by calcification of a bicuspid valve (often presenting in the fifth or sixth decade of life) or by degenerative calcification when the patient is over 70 years. Patients with a significant gradient across the valve may complain of syncope or dizziness on exertion, classical angina or shortness of breath with and without exertion. They may present with CHF findings, arrhythmias with or without syncope, chest pain or MI, and sometimes with embolic stroke. These patients are very labile and can develop pulmonary oedema with minimal exertion or stress. If there is significant delay before the valve is replaced, myocardial function will become depressed, raising the surgical risks. The only treatment is timely valve replacement: the natural history without valve replacement is horrendous, with a 50% 2–3 year mortality from the onset of symptoms. There is no medication that will retard the process or change the prognosis.[109,110] The mortality and morbidity with surgery have been very low, with excellent quality of life afterwards.[111–113] Balloon valvuloplasty looked promising but has been a failure as a long-term treatment for aortic stenosis, with most patients restenosing in less than 6 months.[114] Most elderly patients will receive a bioprosthetic or tissue valve rather than a mechanical valve because anticoagulation with ASA rather than warfarin is usually sufficient and has a lower thromboembolic complication rate.

A leaking aortic valve, aortic insufficiency, is less common and much more difficult to treat. Symptoms are less dramatic and this valvular lesion has a longer and more benign course. If there is an associated thoracic aortic aneurysm which needs replacement together with the valve, the morbidity and mortality are significantly higher. Unless there is progressive cardiac dilatation due to severe aortic insufficiency, aortic valve replacement may be delayed. Timing for valve replacement is a difficult decision.

Mitral insufficiency is also a very common disease in the elderly. Rheumatic disease or mitral valve prolapse with or without endocarditis may be the cause, but it is more likely to be due to papillary muscle dysfunction from ischaemia associated with CAD. For severe mitral regurgitation not due to CAD, mitral valve replacement slows the progression of left ventricular failure and reduces symptoms. There is a higher mortality and morbidity than with aortic valve replacement, but still at an acceptable level, even in the elderly.

Although, with the introduction of sulfa and penicillin in the 1940s, the incidence of rheumatic fever fell sharply, there is still a small elderly population being followed with rheumatic heart disease, mainly mitral stenosis, and mitral and aortic insufficiency. New cases are diagnosed more frequently in the immigrant population. Mitral stenosis can be treated successfully in the young and elderly populations with balloon valvuloplasty if the leaflets are not heavily calcified. There is a high incidence of atrial fibrillation in the elderly, especially in those with mitral stenosis and insufficiency who may have enlarged left atria. Anticoagulation is essential in these patients.[115]

Summary

Ageing causes predictable changes in the heart. Hypertension, diabetes, hypercholesterolaemia and obesity, risk factors that are increasingly prevalent with older age, affect the heart adversely, leading to disease of the coronary arteries, nerve conduction system, heart valves and, ultimately, the heart muscle. The ageing compromised heart cannot compensate, causing morbidity and mortality. Risk modification and prompt treatment using evidence-based medicine may slow the progression and relieve the symptoms of the disease.

References

1 Wilson PW, d'Agostino RB, Levy D *et al.* Prediction of coronary heart disease using risk factor categories. Circulation 1998; 97: 837–847.

2 Hillis LD, Forman S, Braunwald E, Thrombolysis in Myocardial Infarction (TIMI) Phase II Co-Investigators. Risk stratification before thrombolytic therapy in patients with acute myocardial infarction. J Am Coll Cardiol 1990; 16: 313–315

3 US National Center for Health Statistics. 1999 data.

4 Johanson H, Nair C, Bond J. Who goes to hospital? An investigation of high users of hospital days. Health Report 1999; 6: 253–69; Statistics Canada Catalog No H82003.

5 Patterson SW, Piper H, Starling EH. J Physiol 1914; 48: 465.

6 Lewis T. J Exp Med 1912; 16: 395.

7 Wiggers CJ, Katz LN. Am J. Physiol 1922; 58: 439.

8 Yellin EL, Nikolic D. Diastolic suction and the dynamics of left ventricular filling. In: Gash WH, LeWinter MM, eds. Left Ventricular Diastolic Dysfunction and Heart Failure. Philadelphia, PA: Lea and Febiger, 1994: 89–102.

9 Libonati JR. Myocardial diastolic function and exercise. Med Sci Sports Exercise 1999; 31: 1741.

10 Lakatta EG. Catecholamines and CV function in aging. In: Sacktor B, ed. Endocrinology and Metabolism Clinics, Vol. 16, Endocrinology and Aging. , Philadelphia, PA: WB Saunders, 1987: 877–891.

11 Cohn J, Levine B, Olivari M *et al.* Plasma norepinephrine as a guide to prognosis in patients with chronic congestive heart failure. N Engl J Med 1984; 311: 819–823.

12 Kaye D, Lefkovits J, Jennings G *et al.* Adverse consequences of high sympathetic nervous system activity in the failing human heart. J Am Coll Cardiol 1995; 26: 1257–1263.

13 Jackson EK, Garrison JC. Renin and angiotensin. In: Hardman JG, Limbird LE, Molinoff PB *et al.*, eds. Goodman & Gilman's The Pharmacological Basis of Therapeutics. 9th edn. New York: McGraw-Hill, 1996: 733-759.

14 Johnston CI *et al.* Preclinical pharmacology of angiotensin II receptor antagonists. Am J Hypertens 1997; 10: 306S–10S.

15 Rubanyi GM. J Cardiovasc Pharmacol 1993; 22 (Suppl 4): S1–S14.

16 Pouleur H, Rousseau MF, van Eyll C *et al.* Cardiac mechanics during development of heart failure. Circulation 1993; 87: IV–14.

17 Strandell T. Circulatory studies on healthy old men. Acta Med Scand 1964: 175: 1.

18 Canadian Provincial Heart Health Surveys, 1986–1992.

19 Rockwood K, Awalt E, MacKnight C *et al.* Incidence and outcomes of diabetes mellitus in elderly people: report from the Canadian Study of Health and Aging. Can Med Assoc J.2000; 162: 769–772.

20 American Diabetes Association. Management of dyslipidemia in adults with diabetes. Diabetes Care 2000; 23(Suppl 1): S57–S60.

21 Walters V: Women's views of their main health problems. Can J Public Health 1992; 83: 371–374.

22 Statistics Canada, 1999.

23 Hayes O. Fact sheet: cardiovascular disease (ICD – 9 390-448) and women. Chronic Dis Can 1996; 17: 28–30.

24 Malacrida R, Genoni M, Maggioni AP *et al.* A comparison of the early outcome of acute myocardial infarction in women and men. N Engl J Med 1998; 338: 8–14.

25 Ross R. Atherosclerosis – an inflammatory disease. N Engl J Med 1999; 340: 115–126.

26 Toig E, Castaner A, Simmons B *et al.* In-hospital mortality rates from acute myocardial infarction by race in US hospitals: findings from the National Hospital Discharge Survey. Circulation 1987; 76: 280–288.

27 McGovern PG, Pankow JS, Shahar E *et al.* Recent trends in acute coronary heart disease – mortality, morbidity, medical care, and risk factors. N Engl J Med 1996; 334: 884–890.

28 GUSTO Investigators. An international randomized trial comparing four thrombolytic strategies for acute myocardial infarction. N Engl J Med 1993; 329: 673–682.

29 ISIS-2 (Second International Study of Infarct Survival) Collaborative Group. Randomised trial of intravenous streptokinase, oral aspirin, both, or neither among 17,187 cases of suspected acute myocardial infarction: ISIS-2. Lancet 1988; ii: 349–360.

30 PURSUIT Trial Investigators. Inhibition of platelet glycoprotein IIb/IIIA with eptifibatide in patients with acute coronary syndromes. N Engl J Med 1998; 339: 436–443.

31 GUSTO IV. ACS – European Heart Meeting, Amsterdam, August 2000.

32 Theroux P, Ouimet H, McCann J *et al.* Aspirin, heparin, or both to treat acute unstable angina. N Engl J Med 1988; 319: 1105.

33 Eikelboom J, Anand S, Malmberg K *et al.* Unfractionated heparin and low-molecular-weight heparin in acute coronary syndrome without ST elevation: a meta-analysis. Lancet 2000; 355: 1936–1942.

34 Heart Outcomes Prevention Evaluation Study Investigators. Effects of an angiotensin-converting-enzyme inhibitor, ramipril, on cardiovascular events in high-risk patients. N Engl J Med 2000; 342: 145–153.

35 Norwegian Multicenter Study Group. Timolol-induced reduction in mortality and reinfarction in patients surviving acute myocardial infarction. N Engl J Med 1981; 304: 801.

36 Zijlstra F, Hoorntje JCA, de Boer M-J *et al.* Long-term benefit of primary angioplasty as compared with thrombolytic therapy for acute myocardial infarction. N Engl J Med 1999; 341: 1413–1419.

37 Tu JV, Pashos CL, Maylor CD *et al.* Use of cardiac procedures and outcomes in elderly patients with myocardial infaction in the United States and Canada. N Engl J Med: 199X; 336: 1500.

38 Langer A, Fisher M, Califf R *et al.* Higher rates of coronary angiography and revascularization following myocardial infarction may be associated with greater survival in the United States than in Canada. Can J Cardio 1999; 15.

39 European Cardiac Surgery Study Group. Coronary artery bypass surgery in stable angina pectoris: survival at 2 years. Lancet 1979; i: 889.

40 CASS Principal Investigators and their Associates. Coronary Artery Surgery Study (CASS): a randomized trial of coronary artery bypass surgery; survival data. Circulation 1983; 68: 939.

41 Veterans Administration Coronary Artery Bypass Surgery Cooperative Study Group. Eleven-year survival in the Veterans Administrative randomized trial of coronary bypass surgery for stable angina. N Engl J Med 1984; 311: 333.

42 Bypass Angioplasty Revascularization Investigation (BARI) Investigators. Comparison of coronary bypass surgery with angioplasty in patients with multivessel disease [Erratum appears in N Engl J Med 1997; 336: 147]. N Engl J Med 1996; 335: 217–225.

43 Berger AK, Radford MJ, Wang Y *et al.* Thrombolytic therapy in older patients. J Am Coll Cardiol 2000; 36: 366–374.

44 Akins CW, Daggett WM, Vlahakes GJ et al. Cardiac operations in patients 80 years old and older. Ann Thorac Surg 1997; 64: 606–614.

45 Freeman WK, Schaff HV, O'Brien PC et al. Cardiac surgery in the octogenarian: perioperative outcome and clinical follow-up. J Am Coll Cardiol 1991; 18: 29–35.

46 Wajngarten M, Grupi C et al. Frequency and significance of cardiac rhythm disturbances in healthy elderly individuals. J Electrocardiography 1990; 23: 171.

47 Cardiac Arrhythmia Suppression Trial (CAST) Investigators. Preliminary report: effect of encainide and flecainide on mortality in a randomized trial of arrhythmia suppression after myocardial infarction. N Engl J Med 1989; 321: 406–412.

48 Phillips SJ, Whisnant JP, O'Fallon WM, Frye RL. The prevalence of cardiovascular disease and diabetes mellitus in Rochester, Minnesota. Mayo Clin Proc 1990; 65: 344–359.

48 Stroke Prevention in Atrial Fibrillation Investigators. Predictors of thromboembolism in atrial fibrillation: clinical features of patients at risk. Ann Intern Med 1992; 1161: 1.

50 Prystowsky EN, Benson W Jr, Fuster V et al. Management of patients with atrial fibrillation. A statement for health care professionals from the subcommittee on electrocardiography and electrophysiology. Am Heart Assoc 1996; 93: 1262–1277.

51 Cairns JA, Connolly SJ. Nonrheumatic atrial fibrillation: risk of stroke and role of antithrombotic therapy. Circulation 1991; 84: 469–481.

52 Boston Area Anticoagulation Trial for Atrial Fibrillation Investigators. The effect of low-dose warfarin on the risk of stroke in patients with nonrheumatic atrial fibrillation. N Engl J Med 1990; 323: 1505.

53 Petersen P, Godtfredsen J et al. Placebo-controlled, randomized trial of warfarin and aspirin for prevention of thromboembolic complications in chronic atrial fibrillation. Lancet 1989; i: 175.

54 Roy D, Talajic M, Dorian P et al. Amiodarone to prevent recurrence of atrial fibrillation. N Eng J Med 2000; 342: 913.

55 Connolly SJ, Kerr CR, Gent M et al. Effects of physiologic pacing versus ventricular pacing on the risk of stroke and death due to cardiovascular causes. N Engl J Med 2000; 342: 1385.

56 Medtronic company data, 1999.

57 Hospital Morbidity Database, Canadian Institute for Health Information, 1996/97.

58 MacMahon S et al. Blood pressure, stroke and coronary heart disease. Part 1, Prolonged differences in blood pressure: prospective observation studies corrected for regression dilution bias. Lancet 1990; 335: 765–774.

59 Stamler J, Stamler R, Riedlinger WF et al. Hypertension screening of 1 million Americans: Community Hypertension Evaluation Clinic (CHEC) program, 1973–1975. JAMA 1976; 235: 2299–2306.

60 Incremental Risk – Joint National Committee on Prevention, Detection, Evaluation, and Treatment of High Blood Pressure. The Sixth Report. Arch Intern Med 1997; 157: 2413–2446.

61 1999 World Health Organization–International Society of Hypertension Guidelines for the Management of Hypertension. Guidelines Subcommittee. J Hypertens 1999; 17: 151–183.

62 SHEP Co-operative Research Group. Prevention of stroke in older persons with isolated systolic hypertension: final results of the Systolic Hypertension in the Elderly Program (SHEP). JAMA 2001; 256: 3255–3264.

63 Dahlof B, Lindholm LH et al. Morbidity and mortality in the Swedish Trial in Old Patients with Hypertension (STOP-Hypertension). Lancet 1991; 338: 1281–1285.

64 Byyny R. Hypertension in the elderly. In: Laragh JH, Brenner BM, eds. Hypertension: Pathophysiology, Diagnosis, and Management. New York: Raven 1990: 1869–1887.

65 (NHANES) National High Blood Pressure Education Program Working Group. Report on hypertension in the elderly. Hypertension 1994; 23: 275–285.

66 Spence JD, Sibbald WJ, Cape RD. Pseudohypertension in the elderly. Clin Sci Mol Med 1978; 55: 399s.

67 Veteran Administration Co-Operative Study on Antihypertensive Agents. Effects of treatment on morbidity in hypertension. III: Influence of age, diastolic pressure and prior cardiovascular disease. Circulation 1972; 45: 991–1004.

68 MacMahon S, Rodgers A. The effects of blood pressure reduction in older patients: an overview of five randomized controlled trials in elderly hypertensives. Clin Exp Hypertens 1993; 15: 967–978.

69 American Diabetes Association. Clinical Practice Recommendations 1998. Diabetes Care 1998; 21(Suppl 1): S23–S32.

70 Higgins M, Kamel W, Garrison R et al. Hazards of obesity – the Framingham experience. Acta Med Scand 1998; 723(Suppl): 23–36.

71 Cutler JA, Follmann, D, Allender PS. Randomized trials of sodium reduction: an overview. Am J Clin Nutr 1997; 65(suppl): 643S–651S.

72 Cappuccio FP, Elliott P et al. Epidemiologic association between dietary calcium intake and blood pressure: a meta-analysis of published data. Am J Epidemiol 1995; 142: 935–945.

73 Johnson AG, Nguyen TV, Day RO. Do nonsteroidal anti-inflammatory drugs affect blood pressure? A meta-analysis. Ann Intern Med 1994; 121: 289–300.

74 Hansson L, Lindholm LH, Ekhorn T et al. Randomised trial of old and new antihypertensive drugs in elderly patients: cardiovascular mortality and morbidity. The Swedish Trial in Old Patients with Hypertension-2 Study. Lancet 1999; 354: 1751–1756.

75 Cramer JA, Mattson RH, Prevey ML et al. How often is medication taken as prescribed? A novel assessment technique. JAMA 1989; 261: 3273–3277.

76 Norell SE. Accuracy of patient interviews and estimates by clinical staff in determining medication compliance. Soc Sci Med 1981; 15E: 57–61.

77 Myers M. Compliance in hypertension: why don't patients take their pills? Can Med Assoc J 1999; 160: 64–65.

78 National Heart Lung and Blood Institute. Congestive heart failure in the United States: a new epidemic. Bethesda, MD: US Department of Health and Human Services, 1996.

79 Graves EJ, Owing MF. 1995 Summary: National Hospital Discharge Survey. Advance data from vital and health statistics, No. 291. Hyattsville, MD: National Center for Health Statistics, 1997.

80 Graves EJ. Detailed diagnoses and procedures. National Hospital Discharge Survey, 1990. Vital and health statistics, Series 13, data from the National Health Survey. Hyattsville, MD: National Center for Health Statistics 1992; 113: 1–225.

81 Zile MR. Diastolic dysfunction: detection, consequences and treatment. Part 1: Definition and determinants of diastolic function. Mod Concepts Cardiovasc Dis 1989; 58: 67.

82 Vinson JM, Rich MW, Sperry JC et al. Early readmission of elderly patients with congestive heart failure. J Am Geriatr Soc 1990; 38: 1290

83 Digitalis Investigation Group. The effect of digitalis on mortality and morbidity in patients with heart failure. N Engl J Med 1997; 336: 525.

84 CONSENSUS Trial Study Group. Effects of enalapril on mortality in severe congestive heart failure N Engl J Med 1987; 316: 1429.

85 SOLVD Investigators. Effect of enalapril on mortality and the development of heart failure in asymptomatic patients with reduced left ventricular ejection fractions. N Engl J Med 1992; 327: 685–691.

86 Pfeffer M, Braunwald E, Moye L *et al.* for the SAVE Investigators. Effect of captopril on mortality and morbidity in patients with left ventricular dysfunction after myocardial infarction: results of the Survival and Ventricular Enlargement trial. N Engl J Med 1992; 327: 669–677.

87 Cohn JN, Archibald DG, Ziesche S *et al.* Effect of vasodilator therapy on mortality in chronic congestive heart failure (VHeFT I). N Engl J Med 1986; 314: 1547–1552.

88 Cohn JN, Johnson G, Ziesche S *et al.* A comparison of enalapril with hydralazine-isosorbide dinitrate in the treatment of chronic congestive heart failure (VHeFT II). N Engl J Med 1991; 325: 303–310.

89 CIBIS Investigators and Committees. A randomized trial of blockade in heart failure: the Cardiac Insufficiency Bisoprolol Study (CIBIS). Circulation 1994; 90: 1765–1773.

90 Waagstein F, Bristow MR, Swedberg K *et al.* for the Metoprolol in Dilated Cardiomyopathy (MDC) Trial Study Group. Beneficial effects of metoprolol in idiopathic dilated cardiomyopathy. Lancet 1993; 342: 1441–1446.

91 Packer M, Bristow MR, Cohn JN *et al.* The effect of carvedilol on morbidity and mortality in patients with chronic heart failure. N Engl J Med 1996; 334: 1349–1355.

92 Australia/New Zealand Heart Failure Research Collaborative Group. Randomised, placebo-controlled trial of carvedilol in patients with congestive heart failure due to ischaemic heart disease. Lancet 1997; 349: 375–380.

93 Colucci WS, Packer M, Bristow MR *et al.* for the US Carvedilol Heart Failure Study Group. Carvedilol inhibits clinical progression in patients with mild symptoms of heart failure. Circulation 1996; 94: 2800–2806.

94 Anderson JL, Lutz JR, Gilbert EM *et al.* A randomized trial of low dose beta-blockade therapy for idiopathic dilated cardiomyopathy. Am J Cardiol 1985; 55: 471–475.

95 Packer M. COPERNICUS (Carvedilol Prospective Randomized Cumulative Survival). Presented to the European Society of Cardiology, Amsterdam, The Netherlands, Aug. 2000.

96 Leier CV. Comparative systemic and regional hemodynamic effects of dopamine and dobutamine in patients with cardiomyopathic heart failure. Circulation 1978; 58: 466–475.

97 Elis A, Bental T, Kimchi O *et al.* Intermittent dobutamine treatment in patients with chronic refractory congestive heart failure: a randomized, double-blind, placebo-controlled study. Clin Pharmacol Ther 1998; 63: 682–685.

98 Packer M, Carver J, Rodeheffer R *et al.* Effect of oral milrinone on mortality in severe chronic heart failure. N Engl J Med 1991; 325: 1468–1475.

99 Lipkin DP. Sleep-disordered breathing in chronic stable heart failure. Lancet 1999; 354: 531–532.

100 Tkacova R, Rankin F, Fitzgerald F *et al.* Effects of continuous positive airway pressure on obstructive sleep apnoea and left ventricular afterload in patients with heart failure. Circulation 1998; 98: 2269–2275.

101 Cazeau S. MUSTIC (Multisite Stimulation in Cardiomyopathy). Presented to the Heart Failure Society of America, Boca Raton, FL, Sept. 2000.

102 Antiarrhythmic Versus Implantable Defibrillators (AVID) Investigators. A comparison of antiarrhythmic drug therapy with implantable defibrillators in patients resuscitated from near-fatal ventricular arrhythmias. N Engl J Med 1997; 337: 1576–1583.

103 Connolly S, Gent M, Roberts R *et al.* for the CIDS Investigators. Canadian Implantable Defibrillator Study (CIDS): a randomized trial of the implantable cardioverter defibrillator against amiodarone. Circulation 2000; 101: 1297–1302.

104 Kuck K-H, Cappato R, Siebels J, Ruppel R, for the CASH Investigators. Randomized comparison of antiarrhythmic drug-therapy with implantable defibrillators in patients resuscitated from cardiac arrest: the Cardiac Arrest Study Hamburg (CASH). Circulation 2000; 102: 748–754.

105 Shara M, Chapman DB. The impact of a specialized heart failure care clinic on patient outcomes (Abstract). Pharmacotherapy 1997; 17: 1085.

106 Lasater M. The effect of a nurse-managed CHF clinic on patient readmission and length of stay. Home Health Nurs. 1996; 14: 351–356

107 Rich MW, Beckham V, Wittenberg C *et al.* A multidisciplinary intervention to prevent the readmission of elderly patients with congestive heart failure. N Engl J Med 1995; 333: 1190–1195.

108 Nanevicz T, Piette J, Zipkin D *et al.* The feasibility of a telecommunication service in support of outpatient congestive heart failure care in a diverse patient population. Congest Heart Fail 2000; 6: 140–145.

109 Ross J Jr, Braunwald E. Aortic Stenosis. Circulation 1968; 38(Suppl V): V-61–V-67.

110 Pomerance A. Cardiac pathology in the elderly. In: Noble RJ, Rothbaum DA, eds. Geriatric Cardiology, Cardiovascular Clinics. Philadelphia, PA: FA Davis, 1981: 9.

111 Elyada MA, Hall RJ *et al.* Aortic valve replacement in patients 80 years and older: operative risk and longterm results. Circulation 1993; 88(Suppl II): II-11–II-16.

112 Ralph-Edwards AC, Robinson AG *et al.* Valve surgery in octogenarians. Can J Cardiol 1999; 15: 1113–1119.

113 Gehlot A, Mullany C, Ilstrup D *et al.* Aortic valve replacement in patients aged 80 years and older: early and longterm results. J Thoracic Cardiovasc Surg 1996; 111: 1026–1036.

114 Otto CM, Mickel MC, Kennedy JW *et al.* Three year outcome after balloon aortic valvuloplasty: insights into prognosis of valvular aortic stenosis. Circulation 1994; 89: 642–650.

115 Carabello B, Crawford F. Medical progress: valvular heart disease. N Engl J Med 1997; 337: 32–41.

16

Neck pain, hypertension, stroke and cervical manipulation

Brian J Gleberzon

Among the most powerful and effective spinal corrections, often resulting in dramatic clinical results, are those achieved by cervical adjustments. The roots of chiropractic trace back to a thoracic adjustment delivered by DD Palmer which reportedly restored hearing in a deaf janitor in 1895. Years later, BJ Palmer continued and expanded the philosophy of health care first purported by his father, emphasizing the importance of cervical adjustment. In his words, BJ Palmer believed that adjusting the atlas would 'emancipate the imprisoned rivulets of entrapped life force'.[1]

Today, a small group of chiropractors continues to embrace a philosophy that places primacy on cervical (particularly atlas) corrections, identifying the atlas as 'the cause of the cause' of many somatovisceral symptoms and dis-ease, which can be defined as the body's inability to understand and adapt to its surrounding environment. For these 'principled' or 'subluxation-based' chiropractors, health comes from Above, Down, Inside–Out (the ADIO principle). Indeed, the Sherman College of Straight Chiropractic in South Carolina predominantly instructs students in upper cervical techniques.

Even in the absence of philosophical overtones, most chiropractors use adjustive strategies to restore normal function of the cervical spine in order to diminish neck pain and to reduce the severity, intensity and frequency of certain types of headache.[2] A recent study of the economic impact of headaches in the USA estimated that the cost in lost productivity and health-care expenditure was between $5 billion and $17 billion annually, and the impact that headaches have on a patient's quality of life was found to be considerably greater than the impact of other chronic illnesses such as osteoarthritis, hypertension and diabetes.[2–4]

A qualitative review by Nelson[2] reported that, although some variation exists in headache management techniques, several management principles are supported by the literature. Such principles include that the cervical spine is involved in the aetiology of most chronic headaches, and that manipulation is an effective prophylactic therapy for cervicogenic, migraine and tension-type headaches.[2] Nelson concluded that manipulation is best applied in a 'therapeutic trial' basis.[2]

Regrettably, cervical adjusting can result in serious injury, including stroke and death, although this is exceedingly rare. Many intrinsic and extrinsic risk factors may increase a patient's likelihood of experiencing a vertebrobasilar accident or injury. This chapter will discuss those factors that contribute to stroke, particularly considering the management of hypertension. A review of the literature will accurately recount the incidence, prevalence and risk of stroke following cervical adjustments, and will provide strategies to reduce the risk of stroke in general, and specifically during the administration of manual therapies.

Neck pain in the older patient

A recent article by Kriss and Kriss detailed the primary causes of acute or chronic neck pain in older patients and reviewed the models of allopathic management.[5] The authors stated that it is imperative to detect and differentiate between the presence of radiculopathy (indicated by signs and symptoms of single nerve root involvement such as neck pain radiating to the arm) and myelopathy (recognizable by changes in gait, clumsy or weak hands or, occasionally, loss of bladder and bowel function). Radiculopathy is the result of nerve impingement (commonly the result of a disc bulge or herniation), whereas myelopathy may result from discal pathologies, degenerative arthritides or, rarely, metastatic disease.[5]

According to Kris and Kris, common aetiologies of neck pain are trauma, discal disease and rheumatic disorders.[5] Neck pain arising from degenerative arthritides of the cervical spine is thought to affect approximately 60–80% of older patients (see Chapter 10, Spectrum of rheumatic syndromes in the elderly).[5] Neck pain of discal origin often presents with intermittent neck pain gradual onset of arm pain, suboccipital headaches, interscapular pain and numbness or tingling along a characteristic dermatome.[5] Neck pain may also be secondary to depression or stress, or for secondary gains.[5]

Common allopathic treatment includes non-prescription non-steroidal anti-inflammatory drugs (NSAIDs), opioids and corticosteroids.[5] Kris and Kris maintain that there is no evidence to support the use of local injections of corticosteroids for the management of neck pain, and the authors suggested that powerful opioids, such as hydrocodone or oxycodone, should be avoided because of the potential risk of tolerance and addiction.[5] The authors commented that some patients find home traction kits effective, while others may benefit from physical therapy and massage.[5] Spinal manipulative therapy was not mentioned.

Hypertension

Heart disease and stroke are, respectively, the first and third leading causes of death in the USA.[6] This places an enormous financial and social burden on Americans, with direct and indirect costs estimated to exceed $259 billion annually.[6] As hypertension is recognized to be a major contributory factor to heart disease and stroke, its successful management is of vital concern to all health-care providers.

Hypertension affects approximately 50 million men and women in the USA, and hypertension is more common and severe among African-Americans.[6,7] Hypertension is present in over 45% of older patients, representing their most frequent chronic health problem.[7] In Canada and the USA, hypertension is the most common reason for office visits to physicians and for the use of prescription drugs.[7] Between 1976–1980 and 1988–1991, the percentage of Americans who were aware that they had high blood pressure increased from 51% to 73%.[6] Among those

with hypertension, treatment had increased during the same period from 31% to 55%.[6] This has contributed to an age-adjusted decline in death rate from stroke of nearly 60%, and from coronary heart disease by 53%.[6] These trends are more evident among men than women, and among African-Americans more than Caucasians.[6] Beyond 1993, however, these dramatic improvements have slowed, with a current slight increase in the age-adjusted rate of stroke.[6] Similar statistics exist in Canada. It is estimated that 4.1 million Canadians are hypertensive, but only 16% are treated and controlled, and 42% are unaware that they are hypertensive at all.[7]

Unique to North Americans is a gradual increase in systolic blood pressure with age.[7] This is despite the fact that an increase in blood pressure is *not* a normal consequence of the ageing process.[6] Hypertension is defined as a systolic blood pressure (SBP) of 140 mmHg or greater and a diastolic blood pressure (DBP) of 90 mmHg or greater, or taking antihypertensive medication.[6] There is a positive relationship between elevated SBP and DBP and cardiovascular disease.[6]

Among older patients, SBP is a good predictor of cardiovascular disease, heart failure, stroke, end-stage renal failure and all-cause mortality.[6] Recently, it has become apparent that an elevated pulse pressure (the difference between SBP and DBP) may be an even better indicator of future cardiovascular disease than either SBP or DBP alone.[6]

A diagnosis of hypertension is established if a patient demonstrates an average elevated blood pressure on two or more readings taken on two or more visits.[6] However, pseudohypertension (falsely high sphygmomanometer readings) may occur in older patients owing to excessive vascular stiffness, and older women may demonstrate white-coat hypertension (this is a condition noted in patients whose blood pressure is consistently elevated in a practitioner's office but is normal at other times).[6]

Isolated systolic hypertension (ISH) is another abnormal phenomenon of ageing, and is associated with an increase in morbidity and mortality.[6] ISH is more common among older persons, occurring in 15% of elderly men and 25% of elderly women.[6] Like other forms of hypertension, ISH must be treated aggressively.[6]

A practitioner may consider arranging for routine laboratory tests that may demonstrate pathology to target organs. Routine tests include urinalysis, complete blood cell count and blood chemistry.[6] More often than not, there are no presenting signs or symptoms of hypertension. For this reason hypertension is often called 'the silent killer'.

Although high blood pressure does not follow a classic mendelian form of inheritance, hypertension does have a familial predisposition.[6] Among older patients, primary hypertension is by far the most common form of hypertension.[6] Lifestyle choices, therefore, play a significant role in the development of hypertension and lifestyle modification is essential for its successful management.

Lifestyle modifications that may be implemented for the successful management of hypertension include weight loss, moderation of alcohol intake, increase in physical activity, a moderation of sodium intake, increase in dietary potassium and calcium, reduced intake of fats, smoking cessation, as well as relaxation and biofeedback training.[6,7]

There is a strong correlation between increased blood pressure and a body mass index that exceeds 27.[6] A weight reduction of little as 4.5 kg (10 lb) has a significant positive effect on the majority of overweight persons with hypertension.[6] According to some recent studies, even a 1 kg drop in weight can produce a 1 mmHg drop in blood pressure.[7] It is for this reason that weight control to within 15% of a person's ideal weight is generally encouraged.[7]

There is controversy surrounding the relationship between salt and high blood pressure.[7] However, there is some evidence to indicate that limiting salt intake to more no than 2–3 g/day is effective in lowering blood pressure among hypertensive patients.[7] In addition, epidemiological studies have demonstrated that blood pressure varies inversely with dietary potassium, calcium and magnesium intake.[7] Excessive alcohol consumption is an important risk factor for high blood pressure and stroke, and it causes resistance to antihypertensive therapy.[6] Some studies have demonstrated that a diet restricting alcohol intake to about 30 ml of ethanol a day can result in a reduction in SBP by 5 mmHg and DBP by 3 mmHg.[7] Likewise, smoking is a powerful risk factor for cardiovascular disease of all kinds, including hypertension.[6]

When compared with their more physically active peers, sedentary individuals with normal blood pressure have a 20–50% increased risk of developing hypertension.[6] According to Petrella, a sedentary lifestyle doubles the risk of cardiovascular disease, and it is as risky to a person's health as smoking 20 cigarettes a day, having an elevated cholesterol level or even having mild high blood pressure.[7] There is also evidence that a reduction in the level of a person's stress level can reduce high blood pressure, with some studies indicating that stress management can reduce a hypertensive patient's blood pressure by 6–26 mmHg (systolic) and 5–15 mmHg (diastolic).[7] Lifestyle modifications recommended for the successful management of hypertension are:

• Maintain body weight to within 15% of ideal weight
• Limit alcohol intake to no more than 30 ml/day
• Increase aerobic exercise to at least 30 min 3–5 days/week, at moderate intensity.
• Restrict sodium intake to 2–3 g/day
• Maintain an adequate intake of potassium, calcium and magnesium.
• Consider stress-management strategies.

Several antihypertensive medications demonstrate strong efficacy in reducing cardiovascular morbidity and mortality.[6] Among the most commonly used antihypertensive medications are diuretics, β-blockers and angiotensin-converting enzyme (ACE) inhibitors.[6] However, the management of high blood pressure for older patients is made more difficult by several physiological factors. Among these are increased susceptibility to orthostatic hypotension, decreased hepatic and renal function (which alters the bioavailability of many drugs), and decreased regional blood flow can result in an impaired perfusion of vital organs if blood flow is rapidly reduced.[6] For these reasons the management of an older patient with high blood pressure should begin with lifestyle modifications. In the event that the target blood pressure is not achieved, then pharmacological agents may be used. Large trials of patients over the age of 60 years have shown that antihypertensive therapies reduce cardiovascular disease, chronic heart disease, heart failure and stroke (see also Chapter 6).[6]

Stroke

In the USA, it is estimated that there are 731 000 fatal strokes and 4 million stroke survivors annually.[8] Fifty-five per cent of strokes occur in those persons 75 years of age or older.[8] In the USA, annual direct and indirect costs of stroke care total an estimated $40 billion.[8]

Strokes are the third leading cause of death in the elderly, and are most common among African-

American men.[8,9] The most important risk factor for a stroke is uncorrected hypertension, and it is the most preventable and modifiable risk factor for stroke.[8,9]

One of the harbingers of a stroke is a transient ischaemic attack (TIA).[9] A TIA is often called 'a stroke in progress' and is characterized by numbing or tingling sensations in the face or limbs, visual changes, headache, vertigo, loss of limb strength and amourosis fugax.[9]

Post-stroke recovery reaches its maximum within 3 months.[9] Complications resulting from a stroke include dehydration, depression, infection and immobility-induced pathologies.[9] Post-stroke treatment includes rehabilitative exercises, anticoagulant therapy and self-help groups for both the patient and family members to help to develop methods of coping with the change in family dynamics and lifestyle.[9]

Six general strategies to prevent stroke

The six most important risk factors for stroke are hypertension, myocardial infarction (MI), atrial fibrillation, diabetes, asymptomatic carotid artery disease and certain lifestyle habits (e.g. smoking and excessive alcohol consumption).[8] For patients with a history of a previous MI, antiplatelet agents reduce the odds of a non-fatal stroke by 39%, a non-fatal MI by 31% and cardiovascular death by 13%.[8] Lipid-lowering agents are also effective at reducing the chances of stroke and the complications that often follow a stroke.[8,9] Among patients with atrial fibrillation, warfarin has been shown to reduce the risk of stroke by 68% and aspirin by 21%.[8]

Among patients with hypertension and type II diabetes, control of blood pressure has been shown to reduce the risk of fatal and non-fatal stroke by 44% compared with a group of patients with less tight control.[8]

'Prevention of a First Stroke', a new set of guidelines for the American National Stroke Association, has identified six key stroke risk factors and has developed recommendations for their prevention.[8] These are:

(i)   For those patients with high blood pressure, decrease diastolic blood pressure by 5–6 mmHg, which can reduce stroke by 42%.

(ii) In a patient with a history of myocardial infarct, ensure that the patient is on anticoagulants, antiplatelet agents and cholesterol-lowering agents.

(iii) For patients over the age of 75 with a history of atrial fibrillation, the medical physician should prescribe warfarin; patients under the age of 75 can be prescribed warfarin or aspirin.

(iv) In those patients affected by diabetes, strive for tight glycaemic control.

(v)   If a patient has high cholesterol and coronary heart disease, a medical doctor may prescribe simvastatin (Zocor); in those patients with normal cholesterol but a previous history of MI, pravastatin (Pravachol) is recommended.

(vi) For patients with asymptomatic carotid artery disease, surgical intervention is recommended for those patients with a life expectancy of 5 years or more who have a 60% or greater occlusion of the carotid artery and less than a 3% surgical risk.

In addition, the guidelines recommend that practitioners help patients to quit smoking, consume only moderate amounts of alcohol, engage in regular physical activity and maintain a proper diet.

Stroke and cervical manipulations

There have recently been several high-profile legal cases in Canada involving the allegation of stroke following cervical manipulation, particularly following chiropractic adjustments. The case in Saskatchewan of a young women who died shortly after a chiropractic adjustment led to an inquest, which provided several recommendations. These included: (i) that the chiropractic profession develop prototype patient and family history forms; (ii) that the chiropractic associations ensure that the consent to treatment form is discussed by the chiropractor and the patient on the initial visit; (iii) an increase in communication and collaboration among all specialities in health care; and (iv) the development of screening tests which must be administered prior to cervical spinal manipulation.[10] In a response letter to the presiding coroner, Drs David Leprich and Paul Carey, of the Canadian Chiropractic Association and the Canadian Chiropractic Protection Association, respectively, noted that the first three recommendations either have already been implemented or are in common use. The authors also wrote that they would welcome the implementation of a reliable screening test, were one to be developed.[10]

However, both chiropractic representatives took umbrage with another recommendation made by the jury.[10] Specifically, the jury suggested that literature indicating the risk of stroke and other inherent risks that are (allegedly) associated with chiropractic treatment be visible and available in the reception area of every chiropractic facility. Drs Leprich and Carey pointed out that this view presupposed that chiropractic therapy is inherently more risky or dangerous than medical or physiotherapeutic procedures, medications or everyday events in the course of a person's life. Instead, the authors emphasized that chiropractic therapy is basically a safe procedure, although not completely risk free. The authors questioned the fairness of requiring chiropractors to do what medical doctors and other health-care professionals are not required to do, and they also wondered aloud why the chiropractic profession should be treated differently from other health-care providers.[10]

Another pending case in Ontario had named not only the chiropractor in the suit but also the president of the Canadian Memorial Chiropractic College (CMCC), the former registrar of the College of Chiropractors of Ontario (CCO) and the president of the Canadian Chiropractic Protection Association (CCPA). Ontario Superior Court Judge John Cavarzan dismissed the case against the three chiropractic organizations and their representatives named in the suit. The judge further awarded costs to the CMCC, CCO and CCPA, respectively. However, in June 2000, Judge Cavarzan reversed his original decision and called for an inquest into the case. The inquest was scheduled to take place in autumn 2001. This is despite the fact that two other cases alleging stroke and other injuries following chiropractic adjustments were dismissed in August 2000.

Stroke following manipulation is a tragic, yet fortunately rare, event. The stroke is usually the result of a dissection of the vertebrobasilar artery. Current and accepted estimates of the frequency of stroke resulting in serious neurological complications or death following manipulation are 1–3 million adjustments and 400 000 patients.[11,12] The most commonly accepted estimate of risk of serious injury from cervical adjustment is 1 in 1 million patients.[13,14] This is roughly the same likelihood that an individual has of being struck by lightning. A study by RAND[14] further estimated that the rate of serious complications from spinal manipulation to be 5–10 in 10 million for vertebrobasilar reactions and 3–6 in 10 million for major impairments, with an incidence of fewer than 3 fatalities per 10 million manipulations. Nonetheless, a great

deal of attention has recently been focused on this issue in both the media and public domain, much of it fuelled by an article by Norris et al. published in the Canadian Medical Association Journal.[15]

In that article, Norris et al. discussed the preliminary results of a study that sought to gather information on the aetiology of patients who sustained a stroke. The authors reported that they were able to identify 74 cases of patients who had suffered a stroke. Of these, 81% were associated with 'sudden neck movements', following activities ranging from therapeutic manipulation (not always delivered by a chiropractor), major exertion (playing volleyball) and even mild exertion (lifting a pet dog or coughing).[15] The other 19% of the cases of stroke were classified as 'spontaneous'.[15]

The authors of this study claimed that 28% (21/74) of the cases of stroke were attributable to neck manipulation.[15] However, the Canadian and Ontario Chiropractic Associations reminded those in the media and the public that between 30 and 40 million cervical adjustments are performed in Ontario annually. With estimates of the material risk of cervical adjusting ranging from 1 in 1 million to 1 in 2.5 million procedures, the identification of 21 cases of stroke allegedly attributable to neck manipulation is not surprising; In the words of Dr Edward Barisa, executive director of the Canadian Chiropractic Association '... I can only conclude that Dr. Norris has discovered nothing new. His work to date is showing a lower risk of stroke than we are currently managing'.[16]

An extensive review by Haldeman et al. sought to identify the risk factors associated with stroke following spinal manipulation.[11] Their review revealed that identified risk factors include age, gender, migraine, hypertension, diabetes, smoking, oral contraceptives, syphilis, cystic medial degeneration, fibromuscular hyperplasia and Marfan's syndrome.[11] The most commonly discussed risk factors were migraine, hypertension, oral contraceptive use and smoking.[11] However, most of the patients with these risk factors were reported to have had a stroke either spontaneously or following trivial trauma.[11]

The authors of the article concluded they could not definitively state which of the factors were in and of themselves absolute risk factors for stroke.[11] For example, strokes seem to occur more commonly in younger adults; however, younger adults are the group most likely to receive chiropractic manipulation, or to be exposed to major or minor trauma. This may explain the apparent predominance of stroke in this age group.[11] Furthermore, the authors ultimately concluded that, because the event is so rare, and the literature reviewed is often lacking critical details, it is impossible to advise patients or practitioners about how to avoid the risk of stroke during manipulation, nor could they be specific as to which sports or exercise activities result in neck movements or trauma of the greatest potential risk.[11]

The literature provides examples of major and minor traumas which preceded the occurrence of strokes.[11,12] Major traumas associated with stroke include motor vehicle accidents, falls, sports injuries (football, skiing, bicycling), being struck by a tree, struck by a car and lifting such heavy objects as railroad ties, rails and weights. Minor traumas associated with stroke include sports activities (swimming, softball), walking, sustained rotation with extension (yoga, archery, stargazing, sleeping position, having hair washed at a salon, wallpapering, washing walls or ceilings), quick head rotations (checks over shoulder while driving) and sudden head movements (sneezing, coughing). Strokes have also been recorded after kneeling at prayer, following household chores and during sexual intercourse.[11,12]

Spinal manipulation, although important, does not appear to be the precipitating cause in most cases of stroke.[11] Rotation out of all the head positions during manipulation, has been implicated as the position with highest association of stroke.[11,12] However, the sparse data that exist indicate that traction, passive mobilization and range of motion movements have also resulted in stroke, thus making it difficult to determine whether rotation is the primary movement at fault. Because chiropractors perform over 90% of all therapeutic cervical manipulations, it is to be expected that the majority of injuries sustained are more commonly associated with chiropractors.[11]

Identifying the onset of stroke: the 5Ds and 3Ns

In those cases of stroke associated with cervical manipulations, the onset of ischaemic signs or symptoms is usually within minutes of the treatment, although there can be a delay of symptom onset for several days.[12]

A stroke should be suspected if the patient reports severe head or neck pain unlike any pain the patient has suffered before.[12] The other important signs or symptoms of a stroke are:

- Dizziness (vertigo, lightheadedness)
- Drop attacks
- Diplopia
- Dysarthria
- Dsyphagia
- Ataxia
- Nystagmus
- Nausea
- Numbness.

The major problem, however, from a clinical perspective is that the majority of migraine headaches, cervicogenic headaches and cases of mechanical head and neck pain respond very well to cervical adjustments.[2,12] It must therefore be emphasized that practitioners with the proper training should not abandon upper cervical adjustments, even in the light of remote or rare risks. Compared with the relative safety of cervical adjustments, about 100 000 people die from adverse drug reactions annually (see Chapter 22, Iatrogenic drug reactions), 1000 people will die this week from the complications of unnecessary surgery and 1600 children will die this year from allergic reactions to aspirin.[12]

Tests prior to cervical adjustments

To attempt to identify those patients at a greater risk of injury during cervical manipulation, a clinician must take a complete and thorough history, taking special consideration of previous history of stroke or contraindications to cervical adjustments (e.g. acute onset of rheumatoid arthritis). A clinician should also take a patient's blood pressure, especially noting any significant difference between left and right sides. Auscultation of the head and neck for bruits can also be performed. There are two specific tests that may identify vertebrobasilar insufficiency. George's or Houle's test (sometimes referred to as DeKleyn's test) has the patient supine, with his or her head extended and rotated over the examination table. The patient is asked to follow the examiner's finger as it describes an 'H' pattern for 60 s; the examiner looks for nystagmus and asks the patient whether he or she feels dizzy. Other possible indications of impeded vertebrobasilar blood flow include vertigo, nausea, tinnitus, lightheadedness, sensory deficits, nystagmus, vomiting, visual disturbances or loss of consciousness.[17] The second vertrobasilar test, called Hautant's test, is performed with the patient seated. Both arms are extended forwards and supinated. The eyes are shut and the head is moved into extension and rotation. The development of symptoms or the falling of a hand (pronator drift) is considered positive and may indicate vascular insufficiency.[12]

Both of these tests unfortunately lack sensitivity and specificity.[17] For example, if a patient is in a left Houle's position (patient supine with head turned to the left and extended) and a sense of dizziness ensues, the practitioner cannot be certain whether the left vertebral artery is compressed, the right vertebral artery is stretched, or the patient is experiencing a bout of cervicogenic vertigo as the result of imbricated cervical facet joints. Moreover, provocative of symptoms by this head position may indicate benign paroxysmal positional vertigo, Ménierè's syndrome, labyrinthitis or vestibular neuronitis.[17]

A recent study by Cote *et al.* sought to determine the validity of neck extension-rotation tests as a routine screening procedure to detect decreased vertebrobasilar blood flow.[17] The researchers concluded that the sensitivity of the test for increased impedance to blood flow was 0% and the positive predictive value of the test was 0%.[17]

The authors also questioned the underlying wisdom of performing this test.[17] They challenged the concept that head extension–rotation could lead to arterial dissection [one of the pathophysiological mechanisms of stroke following cervical manipulation proposed by Norris *et al.*[15]]. They also questioned the ethics and wisdom of performing this test in light of the fact that another proposed mechanism of stroke is the development of an embolism as the result of dislodging a vertebral artery thrombus;[17] that is, the test potentially puts the patient at increased risk by placing him or her in the exact position that should be avoided.[17] Lastly, their study was unable to support the hypothesis that a stroke is caused by the occlusion of vertebral artery blood flow. The authors concluded that performing this test may be unethical because it may unnecessarily alarm a patient about the potential risk of stroke despite the unsupported link between stroke and cervical manipulation.[17]

The results of the study by Cote *et al.* notwithstanding, it is considered to be prudent and reasonable, in both legal and insurance circles, to conduct these tests prior to administering a cervical adjustment.[18] It is also imperative that the practitioner obtain informed consent prior to performing a cervical adjustment. The risks, benefits and alternatives should be specifically reviewed with the patient, in terms that they can understand. Although not mandated by law, many organizations, such as the Canadian Chiropractic Protective Association (a malpractice carrier), highly recommend that the practitioner obtain written informed consent. This recommendation is made because it is then much easier to defend a practitioner in the case of a dispute between the practitioner and the patient as to whether or not informed consent was obtained.

If a patient is suspected of having a stroke during an adjustment, the practitioner should stop performing the adjustment and, above all, should not try and 'solve' the problem by adjusting the other side.[12] Instead, the practitioner must institute emergency care protocols. These include not panicking, ensuring that the patient is in a safe environment (made more difficult if the patient is on an adjusting table) and beginning the ABC status-check (airway, breathing and circulation). The practitioner must also immediately contact the emergency medical services.

Treatment suggestions

In order to minimize any potential risk of injury during cervical adjusting, consideration should be given to using preferentially those methods that minimize rotation and extention. If circumstances dictate, other low-force techniques (Activator, Logan basic, SacroOccipital technique) and other forms of manual therapy (soft-tissue techniques, long-axis traction, mobilization) can be used.[19] (see Chapter 25. Chiropractic techniques in the care of the geriatric patient). Training in cervical adjusting at CMCC and other accredited chiropractic colleges emphasizes procedures that minimize rotation and extension wherever possible. This can be stated with certainty because the author has participated in curriculum development in psychomotor skills at CMCC, and in the compilation of Part IV (psychomotor skills) of the National Board of Chiropractic Examiners' test. During these meetings, the description of a competent cervical adjustment emphasized the importance of minimizing cervical extension and rotation during the procedure. The author is also the acting chair of the

Technique Consortium of the Association of Chiropractic Colleges. During the meetings of the Consortium, a great deal of discussion describes the manner in which instruction is provided for students to ensure safe and effective cervical adjustment throughout the chiropractic profession.

It should be noted that many recent studies have demonstrated the efficacy, cost-effectiveness and high margin of safety of spinal manipulative therapy for the treatment of certain types of headache, neck pain and low back pain.[2,20]

Medical bias, prejudice and ignorance

A disturbing article by Carey and Townsend describes documented cases of legal reports filed by medical physicians that demonstrated examples of bias, prejudice and ignorance.[21] Most disturbing of all, in not a single case cited was there any evidence of communication between the medical doctor filing the report and the chiropractor towards whom allegations of negligence were aimed.[21]

The article provides examples of inaccurate and misleading reports in the areas of standards of care, misconceptions about the intent of chiropractic treatment, questioning appropriate plans of management, evaluating a case without the facts, the physicians' citing questionable references and describing the risk of chiropractic treatment outside a proper perspective.[21] The authors presented examples of a medical physician commenting on an aspect of chiropractic care that was clearly out of context, and other times when the physician attempted to establish a cause–effect relationship between two events when such a relationship clearly did not exist. Often, an injury, such as a stroke or disc herniation, was solely attributed to a chiropractic adjustment, despite the fact that other interventions were more likely to be causative or that such injuries were accidents in waiting.[21]

Putting risks in perspective

Many field practitioners often find themselves operating with some degree of clinical uncertainty.[22] It is important for the inexperienced complementary and alternative medicine provider not to become paralysed by this uncertainty and to remember that the standard to which any health-care provider is ultimately held is reasonableness (see Chapter 31). That is, did the prac-

titioner act in a manner that a group of his or her peers would have considered to be reasonable? Failure to act reasonably is negligence, defined as conduct falling below accepted professional standards. However, the average or reasonable practitioner is not expected to be a super hero. Field practitioners are not expected to have X-ray vision, nor are they expected to be able see into the future with clairvoyance. A complete history, a thorough examination and a plan of management based on the best available research, which can include clinical experience, are all that can be reasonably expected of a field practitioner. Unfortunately, although exceedingly rare, injuries may unexpectedly occur, despite the best clinical efforts to avoid them. An intern who wishes to become a field practitioner must become comfortable with this clinical uncertainty.

References

1 Palmer BJ. The Truth. Davenport, IA: Palmer School of Chiropractic, c. 1935.
2 Nelson C. Principles of effective headache management. Top Clin Chiropractic 1998; 5(1): 55–61.
3 Osterhaus JT, Gutterman DL, Plachetka JR. Health care resource and lost labor costs of migraine headaches. Pharmacoeconomics 1992; 2: 67–76.
4 Osterhaus JT. Measuring the functional status and well-being of patients with migraine headaches. Headache 1994; 34: 337–343.
5 Kriss T, Kriss V. Neck pain. Primary care work-up of acute and chronic symptoms. geriatrics 2000; 55: 47–57.
6 JNV-VI: The Sixth Report of the Joint National Committee on Prevention, Detection, Evaluation, and Treatment of High Blood Pressure. Arch Intern Med 1997; 157: 2413–2446.
7 Petrella RJ. Lifestyle approaches to managing high blood pressure. Can Fam Pract 1999; 45: 1750–1755.
8 Gorelick PB, Sacco RL, Smith DB et al. Prevention of a first stroke. A review of guidelines and a multidisciplinary consensus statement from the National Stroke Association. JAMA 1999; 281: 1112–1120.
9 Ferri F, Fretwell M, Watchel T. Practical Guide to the Care of the Elderly Patient. 2nd edn. St Louis, MO: Mosby-Year Books, 1997.
10 Leprich D, Carey P. Response letter by the CCA and CCPA to a letter dated October 2, 1998 from Dr. John Nyssen, Chief Coroner for the Province of Saskatchewan. INFOCHIRO Vol. 3, No. 1, Dec. 17, 1998.
11 Haldeman S, Kohlbeck FJ, McGregor M. Risk factors and precipitating neck movements causing vertebrobasilar artery dissection after cervical trauma and spinal manipulation. Spine 1999; 24: 785–794.
12 Terrett A. Vertebrobasilar Stroke Following Manipulation. West Des Moines, IA: National Chiropractic Mutual Insurance Company, 1996.
13 Carey PF. A report on the occurrence of cerebral vascular accidents in chiropractic practice. J Can Chiropractic Assoc 1993; 37:104–106
14 Hurwitz EL, Aker PD, Adams AH et al. Manipulation and mobilization of the cervical spine. A systematic review of the literature. Spine 1996; 21: 1746–1759, Discussion 1759–1760.

15 Norris, JW, Beletsky V, Nadareishvilli ZG. Sudden neck movement and cervical artery dissection. Can Med Assoc J 2000; 163: 38–40.

16 Barisa, E. Letter to the Editor. National Post Newspaper, July 11, 2000.

17 Cote P, Kreitz BG, Cassidy JD, Thiel H. The validity of the extension–rotation test as a clinical screening procedure before neck manipulation: a secondary analysis. J Manipulative Physiol Ther 1996; 19: 159–163.

18 Carey PF. A suggested protocol for the examination and treatment of the cervical spine: managing the risk. J Can Chiropractic Assoc 1995; 39: 35–39.

19 Bregmann TF, Larson L. Manipulative care and older persons. Top Clin Chiropractic 1996; 3(2): 56–65.

20 Vernon H. Spinal manipulation for chronic low back pain; a review of the evidence. Top Clin Chiropractic 1999; 6(2): 8–12.

21 Carey PF, Townsend GM. Bias and ignorance in medical reporting. J Can Chiropractic Assoc 1997; 41: 105–115.

22 Quill T, Suchman A. Uncertainty and control: learning to live with medicine's limitations. Hum Med 1994; 9: 109–120.

17

Gastrointestinal disorders

Robert Annis and Odette Tunks

Several important questions will be addressed in this chapter concerning the chiropractic management of gastrointestinal disorders in the elderly. What is the role of chiropractic in the management of gastrointestinal disorders? What are the normal physiological age-related changes in the gastrointestinal system? How does the autonomic nervous system control gastrointestinal processes, and is there evidence that spinal manipulation can affect autonomic function? Finally, in the most practical sense, what are the most common gastrointestinal disorders and how should they be appropriately investigated and managed?

The role of chiropractic in the management of gastrointestinal disorders

As primary health-care providers and portals of entry to the health-care system, chiropractors play a very important role in recognizing gastrointestinal pathology, for early intervention through treatment or referral if necessary. Functional gastrointestinal disorders have a significant impact on quality of life, associated with impaired mental and physical functioning, including vitality, sexual relations, sleep, social functioning, mental health and diet.[1] Management strategies should focus on minimizing and reducing morbidity, while optimizing opportunities for activity and function.[2] Chiropractic treatments are unquestionably beneficial in the alleviation of musculoskeletal symptoms, as well as disease prevention and management through patient education regarding lifestyle and diet. This chapter will also discuss some early research on somatovisceral and somatoautonomic reflexes, which has exciting implications for the management of visceral disorders with physical manipulations.

Spinal manipulation is not meant to replace allopathic remedies, but rather to enhance and restore the body's natural function (homoeostasis). The chiropractor is not intended to interfere with a patient's medication regimen, nor replace essential surgeries or other necessary medical interventions. The chiropractor's primary therapeutic goal is subluxation correction. Initial care is to provide alleviation of symptoms and the ultimate goal is a patient with fewer subluxations.[3] In keeping with the wellness and holistic approach of chiropractic, the chiropractor is in an ideal position to educate the patient, as diet and lifestyle have a profound impact on the prevention and management of gastrointestinal disorders.

Age-related changes in the gastrointestinal system

Recent literature suggests that the gastrointestinal system does not undergo major changes with age. Many changes are thought to be related to other factors seen in the elderly, including medications and disease processes.[4] However, as with most other body systems, the gastrointestinal system undergoes several important age-related anatomical and physiological changes, and it is important for chiropractors to understand these age-related changes and to have knowledge of the various disorders of the gastrointestinal system (Figure 17.1 and Table 17.1).

Oral cavity

Several anatomical and physiological changes occur in the oral phase of the aging gastrointestinal system. Elderly patients often have difficulty with swallowing, which may in part be due to an age-related decrease

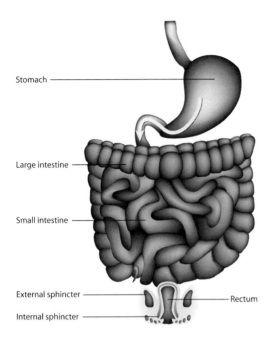

Figure 17.1 Anatomy of the gastrointestinal system.

Table 17.1 Age-related changes in the gastrointestinal system

Area	Changes
Oral cavity	Difficulty swallowing
	Decreased skeletal muscle
	Decreased salivation
	Decreased sense of smell and taste
	Dental changes
Oesophagus	Decreased skeletal muscle
	Thickening of smooth muscle
	Decrease in ganglion cells
	Abnormal peristalsis
	Incomplete lower oesophageal sphincter relaxation
Stomach	Delay of gastric emptying of liquids and mixed liquid–solids
	Gastritis common, increased prevalence of *Helicobacter pylori*
	Decreased pepsin
	Impaired mucosal immunity
Small intestine	Small changes in amplitude of small-bowel contractions
	Atrophy of villi
	Possibly malabsorption of fats, lactose and calcium
	Possible motility problems
Large intestine	Increased incidence of colorectal cancer
	Increased incidence of diverticular disease
	Increased deposits of collagen, elastic, oxytalan and elaunin fibres
	Diminished rectal elasticity
	Constipation more common
Immune system	Decline in mucosal immunity
Nutrition	Decreased lean body mass (–1%/year after the age of 55 years)
	Decreased activity due to pain and decreased postprandial hunger
	Frequent malnutrition

in skeletal muscle fibre density and hypertrophy of individual muscle fibres in the tongue, pharynx and mouth.[5] A decrease in secretory cells in the major salivary gland results in diminished salivary flow, which may lead to dry mouth and difficulty swallowing. Other changes in the oral phase may include diminished sense of smell and taste, and dental changes, such as increased tooth sensitivity, teeth yellowing, fragile roots, and worn and lost teeth.[4]

Oesophagus

The skeletal muscle of the proximal oesophagus undergoes changes similar to those seen in the pharynx (decrease in muscle fibre density, and muscle fibre hypertrophy). Research has also demonstrated a thickening of smooth muscle in the oesophagus and a decrease in ganglion cells. Abnormal peristalsis is found more frequently in otherwise healthy older persons. Patients may have various types of oesophageal dysfunction, including weakened peristaltic contractions, delayed emptying of the oesophagus, incomplete lower oesophageal sphincter relaxation and dilatation of the oesophagus. Defective oesophageal peristalsis may explain the higher incidence and greater severity of reflux oesophagitis in older people.[6]

Stomach

One of the significant documented changes in the ageing stomach is a delay in gastric emptying of liquids and mixed liquid–solids; however, solid emptying remains unchanged.[7,8] Gastric acid secretion does not normally decrease with age, unless associated with gastrointestinal problems such as atrophic gastritis.[9] Gastritis is an inflammation of the mucosal lining of the stomach and is very common in the ageing population. Its clinical significance will be discussed in more detail later in this chapter.

Perhaps one of the most important age-related findings is an increased prevalence of *Helicobacter pylori* (*H. pylori*) colonization in the older patient.[5,10] It is well documented that *H. pylori* is associated with gastritis and peptic ulcer disease[11,12] and it has more recently been associated with gastric malignancies.[13,14] Increased prevalence of *H. pylori*, atrophic gastritis and metaplastic changes in the stomach may affect drug absorption and may play a role in gastrointestinal diseases seen in the older patient.[15]

The natural ageing process of the gastrointestinal system also results in a decrease in stomach mucus neck cell mass or cell function, and a decrease in pepsin output. This decrease in pepsin output has been shown to be independent of atrophic gastritis, smoking and *H. pylori* colonization.[16]

Furthermore, certain age-related changes are postulated to impair the stomach's mucosal defence, thereby increasing the risk of gastrointestinal infections and inflammatory diseases in the elderly. Namely, there is a general decrease in immune function with ageing (which would diminish mucosal immunity) and some studies have shown decreased blood flow to the basal gastric mucosa, which would diminish the supply of oxygen, nutrients and other repair molecules for the gastric mucosa.[17] There is also a documented decrease in gastric mucosal prostaglandin, which is involved in the inflammatory response to injury. All of these changes in the gastric mucosal defence system may weaken the mucosa, leaving the elderly patient more vulnerable to mucosal injury, including increased frequency of ulcers, injury from non-steroidal anti-inflammatory (NSAID) use and susceptibility to *H. pylori* colonization.

Small intestine

Few physiological and anatomical changes are documented in the ageing small intestine. In healthy individuals, the overall structure, motility and absorptive functions do not change significantly. Arora *et al.*[18] reported that there may be small changes in the amplitude of small-bowel contractions. More recent studies suggest that the villi of the small intestine atrophy with age and the intestinal cells themselves may change, possibly resulting in problems such as diarrhoea, malabsorption and impaired barrier function.[19] Some studies show impaired absorption of fats, lactose and calcium with age. Motility and malabsorption problems may also be associated with systemic diseases and/or various medications.

Large intestine

Studies have shown an increased incidence of colorectal neoplasia in the elderly population. There are several explanations for this age-dependent rise in cancer incidence, including altered carcinogen metabolism, cumulative effects of long-term exposure to carcinogens and alterations in cellular proliferation.[20] There is also an age-related increase in diverticular disease. This increased incidence of diverticular disease may be due to a reduction in the colon's tensile strength and ability to resist intraluminal pressure, as a result of increased deposits of collagen, elastic, oxytalan and elaunin fibres.[17] This change in colon structure, along with diminished rectal elasticity, may also increase the risk for faecal incontinence in the elderly. The chiropractic literature suggests that chiropractic adjustments combined with pelvic-floor muscle exercises successfully reduce faecal incontinence in certain elderly patients.[21]

Constipation is also a very common complaint in older patients: the prevalence of self-reported constipation is three times greater over the age of 65 than in the 45–64-year-old age group.[22] Constipation may be in part due to structural changes, such as changes in the colon and rectum. Most commonly it is caused by certain medications, insufficient fluid intake, insufficient dietary fibre, irregular toilet habit and insufficient exercise.[17] Constipation has a significant impact on quality of life and can have some serious complications. In many cases, the chiropractor can play an important role in improving constipation through good dietary and lifestyle advice. This will be discussed in more detail later in the chapter.

Mucosal immune system

Mucosal immunity is the first line of defence against pathogens and plays a vital role in the immune system. Very importantly, the surface of the gastrointestinal tract is the largest single immunological organ, accommodating more than 70% of the body's immunoglobulin-producing cells. There is considerable evidence that the mucosal or secretory immune response in the gastrointestinal tract diminishes with age. These changes include deficits in the differentiation and/or migration of immunoglobulin A (IgA) immunoblasts, and the initiation and/or regulation of local antibody production.[23] This diminished immune response in the elderly has a very significant impact. A study by the World Health Organization showed a 400-fold increase in mortality rate due to gastrointestinal infections in the elderly, compared with young adults.[17]

Ageing and nutrition

Because of a gradual decrease in lean body mass in the elderly (declining by approximately 1%/year after the age of 55), the nutritional requirements for energy decrease. Consequently, the elderly tend to eat less food and are more likely to become malnourished. Further increasing their risk of malnutrition is the fact that older patients typically have reduced physical activity due to pain and disability, and diminished postprandial hunger. Unfortunately, poor nutrition is very common in debilitated or institutionalized elderly people.[24]

Chiropractic and the autonomic nervous system

Autonomic control of the gastrointestinal system

Chiropractors specialize in the diagnosis and management of disorders of the neuromusculoskeletal system. Therefore, practitioners require a solid understanding of human anatomy, including the roles of the central nervous system (CNS), peripheral nervous systems (PNS) and autonomic nervous system (ANS). The ANS is a system of nerves and ganglia concerned with monitoring and control of the heart, smooth muscle, glands and blood vessels. The ANS is made up of the sympathetic nervous system (SNS) and the parasympathetic nervous system (PNS). The SNS stimulates activities for emergency and stress situations (i.e. fight, fright and flight situations). For example, in an emergency situation the SNS will increase blood pressure and heart rate, while decreasing the motility of the stomach and intestines, and decreasing digestive function. Meanwhile, the SNS stimulates activities that conserve and restore body resources. For example, the PNS will slow the heart rate and promote motility of the digestive system, promoting digestion (25).

The SNS has connections with the spinal cord from T1 to L2 or L3 segments. The PNS has a cranial part connected with the brain through cranial nerves III, VII, IX and X, and a sacral part connected through spinal nerves S2 to S4.[25]

Although there are more complicated interconnections between the ganglia and nerves, the basic autonomic connections for the gastrointestinal tract are outlined in Table 17.2.

The PNS promotes digestive functions by increasing motility in the stomach and intestine, and stimulating secretion of gastric juices, bile and other digestive juices. The proximal part of the gastrointestinal system, innervated by the vagus nerve, has the primary function of storage and absorption. The distal portion of the gastrointestinal system has the primary role of expulsion and is controlled by the pelvic parasympathetic nerves.[25]

Table 17.2 Autonomic connections for the gastrointestinal system

Sympathetic nervous system	

T5–T9
  (Form greater splanchnic nerve
  and converge in coeliac ganglion)
	Liver, oesophagus, stomach, suprarenal gland, proximal colon

T10–L1
  (Form lesser splanchnic nerve and
  converge in superior mesenteric ganglion)
	Small intestine, proximal colon

L1–L2	Distal colon and rectum
Parasympathetic nervous system	
CN VII (Pterygopalatine ganglion)	Palate and pharynx
CN X	Oesophagus, stomach, upper intestine
S2–S4 (Form pelvic splanchnic nerves)	Distal colon and rectum

The SNS is opposite in effect to the PNS and inhibits digestive functions. SNS functions include the inhibition of motility and gastrointestinal secretions, vasoconstriction, constriction of the pyloric and anal sphincters and relaxation of the gallbladder.

Somatovisceral reflex

Can somatic manipulation affect the viscera? Some research suggests that there are cases where somatic stimulation or changes can reflexively influence organs. The somatovisceral reflex involves somatic sensory afferent fibres and autonomic efferent nerve fibres. Research has shown that stimulation of skin or muscle can produce changes in visceral function. Several reflexes of this type have been identified, including the ciliospinal reflex (pupillary dilation following noxious stimulation of the neck), cold pressor test (immersion of a hand in ice water results in a reflex increase in heart rate and blood pressure that is dependent on intact sympathetic nerves), the somatovesical reflex (stimulation of the skin of the perineum initiates micturition in patients with chronic spinal cord injury) and somatointestinal reflex (in cases of abdominal pain due to spasmodic intestinal contractions, warming the area of skin innervated by the same segment of spinal cord will inhibit intestinal movements and relieve pain). The physiological mechanisms underlying somatovisceral reflexes are gradually being elucidated by experiments.[26,27]

Most relevant to this chapter is the somatogastrointestinal reflex. The influence of somatic afferent stimulation on gastrointestinal motility has been reported for dogs, cats, monkeys and humans. Studies on anaesthetized rats have shown that pinching the abdominal skin usually inhibits gastric motility via the sympathetic nerves. Pinching the skin of the head, tail, legs and paws results in increased gastric motility, postulated to occur via the vagal and pelvic parasympathetic nerves.[28]

Wiles[29] published a short report demonstrating a relationship between upper cervical manipulation and changes in gastric motility. Lewit and Rychlikova[30] found a characteristic subluxation pattern in peptic ulcer patients, with increased percentages of subluxations at T5–T6, sacroiliac and Occ–C1. Only 11.4% of patients with peptic ulcer were found to have normal thoracic spines, compared with 63.8% of patients without ulcers. Also in 1975, Nicholas found that T7–T12 subluxations predominated in patients with gastrointestinal disease.[3] In summary, most research has shown that patients with peptic ulcers tend to exhibit subluxation patterns in the mid-thoracic and upper cervical spine.

Several early studies examined the link between spinal subluxations and gastrointestinal dysfunction. A very early work describes the importance of manipulation of the lumbar spine and pelvis for colon dysfunction, including constipation.[31] Later, based on clinical experience, another researcher listed specific areas of the spine typically involved in gastrointestinal dysfunction: the stomach (T5–T9), small intestine (T5–T9) and colon (T11–T12).[32] Masterton[33] studied on irritable bowel syndrome (IBS), finding typical patterns of spinal involvement. She reported that T4–T8 subluxations can cause venous congestion of the small bowel and gas, T6–T8 lesions can cause disturbed splanchnic secretion, atonic bowel and diarrhoea, and T10–T12 lesions can produce gas, decreased peristalsis, constipation and atonic bowel.

This research has not been tested thoroughly by randomized control trials, and it is not possible to draw any scientifically significant conclusions. However, clinically the results are important, and patients should be monitored and treated when subluxations are found at these levels.

Effects of spinal manipulation on autonomic function

The existence of somatovisceral and somatoautonomic reflexes has exciting implications for the management of visceral disorders with physical manipulations. Recently, a randomized control trial compared the treatment of colic using drug therapy (dimethecon) versus chiropractic adjustments. The study found that the manipulation group fared significantly better than the drug group.[34] Since chiropractic adjustments have now been shown to improve colic symptoms significantly, the potential beneficial effects for gastrointestinal symptoms in adults also warrant further investigation. Future studies could also determine whether these positive effects of manipulation on different organs and organ systems are due to autonomic changes or the mechanical effects of spinal manipulation.

Disorders of the upper gastrointestinal system

Oropharyngeal and oesophageal disorders

Oropharyngeal dysphagia

Swallowing is a complicated act that requires proper interaction of the CNS, striated muscle of the pharynx and hypopharynx, and the upper oesophageal sphincter. Therefore, it is not surprising that oropharyngeal dysphagia is a relatively common disorder among the debilitated elderly. One study found that 30–40% of nursing-home residents had eating and swallowing difficulties.[35]

Investigations

Common symptoms of oropharyngeal dysphagia include dysphagia for liquids and solids, nasal regurgitation, inability to handle saliva, chronic dehydration and weight loss. Very importantly, misdirection of liquids often leads to aspiration, which may cause symptoms of chronic cough and recurrent pulmonary infections.[36]

Neurological causes of swallowing disorders include cerebrovascular disease (through cranial nerve damage and afferent nerve damage), diabetes with peripheral neuropathy, Parkinson's disease, multiple sclerosis, amyotrophic lateral sclerosis (ALS) and cervical spine disease with impingement on the efferent nerve fibres.[37,38]

Muscular causes of oropharyngeal dysphagia include diseases of the striated muscle, such as polymyositis and dermatomyositis. Other muscular disease processes, which present insidiously in the elderly, include metabolic myopathies (e.g. hypothyroidism or hyperthyroidism) and oculopharyngeal muscular dystrophy, which is characterized by dysphagia and ptosis.[15] Dysfunction of the cricopharyngeal muscle (the main component of the oesophageal sphincter) can contribute to dysphagia. Normally it relaxes quickly with swallowing to let the bolus through, and then contracts as the bolus passes the sphincter. Dysphagia may result from cricopharyngeal achalasia (incomplete relaxation), asynchronous relaxation (delayed relaxation) or incomplete closure of the sphincter.

Goals of therapy

The aims are to alleviate symptoms and prevent complications, such as pulmonary infections due to aspiration of liquids.

Treatment

Treatment should include chiropractic adjustments of symptomatic areas of the spine and/or musculature. General lifestyle and diet should be evaluated and advice may be given (e.g. take daily exercise, eliminate or reduce alcohol intake and smoking, receive proper nutrition and lose weight if necessary).

Patients should be referred for concurrent medical assessment and treatment, and possible treatment of underlying neurological or metabolic disorders. Patients may benefit from careful oesophageal dilatation and in extreme cases may require a cricopharyngeal myotomy.[37]

Oesophageal dysmotility/transport dysphagia

It has been reported that oesophageal peristalsis is decreased in the elderly, which can lead to complaints of dysphagia. Disorders of peristalsis include presbyoesophagus, achalasia and diffuse oesophageal spasm.

Studies of presbyoesophagus (natural ageing of the oesophagus) have varied results. Very early research into chronically ill elderly patients showed a decrease in primary peristalsis, as well as an increase in nonpropulsive contractions following swallows.[39] A later study of healthy elderly subjects showed a decrease in the amplitude of the peristaltic contraction, with no change in the initiation, speed or duration of waves compared with younger subjects.[40]

Individuals with achalasia have aperistaltic waves in the oesophagus, an increased lower oesophageal sphincter pressure and incomplete relaxation of the lower oesophageal sphincter in response to swallows.

Investigations

Patients with diffuse oesophageal spasm present with dysphagia and chest pain, and this condition is often associated with a 'corkscrew' oesophagus. This typically presents in younger adults, but may present in the elderly. Ischaemic heart disease should be ruled out.

Diagnosis is made by oesophagraphy, oesophageal manometry and endoscopy. Differential diagnosis in the elderly patient should include peptic strictures and neoplasms of the lower oesophageal sphincter.[41] Chronic achalasia may increase the risk of cancer of the oesophagus.

Goals of therapy

The aims are to improve symptoms, and rule out underlying pathology.

Treatment

Chiropractic adjustments are used to treat symptomatic areas of the musculoskeletal system, with special attention being paid to segments in the mid-thoracic spine. Lifestyle and diet should be evaluated and addressed.

Patients should be referred for medical assessment and to rule out underlying pathology.

Gastro-oesophageal reflux disease

Gastro-oesophageal reflux disease (GERD) is one of the most common upper gastrointestinal problems seen in the elderly. A 1988 US Gallup poll revealed that 44% of adults experienced heartburn (the most common GERD symptom) at least once per month.[42] GERD presents with a range of clinical symptoms and varying severity. The incidence of GERD increases with age, particularly increasing in incidence after the age of 40, then again at the ages of 60 and 70 years.[43] Normal individuals may have gastric acid reflux into the oesophagus; however, unlike GERD sufferers, normal individuals will not have signs or symptoms of mucosal damage due to the acid reflux.

Most acid reflux events are due to transient relaxation of the lower oesophageal sphincter.[44] GERD sufferers have a higher frequency of transient lower oesophageal sphincter relaxation and more acid reflux associated with these transient relaxations (Figure 17.2). Another mechanism of GERD is dysfunctional oesophageal peristalsis, resulting in improper clearance of acid refluxate. Increased acid exposure will increase injury to the oesophagus.[45] A third mechanism for the development of GERD is decreased oesophageal mucosal resistance, which makes the epithelium more susceptible to acid damage.[44] It has also been postulated that the ageing oesophagus has a diminished ability to regenerate epithelial cells, resulting in more severe mucosal disease in the elderly.[46]

GERD may be classified according to symptom severity:[47]

(i) mild GERD:
  - reflux symptoms less than three times/week
  - symptoms for more than 6 months
  - symptoms do not interfere with daily activities
  - no major complications
  - heartburn pain severity rated 1–3 out of 10;
(iii) moderate GERD
  - same as mild GERD except heartburn pain severity rated 4–6 out of 10;

(iii) severe GERD
  - daily reflux symptoms
  - symptoms for less than 6 months
  - symptoms regularly interfere with daily activity and can awaken the patient at night
  - complications
  - heartburn pain severity rated 7–10 out of 10.

Investigations

The most common symptoms of GERD are heartburn, regurgitation of acid or bile, or dysphagia. The older patient may present with other symptoms, including chest pain (cardiac disease or peptic ulcer disease must be ruled out), difficulty swallowing, regurgitation, postprandial fullness and belching, and vomiting. Owing to inhalation of refluxate, the elderly patient often presents with respiratory symptoms, such as coughing, wheezing or a hoarse voice.[46] All patients tend to have worse GERD symptoms if they sleep, lie down or exercise after eating.

The physical examination is generally unremarkable, except in more severe cases with complications, such as respiratory symptoms, anaemia due to haemorrhage or weight loss due to peptic strictures.

Special diagnostic evaluations may include oesophogastroscopy, barium swallow, Bernstein test,

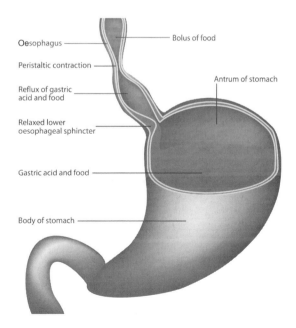

Oesophagus

Peristaltic contraction

Reflux of gastric acid and food

Relaxed lower oesophageal sphincter

Gastric acid and food

Body of stomach

Bolus of food

Antrum of stomach

Figure 17.2 Gastro-oesophageal reflux disease.

oesophageal manometry and pH monitoring. These tests are generally not required in mild cases of GERD with no complications. However, patients should be referred for special testing in the following situations: heartburn refractory to 4–8 weeks of conservative treatment, dysphagia, atypical chest pain, odynophagia, extraoesophageal symptoms (e.g. respiratory or oropharyngeal) or gastrointestinal bleeding.[47]

Goals of therapy
Goals of therapy for GERD include the alleviation of symptoms (particularly heartburn), promotion of healing of oesophagitis, prevention of complications (e.g. stricture formation, bleeding, progression to Barrett's epithelium) and prevention of recurrences.[47]

Treatment
In milder or infrequent cases of GERD, chiropractors may play a very significant role. Conservative treatment should be initiated immediately, with lifestyle changes, dietary modifications and over-the-counter antacids. If symptoms are significantly reduced or eliminated, further diagnostic tests are not required. Dietary and lifestyle changes for GERD management include:

- losing weight if 20% greater than ideal body weight
- avoiding foods that cause symptoms (often fatty or greasy foods, spices, caffeine, chocolate, acidic citrus juices)
- not overeating or eating large meals
- reducing alcohol intake
- quitting smoking
- avoiding sleeping or lying down until 3 h after eating
- elevating the head of the bed or sleep with multiple pillows
- avoiding exercise until 2–3 h after eating
- avoiding girdles or tight-fitting clothes
- avoiding certain medications (consult with doctor or pharmacist).

The patient can also be managed with a course of chiropractic adjustments of symptomatic regions of the musculoskeletal system, with special attention being paid to T5–T9 if subluxations or fixations are found at these levels.

In patients with persistent symptoms, and in patients with more severe or frequent GERD symptoms, referral for special diagnostic testing is required

Table 17.3 Red flags when assessing patients with gastro-oesophaged reflux disease

Red flag	Rule out
Pain radiation to back, neck, left shoulder, left arm, jaw	Cardiac disease
Black stools, vomiting blood, fatigue, anaemia	Bleeding ulcer
Gastrointestinal symptom onset over the age of 40 and sudden unintentional weight loss	Cancer
Persistent postprandial or nocturnal pain	Ulcer or cancer
Abdominal mass, hepatomegaly, jaundice	Cancer
Recurrent chest infections, chronic cough, laryngitis, bronchospasm	Signs of aspiration
Pain or difficulty swallowing	Peptic stricture

to rule out complications, such as oesophageal ulceration, columnar metaplasia (Barrett's oesophagus) or oesophageal stricture formation.[48] New-onset symptoms in the elderly must be carefully assessed to rule out pathology. Patients who exhibit certain 'red flag' symptoms should be referred immediately for medical assessment (Table 17.3).

Patients with more frequent or severe GERD symptoms who have failed to respond to conservative management often require medications. Medications may include H_2-receptor antagonists (e.g. cimetidine, famotidine, inizatidine, ranitidine) and/or prokinetic agents (e.g. cisapride, metoclopramide).[46] Recent studies have shown that the best overall medications for GERD are proton pump inhibitors (PPIs; e.g. omeprazole, iansoprazole, pantoprazole). Research has shown that this type of medication alleviates symptoms more rapidly and more effectively, has few side-effects and promotes healing of erosive oesophagitis.[49] However, PPIs are relatively expensive and often not used unless other medications fail.

Surgery is indicated when conservative management fails to control the disease, when the patient is unable to tolerate medical management or when there is a risk of disease complications. New laparoscopic or minimally invasive surgeries allow for less morbidity and faster recovery than older surgical methods (48).

Oesophageal infections
Investigations
Oesophageal infections occur most commonly in patients with underlying illnesses such as cancer,

diabetes, malnutrition or autoimmune disorders. Patients being treated with antibiotics, corticosteroids or cytotoxic agents are also at higher risk of oesophageal infections.[50] *Candida albicans* and herpes simplex are the most common infectious agents found in the oesophagus, and symptoms include odynophagia and dysphagia.

Goals of therapy
The patient should be referred to a medical doctor to eliminate infection. The aim is for chiropractic treatment of associated somatic dysfunction.

Treatment
Immediate referral to a medical doctor is necessary. Any somatic dysfunction may be treated with chiropractic techniques (with special attention being paid to mid-thoracic vertebrae T5–T9 if dysfunction is found at those levels) and lifestyle advice.

Cancer of the oesophagus
Investigations
Carcinoma of the oesophagus is not common in the USA; however, it is much more common in other countries, including China and Iran. It is most commonly found between 50 and 70 years of age, and risk factors include smoking and alcohol use, achalasia, history of Barrett's oesophagus or history of lye ingestion. Symptoms usually include dysphagia. Diagnosis is usually made late and prognosis is poor (<10% 5-year survival); therefore, palliative care is often required.[15]

Goals of therapy
The aims are early detection so that medical treatment can be initiated, and palliation of symptoms.

Treatment
Immediate referral to a medical doctor is necessary in these cases. Patients may often benefit from palliative care of musculoskeletal symptoms. Adjustments are contraindicated in patients with metastatic disease to bone; therefore, treatments should be gentle, perhaps focusing on soft tissues only, and no manual adjustments should be made in cases where metastatic disease is suspected.

Pill-induced oesophageal injury
Many medications produce injury of the oesophageal mucosa by prolonged contact with a caustic drug.

Elderly patients and people with pre-existing oesophageal disease are at increased risk for delayed pill transit.[51] The risk of injury can be reduced by taking adequate liquids with solid medications, avoiding taking pills in the supine position and crushing or breaking pills that are too large.

Stomach disorders
Dyspepsia
Dyspepsia describes upper abdominal discomfort arising from the upper gastrointestinal tract.[52] It is a very common problem, with a prevalence of up to 40% of the population. According to one study, an estimated 7.3% of all doctor visits were attributable to dyspeptic symptoms.[49]

Investigations
As chiropractors, it is important to recognize the commonly presenting symptoms, which include heartburn, epigastric pain, bloating, gaseous distension and a sense of indigestion or meal-related fullness.[52]

Goals of therapy
The goals of therapy are to relieve symptoms, prevent recurrences and prevent complications by early diagnosis of the underlying pathology (e.g. *H. pylori*, ulcer).

Treatment
In patients with mild to moderate symptoms, it is reasonable to discuss lifestyle and dietary issues. Chiropractic care should also focus on the management of any associated musculoskeletal dysfunction. Some research suggests that increased dysfunction may be found in the upper cervical and mid-thoracic spine; however, proper research is required to substantiate this suggestion.

As in gastro-oesophageal reflux, certain foods may precipitate dyspepsia and should be avoided. Irritants may include caffeine, alcohol, rich fatty foods and possibly certain spices. Lifestyle issues should also be discussed, including quitting smoking, avoiding large meals, and avoiding eating within 1–2 h of bedtime or lying down.

It is important to always refer patients to the family doctor or specialist to check for possible *H. pylori* infection, which is effectively treated with antibiotics. In cases of dyspepsia without *H. pylori* infection, medical treatment is similar to the treatment of gastro-oesophageal reflux, using H_2-receptor antagonists, prokinetic agents or PPIs.

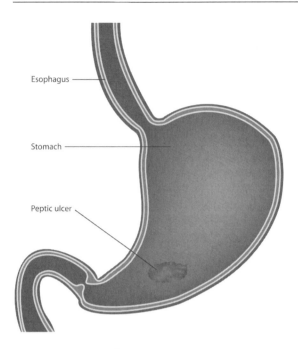

Figure 17.3 Peptic ulcer.

It is also important for the chiropractor to refer the patient for further investigations in cases where conservative management fails to control symptoms, in patients with anaemia, dysphagia, weight loss or evidence of gastrointestinal bleeding, and in those aged over 45–50 years with new-onset dyspepsia.

Peptic ulcer disease

Peptic ulcer disease is very common, with a lifetime prevalence of 10% in males, and is more commonly seen in people over 60 years old.[15] Most patients with duodenal ulcers and many patients with gastric ulcers are chronically infected with *H. pylori* and patients recover dramatically if given medication to eradicate the bacteria (Figure 17.3). In approximately 85% of cases, medications, including antibiotics, fully eradicate the bacteria within 1 week.[52]

Risk factors for peptic ulcer disease include associated disease, smoking and medication usage (particularly NSAIDs). One study revealed that 40% of patients with bleeding ulcers and 30% of patients with perforated ulcers were taking NSAIDs at the time of admission to hospital.[53] A recent study by Suadicani *et al.*[54] showed significant or nearly significant associations of peptic ulcers with history of smoking, sugar

intake in coffee or tea, low social class and low leisure-time physical activity level.

Investigations

Symptoms in older patients with ulcers may include anorexia, weight loss, epigastric pain (may be absent) and anaemia.[55] ASA or NSAID use, should be determined, as there is a high correlation with ulcers in patients using these medications. It is important to know that NSAID ulceration and bleeding may occur in some patients without symptoms. Physical examination is usually unremarkable, except that some patients may have epigastric tenderness. Definitive diagnosis is made with endoscopy, and in some cases patients may have other tests such as an upper gastrointestinal barium series of X-rays or blood tests.[56] Certain patients should be referred out immediately:

- patients with new onset of symptoms: require special diagnostic tests
- patients over 45 years of age
- patients with severe frequent and/or persistent symptoms
- patients with 'alarm symptoms': perforation is a common complication and can be fatal; patients showing signs or symptoms of bleeding (e.g. black blood in stool, vomiting of blood) may require transfusion surgery.

Goals of therapy

Goals of therapy for peptic ulcer disease include alleviation of symptoms, acceleration of healing of the ulcers, prevention of complications, prevention of recurrence of the ulcers and curing the disease.

Treatment

Chiropractors play an essential role in the management of patients with peptic ulcer. One of the main contributions that the chiropractor makes is in educating the patient about lifestyle and dietary changes. Patients should avoid any foods that aggravate the condition (often including caffeine, citrus or acidic foods or juices, and alcohol), and patients should be advised to quit smoking (smoking increases the likelihood of ulcer recurrence in patients affected by *H. pylori*). Although stress has never been shown to have a direct effect on ulcers, it has been shown to affect the immune system and may diminish the body's inflammatory response to *H. pylori*. Chiropractors should treat presenting musculoskeletal dysfunction, including spinal manipulative therapy to the upper cervical and mid-thoracic regions, if dysfunction is found at these levels.

All patients should also be referred to a medical doctor to test for and treat any *H. pylori* involvement.

NSAID-associated mucosal injury

The use of NSAIDs is said to increase the risk of peptic ulcer complications by three- to five-fold. The elderly are at increased risk for NSAID-induced mucosal damage owing to several factors, including increased medication usage, decreased mucosal resistance and repair mechanisms, delayed drug metabolism leading to increased blood levels of the drug, gastric atrophy and delayed gastric emptying. Injury may occur through direct local irritation of the mucosa or indirectly by the systemic effects of prostaglandin inhibition.[57] Management should include discontinuation of the NSAID, treatment with certain medications, and the recommendation to discontinue alcohol and tobacco use.

Gastritis

Acute gastritis is often caused by ingestion of damaging agents, the most common culprits being NSAIDs.[58] Chronic gastritis may be related to *H. pylori* infection and certain forms of chronic gastritis are thought to be premalignant conditions.[59] Hypertrophic gastritis is characterized by giant gastric folds, and the peak incidence is 40–60 years of age.

Investigations
Symptoms of hypertrophic gastritis include dyspepsia, epigastric pain, nausea, vomiting, peripheral oedema and diarrhoea.

Medical referral is necessary for the assessment and treatment of *H. pylori*.

Goals of Therapy
Goals of therapy are to determine and remove the source of gastritis when possible and to alleviate symptoms.

Treatment
Chiropractic treatment should include dietary and lifestyle advice similar to that given for dyspepsia and gastric ulcers, and chiropractic adjustments and manipulation of musculoskeletal symptoms (with attention being paid to any upper cervical or mid-thoracic subluxations or fixations).

All patients should also be referred to a medical doctor to test for and treat any *H. pylori* infection. Treatment may also include H2-receptor agonists, anticholinergics and sometimes surgery.[60]

Gastric cancer
Most commonly found in patients older than 60 years, an estimated 25 000 new cases of gastric cancer are reported per year in the USA.[61] Patients often have non-specific symptoms and diagnosis is often delayed. Atrophic gastritis, gastric polyps and intestinal metaplasia are thought to be premalignant conditions.[58] Surgery is the only potential cure, and still has a very low 5 year survival rate (only 15–25% survival). Untreated gastric cancer patients have an extremely low survival rate (only 5% survive for 1 year). Palliative treatments include radiation, chemotherapy and laser therapy.[15]

Medical referral is absolutely necessary in these patients. As in other types of cancer, patients may benefit from palliation of musculoskeletal symptoms. Adjustments are absolutely contraindicated in patients with suspected metastatic disease to bone. It is imperative to treat all cancer patients very gently and cautiously, focusing on the soft tissues, exercises and gentle mobilizations if necessary, avoiding manual adjustments.

Disorders of the lower gastrointestinal system

Diverticular diseases

Diverticular disease is the most common condition affecting the intestine. Diverticular disorders include diverticulosis, diverticulitis and diverticular bleeding (Figure 17.4). A diverticulum is a finger-like projection in the colon wall caused by herniation of the mucosa and submucosa through the muscularis mucosa of the colon wall. The incidence of diverticular disease increases with age, from 9% in people less than 50 years of age to 50% in people older than 70 years. It is more common in people with low-fibre diets and less common in vegetarians or people with high-fibre diets.

Diverticulosis
Diverticulosis is the existence of diverticula in the colon. It is thought that these herniations are partly due to decreased tensile strength in the ageing colon, as well as smooth-muscle hypertrophy and narrowing of the

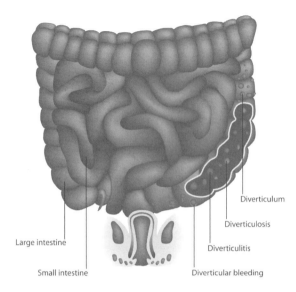

Diverticulum

Diverticulosis

Large intestine

Diverticulitis

Small intestine

Diverticular bleeding

Figure 17.4 Diverticular disease is the most common condition affecting the intestine. Diverticular disorders include diverticulosis, diverticulitis and diverticular bleeding.

lumen in many cases. Low-fibre diets are thought to increase the incidence of diverticulosis as a result of increased intraluminal pressure. Each diverticulum may be up to 1 cm in diameter and patients may have groups of several hundred diverticula. Most cases of diverticulosis involve the sigmoid colon, but they do not tend to involve the rectum.[62]

Investigations
Approximately 70% of cases of diverticulosis are asymptomatic. Some patients may experience cramping, bloating, flatulence or irregular defecation. Diagnosis may be made through barium enema examination and/or colonoscopy.[63]

Goals of therapy
Of the people with diverticulitis, approximately 15–25% develop diverticulitis and approximately 5–15% diverticular bleeding. Therefore, the primary goals of therapy are to prevent the development of diverticulitis and diverticular bleeding, and to alleviate symptoms.

Treatment
Treatment of diverticulosis should include a high-fibre diet and referral to a medical doctor for the prescription of certain medications (anticholinergic and antispasmodic agents).[63]

Chiropractic treatment should include lifestyle advice (including exercise and a high-fibre diet) and spinal manipulative therapy for presenting musculoskeletal dysfunction. Patients with diverticular disorders may have associated dysfunction of the lumbar spine and pelvis, which will require treatment.

Diverticulitis
As indicated earlier, approximately 15–25% of people with diverticulosis will develop diverticulitis, which is an inflammation of the wall of the diverticulum and the surrounding tissue. Most cases (approximately 75%) are mild and patients may complain of abdominal pain, which often resolves spontaneously. If the inflammation is more extensive, the inflamed surface of the colon may adhere to surrounding organs, which may result in obstructions or fistulae. In severe cases there may be perforation of the diverticulum resulting in peritonitis. Perforation may be very serious, and can result in sepsis and even death.[62]

Goals of therapy
Goals of therapy for diverticulitis are to alleviate symptoms, reduce inflammation and prevent complications, including diverticular bleeding, obstructions or fistulae.

Investigations
The patient with diverticulitis typically presents with abdominal tenderness and constant, non-colicky pain in the left lower quadrant of the abdomen. In some cases pain may extend to the right lower quadrant, the suprapubic area or the whole abdomen. The pain is generally gradual in onset, unlike acute abdominal presentations. In cases with partial or complete obstruction, patients may present with nausea, vomiting, anorexia, diarrhoea and constipation. Patients with bowel obstruction usually have a palpable abdominal mass and possible abdominal distension.[63]

Differential diagnoses include colon cancer, Crohn's disease, ulcerative colitis and ischaemic colitis. It is not recommended to perform contrast studies with barium or water-soluble contrast with colonoscopy because of the risk of rupture of diverticula or an increased inflammatory response. The preferred diagnostic tools are computed tomographic (CT) scans and high-resolution abdominal ultrasound.

Treatment

Management of mild cases includes a liquid diet and antibiotics. In moderate to severe cases, patients may require bowel rest, intravenous fluids and parenteral antibiotics. When conservative management is not successful, surgery may be required to drain abscesses or remove the affected segment of the colon.[62]

> The use of certain laxatives or large enemas may be dangerous, as they will increase intraluminal pressure of the intestine, and may cause perforation and bleeding.

As in the treatment of diverticulosis, chiropractors should treat any musculoskeletal symptoms, particularly dysfunction found in the lumbar spine and pelvis, and lifestyle and dietary advice should be given.

Diverticular bleeding

Diverticular bleeding is thought to be caused by injury of the blood vessels due to inflammation and/or increased intraluminal pressure of the colon. Approximately 5–15% of patients with diverticulosis will develop diverticular bleeding. Patients are usually between 68 and 77 years of age, and are often asymptomatic until they pass bright red or maroon-coloured blood from the rectum. Fortunately, in most cases diverticular bleeding is self-limiting. However, approximately 30% of patients have massive bleeding, requiring hospitalization to replace fluids, find the bleeding site and control the bleeding. In severe cases emergency surgery is necessary.[62]

Patients must be referred out immediately if they show signs of intestinal bleeding.

Table 17.4 Summary of Crohn's disease versus ulcerative colitis

	Crohn's disease	Ulcerative colitis
Peak ages of onset	Male and Female: 20–29, 50–59, 70–79	Male: 20–29, 70–79 Female: 30–39, 70–79
Pathology and location	Inflammation affects all layers of tissue May involve any part of gastrointestinal tract (most commonly small intestine in younger patients and large intestine in elderly patients) Usually gradual onset (sometimes acute)	Inflammation of inner lining of colon and rectum Involves only the large bowel and rectum Can be gradual onset (months, years) or acute onset (within days or weeks)
Signs and symptoms	Abdominal pain Diarrhoea (with or without blood) Weight loss Fatigue Possible low-grade fever	Abdominal pain (most cases) Bloody diarrhoea (most cases) and may have mucus in stool Weight loss Possible fever
Associated extraintestinal disorders	Iritis, arthritis, erythema nodosum, gallstones, urinary stones, pyoderma gangrenosum	Iritis, arthritis, erythema nodosum, liver abnormalities, pyoderma gangrenosum
Possible complications	Strictures, abscesses, fistulae, intestinal obstruction, perianal disease	Perforation, toxic megacolon, colon cancer, massive bleeding
Precise diagnosis	Biopsy/histopathology and Small-bowel X-rays	Biopsy/histopathology and small-bowel X-rays
Medical management	May include medications (e.g. corticosteroids) Surgery for abscesses, fistulae, strictures Tends to recur after surgery	May include medications (e.g. aminosalicylates) Colonoscopic surveillance in patients at high risk for cancer Colectomy in more severe cases: does not tend to recur
Lifestyle and dietary changes	Nutritious diet Sometimes parenteral nutrition or supplements are necessary Psychological and social support Quit smoking	Nutritious diet Sometimes parenteral nutrition or supplements are necessary Psychological and social support Quit smoking Folate supplements may reduce risk of colon cancer

Inflammatory bowel disease

The idiopathic inflammatory bowel diseases (IBDs) are chronic disorders causing inflammation or ulceration of the gastrointestinal system. They can be classified as ulcerative colitis, ulcerative proctitis and Crohn's disease (Table 17.4). Crohn's disease affects all layers of tissue and may involve any part of the gastrointestinal tract from the mouth to the rectum (Figure 17.5). Ulcerative colitis is an inflammation of the inner lining of the colon and rectum (Figure 17.6). Ulcerative proctitis is a variant of ulcerative colitis involving less than 30 cm of the distal colon.[64]

IBD may develop at any age, but the peak incidence for elderly patients is between 60 and 80 years. Ulcerative colitis is three times more common than Crohn's disease in the elderly. Although the aetiology of IBD is unknown, it is theorized that the inflammatory conditions are due to viral or bacterial infections, and some studies have shown abnormal immune responses in patients with ulcerative colitis.[65] Most patients have periods of remission and exacerbations requiring treatment.[66]

Crohn's disease

In patients with Crohn's disease, lifestyle and dietary advice should include eating a well-balanced diet (supplements or parenteral nutrition may be necessary in selected patients), and quitting smoking (some studies suggest that smoking worsens Crohn's disease), and psychological and social support should be available. Medically, patients may require medications (e.g. corticosteroids) or surgery in cases of strictures, abscesses or fistulae, or in patients not responsive to treatments.

Ulcerative colitis

Similarly, in patients with ulcerative colitis, lifestyle and dietary advice should include eating a well-balanced diet (a small number of cases require supplements or parenteral nutrition) and there is some evidence to support that folate supplements may reduce the risk of colon cancer. Medically, patients may require medications (e.g. aminosalicylates), colonoscopic surveillance (in patients at high risk for cancer) and surgery in more severe cases.

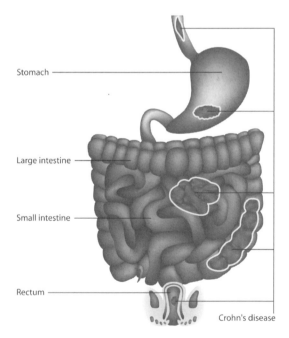

Figure 17.5 Crohn's disease affects all layers of tissue, and may involve any part of the gastrointestinal tract from mouth to rectum. In younger patients it is more likely to affect the small intestine, while in elderly patients it is more likely to be linked to the large intestine.

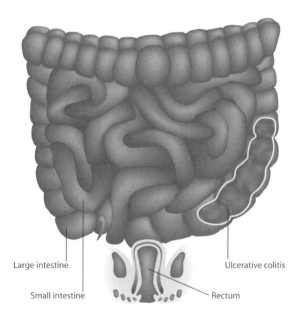

Figure 17.6 Ulcerative colitis is three times more common in the elderly than Crohn's disease. Ulcerative colitis is an inflammation of the inner lining of the colon and rectum.

Ulcerative proctitis

Ulcerative proctitis is limited to the rectum and sigmoid colon; therefore, treatment consists of topical medications through suppositories or enemas. If these fail, oral medications can be used. Surgery is required in a small percentage of cases.[64]

Investigations

A good history, physical examination and laboratory tests are required for the diagnosis of IBDs. In terms of history, the most common symptoms are diarrhoea, abdominal pain, rectal bleeding and weight loss. Patients may also exhibit extraintestinal manifestations, such as arthritis, iritis, fever, perianal disease, aphthous ulcers and erythema nodosum. IBDs are more common in Ashkenazi Jews and patients with a family history of IBD. The doctor's assessment should include asking the patient whether he or she has had a previous diagnosis of IBD and/or treatment for IBD.

Physical examination may reveal abdominal tenderness, an abdominal mass, malnutrition (and in children failure to grow), perianal disease such as abscesses or fistulae, and extraintestinal manifestations.

Definitive diagnosis may only be made through biopsy and small bowel X-rays. Laboratory tests are used to measure levels of inflammation and examine stool cultures. It is important to definitively diagnose the IBD and precisely locate the disease, so that proper treatment can be rendered. Ulcerative colitis may be cured by colectomy, while Crohn's disease tends to recur after surgery.

Goals of therapy

Primary goals of therapy are to relieve symptoms, improve quality of life and prevent disease recurrence. In patients with ulcerative colitis, treatment may prevent the development of colon cancer. (In children the treatment goal is to improve nutritional status and growth.)

Treatment

In all cases of IBD patients require co-operative efforts between the chiropractor and medical specialists. As usual, chiropractors play an essential role in educating the patient. All patients should be given lifestyle and dietary advice. This advice will help in the relief of symptoms, improvement in quality of life and possibly the prevention of disease recurrence. Medications may include aminosalicylates, corticosteroids, immunosuppressives, antibiotics, antidiarrhoeals and opioid analgesics.

As in the treatment of diverticular disorders, chiropractors should treat any musculoskeletal symptoms, particularly dysfunction found in the lumbar spine and pelvis.

Irritable bowel syndrome

Irritable bowel syndrome (IBS) is the most common gastrointestinal problem seen in general practice, comprising 50% of referrals to gastrointestinal specialists. Surveys show that approximately 15% of adult North Americans suffer from symptoms of IBS, one-quarter of whom seek medical attention. In North America IBS is twice as common in females as in males. The aetiology of IBS is still unknown and it is likely to have variable causes.[67] Most patients experience IBS before the age of 50 (50% before 35 and 40% between 35 and 50 years of age). First-time development of IBS is uncommon in the elderly and a thorough investigation must be conducted to rule out any underlying pathology.[68]

Investigations

Typically, IBS patients present with abdominal pain, bloating, and constipation and/or diarrhoea. The most commonly accepted formal diagnostic criteria for IBS are the Rome criteria (Table 17.5) Physical examination is typically unremarkable.

For patients with a classic history of IBS, it is

Table 17.5 Rome criteria for diagnosis of irritable bowel syndrome

A patient with at least 3 months' continuous or recurrent symptoms of abdominal pain, which is: • relieved by bowel movement • or associated with a change in consistency of stool • or associated with a change in stool frequency
The patient must also exhibit two of the following symptoms at least 25% of the time: • Change in stool frequency (>3 times/day or <3 times/week) • Change in stool form • Change in stool passage (straining, urgency, incomplete evacuation) • Passage of mucus • Abdominal bloating

usually effective to defer usually detailed investigations and begin a course of therapy. If the patient's symptoms do not improve, then further testing can be done (e.g. stool culture, biopsy, sigmoidoscopy, colonoscopy, air-contrast barium enema, thyroid function).

> Patients must be referred for further investigations when they present with 'red flags', including new onset of IBS in patients over the age of 50 years, rectal bleeding, fever, weight loss and steatorrhea.[67]

Goals of therapy
Goals of therapy include alleviation of symptoms and reduction in recurrences of symptoms.

Treatment
First of all, the patient should be reassured that IBS will not develop into other illnesses, and it does not shorten life expectancy. As with most other disorders of the gastrointestinal system, diet and lifestyle play crucial roles in the management of IBS. Patients should be encouraged to eat slowly and have regular meals. Patients should avoid common offending foods (at least temporarily), such as alcohol, caffeine, lactose and gas-forming foods. Evidence also shows that regular use of psyllium fibre can be very effective for both diarrhoea and constipation.[67] Since many patients report aggravation of their symptoms with certain stresses, the doctor may educate the patient on stress management.

Spinal manipulative therapy should be used to treat any associated somatic dysfunction.

Although most cases of IBS can be managed conservatively with dietary and lifestyle advice, certain patients may find benefit from the use of certain medications, such as antispasmodics, antidiarrhoeals and antidepressants.[67]

Constipation

Constipation is a very common complaint, responsible for an estimated 2.5 million doctor visits a year in the USA.[69] The prevalence of self-reported constipation increases with age, and is three times higher after the age of 65 than in the 45–64 age group. Constipation is most commonly defined as the infrequent, difficult passage of hard, dry stool, usually accompanied by a feeling of incomplete evacuation.[22] The normal range of bowel movements is between three times per day and three times per week. A patient may be diagnosed with constipation if they have no more than two bowel movements per week and/or straining on more than 25% of occasions.

Constipation not only leads to diminished quality of life, but also may lead to very serious complications, including faecal impaction, faecal incontinence, and dilatation and perforation of the colon.

Investigations
A good history is essential for the proper assessment and management of constipation. The most common causes of constipation are insufficient fluid intake, insufficient fibre in the diet, insufficient exercise, irregular toilet habit and the use of certain medications (e.g. antihistamines, diuretics, narcotics, aluminium antacids, calcium-channel blockers, iron supplements).

It is important for the doctor to be aware that underlying diseases or disorders may also cause constipation. Disorders may be neurological (e.g. Parkinson's disease, multiple sclerosis, dementia, ALS, stroke, spinal cord injury, autonomic neuropathy), gynaecological (e.g. endometriosis, rectocele, cystocele), endocrine (e.g. diabetes mellitus, hypothyroidism), gastrointestinal (e.g. obstructions, anorectal lesions, strictures, adhesions, rectal prolapse, hypomotility disorders), psychiatric (e.g. depression, chronic psychosis, anxiety disorders) or metabolic (e.g. hypercalcaemia, hypokalaemia).[22] Many patients use laxatives; however, habitual use of laxatives is a common cause of chronic constipation.

Physical examination may reveal a palpable mass in the descending colon. Laboratory tests may be required to diagnose underlying metabolic or endocrine disorders. If blood is found in the stool or the patient has anaemia, then the patient may have an obstruction or possibly colon cancer and should be assessed further.

Goals of therapy
The primary goals of therapy are to reduce constipation, improve quality of life for the patient and prevent complications.

Treatment
Most cases of clinical constipation can be treated very effectively with proper education, and dietary and lifestyle changes:[22]

- Establish a regular time to go to the toilet each day. The best time to defecate is approximately 30 min after eating because this maximizes the gastrocolic reflex (reflex where the stretching of the stomach results in contractions of the rectum and the desire to defecate.)

- Eat a well-balanced diet with a minimum of 25 g of fibre per day.
- Drink more fluids (approximately 8 glasses per day).
- Avoid caffeine (cause dehydration).
- Exercise daily (promotes colonic motility).
- Avoid stimulant laxatives (can lead to chronic constipation).

The patient should be educated on normal bowel movement frequencies and function. Constipation is a very common age-related problem, and in the majority of cases may be effectively treated with proper dietary and lifestyle advice. The chiropractor should always assess and treat each patient for musculoskeletal dysfunction, paying special attention to the lumbar and sacroiliac joints, which may play a role in easing constipation.

In some cases, conservative treatment alone fails and it may be necessary to refer the patient for pharmacological treatment (Table 17.6). These should be carefully selected and used, as long-term use may lead to other complications, such as malabsorption, dehydration, electrolyte imbalance and faecal incontinence.[70]

Summary

The elderly patient provides unique challenges in chiropractic care, in part because of increased frequencies of various pathological processes associated with ageing. Gastrointestinal disorders have been shown to have a significant impact on quality of life, associated with impaired mental and physical functioning, including sleep, diet, vitality, sexual relations, social functioning and mental health.

As a portal of entry to the health-care system, the chiropractor plays a very important role in recognizing pathology, that patients may receive appropriate early interventions. Often patients will initially present with somatic complaints, and a thorough history and examination will reveal underlying or concomitant

Table 17.6 Summary of laxatives used in treatment of constipation

Most effective laxatives	
Lactulose and sorbitol (hyperosmolar agents)	Laxatives of choice for older adults, because they are effective and safe for long-term use
Olive oil	An effective stool softener, which promotes healing of rectal fissures. It is a nutrient, demulcent and mild purgative
Bulk-forming laxatives	Effective if taken with enough water. However, faecal impaction may occur if the patient is already impacted or dehydrated
Enemas	All enemas carry a risk and should only be used if all other measures fail. The safer enemas include tap-water enemas or sodium citrate enemas
Laxatives to avoid using	
Over-the-counter stimulant laxatives	Chronic use may lead to chronic constipation, malabsorption (of fats, calcium, potassium) and a cathartic colon
Prokinetic agents (e.g. cisapride)	May be helpful; however, may be dangerous in combination with certain drugs or in patients with certain health conditions
Mineral oils	Should be completely avoided, because they cause malabsorption of fat-soluble vitamins and put the patient at risk of lipid pneumonia, which can be fatal
Docusate salts	Not useful in the treatment of constipation in older adults
Saline laxatives (e.g. milk of magnesia)	Works rapidly (1–3 h), but should only be used for acute bowel evacuation and not for long-term management, owing to a high risk of faecal incontinence, dehydration and hypermagnesaemia
Large soap-and-water enemas	Should not be used in older adults, because large enemas may cause the colon to distend, causing distress and sometimes perforation (elderly patients have higher risk of perforation owing to a greater incidence of diverticula)

gastrointestinal disorders. Patients should be given chiropractic care, including spinal manipulative therapy for somatic dysfunction, lifestyle and dietary advice, and appropriate medical referral if necessary. The chiropractor is in an ideal position to educate the patient, to manage the patient with a holistic view, and to have a profound impact on the prevention and management of gastrointestinal disorders.

Acknowledgement

Special thanks to Propaganda Studios, Hamilton, ON, Canada (Adam Antoszek-Rallo, owner: 545–9794) for graphic design.

References

1 Koloski N, Talley N, Boyce P. The impact of functional gastrointestinal disorders on quality of life. Am J Gastroenterol 2000; 95: 67–71.

2 McCarthy K. Management considerations in the geriatric patient. Top Clin Chiropractic 1996; 3(2): 66–75.

3 Wiles M. Visceral disorders related to the spine. In: Gatterman M. ed. Chiropractic Management of Spine-related Disorders. Baltimore, MD: Williams & Wilkins, 1990.

4 Sedmihradsky J. Good prospects for the aging gastrointestinal system: normal function is retained despite age-related changes. Geriatr Aging 2000; 3(2): 1, 20.

5 Nelson J, Castell D. Aging of the gastrointestinal system. In: Hazzard W, Andres R, Bierman E, Blass J, eds. Principles of Geriatric Medicine and Gerontology. 2nd edn. New York: McGraw-Hill, 1990: 593–608.

6 Ferriolli E, Oliveira R, Matsuda F et al. Aging, oesophageal motility, and gastroesophageal reflux. J Am Geriatr Soc 1998; 46: 1534–1537.

7 Altman D. Changes in gastrointestinal pancreatic, biliary, and hepatic function with aging. Gastroenterol Clin North Am 1990; 19(2): 227–234.

8 Steinheber F. Aging and the stomach. Clin Gastroenterol 1985; 14: 657–688.

9 Green L, Graham D. Gastritis in the elderly. Gastroenterol Clin North Am 1990; 19(2): 273–292.

10 Saltzman J, Russell R. The aging gut. Gastroenterol Clin North Am 1998; 27(2): 309–324.

11 Warren J, Marshall B. Unidentified curved bacilli on gastric epithelium in active chronic gastritis. Lancet 1983; i: 1273–1275.

12 Marshall BJ. *Helicobacter pylori* (Review). Am J Gastroenterol 1994; 89: S116–S128

13 Eurogast Study Group. An international association between *Helicobacter pylori* infection and gastric cancer. Lancet 1993; 341: 1359–1362.

14 Parsonnet J, Hansen S, Rodriguez L et al. *H. pylori* infection and gastric lymphoma. N Engl J Med 1994; 330: 1267–1271.

15 Bozymski E, Isaacs K. Special diagnostic and therapeutic considerations in elderly patients with upper gastrointestinal disease. J Clin Gastroenterol 1991; 13(2): S65–S75.

16 Feldman M, Lee M. The aging stomach: implications for NSAID gastropathy. Gut 1997; 47: 425–426.

17 Blechman M, Gelb A. Aging and gastrointestinal physiology. Clin Geriatr Med 1999; 15(3): 429–438.

18 Arora S, Kassarjian Z, Krasinski S et al. Effect of age on tests of intestinal and hepatic function in healthy humans. Gastroenterology 1989; 96: 1560–1565.

19 Thomson ABR, Wild G. Small bowel review: Part II. Can J Gastroenterol 1997; 11(7): 607–618.

20 Majumdar A, Jaszewski R, Dubick M. Effect of aging on the gastrointestinal tract and the pancreas. Proc Soc Exp Biol Med 1997; 215: 134–144.

21 McDonald C. Changing the quality of life for the elderly through chiropractic and wellness care. Inter Chiropractic Assoc Rev 1997; Sept./Oct.: 36–40.

22 Quail F. Easing the strain of constipation. Can J CME 1998; 10(12): 117–125.

23 Schmucker D, Heyworth M, Owen R, Daniels C. Impact of aging on gastrointestinal mucosal immunity (Review article). Dig Dis Sci 1996; 41: 1183–1193.

24 Lovat L. Age related changes in gut physiology and nutritional status. Gut 1996; 38: 306–309.

25 Moore K. Clinically Oriented Anatomy. 3rd edn. Baltimore, MD: Williams & Wilkins, 1992.

26 Haldeman S. Principles and Practice of Chiropractic. 2nd edn. Stamford, CT: Appleton & Lange, 1992.

27 Sato A. Spinal reflex physiology. In: Haldeman S, ed. Principles and Practice of Chiropractic. 2nd edn. Stamford, CT: Appleton & Lange, 1992: 87–114.

28 Sato A, Sato Y, Shimado F, Torigata Y. Change in gastric motility produced by nociceptive stimulation of the skin in rats. Brain Res 1975; 87: 155–159.

29 Wiles M. Observations on the effects of upper cervical manipulation on the electrogastrogram. J Manipulative Physiol Ther 1980; 3: 226–228.

30 Lewit K, Rychlikova E. Reflex and vertebrogenic disturbances in peptic ulcer. In: Lewit K, Gutmann G, eds. Rehabilitacia: Proceedings of the IV Congress, Prague. International Federation of Manual Medicine, 1975.

31 Strong W. Disorders of the digestive system. In: Hoag J ed. Osteopathic Medicine. New York: McGraw-Hill, 1969.

32 English W. The somatic components of colon disease. Osteopathic Annual 1976; 7: 24–27.

33 Masterton E. Irritable bowel syndrome: an osteopathic approach. Osteopathic Annual 1984; 12: 21–31.

34 Wilberg J, Nordsteen J, Nilsson N. The short-term effect of spinal manipulation in the treatment of infantile colic: a randomised controlled trial with blinded observer. J Manipulative Physiol Ther 1999; 22: 517–522.

35 Siebens H, Trupe E, Siebens A et al. Correlates and consequences of eating dependency in institutionalized elderly. J Am Geriatr Soc 1986; 34: 192–198.

36 Pelemans W, Vantrappen G. Oesophageal disease in the elderly. Clin Gastroenterol 1985; 14: 635–656.

37 Sodeman W, Saladin T, Boyd W. Geriatric Gastroenterology. Philadelphia, PA: WB Saunders Co., 1989.

38 Hollis J, Castell D, Braddom R. Oesophageal function in diabetes mellitus and its relation to peripheral neuropathy. Gastroenterology 1984; 73: 1098–1102.

39 Soergel K, Zboralske F, Amberg J. Presbyesophagus: oesophageal motility in nonagenarians. J Clin Invest 1986; 43: 1472–1479.

40 Hollis J, Castell D. Oesophageal function in elderly men. A new look at apresbyesophagus. Ann Intern Med 1974; 80: 371–374.

41 Kahrilas P, Kisak S, Helm J. Comparison of pseudoachalasia and achalasia. Am J Med 1987; 82: 439–446.

42 Mittal R, Holloway R, Penagini R et al. Transient lower oesophageal sphincter relaxation. Gastroenterology 1995; 109: 601–610.

43 Carruthers-Czyzewski P. GERD in older adults. Can Pharmacol J 1999; 132(2): 28–32.

44 Orlando R. The pathogenesis of gastroesophageal reflux disease: the relationship between epithelial defense, dysmotility, and acid exposure. Am J Gastroenterol 1997; 92: S3–S5.

45 Kahrilas P, Dodd W, Hogan W *et al*. Oesophageal peristaltic dysfunction in peptic esophagitis. Gastroenterology 1986; 91: 897–904.

46 Tack J, VanTrappen G. The aging oesophagus. Gut 1997; 41: 422–424.

47 Shaffer E. Gastroesophageal reflux disease. In: Gray J, ed. Therapeutic Choices. 2nd edn. Canadian Pharmacists Association, 1998: 326–334.

48 Henteleff H. Minimally invasive surgery for gastroesophageal reflux disease. Can J CME 2000; 12(1): 78–86.

49 Chiba N, De Gara C, Wilkinson J, Hunt R. Speed of healing and symptom relief in grade II to IV gastroesophageal reflux disease: a meta analysis. Gastroenterology 1997; 112: 1798–1810.

50 Wheeler R, Peacok J. Esophagitis in the immunocompromised host: role of esophagoscopy in diagnosis. Rev Infect Dis 1987; 9: 88–96.

51 Kikendall J, Friedman A, Oyewole M *et al*. Pill-induced oesophageal injury: case reports and review of the medical literature. Dig Dis Sci 1983; 28: 174–182.

52 Bursey R. Investigating acid-related disorders. Can J CME 1998; 10(11): 111–118.

53 Watson R, Hooper T, Ingram G. Duodenal ulcer disease in the elderly. A retrospective study. Age Ageing 1985; 14: 225–229.

54 Suadicani P, Hein O, Gyntlberg F. Genetic and life-style determinants of peptic ulcer. A study of 3387 men aged 54 to 74 years: the Copenhagen Male Study. Scand J Gastroenterol 1999; 34: 12–17.

55 Gilinsky N. Peptic ulcer disease in the elderly. Gastroenterol Clin North Am 1990; 19: 255–272.

56 Hunt R. Peptic ulcer disease and upper gastrointestinal bleeding. In: Gray J, ed. Therapeutic Choices. 2nd edn. Canadian Pharmacists Association, 1998: 346–357.

57 Moore J, Bjorkman D. NSAID-induced gastropathy in the elderly: understanding and avoidance. Geriatrics 1989; 44: 51–57.

58 Kerr R. Disorders of the stomach and duodenum. In: Hazzard W, Andres R, Bierman J, Blass J, eds. Principles of Geriatric Medicine and Gerontology. 2nd edn. New York: McGraw-Hill, 1990: 619–629.

59 Sipponen P. Atrophic gastritis as a premalignant condition. Ann Med 1989; 21: 287–290.

60 Cooper B. Menetrier's disease. Dig Dis Sci 1987; 5: 33–40.

61 Keppen M. Upper gastrointestinal malignancies in the elderly. Clin Geriatr Med 1987; 3: 637–648.

62 Young-Fadok T, Sarr M. Diverticular diseases of the colon. In: Yamada T, Alber D, Laine L *et al*. eds. Textbook of Gastroenterology. Lippincott, William & Wilkins, 1999: 1926–1945.

63 Malik N. Diverticulitis, diverticulosis and diverticular bleeding – managing these afflictions of the colon. Geriatr Ageing 2000; 3(2): 4, 40–41.

64 Feagan B. Inflammatory bowel disease. In: Gray J, ed. Therapeutic Choices. 2nd. edn. Canadian Pharmacists Association, 1998: 335–345.

65 Garland C, Lilienfeld A, Mendeloff A *et al*. Incidence rates of ulcerative colitis and Crohn's disease in fifteen areas of the United States. Gastroenterology 1981; 81(6): 15–1124.

66 Horn L. Inflammatory bowel disease (Crohn's and colitis) is harder to diagnose in older patients. Geriatr Aging 2000; 3(2): 7, 16, 44.

67 Gray J. Treating irritable bowel syndrome. Can J CME 1999; 11(5): 83–88.

68 Lavine E. Irritable bowel syndrome is not just a psychosomatic illness – it warrants medical investigation and treatment. Geriatr Aging 2000; 3(2): 9, 42–43.

69 Sonnenberg A, Koch T. The physician visits in the United States for constipation: 1958–1986. Dig Dis Sci 1989; 34: 606–611.

70 Singh S. Constipation: there may be a number of underlying causes. Geriatr Aging 2000; 3(2): 8, 37.

18

Urinary incontinence in the elderly patient

Keith Wells

Urinary incontinence (UI) is an embarrassing and demoralizing problem often experienced in the elder population. For cultural and social reasons as well as undereducation of health providers, it is underreported, underdiagnosed, and mistakenly believed to be an inevitable, irreversible and untreatable consequence of ageing.[1–5] UI is also a common precipitant to placing elderly patients in nursing homes. This is usually unnecessary, but is often done because of the social consequences of UI, reluctance of family members to assist the patient in going to the toilet and possibly the reluctance of the patient to accept assistance.[1,2,6]

UI is defined as the involuntary loss of urine.[7] The International Continence Society (ICS) defined UI as the 'involuntary loss of urine which is objectively demonstrable and a social and hygienic problem'.[8] The definition does not account for the type or cause of UI or whether the problem is transient or chronic. The amount of urine loss per incontinence episode may be from a few drops to a clothing and floor-soaking discharge, depending on the underlying cause or causes.

The prevalence of UI is difficult to determine. Factors inhibiting an accurate prevalence estimate include the use of different study populations, different criteria to define incontinence and the reluctance of patients to report incontinence. In light of these limitations, the prevailing data emerging through the 1990s show that at least 13–15 million persons in the USA have experienced some form of UI, 11 million of whom are women.[4,6,8,9] Weiss[6] summarized prevalence estimates of UI in the USA for a variety of populations in 1998. Nursing-home residents over 65 years of age had a prevalence of 50%, as did homebound elderly people over 65. Persons over the age of 65 hospitalized for acute conditions had a prevalence of 25–30%. Community-dwelling women over 60 had a range from 25 to 35%. Raz et al.[10] reported that the prevalence of UI in community-dwelling women over 60 ranged from 17 to 46%.

The estimated costs of diagnosis and management of UI also vary. Weiss[6] reported an annual cost of managing UI and its complications at $1.5 billion per year in the USA. Burgio et al.[11] reported an estimated cost at $16 billion per year and Resnick[4] reported a projected cost of $26 billion per year in the USA. The differences may be based on how UI is defined and what data are included in the cost analysis, e.g. diagnosis, treatment, assessment of complications and treatment of complications. The complications of UI include cystitis, perineal rashes, pressure sores, urosepsis, falls (from attempting to reach to the bathroom in time) and fractures. In addition, patients may experience embarrassment, restriction of social and sexual activity, isolation and depression, and may be institutionalized.[6,12,13]

Review of anatomy and physiology

The urinary bladder is primarily composed of the interlacing fibres of the multilayered detrusor muscle. The detrusor is smooth muscle innervated by the parasympathetic nervous system via cholinergic receptors, which cause the detrusor to contract and empty the bladder. The parasympathetic innervation of the detrusor arises from the sacral plexus (S2–S4). The bladder base, neck and proximal smooth-muscle urethral sphincter (internal sphincter) are innervated by α-adrenergic fibres of the sympathetic nervous system, which cause the internal sphincter to contract and maintain continence.[12] There is also β-adrenergic innervation to the internal sphincter that causes the sphincter to relax during urination.[12] The distal urethra is encircled by voluntary striated muscle, forming the external sphincter, and is innervated by the pudendal nerves. The external sphincter has greater competence in men but is not necessary for normal continence.[14] The complete emptying reflex due to the stretch receptor response to bladder distension is found in the spinal cord; however, the overall normal mechanism of filling and emptying the bladder involves higher centres. As the bladder fills, neural impulses follow the sacral nerves to the spinal cord and then travel to subcortical centres found in the basal ganglia and cerebellum. These centres cause subconscious relaxation of the bladder without the urge to void.[6] In addition, the bladder mucosa lies in folds that allow both relatively tension-free expansion of the bladder and slowly increasing intravesical pressure until a volume of 250–450 ml is reached.[7,14] The pressure then rises rapidly and the urge to void reaches consciousness. Frontal lobe centres then permit voluntary delay of urination until desired. To void, cerebral (conscious) disinhibition of the autonomic reflex allowing detrusor contractions occurs simultaneously with voluntary relaxation of the pelvic floor. Voiding requires co-ordination between detrusor contraction and sphincter relaxation. This relationship is mediated by a micturition centre in the pons.[7,12] Without cerebral inhibition, voiding would be a simple reflex mediated in the spinal cord, which may happen if there is interference with higher function, such as dementia and spinal cord injury or lesions.

Changes with age

The changes in urinary function with age are:[12,13]

(i) decreased:
- bladder contractility
- bladder capacity
- bladder compliance
- ability to postpone voiding
- urethral closure pressure, especially in women
- urinary flow rate, especially in men with benign prostatic hypertrophy (BPH);

(ii) increased:
- postvoid residual volume (50–100 ml)
- occurrence of uninhibited detrusor contractions (detrusor instability).

In addition to anatomical and physiological changes that may alter urinary function, elderly persons often undergo cognitive and mobility changes that can affect continence. Some patients are mistakenly thought to be pathophysiologically incontinent, but they have otherwise normal lower urinary tract function. In reality, their accidents are happening, for example, as a result of dementia and lack of conscious ability to go to the toilet, or severe arthritis restricting rapid access to the bathroom. Elderly persons also excrete most of their fluids at night and may have sleep disorders, leading to possible nocturnal UI.[13]

Review of terminology and classification of urinary incontinence

A review of the literature reveals many different terms describing UI, which are often synonymous with one another. No single classification system is in use. The ICS recognizes four types of UI, including urge, stress, mixed and overflow incontinence (15). The Agency for Health Care Policy and Research (AHCPR) of the USA recognized these four types as well as functional UI (5, 9). In addition to these systems, transient incontinence has been used to describe incontinence that is amenable to non-surgical treatment and is caused by other than anatomical or physiological lower urinary tract dysfunction, such as delirium or urinary tract infection (UTI).[12,13,16] Established incontinence has been used to describe causes of UI that result from primary or secondary lower urinary tract dysfunction once other causes such as reduced mobility and pharmaceuticals have been addressed.[12,13] Functional incontinence is used when the cause is altered mentation or mobility, such as Alzheimer's dementia or severe arthritis. Sirls and Rashid[13] were careful to point out that elderly patients with mentation or mobility problems may also have lower urinary tract dysfunction. UI may also be classified in terms of dysfunction of the filling and storage phase and/or the emptying phase of micturition. Patients may have dysfunction of both phases in addition to non-lower urinary tract causes of UI.[8,13] McInerney and Mindy[7] distinguished between non-neuropathic and neuropathic causes of UI such as strokes (affecting mentation and mobility), suprapontine tumours, spinal cord lesions and diabetes mellitus leading to peripheral autonomic neuropathy. The terminology for specific types of UI and the various synonyms are:[1,2,5–8,12,13,15,16]

- urge incontinence: detrusor or bladder instability, hyperreflexia, overactivity or hypersensitivity
- detrusor-sphincter dyssynergia:[1] detrusor contractions against a closed sphincter; a stand-alone term that combines urge incontinence with inappropriate sphincter contraction
- detrusor hyperactivity with impaired contractility:[13] a combination of urge incontinence and failure to empty
- stress incontinence
- mixed incontinence: typically a combination of urge and stress incontinence
- overflow incontinence: paradoxical incontinence, neurogenic bladder
- functional incontinence: caused by mentation or mobility disturbance
- transient incontinence: caused by non-lower urinary tract dysfunction; reversible and amenable to non-surgical treatment
- chronic incontinence: established incontinence
- insensible incontinence:[7] the patient notices incontinence only when underwear is wet; caused by stress leakage or detrusor contractions.
- total incontinence:[7] constant dribbling with no voiding episodes.

Types of urinary incontinence

For this chapter the ICS terminology will be used to define the types of UI, including urge, stress, mixed and overflow incontinence. Other terms will be discussed within the context of the particular subject. The first three types of UI are disorders of the filling and storage phase of micturition. Overflow incontinence is a disorder of the emptying phase.

Urge incontinence

Urge incontinence has been reported as the most prevalent type of UI in the elderly population.[2,13] Weiss[6] disagrees and states that stress incontinence is the most prevalent type owing to the number of older women who have this type. Urge incontinence typically involves involuntary detrusor contractions (hence the use of terms such as instability, hyperreflexia and hyperactivity) accompanied by an abrupt and strong urge to void. Cerebral inhibition of these contractions is lost or ineffective depending on the underlying pathophysiology. The amount of urine leakage per episode may vary but may be moderate to large.[12] If the patient has learned to attempt voiding frequently

to keep the bladder empty the urine loss may be minimal. Patients may experience nocturia, urgency and frequency.

Urge incontinence can be described as sensory or motor.[2,13] Motor urgency results from demonstrable uninhibited detrusor contractions resulting in urine leakage. These contractions may be idiopathic or may be caused by central nervous system (CNS) disorders which affect the brain centres that inhibit bladder contractions. Examples include stroke, Parkinson's disease and tumours. Spinal cord lesions may cause urge incontinence.[12] Keating et al.[2] cited 'deconditioned' voiding reflexes due to chronic low-volume voiding as a possible cause of detrusor instability, as well as negative emotional states. Anxiety induced by incontinence may indirectly contribute to further incontinence by encouraging frequent small voids, which then may lead to reduced bladder capacity and increased detrusor tone and instability.[2] Beal[17] cited a possible connection between bladder function and mechanical lumbar/sacroiliac dysfunction in his review of viscerosomatic reflexes. It is not known whether bladder dysfunction leads to lumbar/sacroiliac dysfunction or vice versa. Controlled trials have not been performed to determine whether there is a meaningful clinical relationship involving viscerosomatic reflexes. Eisenstein et al.[18] identified 16 patients among 5000 in a spinal practice who had urge incontinence with no apparent conventional explanation after extensive investigations. In all cases incontinence was related to increasing low back pain and could not be attributed to other causes. Surgery to relieve the pain was performed in 12 of 16 patients. One patient had no reduction in pain. The pain was cured in one patient and described as 'much better' in 10. Nine of these improved patients stated that their incontinence was cured and one declared that it was 'much better'. Urge incontinence did not improve in the one patient whose surgery was unsuccessful in pain relief, and the four patients who did not receive surgery reported their incontinence as unchanged. It was hypothesized that there is a possible causal relationship between chronic low back pain and urge incontinence. Stimulation of the sacral plexus by pain neuropeptides was suggested as a possible explanation of the hypothesis, as was the influence of pain on the micturition control centres in the CNS. Increased intra-abdominal pressure may also cause detrusor instability and resulting involuntary contractions.

The sensory type of urge incontinence occurs when the patient has the strong urge to urinate but there is no involuntary detrusor contraction. Sensitivity to bladder stones, UTI, bladder tumour, and other bladder pathologies causes this dysfunction.[7,13] Patients are not often actually incontinent in these cases, but are usually plagued with urgency and frequency.

Stress incontinence

Stress urinary incontinence (SUI) is defined as small to moderate urine losses resulting from stressors that raise intra-abdominal pressure, such as laughing, coughing and sneezing. In SUI the increased intra-abdominal pressure exceeds the bladder outlet pressure, resulting in leakage. Changing body positions, lifting and a variety of exercises may also cause leakage.[2,5–8,12,13,19] The predisposing factors are usually urethral hypermobility and alteration of the angle between the bladder and the urethra. These factors allow increased intra-abdominal pressure to exceed urethral sphincter pressure during the aforementioned stressors. SUI is most common in women, but may result in men after prostatectomy.[6,12,13,20]

Sirls and Rashid[13] distinguish between anatomical and intrinsic SUI. Anatomical (simple) SUI is the loss of small amounts of urine during laughing, coughing and sneezing. Intrinsic SUI is caused by urethral sphincter damage resulting from bladder or pelvic surgery, neurological disease, trauma and pelvic radiation. Urine loss is more severe in these cases.

There are probably multiple factors leading to change in the urethral angle and urethral hypermobility. Vaginal childbirth may damage pelvic muscles and nerves, compounded by any other pelvic trauma and ageing.[8,19] Elia[8] cited the 'hammock hypothesis' in which the normal support of the urethra by compression from the pelvic fascia, levator ani muscle and vaginal wall is lost by weakening of these structures. This allows incontinence with increased intra-abdominal pressure. It is also proposed that some women have weaker collagen in pelvic support structures, possibly mediated by a genetic predisposition and/or lack of oestrogen in the postmenopausal patient, but this hypothesis requires more study.[8] Chronic constipation can lead to weakened pelvic-floor muscles from prolonged straining, and a variety of gynaecological problems such as cystocele, vaginal prolapse and uterine prolapse can contribute to SUI.[19] Decreased oestrogen levels in postmenopausal women lead to atrophic vaginitis and loss of urethral closure pressure, and the perineal tissues lose bulk with age.[2,19] These factors also contribute to SUI. Other causes of SUI include drugs that block α-adrenergic function to the internal sphincter, urethral damage and irritation from radiation, surgical trauma and infection.[2,6]

Patients with true SUI leak urine simultaneously with the mechanical stressors that raise intra-abdominal pressure, and nocturnal incontinence is unusual. Increased intra-abdominal pressure can stimulate detrusor contraction, but there is a time delay of a few seconds between the stressor and the urine leakage. In addition urine loss with detrusor instability is greater than in simple SUI and the patient has nocturnal incontinence.[5,6,12] Overflow incontinence may be caused by mechanical stress, but occurs at other times as well.

Mixed incontinence

This form is usually a mixture of urge and stress incontinence; however, there may be a combination of other types of UI, such as urge incontinence with bladder outlet obstruction in a man with benign prostatic hypertrophy (BPH). The challenge is to determine whether the patient has more than one mechanism of incontinence. This begins with a careful history and may require urodynamic studies to confirm the diagnoses.

Overflow incontinence

Overflow urinary incontinence (OUI) usually results from neurological problems or bladder outlet obstruction or both. The term 'neurogenic bladder' 'may be used to describe this type, but this term does not include outlet obstruction and other causes, and therefore overflow is a better term. The factors that cause OUI lead to urinary retention, which distends the bladder. The intravesical pressure then rises to a point that exceeds the outlet resistance. Urine frequently dribbles out in small amounts around the clock, the urine flow rate is reduced, and urinary retention may be great enough to reveal a percussible and palpable bladder on examination.[2] Bladder contractions are weak or absent. Manfrey and Finkelstein[1] identified three categories of OUI, which they termed paradoxical incontinence. The first is overdistension atony from chronic voluntary holding of urine, in which patients were unable to use the bathroom or receive assistance frequently enough to void properly. This category is reversible by bladder decompression allowing normal tone to return, occasionally assisted by pharmaceuticals. The second category is overdistension atony from outlet obstruction, typically in men with BPH. Urethral stricture, faecal impaction and urethral constriction from α-adrenergic agonists can also contribute to outlet obstruction.[6] Spinal cord lesions between the micturition centre at the pons and the sacral parasympathetic supply to the bladder may cause simultaneous uncoordinated detrusor contractions and sphincter contraction, leading to high-pressure outlet obstruction, also called detrusor–sphincter dyssynergia.[7] Outlet obstruction is unusual in women.[12]

The third category is detrusor atony from neurogenic problems. These may be neuropathies such as autonomic neuropathy from diabetes mellitus or neuropathy from disc herniation or cauda equina compression. Damage to bladder innervation from radiation, surgery, trauma and tumours may also cause overflow.[1,6,7,12] Overflow bladder can be complicated by UTI urosepsis, vesicoureteric reflux, impaired renal function and renal failure.[7,12]

Diagnosis

The importance of history in UI cannot be overstated, as determining the source of UI can be challenging. Johnson and Busby-Whitehead[5] note that the history for urge incontinence is neither sensitive nor specific, and the history for stress incontinence is sensitive but not specific. Even though the underlying cause or causes may not be discernible from history alone, the history provides a direction for further investigation that allows the more judicious use of expensive and invasive diagnostic procedures. In addition to a careful history, the patient may be asked to provide a voiding diary.[2,13] The diary includes information on the number of accidents, time of day, intensity of urge to void and volume loss during each void (if the patient is able to reach the toilet), and comments on the circumstances of each void. This information may disclose a pattern suggestive of a particularal etiology of UI.

Table 18.1 Drugs that affect continence[5–7]

Influence on urinary system	Drug class	Mechanism or effect
Reduction of bladder contractility/urinary retention	Anticholinergics	Inhibit parasympathetic activity
	Antidepressants	Anticholinergic effects
	Antihistamines	Anticholinergic effects
	Antipsychotics	Anticholinergic effects
	Calcium-channel blockers	Urinary retention
	Narcotics	Urinary retention
	Sedatives/hypnotics	Urinary retention
Internal sphincter contraction	α-Adrenergic agonists	Sphincter contraction with retention
	β-Adrenergic blockers	Sphincter contraction with retention
Internal sphincter relaxation	α-Adrenergic blockers	Sphincter relaxation with leakage
	β-Agonists	Sphincter relaxation with leakage
Diuresis	Alcohol	Diuretic effect
	Caffeine	Diuretic effect
	Diuretics	Diuretic effect
Altered state of consciousness or sedation	Alcohol	Delirium, sedation
	Antidepressants	Sedation
	Antipsychotics	Sedation
	Narcotics	Sedation
	Sedative/hypnotics	Delirium, sedation
Immobility	Alcohol	Immobility from acute toxicity
	Antipsychotics	Immobility and rigidity
Faecal impaction	Anticholinergics	Reduced gastrointestinal motility, impaction compresses outlet
	Narcotics	Reduced gastrointestinal motility, impaction compresses outlet

The history should be directed to determine whether the cause of UI is transient, established or a combination of both.[6] If it seems that the cause is established, further history helps to determine the types of investigational procedures needed to determine the diagnosis. When considering transient causes of UI special attention should be paid to medications. Table 18.1 summarizes various drugs that affect the bladder and sphincter mechanisms. Various causes of transient incontinence should be routinely considered in the diagnosis of UI:[5,7,12,13]

- Functional causes (mental/mobility): delirium, dementia, confusion, arthritis, myopathy, neuropathy, obstacles in the home, general difficulty with activities of daily living (may give an impression of mobility)
- Medicines
- Urinary tract infection
- Atrophic vaginitis/urethritis
- Psychological factors: depression, patient's attitude towards incontinence, relatives' attitudes toward patient

Table 18.2 Lower urinary tract symptoms

Symptom	Possible source
Dysuria	UTI
Frequency	UTI, BPH, urge incontinence, overflow incontinence
Urgency	UTI, bladder pathology, BPH, urge incontinence
Difficulty starting stream (hesitancy)	BPH, urethral stricture, urethral constriction, other obstructive causes
Dribbling (without voiding or after voiding)	Overflow incontinence, BPH
Slow stream	BPH, faecal impaction, other obstructive causes
Feeling of fullness (incomplete emptying)	BPH, faecal impaction, other obstructive causes, overflow incontinence, drugs
Nocturia	BPH, UTI, bladder pathology, e.g. tumour, stone
Haematuria	Bladder tumour, occasionally severe UTI, kidney pathology
Polyuria	Diabetes mellitus, diabetes insipidus

UTI: urinary tract infection; BPH: benign prostatic hypertrophy.

- Endocrine (polyuria): diabetes mellitus, hypercalcaemia
- Faecal impaction.

In addition, UI should be considered as one of a cluster of lower urinary tract symptoms that the patient may be experiencing.[13] Table 18.2 summarizes the lower urinary tract symptoms that should be considered with every incontinent patient.

The patient should be questioned about any changes in the urine, in addition to urinary symptoms, such as the odour and colour, and whether there is visible blood or pus. Precipitating events such as laughing and coughing suggest SUI, whereas the sudden strong urge to void suggests urge incontinence. Another important historical factor is the amount of daily fluid intake and at what time during the day fluids are ingested. Large amounts of fluid taken before bed may cause diuresis and contribute to nocturnal incontinence, especially if the fluid is alcoholic. Conversely, the patient may ingest too little fluid in an attempt to avoid incontinence and become dehydrated. Polyuria with polydipsia suggests diabetes mellitus.

The patient should also be assessed during the history as to their mental status and psychological factors such as depression.[7]

The history should include any pelvic radiation treatment, pelvic surgery including prostatectomy and previous attempts to correct incontinence, spinal surgery and bladder pathologies such as UTI. Raz et al.[10] found UI to be strongly associated with recurrent UTI. It appears that the relationship between UI and UTI is bidirectional, i.e. UTI can cause detrusor instability as a transient cause of UI, and in reverse UI may be a causative factor in recurrent UTI. Finally, an essential factor to remember is the older patient may have more than one cause of UI. Even if a transient cause is identified, the examiner should still consider causes of chronic UI.

The physical examination may give strong clues to the type of UI. Chiropractors may elect to forgo certain elements of the examination, depending on the scope of practice laws in their region. Nevertheless, all elements of the examination are necessary. Referral and comanagement with a urologist provide a reasonable approach to patients with UI. Table 18.3 summarizes the focused physical examination elements and their purpose in the assessment of UI. The anal reflex is performed by stroking the mucocutaneous junction of the anal skin with a cotton applicator, and the anus should contract in response. The clitoral reflex is performed by gently tapping or stroking the clitoris with a cotton applicator. The pelvic-floor muscles should contract in response.[8] The bulbocavernosus reflex is performed by squeezing the glans penis in men or tapping the clitoris in women, resulting in the contraction of the external anal sphincter. The anal reflex may be absent in a healthy older patient, otherwise absence suggests disease at the S2–S4 nerve root level. The bulbocavernosus reflex may be absent in 20% of normal women.[13] The stress test is used to confirm SUI. The patient stands with a full bladder and coughs as the examiner inspects the genitalia. Immediate urine leakage suggests SUI.[6,12,13]

Table 18.3 Physical examination for assessment of urinary incontinence[2,5,6,8,12,13]

Procedure	Purpose/finding
Inspection	Surgical scars on abdomen or back
	Obesity (risk factor for urinary incontinence)
	Abdominal or inguinal hernia
	Oedema (kidney pathology, congestive heart failure)
	Spinal deformity
	Gait, mobility, frailty
Percussion	Distended bladder, pelvic mass
Palpation	Distended bladder, pelvic mass
Neurological examination	
Mini-mental status exam	Dementia, confusion, delirium
Posterior column exam	Cord pathology
Assess lumbosacral plexus (motor, sensory, deep tendon reflex)	Radiculopathy, cord pathology
Anal reflex	All three help to assess the
Clitoral reflex	integrity of S2–S4 nerve roots
Bulbocavernosus reflex	
Digital rectal examination	Benign prostatic hypertrophy, prostate nodules, faecal impaction, rectal mass, sphincter tone
Pelvic examination	Atrophic vaginitis/urethritis, pelvic floor laxity, pelvic masses, cystocele, uterine/vaginal prolapse
Stress test	Urine leakage when bladder is full

Laboratory analysis of UI should include urinalysis, urine culture and a renal panel (at least serum creatinine and blood urea nitrogen). The urinalysis reveals possible microscopic haematuria (suggestive of bladder cancer), pyuria and/or bacteriuria, and the urine culture identifies the organism if present. It should be remembered that elderly women may have asymptomatic bacteriuria, which can lead to detrusor instability even in the absence of typical UTI symptoms.[5] The renal panel gives a baseline assessment of renal function. Serum glucose should be measured if there is suspicion of diabetes mellitus. Measurement of serum electrolytes and calcium should be obtained if there is evidence of confusion or suspicion of metabolic disease.

Postvoid residual (PVR) volume is measured to determine whether there is urinary retention, because history and physical examination are insensitive to retention unless there is a greatly distended bladder.[5] This can be determined after the patient has attempted to empty the bladder, either by simple 'in-and-out' catheterization or by ultrasonography. Normally there is less than 50 ml of urine left in the bladder after voiding. More than 200 ml is definitely abnormal, and between 50 and 250 ml must be interpreted in light of the patient's history.[6] If there is urinary retention the diagnosis is at least overflow bladder.

Office cystometry is a method used to evaluate lower urinary tract function, and can be helpful in establishing the diagnosis of urge incontinence. A catheter is inserted into the patient's empty bladder and sterile water is incrementally added into the bladder via a 50 ml syringe, which the examiner holds upright until the patient has the urge to void. At that point water is added in smaller increments until the patient has severe urgency or the fluid level in the syringe begins to fluctuate, indicating detrusor contractions. If the urgency or the contractions occur at less than 300 ml of added water the presumptive diagnosis is urge incontinence. This test cannot differentiate between subtypes of urge incontinence, and may not be helpful if the patient has a combination of detrusor instability with poor contractility.[5,6,13] Gas cystometry may be used in place of water cystometry.

Other urodynamic studies include the measurements of volume, pressure and flow rate in the lower urinary tract.[16] These are performed, for example, when the cause of UI is unclear, when there may be more than one cause (mixed incontinence) and in the case of neuropathy.[7] Sophisticated cystometrography (as distinguished from simple office cystometry, above) may be performed with synchronous video-cystourethrography in cases of neurogenic bladder disease. Cystourethroscopy is performed to look for the source of sensory urgency (e.g. tumour) and to assess and/or possibly treat the cause of outflow obstruction. Uroflowmetry is performed to estimate the urine flow rate and volume of a patient's void in suspected outflow obstruction, as one example. Cystourethrography may be performed to identify abnormal anatomy (e.g. an ectopic ureter) or intravesical pathology, as well as to assess bladder contractility and urethral function.[21] Pelvic-floor sphincter electromyography evaluates the function of the urethral and/or anal sphincter.[21]

Advanced urodynamic studies are in the purview of the urologist or urogynaecologist and their use should be based on the judgement of these specialists.[6]

Management

In most cases UI in the elderly will be managed by a urologist, assuming it is not overlooked or ignored. Most chiropractors will probably refer the patient after the history and limited physical examination (i.e. non-invasive procedures). Treatment methods depend on the source of UI and the motivation and ability of the patient to use conservative therapies when appropriate. Retzky[19] speculates that more than 90% of cases of UI can be cured or improved with medical care (without surgery). Manfrey and Finkelstein[1] showed that 132 of 200 UI patients in their study achieved voluntary control of micturition with pharmaceutical treatment, 15 could store urine but required a device or mechanism to empty the bladder, and only 24 could not be helped. Of these 24, only five required indwelling catheters. Many patients fear that surgery is the only answer to UI and therefore remain reluctant to discuss the subject with their doctors. Shame is also a consideration in the patient's unwillingness to disclose UI.

The first step in management of UI for the chiropractor is to question proactively and sensitively older patients about incontinence and inform them that there are effective and non-surgical options for the majority of cases. The need for treatment also depends on the patient's view of how debilitating their symptoms are. If the symptoms are mildly annoying a patient may only wish to be reassured, and UI symptoms may wax and wane or actually remit without treatment. Reassurance and watchful waiting may be the best treatment in some cases.[22,23]

Conservative treatment options

Various non-pharmaceutical and non-surgical treatments are available:

- make the home more 'user friendly'
- reduce risk factors for UI
- behavioural training: bladder drill, habit retraining, timed voiding, prompted voiding, pelvic-floor re-education, biofeedback
- pessaries
- intraurethral inserts
- pelvic-floor electrical stimulation.

Again the success of these options depends on the willingness and the ability of the patient to participate in the methods, as well as the willingness and ability of the health professional to provide them.

Simple steps in the home

One of the easiest aids to reduce accidents is to make the home 'toileting friendly'. Patients can change their bedroom to one closer to a bathroom, or sleep on the side of the bed closer to the toilet. Favourite chairs can also be placed closer to a bathroom. Another option at night is to use a bedside commode (or a urine bottle for men) to save time or make urination easier for an arthritis patient. If the patient has poor eyesight a nightlight or luminous tape guiding the route to the bathroom may help. Any obstacles should be removed from the pathway. In the arthritis patient a riser-type toilet seat and grab-bars may be useful, with a non-skid floor or low-profile carpeting to help prevent tripping and falling.

The use of a urobehavioural diary is a patient-empowering tool that may help to educate elderly persons and increase understanding of their problem. Self-monitoring and improvement of symptoms can boost confidence and willingness to participate in treatment.[2]

Reduction of risk factors

Obesity is a risk factor for UI.[19] Weight loss may improve SUI in particular. In addition, chronic cough from smoking or chronic obstructive pulmonary disease can cause repetitive increases in intra-abdominal pressure and weaken pelvic muscles. Lifting heavy objects and bearing down to urinate (called Valsalva voiding) can also weaken pelvic muscles over time. Avoiding these habits can improve SUI.

Nicotine is a bladder irritant and the patient should be encouraged to stop smoking. Caffeine and alcohol are diuretics and should be reduced or eliminated. Foods and beverages that contain caffeine include many carbonated soft drinks, non-herbal tea and chocolate. Other bladder irritants include citrus fruits, tomatoes, apple juice, cranberry juice, spicy food and the sweetener aspartame.[24] Sirls and Rashid[13] mention fluid restriction to 1000–1200 ml/day in order to reduce the need to void, but are careful to mention that this should not be done with patients at risk for kidney stones or kidney infection, or those who have diabetes mellitus with polyuria. In general, too much fluid restriction may lead to dehydration, which is a problem by itself. In addition, fluid restriction may contribute to UI by decreasing the accommodation of volume by the bladder.[2]

Behavioural training

Several types of behavioural training regimens can be used in the management of SUI and urge incontinence. Hadley[25] preferred to call these scheduling regimens (scheduled voiding) owing to the overlap and confusion of terms.

The first type is bladder training (drill, discipline, re-education, retention control), where the patient learns to extend the time between voids up to 4 h. Sometimes the training is mandatory, meaning that the patient may not use the bathroom until the scheduled time, even if incontinent. The alternative is a self-selected time interval that steadily increases, but the patient may use the bathroom if the urge becomes unbearable. This type of training is best used for urge incontinence and mixed incontinence, but can be used for SUI as well.[6,9,25,26] Bladder training is based on the premise that gradually distending the bladder to greater capacity before voiding increases the threshold of irritability and involuntary contraction.[2]

Habit retraining begins with an assigned voiding schedule, such as every 2 h. The patient does not use the toilet unless absolutely necessary until the scheduled time. Using the bladder (urobehavioural) diary, which records the times of incontinence and the times when the patient has the urge to void, a pattern emerges.[2] The patient's voiding schedule is then adjusted to reflect the pattern. The time between voids

may be lengthened or shortened depending on the need. As with bladder training, the patient is encouraged to lengthen the time between voids.

Timed voiding begins with a fixed schedule that does not change, which differs from bladder training (progressive increases) and habit retraining (adjusting intervals to longer or shorter times as needed). The interval between voids may vary depending on the patient and the institution. This technique was reported as being commonly used in nursing homes and for patients with bladder dysfunction secondary to spinal cord lesions.[25]

Prompted voiding is used for patients with mentation or mobility problems. The patients are regularly asked whether they need to void and assistance is given as needed.

Pelvic-floor re-education and biofeedback

These two methods of conservative treatment are under the category of behavioural training, but differ from scheduling regimens in that they are actual training protocols in the physical control of UI.

Pelvic-floor re-education (exercises) and Kegel exercises are essentially synonymous. The patient must first be trained to become aware of the pelvic-floor muscles. The exercises are then performed by using the pubococcygeus muscles to 'draw in' the vagina and anal sphincter as if to interrupt defecation or urination. This is done without contracting the abdominal, buttock, or inner thigh muscles.[2,27] The exercises can be performed at any time and in any body position without the awareness of others. They are typically begun at 10 contractions for 10 s each and may start at three or four sets per day. The number of sets can be increased as often as desired.

To train patients in the use of the pelvic-floor muscles, examiners often instruct female patients to contract the vagina around the examiner's fingers and give verbal feedback as to accurate muscle contraction. Alternatively, patients can place their own fingers in the vagina. Either method may be inadequate, however. Burgio et al.[27] demonstrated a better outcome in reduction in UI by providing instruction in pelvic-floor exercise using biofeedback (75.9% reduction in UI in the biofeedback group versus. 51% reduction in UI in the verbal instruction group). Kegel used a biofeedback device to instruct patients in the proper contraction of the pelvic-floor musculature, as opposed to contraction of the abdomen or irrelevant muscles such as the gluteus.[27] Biofeedback is used to give audio or visual information to patients on their own bladder, sphincter, pelvic muscle and abdominal contractions. In this way they learn how to recognize what is and what is not contraction of the correct structures.[2,25,27] The use of biofeedback to instruct patients in Kegel exercises has enjoyed success for some time, in young and old people, both men and women.[2,27,28,29] However, the use of biofeedback with Kegel training is labour intensive and ongoing commitment from the patient using these techniques is necessary to provide continuous cure or improvement.[13,30] In some cases UI becomes so severe that more invasive methods become necessary.[16,30] Kegel exercises with biofeedback have been successfully used to rehabilitate incontinent men after radical prostatectomy.[20,31] These techniques may be used alone or in combination with scheduling regimens in managing urge and mixed incontinence as well as SUI.[9,11]

Behavioural training has the added benefit of providing increased confidence and a sense of well-being for the incontinent patient, but patients with low motivation or cognitive impairment are unlikely to gain significant benefit from pelvic-floor exercises.[2,25]

Pessaries

A pessary is a silicone or latex intravaginal insert used to provide pelvic structural support in several gynaecological problems, such as rectocele, cystocele, uterine and vaginal prolapse, and SUI.[32] These devices are made in different shapes and sizes depending on their intended use, but all are made for intravaginal insertion. The premise is that the device provides physical support for drooping or prolapsing structures by compression or by 'propping them up', depending on the anatomical problem. The incontinence pessary compresses the urethra against the upper posterior symphysis pubis and also elevates the bladder neck to a more favourable angle with the bladder. Selection and fitting of the right pessary are a matter of trial and error in the office setting and should be done by those trained in its use. The device can be cleaned with soap and water and may be replaced as necessary due to wear and tear. Although safe, patients with active pelvic or vaginal infection or allergies to silicone or latex should not wear a pessary. Follow-up examinations are necessary to ensure that the pessary is not damaging the vagina, particularly in the elderly woman. If the patient is cognitively impaired or unlikely to be compliant in its use, the pessary should be avoided.[32]

Intraurethral inserts

Narrow liquid and silicone tubes can be inserted into the urethra by the patient, which then conforms to the urethra and creates a seal at the bladder neck to prevent SUI. The device is removed when going to the toilet and is disposable.[33]

Pelvic-floor electrical stimulation

Pelvic-floor electrical stimulation (PFES) has been used since the 1960s as a treatment for SUI and may have clinical efficacy for urge incontinence.[2,9,34] The technique has used anal plugs, intravaginal (transvaginal) devices, transcutaneous electrical nerve stimulation (TENS) and needle electrodes to accomplish sphincter contractions and pelvic-floor strengthening. Sand et al.[34] reported a significantly improved performance over placebo of an intravaginal pelvic-floor stimulator in a double-blind, randomized controlled trial of 35 women over 15 weeks of treatment for SUI. Long-term benefits of PFES have not been studied.

Pharmaceutical, surgical and invasive treatment

Several pharmaceutical, invasive non-surgical and surgical procedures may be used for treating the various forms of UI:

- pharmacological therapy
- periurethral bulking injections
- artificial urinary sphincter
- intermittent and indwelling catheterization
- surgery.

Pharmacological therapy

Pharmaceutical treatment of UI has been a mainstay of management. It may be used alone or preferably in conjunction with conservative care, if used at all. Manfrey and Finkelstein[1] showed that judicious use of drug treatment can bring significant improvement or cure in most cases of UI, based on routine urodynamic evaluation.

Anticholinergic agents such as oxybutynin and dicyclomine hydrochloride are first-line pharmaceuticals in the treatment of urge incontinence. The reduction of detrusor contractions is the goal, without going so far as to inhibit bladder contractility completely. Tricyclic antidepressants such as imipramine and nortriptyline are also used for urge incontinence.[6,9,13]

α-Adrenergic agonists such as phenylpropanolamine are used to enhance urethral sphincter tone in

SUI. Oestrogen creams are used to increase outlet resistance by reversing the effects of atrophic vaginitis and urethritis, although how this is accomplished is not clear.[13]

Periurethral bulking injections

In this cystoscopic procedure a natural collagen is injected just proximal to the internal sphincter until the urethra is coapted. Although the success rate is not as high in men as in women, both genders may benefit from the procedure for SUI from intrinsic sphincter deficiency.[9,13] Men typically undergo the procedure for urethral damage after prostatectomy.

Artificial urinary sphincter

A prosthetic sphincter can be implanted in mentally competent patients with intrinsic sphincter deficiency and severe SUI that will not respond to other methods, including other forms of surgery.[9,13]

Intermittent and indwelling catheterization

These methods are used for patients with overflow bladder from neurogenic causes or temporarily for outflow obstruction.[9] Mentally competent patients can be taught to perform intermittent self-catheterization. Intermittent catheterization generally has a lower risk of complications and infection than indwelling catheters. The longer a catheter remains in the bladder, the risk of irritation, infection and urosepsis increases, and the use of an indwelling catheter must be carefully evaluated. Condom catheters for men are not invasive. A condom sheath attached to a tube and collection bag is worn over the penis and the bag is strapped to the leg under clothing.

Surgery

Various surgical techniques are used to manage SUI.[16] Surgery is also used to relieve outlet obstruction, especially in men. Augmentation cystoplasty is used in cases of refractory detrusor instability.[13] Segments of the stomach, ileum or colon are used to create a larger bladder reservoir that stores urine without pain and at low pressure. Detailed discussion of surgical procedures is beyond the scope of this chapter.

Summary

Although UI is a ubiquitous problem, many cases can be significantly improved or cured using conservative treatment alone or in combination with non-conservative therapies. Chiropractors can contribute to the geriatric population's health and well-being by understanding the problem, proactively facilitating discussion of the problem with patients and making appropriate referrals to specialists for comanagement. Although there have been no randomized controlled trials addressing the efficacy of spinal manipulation and the treatment of various forms of UI, it will be possible in the future to develop a pilot study protocol to determine whether there is a meaningful clinical relationship between manipulation and treatment outcomes.

Acknowledgement

The author would like to thank Joseph Keating Jr, PhD, for his thorough and thoughtful editorial review of this chapter, and for his excellent suggestions.

References

1 Manfrey SJ, Finkelstein LH. Treatment of urinary incontinence in the geriatric patient. J Am Osteopath Assoc 1982; 81: 691–696.

2 Keating JC Jr, Schulte EA, Miller E. Conservative care of urinary incontinence in the elderly. J Manipulative Phys Ther 1988; 11: 300–308.

3 Bowers L. Clinical assessment of geriatric patients: unique challenges. Top Clin Chiropractic 1996; 3(2): 10–22.

4 Resnick NM. Improving treatment of urinary incontinence (Editorial). JAMA 1998; 280: 2034–2035.

5 Johnson TM, Busby-Whitehead J. Diagnostic assessment of geriatric urinary incontinence. Am J Med Sci 1997; 314: 250–256.

6 Weiss BD. Diagnostic evaluation of urinary incontinence of geriatric patients. Am Fam Physician 1998; 57: 2675–2684.

7 McInerney PD, Mundy AR. Incontinence. Medicine 1995; 23: 205–210.

8 Elia G. Stress urinary incontinence in women: removing the barriers to exercise. Phys Sports Med 1999; 27: 39–52.

9 Fantl JA, Newman DK, Coiling J et al. Urinary incontinence in adults: acute and chronic management. Rockville, MD: US Deptartment of Health and Human Services, Public Health Service, Agency for Health Care Policy and Research 1996. Clinical Practice Guidline No. 2, 1996 Update. AHCPR Publication No. 96-0682.

10 Raz R, Gennesin Y, Wasser J et al. Recurrent urinary tract infections in postmenopausal women. Clin Infect Dis 2000; 30: 152–156.

11 Burgio KL, Locher JL, Goode PS et al. Behavioral vs drug treatment for urge urinary incontinence in older women. JAMA 1998; 280: 1995–2000.

12 Resnick NM, Yalla SV. Management of urinary incontinence in the elderly. N Engl Med 1985; 313: 800–805.

13 Sirls LT, Rashid T. Geriatric urinary incontinence. Geriatr Nephrol Urol 1999; 9: 87–99.

14 Plum F. Autonomic disorders and their management. In: Wyngaarden JB, Smith LH, eds. Cecil Textbook of Medicine. Philadelphia, PA: WB Saunders 1988: 2107–2108.

15 Kirschner-Hermanns R, Scherr PA, Branch LG *et al.* Accuracy of survey questions for geriatric incontinence. J Urol 1998; 159: 1903–1908.

16 Galloway NTM. Surgical treatment of urinary incontinence in geriatric women. Am J Med Sci 1997; 314: 268–272.

17 Beal MC. Viscerosomatic reflexes: a review. J Am Osteopath Assoc 1985; 85: 786–801.

18 Eisenstein SM, Engelbrecht DJ, El Masry WS. Low back pain and urinary incontinence: a hypothetical relationship. Spine 1994; 19: 1148–1152.

19 Retzky SS. Incontinence: usually stress or urge. DO 1999; 40(19): 62–65.

20 Burgio KL, Stutzman RE, Engel BT. Behavioral training for post-prostatectomy urinary incontinence. J Urol 1989; 141:303–306.

21 Pagana KD, Pagana TJ. Mosby's Diagnostic and Laboratory Test Reference. 3rd edn. St Louis: Mosby-Year Book, 1997: 305–314, 606–607.

22 Hunskaar S. Fluctuations in lower urinary tract symptoms in women (Editorial). BMJ 2000; 320: 1418–1419.

23 Moller LA, Lose G, Jorgensen T. Incidence and remission rates of lower urinary tract symptoms at one year in women aged 40–60: longitudinal study. BMJ 2000; 320: 1429–1432.

24 Kulpa P. Preventing urinary incontinence in active women. Phys Sport Med 1997; 25(4): 24.

25 Hadely EC. Bladder training and related therapies for urinary incontinence in older people. JAMA 1986; 256: 372–379.

26 Jarvis JG. Controlled trial of bladder drill for detrusor instability. BMJ 1980; 281: 1322–1323.

27 Burgio KL, Robinson JC, Engel BT. The role of biofeedback in Kegel exercise training for stress urinary incontinence. Am J Obstet Gynecol 1986; 154: 58–64.

28 Cardozo LD, Abrams PD, Stanton SL, Feneley RCL. Idiopathic bladder instability treated by biofeedback. Br J Urol 1978; 50: 521–523.

29 Krauss DJ, Schoenrock GJ, Lilien OM.'Reeducation' of urethral sphincter mechanism in postprostatectomy patients. Urology 1975; 5: 533–535.

30 Cardozo LD, Stanton SL. Biofeedback: a 5-year review. Br J Urol 1984; 56: 220.

31 Van Kampen M, De Weerdt W, Van Poppel H *et al.* Effect of pelvic floor re-education and degree of incontinence after radical prostatectomy: a randomised controlled trial. Lancet 2000; 355: 98–102.

32 Viera AJ, Larkins-Pettigrew M. Practical use of the pessary. Am Fam Physician 2000; 61: 2719–2726, 2729.

33 Preboth M. FDA approval of urinary incontinence device (Clinical brief). Am Fam Physician 2000; 61: 894.

34 Sand PK, Richardson DA, Staskin DR *et al.* Pelvic floor electrical stimulation in the treatment of genuine stress incontinence: a multicenter, placebo-controlled trial. Am J Obstet Gynecol 1995; 173: 72–79.

19

Skin disorders of the elderly

Jerry Grod

The skin provides a strong, cosmetic and flexible covering for the body.[1] It is important for chiropractors to recognize major skin conditions. As health professionals chiropractors see exposed skin throughout the day when examining their patients. As primary-contact health professionals, chiropractors should possess the ability to evaluate and, when appropriate, refer any dermatological presentation.

The purpose of this chapter is to discuss and review the important aspects of skin disorders in the elderly. It is not meant to be an all-encompassing treatise of dermatology. A rudimentary review of the skin is followed by a discussion of skin changes in ageing and the more common and important conditions that may be seen in clinical practice.

The incidence of skin disorders rises with age, owing to changes in skin integrity and environmental effects. Approximately 40% of people between 65 and 74 years of age suffer from a skin disease severe enough to warrant at least one visit to a primary-care physician.[2]

The skin is responsible for:

- preventing foreign substances entering the body after trauma
- regulating immune reactions in the skin
- providing sense perception
- slowing fluid loss
- maintaining constant temperature in the body
- manufacturing vitamin D from elements in the skin
- healing and repair
- excretion of metabolites and waste
- blood-pressure regulation through constriction of blood vessels.[1]

The skin is composed of three major layers, starting with the most superficial:[3]

- epidermis, which is thin and lacks blood vessels
- dermis, which provides nutrition for the dermis, is well vascularized, contains sebaceous and sweat glands, hair follicles, components of the immune system and connective tissue
- subcutaneous tissue.

See the Anatomy of the skin website (http://www.telemedicine.org/stamfor1.htm). Click on 'Anatomy' in narrow window on left (http://www.meddean.luc.edu/lumen/MedEd/medicine/dermatology/melton/skinlsn/sknlsn.htm).

The hair, nails, sebaceous and sweat glands are classified as appendages of the skin. Sebaceous glands produce a lipid substance (sebum) which is secreted on to the surface of the skin surface through hair follicles. Sebum protects the surface of the skin and keeps it supple. The sweat glands (eccrine and apocrine glands) provide moisture and temperature control.

Ageing

Normal ageing changes

There are several distinct changes to the skin as people age:

- marked thinning of the outer layers
- wrinkling or loss of elasticity causing fragility
- dryness
- susceptibility to injury.

Both normal ageing and pathological conditions contribute to the risk of chronic health problems. This may lead to open wounds and retarded healing.[4]

Physiological ageing

Physiological ageing is responsible for laxity, loss of turgor and wrinkling in the skin of the elderly. Dermal vascularity decreases and the skin of Caucasians tends to look paler. Blackheads may appear on the face, and the skin on the backs of the hands and forearms looks thin, fragile and lax, with a see-through appearance. Some areas may become depigmented. Occasionally dark macules or patches appear. Pruritic or dry skin is common in the elderly, particularly in cold, dry weather. The skin can be shiny and rough with flakes, cracks or fissures when severe. Liver spots appear on the backs of the hands and forearms and sometimes on the face. They are described as brown macules. These spots do not fade.

Photoageing

Photoageing due to exposure to the sun is responsible for yellowing, blotchiness, leathery quality and roughness of the skin. Lentigines (asymptomatic small, brown macules), benign tumours and preneoplastic lesions result from cumulative sun exposure and are not necessarily due to physiological ageing.[5]

The stratum corneum, which is the outermost portion of the dermis, protects the body against infection and harmful environmental substances, and prevents water loss. The stratum corneum forms the main protective barrier of the skin. Physiological decline due to ageing may diminish the stratum corneum's role as a protective barrier. Noxious substances are cleared less rapidly and may not cause the pain reactions that would serve as an alarm to younger person. This is the reason that many of the common problems of the elderly may appear as subtle and chronic skin irritations. The cell turnover decreases, thus inhibiting repair as well as recovery from trauma.[6]

Sun-induced damage and other photoageing effects are preventable. Some clinical evidence has shown that reduction of sun exposure and regular use of sunscreens prevent this type of damage. Sun protection factor (SPF) is the term used to measure the effectiveness of sunscreens.[7]

History

It is important to investigate the history of the condition. The following are key items to consider in a history:

- skin changes, i.e. rashes, itching, dryness, lumps, texture, colour, moisture and lack of healing
- location of the lesion
- chronology of onset and development
- preceding illness such as infection or fever
- seasonal changes
- occupational or recreational activities
- stress
- history of drugs (prescription, over-the-counter, recreational), cosmetics, environmental exposure and household chemical use
- patient's statement as to the possible cause
- all treatments the patient has attempted
- past medical history
- sensitivities and allergies
- exposure to sunlight
- any systemic disease such as liver disorder or endocrine problems
- changes in sensation
- hair loss, thinning or abnormal distribution
- any fungal problems or discoloration of nails.

Personal habits are important in the history taking, including bathing routines, use of soaps, lotions, cosmetics, perfumes, laundry detergents and fabric softeners, as well as hair care, such as shampoos, dandruff medication and other hair-styling habits.

Family history must also be investigated to seek other clues.

Examination

Physical examination is useful in diagnosing many skin diseases. Such an examination may include examining:[8]

- skin, i.e. the entire skin surface
- nails
- oral mucosa
- anogenital area
- scalp.

The following equipment for examination, as well as good natural or artificial lighting, is appropriate:[1]

- flexible, clear ruler
- flashlight with transillumination
- magnifying glass (10–20×)
- Wood's lamp to fluoresce the lesion.

Evaluation of the skin

- Colour, looking for increased pigmentation (brownness), loss of pigmentation, redness, pallor, cyanosis and yellowing of the skin.
- Moisture, looking for dryness, moisture and oiliness.
- Temperature, using the backs of the fingers assess the temperature to identify warmth or coolness.
- Texture, which can be rough or smooth.
- Mobility and turgor, by lifting a fold of skin noting the ease with which it moves (mobility) and the speed with which it returns into place (turgor).
- Lesions, observing any unusual skin lesions.

Evaluation of the nails

Palpation and inspection of the fingernails and toenails is necessary, looking for unusual colour, shape and lesions.

Evaluation of the hair

Inspection and palpation are important, looking at quantity, distribution and texture.[3]

Skin lesions

Dermatological lesions are divided into primary and secondary skin lesions.

Primary skin lesions

Primary lesions are seen as early changes of the skin. They are described as follows:

- A *macule* is flat, variably shaped and of any size or colour.
- A *patch* is a large macule. This category includes rubella, measles, freckles, tattoos and flat moles.
- A *papule* is a superficial, solid, elevated lesion, usually less than 0.5 cm.
- A *plaque* is a plateau-like lesion above the skin surface that occupies a relatively large surface area in comparison with its height above the skin. Warts, psoriasis, syphilitic chancre, insect bites and skin cancers are examples of this category.
- A *nodule* is a palpable solid lesion which may or may not be elevated. It may involve the epidermis, dermis or subcutaneous tissue. Large nodules are called tumours. Small lipomas, keratinous cysts and lymphomas serve as examples.
- A *vesicle* is a circumscribed, elevated lesion containing serous fluid that is less than 0.5 cm. If it is greater

than 0.5 cm it is known as a *bulla* (*blister*). Conditions characterized by vesicles and bullae include sunburn, allergic dermatitis, insect bites, physical trauma, and viral infections such as herpes simplex, varicella and herpes zoster (HZ).
- *Pustules* are superficial and elevated and contain pus. Conditions characterized by pustules include impetigo, folliculitis, furuncles and carbuncles.
- *Wheals* (*hives*) are elevated and transient lesions caused by local swelling. They are caused by immediate allergic reaction to food, drugs, insect bites, exposure to hot and cold, and pressure or sunlight.
- *Purpura* is a general term for areas of extravasation of blood in the skin. *Petechiae* (< 0.5 cm) are very small centres of extravasation and *ecchymoses* (bruises) are larger focal areas. *Haematoma* refers to severe bleeding into the underlying tissues.
- *Telangiectasia* refers to dilated surface blood vessels. In contrast to petechiae, telangiectasis will blanch on pressure.

Secondary skin lesions

When primary lesions are injured or scratched by the patient or undergo a natural evolution, such as a burst vesicle, they are known as secondary lesions:

- Scales are heaped-up keratinized cells and flaky skin; they are irregular, thick or oily. Examples of scaling disorders are psoriasis, seborrhoeic dermatitis and fungal infection.
- Crusts (scabs) consist of dried serum, blood or pus.
- An erosion is a shallow lesion due to loss of part of the epidermis.
- Ulcers are deep lesions due to a loss of epidermis and dermis.
- An excoriation is a shallow, linear lesion caused by scratching, rubbing or picking.
- Lichenification is a rough and thickened skin area. Lichenification is characteristic of atopic dermatitis and lichen simplex chronicus, and results from scratching of itchy skin.
- Scars are thin to thick fibrous tissue that replaces normal skin following injury such as lacerations, burns or cuts.[1,8]

See Section III: How to Describe a Lesion on the 'Basic lesions (primary & secondary) of the skin' website: http://matrix.ucdavis.edu/tumors/introduction/introduction.html

Benign skin tumours

Seborrhoeic keratoses

These are benign epidermal growths often found in people over the age of 30 years. The lesions are multiple and occur mainly on the trunk, but can occur on other body surfaces. Typically, they are well-defined, flat, brown papules. Some are smooth and some are rough. The size varies from several millimetres to several centimetres. Treatment is usually for cosmetic purposes. Electrodesication or cryosurgery with liquid nitrogen may be used to remove these lesions.

See the Seborrheic Keratosis website (http://tray. dermatology.uiowa.edu/SebK001.htm).

Fibroepitheliomatous polyps (skin tags)

Skin tags are asymptomatic, benign lesions common in the elderly and of unknown aetiology. They are only painful if traumatized. Skin tags are flesh-coloured or hyperpigmented papules which are occasionally pedunculated. They are mostly found around the neck, eyelids, groin and axillary regions. Friction and obesity may be factors in polyp formation. Treatment is electrodesiccation or simple surgical removal.

Click on 'Skin Tags:' in the http://www.meddean. luc.edu/lumen/MedEd/medicine/dermatology/melton /content1.htm website

Cherry haemangiomas

These bright red papules are found mainly on the trunk and are only a few millimetres in size. The condition is asymptomatic. This lesion occurs as a result of increased growth of capillaries and the aetiology is unknown. Treatment is removal or electrodesiccation.

Click on Cherry Angioma:' in the website http:// www.meddean.luc.edu/lumen/MedEd/medicine/ dermatology/melton/content1.htm

Sebaceous hyperplasia

The lesions are described as flesh-coloured, soft yellow papules, which are small, umbilicated and slightly raised on the face. The cause is unknown and the prevalence increases with age. The lesions are multiple and asymptomatic. Treatment is electrodesiccation.

Click on 'Sebaceous Hyperplasia:' on http:// www.meddean.luc.edu/lumen/MedEd/medicine/ dermatology/melton/content1.htm

Solar lentigo

'Liver spot' is the common lay term for this condition. It is a macule, which is tan to dark brown or black. Pigmentation is uniform throughout the lesion, which develops on sun-exposed areas, often in the elderly. It may be up to 2 cm in diameter.

See the Solar lentigo web site: http://www.dermis. net/doia/image.asp?zugr=d&lang=e&cd=6&nr=32 &diagnr=709029

Premalignant skin tumours

Actinic keratoses

Exposure to sun is the main aetiology. These epithelial precancerous lesions are also known as solar keratoses or senile keratoses and they are progressive with age. They are found primarily on sun-exposed parts of the body (forehead, nose, tops of ears, neck). They are poorly circumscribed, reddish-brown macules with some scaling. The main concern is that the lesions can progress to squamous or basal cell carcinoma (SCC or BCC). It is important to identify these lesions early because SCC can metastasize. Differentiation of SCC from other scaling lesions on the skin is paramount. The key observations are that SCC lesions do not heal and slowly enlarge. Treatment involves electrodesication, curettage and nitrogen cryotherapy.

See the Actinic Keratosis website: http://www. meddean.luc.edu/lumen/MedEd/medicine/ dermatology/melton/content1.htm and click on 'Actinic Keratosis'.

Bowen's disease

This condition is SCC *in situ*. It is most commonly seen in middle-aged and elderly people. The main cause is sun exposure. Hyperkeratotic, demarcated erythematous papules may also appear eczematous in nature. The lesions closely resemble those of psoriasis. The treatment is curettage, electrodesiccation and nitrogen cryotherapy, similar to that for actinic keratoses. Large lesions may require excision with radiation therapy.

See the Squamous Cell Carcinoma web site: http:// tray.dermatology.uiowa.edu/SqCCa001.htm and also http://www.meddean.luc.edu/lumen/MedEd/ medicine/dermatology/melton/content1.htm – click on Bowen's disease.

Table 19.1 Treatment of stasis ulcers

Aim	Method
Cleanliness	Surgical débridement
	Hydrogen peroxide
	Burrow's solution
	Silver nitrate
Prevent secondary infection	Vapour-permeable dressings
Arrest stasis alteration	Stockings
	Elevation
	Weight reduction
	Diuretics
Surgical intervention	Skin grafts
Increase oxygen	Benzoyl peroxide
	Hyperbaric oxygen treatment
Pain relief	Proper dressing
	Pain-relief medication

Keratoacanthoma

This benign lesion occurs as an isolated nodule, often on the face and other sun-exposed areas. It is usually seen after the age of 50 and most commonly at 60–70 years of age. This lesion grows rapidly, reaching 2.5 cm within a few weeks. It is typically a flesh-coloured to red papule with a keratotic centre. Keratoacanthoma can be confused clinically and histologically with SCC. Surgical excision, curettage and electrodesiccation are the treatments of choice.

See the Keratocanthoma website: http://tray.dermatology.uiowa.edu/KA-001.htm

Vascular lesions

Venous lakes (senile purpura)

The lesions are violet to black in colour and mostly seen on the head and neck of older individuals. The cause is unknown. The lesion must be differentiated from nodular or metastatic melanoma. In many cases treatment is unnecessary, although laser removal can be used.

See the Venous lake website: http://www.dermis.net/doia/image.asp?zugr=d&lang=e&cd=16&nr=109&diagnr=529905

Stasis dermatitis and ulceration

This condition develops as a complication of varicose veins. Stasis dermatitis occurs in the lower legs, most often on the medial aspect. A common occupational hazard is long periods of sitting or standing. Stasis ulcers are easily identified by the erosion, ulceration, swelling, varicose veins and scaling with dermatitis. Leg ulcers are highly prevalent, affecting approximately 2.5 million individuals in the USA.[10]

Treatment includes supportive stockings, avoidance of standing and sitting, antibacterial soaks, topical steroids, and in severe cases surgical intervention (Table 19.1). The advent of tissue-engineered skin represents an important development in the management of hard-to-heal venous leg ulcers. One study presented the collective clinical experience with the use of human skin equivalent (HSE) for the treatment of venous leg ulcers. The benefits of HSE include substantial pain relief, rapid and complete closure of hard-to-heal ulcers that have not healed with standard compression therapy, and cost savings over standard therapy.[10]

See the Stasis dermatitis website: http://www.pathology.iupui.edu/drhood/stasisdermatitis.html

Skin cancer

Basal cell carcinoma

BCC is the most common type of skin cancer among Caucasians world-wide. It is rare in Africans, Asians and persons under the age of 40. In the USA the incidence is 500–1000 per 100 000, and higher in the sunbelt. There are over 400 000 new patients per year. It is more common in males than females.[9] If untreated, this malignant tumour may be aggressive, highly destructive and invasive.

BCC almost never metastasizes. It appears as slow-growing plaques or waxy, pink translucent nodules with pearly, rolled borders with telangiectasis. It may rarely have a violaceous to black colour. Often there is central ulceration, which is typically referred to as a rodent ulcer.

Treatment of choice is early diagnosis and complete removal of the lesion. Surgical excision or curettage followed by electrodesiccation is the most common treatment. In certain cases ionizing radiation may be required.

See the Basal cell carcinoma (nodular type) website: http://tray.dermatology.uiowa.edu/BCC-005.htm and the Basal cell carcinoma (rodent-ulcer type) website http://tray.dermatology.uiowa.edu/BCC-009.htm

Squamous cell carcinoma

SCC is a malignant tumour of the skin and mucous membranes, and is the second most common type of skin cancer. It occurs through exposure to sunlight or ionizing radiation, or ingestion of arsenic. The lesion is described as erythematous, hyperkeratotic patches or plaques. The tumour may begin as a red papule or plaque with a scaly or crusted surface and it may become nodular. The incidence in the USA is 12 per 100 000 Caucasian males, 7 per 100 000 Caucasian females and 1 per 100 000 African-Americans, and in Hawaii it is 62 per 100 000 Caucasians.[9] Any isolated, slowly evolving, keratotic or eroded papule or plaque persisting for over a month should be considered a carcinoma until this is ruled out.

The prognosis for smaller lesions that are removed early is excellent. Lesions that are not removed may eventually metastasize. The treatment is the same as for BCC.

See the Squamous cell carcinoma website: http://tray.dermatology.uiowa.edu/DIB/SqCCa002.htm

Kaposi's sarcoma

The aetiology of Kaposi's sarcoma (KS) is unknown. Many individuals presenting with KS may be immunocompromised, particularly if the human immunodeficiency virus (HIV) is present.

Classic or European KS is found in elderly males of Mediterranean descent (Italian, Greek, Jewish). This type usually occurs on the legs, lymph nodes and abdominal viscera. For the purposes of this text, the emphasis is mainly on classic KS, since the peak incidence occurs after the sixth decade. The clinical appearance is macular to nodular with a dark blue to purple colour, seen mainly on the lower extremities and feet. Lymph nodes and internal organs may be involved. Local treatment includes excision, laser surgery, cryosurgery and radiotherapy. Systemic involvement includes treatment such as chemotherapy.

Click on the 'Kaposi's sarcoma' website: http://www.meddean.luc.edu/lumen/MedEd/medicine/dermatology/melton/atlas.htm

African-endemic KS (non-HIV-associated) has four patterns:

• nodular: runs a benign course and resembles classic KS
• florid or vegetating: more aggressive, nodular and extends far more deeply into the dermis, muscle and bone

• infiltrative: far more aggressive with visceral involvement
• Lymphadenopathic: often found in the lymph nodes and viscera, affecting children and young adults.

Iatrogenic immunosuppressive drug-associated KS occurs in individuals with kidney transplants and cytotoxic chemotherapy.

HIV-associated KS is more common in males.

Pigmented skin cancer

Malignant melanoma

This cancer occurs most frequently in Caucasians in the 30–60 year-old age group. It is responsible for the most deaths due to skin cancer and the incidence is rising rapidly. Risk factors are sun exposure and family history.

Around 40–50% of malignant melanomas arise from pigmented moles and most of the rest develop from melanocytes in normal skin.[8]

Early recognition of melanoma before it has invaded the dermis and metastasized is essential. The most diagnostic and recognizable features of melanoma follow the ABCD rules:[7]

• asymmetry: one half does not match the other half
• border irregularity: the edges are ragged, notched or blurred
• colour: the pigment is not uniform in colour, but has shades of tan, brown or black, or a mottled appearance with red, white or blue areas
• diameter: the diameter is greater than 6 mm or an increase in size has occurred.

Superficial spreading melanoma

This is the most common form of melanoma. The basic description is a brown lesion, which is small and haphazardly shaped. As time goes by the brown lesion may develop varying shades of red, white and blue. The age range is 30–50 years (median age of occurrence is in the fourth decade).

See the 'Malignant Melanoma' website: http://tray.dermatology.uiowa.edu/DIB/MM-007.htm

Nodular melanoma

This is a fast-growing papule or nodule, usually brown or black. It may be scaly or ulcerated. The distribution may be anywhere on the body. It occurs most often in the fifth or sixth decade.

See the 'Nodular Melanoma' website: http://tray.dermatology.uiowa.edu/MM-003.htm

Lentigo maligna melanoma

This is the least common of these three principal melanomas. It is found in older persons (sixth or seventh decade), beginning with the premalignant condition of lentigo maligna. It is flat with focal areas of papules and nodules, with variations of brown to black. They may also appear as blue, black or pink.

The treatment for malignant melanoma involves surgical excision of the lesion as well as skin grafting when the lesion is larger.

See the 'Lentigo Malignant Melanoma' website: http://tray.dermatology.uiowa.edu/DIB/MM-011.htm

Pruritus (itchiness) and dry skin (xerosis)

Pruritus (itchiness) is a symptom and not a disease. It is an instinctive action to scratch to relieve itchiness or pain. Lesions such as scabies, pediculosis, insect bites, atopic and contact dermatitis, urticaria and lichen planus cause pruritus. In the elderly, this is a common complaint. With age the skin thins and becomes more vulnerable to contact irritants. Dry skin (xerosis) may contribute to these symptoms in the elderly. Xerosis is the most common problem of the aged and is poorly understood. Other causes include excessive hot-water bathing, harsh soaps, prolonged bed rest, nutritional deficiencies, heat and low humidity.

The focus of treatment of dry skin in the aged is relief of symptoms. Rehydrating the epidermis and ensuring that moisture remains in the skin are further aims. Products such as oils, Vaseline and zinc oxide serve to retain moisture that is already in the skin. Bath oils and hydrophobic preparations during bath time will also assist in this problem. A danger with bath oils is that bath surfaces become slippery, so they are better used on the body after bathing or showering. Lotions applied daily will lubricate the skin.[7] Tips for treating pruritus include:

- taking warm baths using bath oils
- wearing soft cotton clothing for absorbency of moisture
- application of emollient creams (hand and body creams) throughout the day
- limiting or avoiding use of topical steroids
- using natural preparations such as aloe vera
- limiting the use of regular soaps
- ensuring proper humidity in the home
- evaluating nutritional status.

Asteatotic dermatitis (eczema craquelatum) is a common pruritic dermatitis. It occurs in the winter in older persons on the legs, arms, and hands and occasionally on the trunk. The eruption is characterized by dry, 'cracked', fissured skin with slight scaling (see http://tray.dermatology.uiowa.edu/DIB/EryCraq-01.htm)

Pressure sores (bedsores, decubitus ulcers, trophic ulcers)

Compressed blood and blood vessels that have been forcibly constricted cause pressure sores. Pressure-sore formation begins with redness, swelling, blister formation and ulceration. The aged seem particularly predisposed to this condition. Persons with poor nutrition, the very thin, those on corticosteroid therapy and wheelchair-bound or immobilized individuals are most susceptible. Persons lying prone for extended periods are affected in the knees, shins and pelvis. The supine position affects the shoulders, lower back and heels. The lateral recumbent position affects the hips and trochanter. On sitting, the buttocks are affected.

Impaired wound healing is a major factor in pressure sores. Tissue hypoxia, fibrin deposits, necrotic tissue, local infection, defective migration of keratinocytes and impaired general circulation prolong wound healing. Five therapeutic principles should be engaged: complete relief of skin surface pressure, débridement of necrotic tissue, treatment of infection using antibiotics, wet and air-permeable wound dressing, and improvement of the patient's general health.[11]

Dermatoses

Bullous pemphigoid

This is an autoimmune disorder presenting as a chronic bullous eruption.[9] Eighty per cent of patients are over 60 years of age at onset.[5] The blisters occur mainly on the flexural aspects of the extremities, especially the calves, and on the central abdomen. They are also found on the medial aspects of the thighs, groins and flexor aspects of the forearms. Oral prednisone is the treatment of choice, with topical steroids to reduce the oral dose of prednisone.

Rosacea

'Rosacea' derives from the Latin for 'like roses'. It is a disorder of the facial pilosebaceous units, along with an increased reaction of capillaries to heat. This leads to flushing and eventually telangiectasis. This condition was previously known as acne rosacea but it is not related to acne. Peak incidence is between 40 and 50 years of age. The lesion is described as chronic confluent erythematous papules and pustules on the forehead, cheeks and nose.

Treatment begins with prevention, which includes elimination of any factors that cause flushing. These include alcoholic and hot beverages such as coffee and tea, and exposure to sunlight. Metronidazole gel or cream and topical antibiotics are effective. In severe cases oral tetracycline or minocycline may be necessary.

Seborrhoeic dermatitis

Seborrhoeic dermatitis (SD) is characterized by redness and scaling and occurs in the regions where the sebaceous glands are most active. The face and scalp are the most commonsites. It is a significant source of pruritus. The lesions are yellowish red and often greasy, or white, dry scaling macules and papules (dandruff). Their size varies. Sticky crusts and fissures are common and involve the scalp, axilla, groin, submammary areas and the external ear. The prevalence of SD increases noticeably in the elderly.

Treatment on the face includes the use of non-fluorinated corticosteroid creams. Shampoos containing tar, sulfur, selenium or salicylic acid are useful.

See the Seborrhoeic dermatitis website: http://www.vh.org/Providers/Lectures/PietteDermattology/BlackTray/19SeborrheicDermatitis.html

Herpes zoster

More than 66% of patients with HZ are over 50 years of age.[9] HZ is an acute skin infection due to reactivation of the varicella-zoster virus in specific dermatomes. It is also known as shingles. The lesions are bullous or vesicular eruptions. New lesions may continue to appear for about 1 week. When the ophthalmic nerve is involved complications such as retinitis, glaucoma and optic neuritis may occur. With this type of complication an ophthalmological consultation is essential. The pain of HZ is usually unilateral. A common complication is postherpetic neuralgia (PHN). The pain of PHN is usually described as lancinating or burning, lasting for weeks to months and occasionally for years.

The goals of treatment are to minimize pain, prevent viral spread and facilitate the healing of the lesions. Analgesics and antiviral agents are used in the pharmacological treatment of HZ. Acyclovir and oral corticosteroids may also be used.

Chiropractic treatment of PHN may include manipulation of the involved dermatomal spinal level as well as ultrasound application at the same level. Anecdotal reports indicate some symptomatic relief. More study is required regarding the use of manual medicine.

See the Herpes zoster website: http://www.pathology.iupui.edu/drhood/herpeszosterinfection.html

Candidiasis

Intertrigo is a candidal infection of the axillae, groins, inframammary regions and any folds of the body. The appearance is bright red and glazed, especially around the folds of the body. Satellite lesions are common and are diagnostic. The major treatment is keeping the area dry and friction free. Loose clothing and talcum powder assist in healing, and zinc oxide creams are useful. Eroded areas will require moist compresses using drying agents such as Burrow's solution. A non-fluorinated corticosteroid cream may also be useful.

Angular cheilitis is common in the elderly as a result of poorly fitting dentures and inadequate nutrition. The corners of the mouth are red, scaly and fissured. Iron and vitamin B deficiencies may have to be ruled out. Treatment consists of refitting dentures and/or addressing the nutritional deficiencies of the individual. Zinc oxide cream or hydrocortisone cream can assist in the healing of the lesion.

Antioxidants and skin ageing

One of the major causes of skin disorders is oxidative damage. The skin is rich in proteins, lipids and DNA; being highly metabolic, it continues to be barraged by oxidative stress such as chemicals and ultraviolet (UV) light throughout life.[12]

Vitamin's C and E are two of the best-known antioxidants. They have been shown to be effective in the prevention and treatment of photoageing. Vitamins C and E have been combined with commercial UV sunscreen (oxybenzone) and one study has shown protection against phototoxic ageing.[13]

UV radiation-induced free-radical formation in a hairless mouse skin has been analysed and evaluated by electron paramagnetic resonance (EPR). The following topically applied antioxidants were applied:

tocopherol sorbate, α-tocopherol and tocopherol acetate. Tocopherol sorbate significantly decreased the UV radiation-induced radical flux of the skin. It was also found to be more protective against skin photoageing than the other topical applications. Tocopherol sorbate as an antioxidant apparently provides some protection against UV-induced damage.[14]

It is becoming evident that photoageing is responsible for development of precancerous lesions or skin cancer. There is good clinical and histological evidence that the skin changes of photoageing can be reversed in some cases by the use of topical retinoids.[15]

Coenzyme Q10 (ubiquinone, CoQ10) levels decline with age. Hoppe *et al.* demonstrated that CoQ10 penetrated into the viable layers of the epidermis and reduced the level of oxidation measured by weak photon emission. There was also a reduction in wrinkle depth following application of CoQ10. The results of this study indicate that CoQ10 may prevent many of the detrimental effects of photoageing.[16]

Recent studies into the structural changes in the telomeric region of the genome have provided new insights into DNA damage mechanisms. This area offers new opportunities to study the molecular mechanisms regulating ageing. In the future, new approaches may be devised to manipulate these molecular events for therapeutic ageing.[17]

Summary

Ageing of the skin is a complex biological process associated with the intrinsic, genetically determined ageing process, as well as extrinsic ageing due to exposure to sunlight. The intrinsic and extrinsic phenomena together affect the sun-exposed areas of skin. This has detrimental effects on the biology of cellular and structural elements of the skin.[18]

Some elderly individuals seem more youthful whereas others seem older than their age. There may be a wide gap between chronological and physiological age. The development of methods to assess physiological ageing is a major concern of gerontology.[6]

The study of the mechanisms involved in skin oxidation and examination of the defence systems may contribute to a better understanding of skin ageing and

of the mechanisms involved in the various pathological processes of the skin. Early recognition, prevention, and treatment of skin disorders by the primary-contact health professional are important elements in the overall care of middle-aged and older patients.

References

1 Seidel H, Ball JW, Dains JE, Benedict GW. Mosby's Guide to Physical Examination. St Louis, MO: Mosby, 1999.
2 Kurban RS, Kurban AK. Common skin disorders of aging: diagnosis and treatment. Geriatrics 1993; 48(4): 30–35.
3 Bates B. A Guide to Physical Examination and History Taking. Philadelphia, PA: JB Lippincott, 1995.
4 Boynton PR, Jaworski D, Paustian C. Meeting the challenges of healing chronic wounds in older adults. Nurs Clin North Am 1999; 34: 921–932, vii.
5 Lonergan ET. Geriatrics: A Lange Clinical Manual. Stamford, CT: Appleton & Lange, 1996.
6 Grove GL. Physiologic changes in older skin. Clin Geriatr Med 1989; 5: 115–125.
7 Ebersole P, Hess P. Toward Healthy Aging. St Louis, MO: Mosby, 1999.
8 Beers MH, Berkow R. The Merck Manual of Diagnosis and Therapy. 17th edn. St Louis, MO: Merck, 1999.
9 Fitzpatrick TB et al. Color Atlas and Synopsis of Clinical Dermatology: Common and Serious Disorders. New York: McGraw-Hill, 1997.
10 Kirsner R et al. Clinical experience with a Human Skin Equivalent for the treatment of venous leg ulcers: process and outcomes. Wounds 1999; 11: 137–144.
11 Seiler WO, Stahelin HB. Decubitus ulcers in geriatrics: pathogenesis, prevention and therapy. Ther Umsch 1991; 48: 329–340.
12 Kohen R. Skin antioxidants: their role in aging and in oxidative stress – new approaches for their evaluation. Biomed Pharmacotherp 1999; 53: 181–192.
13 Darr D, Dunston S, Faust H, Pinnell S. Effectiveness of antioxidants (vitamin C and E) with and without sunscreens as topical photoprotectants. Acta Derm Venereol 1996; 76: 264–268.
14 Jurkiewicz BA, Bissett DL, Buettner GR. Effect of topically applied tocopherol on ultraviolet radiation-mediated free radical damage in skin. J Invest Dermatol 1995; 104: 484–488.
15 Katsambas AD, Katoulis AC. Topical retinoids in the treatment of aging of the skin. Adv Exp Med Biol 1999; 455: 477–482.
16 Hoppe U, Bergemann J, Diembeck W, et al. Coenzyme Q10, a cutaneous antioxidant and energizer. Biofactors 1999; 9: 371–378.
17 West MD. The cellular and molecular biology of aging. Arch Dermatol 1994; 130: 87–95.
18 Uitto J, Bernstein EF. Molecular mechanisms of cutaneous aging: connective tissue alterations in the dermis. J Investi Dermatol Symp Proc 1998; 3: 41–44.

20

Diseases of the thyroid

Irving Rosen and TA Bayley

The thyroid is an endocrine gland which secretes the hormones sodium-L-thyroxine (T_4) and sodium-L-triiodothyronine (T_3) into the circulation, where they travel to many tissues to affect metabolism. The active hormone is T_3. T_4 is converted to T_3 in the peripheral tissues, where it exerts its effect by attaching to receptors in the cell nucleus. Thyroid hormone production of T_4 and T_3 is physiologically under negative feedback regulation from the pituitary gland, which produces thyrotropin (thyroid-stimulating hormone, TSH). This, in turn, is under control of thyrotropin-releasing hormone (TRH) from the hypothalamus.

This chapter will discuss benign thyroid disorders, nodular thyroid disease and malignancy. A brief review is given to provide the practising chiropractor with a basic understanding of thyroid diseases seen in clinical practice, how to suspect and recognize them and how to decide which patients should be referred for more detailed assessment and appropriate therapy. Diseases of the thyroid affect the patient by changes in size, function, or both.

Methods of assessment

Clinical assessment

A history of symptoms of thyroid disease, including a family history, should be obtained. This should be followed by observation and palpation of the neck anteriorly and laterally. Any asymmetry or unusual swelling raises the suspicion of thyroid disease, which should be investigated further by tests of thyroid function.

Diagnostic tests

Thyroid function tests include blood tests, free T_4, free T_3, TSH and thyroid antibodies as well as radionuclide uptake and scans using iodine-131, iodine-123 and technetium-99m-pertechnetate. They are of considerable value in the diagnosis and management of benign thyroid disease, as will be demonstrated later. Ultrasonography is also useful, while fine-needle aspiration biopsy has a more limited use in diffuse than in nodular thyroid disease.

Disorders of thyroid function

It is important for the chiropractor to be aware of the major disorders of thyroid function, hyperthyroidism and hypothyroidism.

Hyperthyroidism (thyrotoxicosis)

Thyrotoxicosis is a disorder caused by excess circulating thyroid hormones. For practical purposes the terms thyrotoxicosis and hyperthyroidism are interchangeable.

Aetiology

Thyrotoxicosis may be due to uncontrolled overproduction of thyroid hormones, as in Graves' disease, toxic adenoma, toxic multinodular goitre and iodine-induced hyperthyroidism, and rarely to other causes such as TSH-secreting pituitary tumours. There are other causes of hyperthyroidism where there is no increased production, but an increased release of thyroid hormones into the circulation due to an inflamed gland, as occurs in transient painless (silent) thyroiditis. In the postpartum state it is known as postpartum thyroiditis. It occurs also in the hyperthyroid phase of a chronic autoimmune thyroiditis (Hashimoto's disease) and in subacute thyroiditis.

More than 90% of cases of hyperthyroidism are due to Graves' disease, in which there is a diffuse overproduction of thyroid hormones by most or all cells of the gland. Hyperthyroidism due to a single nodule or multiple nodules is seen more frequently in elderly people, but is still less common than Graves' disease, even in elderly patients. The prevalence of

Graves' disease overall does not appear to increase with age. This disease is much more common in women than in men, in a ratio of 7:1. Graves' disease is an autoimmune disorder caused by defects in immune surveillance, permitting a forbidden clone of cells, T-lymphocytes, to proliferate and, through a complex series of steps, lead to the production of B-lymphocytes which secrete thyroid-stimulating immunoglobulins (TSI). These immunoglobulins bind to the TSH receptor on the thyroid cell and stimulate an excessive quantity of thyroid hormones.

Other common causes of hyperthyroidism are painless thyroiditis, particularly in its postpartum variant, and less commonly, subacute thyroiditis.

Clinical picture

Symptoms of hyperthyroidism (thyrotoxicosis) include nervousness, irritability, palpitations, heat intolerance and increased sweating, fatigue, shortness of breath, eye complaints, weakness and weight loss despite a good appetite, increased frequency of bowel movements and menstrual irregularities.

On examination, the patient appears restless and may have thyroid enlargement. The heart rate is usually increased. The skin is warm and moist owing to increased sweating. Weakness, particularly of proximal muscles, and weight loss may be evident and there is a fine tremor of the outstretched hands.

The symptoms and signs vary considerably in frequency and severity. In the elderly, the symptoms may be quite mild with only weakness and weight loss, known as apathetic hyperthyroidism. The elderly hyperthyroid patient may present only with atrial fibrillation and congestive heart failure.

Diagnosis

The diagnosis of the different types of thyrotoxicosis (hyperthyroidism) is based on clinical findings and confirmed by laboratory function tests. For example, in Graves' disease, about 50% of patients have a thyroid-associated eye disease in which the patient may have a stare (widening of the palpebral fissures), protrusion of the eyes (proptosis), varying degrees of swelling of the eyelids, and congestion of the scleral and conjunctival vessels. This orbitopathy may also be seen in a few patients without hyperthyroidism and in 3–5% of patients with chronic autoimmune thyroiditis (Hashimoto's disease). The orbitopathy is also an autoimmune disorder associated with antibodies different to those involved in the pathogenesis of the hyperthyroidism. Another autoimmune manifestation occurring in 8% of patients with Graves' disease is an infiltrative dermopathy, pretibial myxoedema, which is a thickening of the skin over the tibiae.

In painless thyroiditis, the thyroid gland is usually normal in size and not tender. In subacute thyroiditis, the patient has significant neck pain and the thyroid gland is quite tender to palpation.

In all patients with thyrotoxicosis, the free T_4 and or free T_3 are elevated and the TSH is fully suppressed. In Graves' disease, the radioiodine uptake is increased and the scan shows a diffusely enlarged hyperactive gland. TSI levels are elevated in active hyperthyroidism but are not usually required for diagnosis. Thyroid autoantibodies, sometimes in significant titre, are also found in patients with Graves' disease. They are, however, non-specific and only confirm the presence of an autoimmune process. They are also found in Hashimoto's disease.

The thyroid scan in a toxic nodular goitre shows 'hot' nodules with greatly increased uptake, while the uptake around the nodules is suppressed. The radioiodine uptake in hyperthyroidism due to thyroiditis is low and there is very low uptake in the scan.

Treatment

Rest, sedation, good nutrition and β-adrenergic blocking agents such as propranolol are useful in all types of thyrotoxicosis.

There is no specific therapy for the underlying hyperthyroidism of Graves' disease, a genetically determined autoimmune disorder. The clinical manifestations, however, can be well controlled. The thionamides, propylthiouracil or methimazole, block the synthesis of thyroid hormones and the patient returns to the euthyroid state on average in 6–9 weeks. These drugs are useful in patients with mild disease and small goitres. Overall, less than 50% of patients who have been treated with thionamides for 1.5–2 years remain in long-term remission. Therefore, the persisting thyrotoxicosis must be treated by thyroidectomy or thyroid cells destroyed with radioactive iodine using [^{131}I]sodium iodide. Radioactive iodine is the most convenient treatment for most adult patients. The only major long-term effect is the rising incidence of hypothyroidism, about 50% in 5 years. There may be some worsening of the orbitopathy, which can be prevented or lessened by glucocorticoid therapy with prednisone for 2 months.

In thyrotoxicosis due to nodular thyroid disease, the thyrotoxicosis will never go into long-term remission with antithyroid drugs alone. Antithyroid drugs are useful to bring the patients to the euthyroid state. They can then be treated by thyroidectomy or with radioiodine.

The hyperthyroidism associated with painless thyroiditis is usually mild and transient lasting from 3 weeks to 3 months. The symptoms and signs can usually be controlled with rest, sedation and propranolol. Usually the patients return to normal, after first going through a hypothyroid phase. Since this is an autoimmune disorder, some patients may go on to develop persistent thyrotoxicosis due to Graves' disease. In subacute thyroiditis, glucocorticoids starting with 20–40 mg prednisone are quite valuable in controlling quickly the symptoms and signs, particularly the acute and sometimes severe neck pain and tenderness. Treatment with decreasing doses, but enough to control symptoms, is usually used for up to 12 weeks. For iodine-induced hyperthyroidism, exogenous iodides have to be stopped immediately if iodides have precipitated the thyrotoxicosis. For patients with underlying Graves' disease or toxic nodular goitre the symptoms may subside but the other usual therapeutic agents may also have to be given. One unusual form of iodine-induced hyperthyroidism due to amiodarone is now being seen more frequently with the increasing use of this drug in patients with cardiac disease. Stopping the drug may not lead to alleviation of the hyperthyroidism. The organic iodine in the amiodarone molecule persists for many months in the body. In some patients it leads to an inflammatory process in the thyroid with increased release of thyroid hormones into the circulation for a long time. Methimazole in large doses of 40 mg daily has been useful. In severe cases of thyrotoxicosis which cannot be controlled, total thyroidectomy has to be performed.

Hypothyroidism

Hypothyroidism is due to an inability of the thyroid gland to produce an adequate supply of thyroid hormones for the body's needs.

Aetiology

The aetiology of hypothyroidism may be primary due to a disorder in the thyroid gland, secondary due to disease of the pituitary gland with decreased TSH, or tertiary due to hypothalamic dysfunction with a decrease in TRH. There may also be resistance to the action of thyroid hormone. The last two categories are rare. Primary hypothyroidism occurs in 95% of cases. Secondary and tertiary hypothyroidism and resistance to thyroid hormone action make up the other 5%.

The most common causes of primary hypothyroidism are chronic autoimmune thyroiditis (Hashimoto's disease), thyroidectomy for Graves' disease or malignancy, radioiodine therapy for Graves' disease, the late phase of a painless thyroiditis or subacute thyroiditis and excess iodine ingestion, including amiodarone. Iodine deficiency as a cause for hypothyroidism is rare in North America but quite common in many areas of the world where there is a deficiency in the iodine required in the synthesis of thyroid hormone. This results also in hypothyroidism at birth and infancy (cretinism). Other antithyroid drugs and congenital defects in thyroid hormone synthesis are quite rare causes of hypothyroidism. Secondary hypothyroidism is due to hypopituitism with destruction of TSH and other pituitary hormones by a pituitary tumour, ablative therapy or intrinsic pituitary disease. These aetiologies also occur in the rare tertiary hypothalamic hypothyroidism.

Clinical picture

Symptoms and signs are related to the severity of the deficiency of the thyroid hormone secretion, which can affect practically all systems in the body in which there is slowing of metabolic processes. In the adult the common symptoms are fatigue, intolerance to cold, dry skin, lethargy, slowing of intellectual function, with impairment of memory, constipation, gain in weight, muscle cramps, weakness, prolonged menses in women and deafness.

On examination, the physical findings include puffiness of the face and eyes, thickened, dry cool skin and non-pitting oedema. The hair is dry and brittle. The thyroid gland varies from being not palpable to a large goitre. The heart may be enlarged owing to an effusion into the pericardium. The heart rate may be slow. There is a decreased cardiac output with increased peripheral resistance. As a result, blood pressure may be elevated. The intellectual function is slowed. There are defects in memory and lethargy. Psychiatric disorders may occur, associated with depression and paranoia. There is a delay in the relaxation phase of the deep tendon reflexes. The full-blown clinical picture of hypothyroidism is known as primary myxoedema. Untreated patients with severe myxoedema go into a coma and die.

Spontaneously occurring hypothyroidism, mainly chronic autoimmune thyroiditis, increases with age and is most prevalent in elderly women, who have varying degrees of hypothyroidism with a prevalence of up to 15%. It can be difficult clinically to recognize hypothyroidism in the elderly. Some of the symptoms of hypothyroidism such as intolerance to cold, gain in weight, constipation, and slowing of mental and physical function in hypothyroidism may also be due to ageing and degenerative diseases, and the hypothyroidism can be mild.

In contrast, hypothyroidism may be present at birth, or occur in infancy and or childhood. Neonatal hypothyroidism is now detected in North America and other well-developed countries by neonatal screening programmes: 1 in 4000 live births will have an elevated TSH, indicative of primary neonatal hypothyroidism. Such infants must be treated immediately to prevent severe mental retardation and other abnormalities of growth and development. Children with hypothyroidism present with retarded growth and sometimes mental retardation.

Diagnostic tests

In primary hypothyroidism, the free T_4 is normal or low and TSH is always elevated. In secondary and tertiary hypothyroidism, TSH is normal or low and free T_4 is also normal or low. Increases in serum thyroglobulin and serum microsomal (peroxidase) antibodies are seen in patients with chronic autoimmune thyroiditis (Hashimoto's disease). Very high levels of antibodies are diagnostic of Hashimoto's disease; however, antibody levels are not elevated in all patients.

Treatment

Hypothyroidism can be effectively treated and fully controlled in practically all patients by replacement thyroid hormones. T_4 is used, since it has a prolonged effect with a half-life of 8 days and produces stable levels of thyroid hormone. The administered T_4 is also converted into T_3, the active hormone, and both are present in the circulation. The mean replacement dose of T_4 is 1.6 µg/kg of ideal body weight. The replacement dose of T_4 is increased gradually until the symptoms and signs of hypothyroidism are controlled, the free T_4 is normalized and on the most sensitive test TSH falls into the normal range and optimally to the mean level seen in the normal population, which is 1.6 mU/l. In older patients, the dose of T_4 has to be increased very slowly, starting with a dose as low as 12.5 µg. This dose is increased by the same amount every 6 weeks.

The total dose needed to control elderly patients is less than in younger patients (75–100 µg daily), whereas in young women the mean daily dose is 110 µg and in young men 125 µg.

Pregnancy is a special situation. Pregnant women with known hypothyroidism should be monitored at the beginning of pregnancy and every 2–3 months since the dose of thyroid hormone infrequently has to be increased to meet the increased metabolic needs of that state. It is important that the hypothyroidism be well controlled in pregnancy. Mothers with subclinical hypothyroidism, i.e. a normal free T_4 and even a slightly elevated TSH, should be treated. There is new evidence that even very mild degrees of hypothyroidism in the mother can produce a significant decrease in the intellectual function of the child. In early foetal life, the foetus receives at least half of its thyroid hormone requirement from the mother. Therefore, a mild deficiency of thyroid hormone supply in the mother can affect the foetus and result in adverse outcomes.

Thyroid nodular disease

Nodular disease of the thyroid gland (TND) that is detectable by palpation affects 5% of the North American population; if one were to include those nodules that are detected by ultrasonographic examination, 50% of patients would be affected. It is therefore apparent that a chiropractor who examines or palpates a patient's neck is bound to come across TND and in that way is in a position to influence appropriate management. Furthermore, what may be construed as a solitary nodular thyroid gland (TND) proves in over 70% of cases to be a multicentric nodular involvement of the thyroid gland. The differential diagnosis of TND can be separated into non-neoplastic and neoplastic causes. The non-neoplastic group includes:

- colloid nodule
- nodular hyperplasia
- thyroiditis that includes a subacute or DeCuervain chronic or Hashimoto's disease, acute or abscess
- cyst formation of an underlying benign nodule
- nodule associated with Graves' toxic disease
- toxic nodular goitre
- thyroid fibrosis secondary to radioactive iodine or radiation
- Reidel's struma.

Neoplastic disease can be divided into benign and malignant. The benign variety includes:

- adenoma
- cystadenoma.

Malignent carcinoma includes:

- papillary carcinoma, which is the most common malignancy
- follicular carcinoma
- Hurthle cell carcinoma
- lymphoma
- anaplastic cancer
- sarcoma
- cancer metastatic to the thyroid gland.

Certain factors favour the formation of TND. These include age, with 50% of men and women in the sixth decade having TND, in contrast to approximately 1% of children not exposed to radiation having TND. Almost twice as many women as men are diagnosed with TND. Other factors need to be recognized. Patients who have undergone radiation to the head and neck area for treatment of benign conditions are of particular concern, but so are patients who have had radiation for malignant disease elsewhere. In about 40% of postradiation cases, the occurrence of nodule formation can be detected. Women are up to two to three times more likely to develop such nodules than men following radiation. Furthermore, radiation has a particular association as a cause for thyroid cancer. In clinical solitary nodules of the thyroid gland with a history of radiation, the frequency is approximately 60%, compared with 30% in people without a history of radiation exposure. Pregnancy and the history of parturition also favour the occurrence of TND and cancer. Certain dietary conditions such as a lack of iron and the ingestion of goitrogenic food stuffs favour TND. Hyperparathyroidism is associated in 50% of cases with TND, although the results of strictly controlled studies have been equivocal.

Family history

A familial incidence of TND is common, whereas a family history of thyroid carcinoma is uncommon except in the infrequent type called medullary cancer. Patients with adenomatous polypi of the colon may have concurrent thyroid disease, which used to be termed Gardiner's syndrome. Several other endocrinological syndromes feature TND, such as Penderith's syndrome. Currently, thyroid

cancer represents the fastest growing malignancy in females and the second fastest growing malignancy in men, according to the 2000 statistical survey issued by the Canadian Cancer Society. This illustrates the need for assessment of TND patients.

Methods of assessment

Thyroid function tests are blood tests that include TSH, free T_4, free T_3 and thyroid antibodies which are essential in the assessment of the patient's thyroid function status with regard to hyperthyroidism or hypothyroidism, as well as the possibility of thyroiditis. Patients who are in an uncontrolled overproductive state are not safe candidates for surgical treatment. Surgery in a patient who is uncontrollably hyperthyroid may induce a thyrotoxic crisis. Similarly, hypothyroid patients do not tolerate surgery as well as euthyroid patients and require prior correction if possible. Thyroid functional status therefore is mandated prior to any active surgical treatment, but it cannot distinguish pathology. Thyroid antibodies can be elevated in chronic thyroiditis. Basal serum calcitonin can be elevated in medullary thyroid cancer. The expense and complexity of this test discourage its routine use.

Radionuclide uptake and scanning

Uptake and scanning by radionuclide is a standard thyroid assessment. The usual isotope that is utilized is technetium-99m, although others such as iodine-131 are also used. Uptake gives a measure of thyroid function. Scanning will divide TND into cold and hot nodules. Congenital abnormalities may also occur. Thirty per cent of cold nodules are associated with malignancy and are certainly construed in that hot nodules are associated with an overfunctioning nodule and not considered as a usual site for cancerous change. Scanning can also demonstrate a substernal goitre and the presence of functioning metastatic thyroid cancer elsewhere in the body. Thyroid scans are not frequently performed in the USA because of controversy, expense and a lack of direct information. Scanning has therefore been downgraded as a diagnostic test but is still of relevance. Its diagnostic implications are limited but have an indirect quality.

Ultrasonography

The projection of ultrasonic sound and its reflection by tissue planes within a mass produce an image of echoes or lack of echoes producing a visible image that can be used in various ways. Sound frequencies range between 5 and 10×10^6 MHz above the range of human hearing. This is a painless and simple test to perform. While some feel that it may provide information regarding the underlying histological nature of a nodule, this is not a commonly accepted phenomenon. Characteristic patterns for multinodular goitre and thyroiditis as well as cancer and basic properties can be distinguished. Essentially, ultrasonography can recognize solid and cystic lesions, again with an indirect implication as far as pathology is concerned, since cystic lesions are less likely to be malignant, but too rigid an acceptance of this phenomenon will turn out to be misleading. False reporting occurs in about 30% of cases, in both a positive and a negative way. Its chief virtues lies in the detection of impalpable nodularity, demonstration of cervical nodal metastatic disease, response of thyroid nodule size to medical treatment and fine-needle aspiration biopsy of occult, obscure or clinically negative aspiration. Other imaging techniques can be used such as computed tomographic (CT) scans and magnetic resonance imaging. This is beyond the scope of this chapter, but in the assessment of common TND this is not a necessary manoeuvre and its expense seems unwarranted.

Fine-needle aspiration

This is the most effective assessment short of operative removal for surgical pathology. This technique is carried out clinically in an office situation, frequently using local anaesthesia. In some clinics local anaesthesia is not used, but it is used frequently. A 10–20 ml syringe is attached to a needle varying in calibre from 22 to 25, but an even larger needle can be used. The needle is then advanced into the nodule and aspiration takes place. Usually a small amount of blood-stained material fills the hub of the needle and a portion of the syringe, which is then usually expressed as in a blood culture and smeared for Papanicolaou staining as well as being placed in an alcohol-containing medium for centrifugation and cytological examination. The cytological interpretation can include cancer or suspected cancer, which is described as either nuclear atypia, follicular or cellular lesions, and cytology can also describe a colloid nodule which is highly benign, thyroiditis or inadequate aspirate, particularly in a cystic lesion or where there is not very much nuclear detail. False-positive and false-negative aspirates do occur, and repeat needle biopsies are part of a patient's assessment. Fine-needle aspiration biopsies have the virtue of being easy, with a lack of significant morbidity, patient acceptability, relative reliability and accuracy. They are far more specific than other diagnostic tests. Other forms of needle biopsy are available, such as coarse-needle biopsy or Vim–Silverman biopsy, which will produce histological rather than cytological sections. Efforts to improve the reliability of cytological results include the use of monoclonal markers, but nothing is currently of widespread use in thyroid cytology.

Clinical presentation

TND classically presents with a lump in the thyroid gland that may be solitary or multiple. In about 90% of patients, it is unassociated with any pressure symptoms, but it can cause dysphagia, dysphonia and respiratory distress, and is significant particularly if the patient has been taking a TSH suppressive dose of thyroxine. This stimulates concern in the clinician that there is an underlying tumour. However, this does not necessarily mean that a growing lesion is a malignant situation. Acute painful swelling of the thyroid is usually associated with degeneration of the lesion and cyst formation, which can show a spontaneous decrease in size and resolution. Needle biopsy of a thyroid nodule may be followed on occasion by its heamorrhagic infarction and disappearance. The presence of lateral nodules in the neck may signal the occurrence of cancer due to metastatic malignant disease. Currently, there is a greater appreciation of the implications accompanying thyroid nodules, some of which may turn out to be a significant problem in the diagnosis of tumour malignancy. Where functional abnormalities are associated with nodular disease, the patient may have a set of symptoms that were described in the sections on hyperthyroidism and hypothyroidism. Aggressive thyroid cancer shows alarming signs, particularly with the findings of tissue fixation or nodule hardness. In such a situation, one must be concerned about the presence of an anaplastic cancer, which is a very serious form of malignancy with a particularly poor outcome.

Indications for surgical treatment include:

- cytology: the presence of cancer
- cytology: the presence of suspected cancer such as cellular atypia or follicular lesion
- pressure symptoms
- growth: particularly if the patient is on TSH suppressive thyroxine
- a toxic nodular goitre
- Graves' disease with nodular formation

- request by the patient because of anxiety
- failure of medical treatment.

Treatment can either conservative or surgical. Conservative treatment involves the utilization of thyroxine as a growth suppressant or the use of antithyroid drug in hyperthyroidism. The thyroid suppressive effect of thyroxine is effective in only one-third of patients so treated and is usually a disappointing modality in most patients' management. Other conservative measures include intralesional injections of alcohol, which are not widely accepted in North America. Repeated aspiration of thyroid cyst formation usually leads to surgical treatment because of a 30% incidence of cancer. The surgical technique varies between a partial thyroidectomy, namely a lobe, and a total or near-total thyroidectomy. Complications include injury to the recurrent nerve, producing voice deficits, and injury to the parathyroid gland, which may be apparent only in a total thyroidectomy. Haematomas, wound infections and problems with healing are other problems. Thyroid cancer is currently treated by near-total or total thyroidectomy, supplemented by radioactive iodine ablation and on infrequent occasions by external radiation. The survival rates are superb. Tumours with disease such as medullary cancer, lymphoma and anaplastic cancer have a far poorer prognosis and are better treated by radiation with or without chemotherapy.

Diseases of the parathyroid

Attached to, but not part of the thyroid gland are usually four small glands, about 5 mm in size and weighing less than 30 mg, which control calcium metabolism. Their dysfunction is usually manifested by overfunction and has become a markedly increasing phenomenon. One or more of these glands can enlarge and produce an excess of parathyroid hormone (normal 1–5). This in turn leads to an increase in calcium (normal 2.2–2.6 mmol/l) which is derived from calcium within bone. This is known as primary hyperparathyroidism and is usually idiopathic, although on occasion it can be caused by familial genetic multiendocrinopathies (MEA-1 and -2 syndromes) or exposure to radiation. In most cases the cause is unknown. This also leads to an increase in urinary calcium. Its manifestations can be rather subtle but classically include:

- body pain affecting all joints of the body which defies easy analgesia
- diffuse osteoporosis
- decrease in height
- pathological fracture
- punctate lytic lesions of bone, known as Von Recklinghausen's disease, that can be mistaken on X-rays for metastatic disease
- renal calculi with abdominal and back pain
- renal failure secondary to calculus obstruction of the genitourinary tract
- hypertension and its consequent vascular degenerative disease
- profound fatigue
- abdominal pain of apparent unknown origin
- gallstones and their consequences
- acute pancreatitis
- oesophagitis manifested by heartburn
- intractable duodenal ulcer and its complications.

Detection lies in a simple blood estimation of serum calcium and parathyroid hormone levels. In dealing with patients with complaints of body aches and pains, a simple blood test can be appropriately diagnostic. Curative treatment lies in surgical excision of one or more parathyroid glands. This is well tolerated by the patient because the surgical treatment is relatively simple, consisting of a night or less in hospital. If patients show symptoms that are too extensive, then the benefit of parathyroidectomy is minimized. Malignancy occurs in 0.5–2% of patients, with adenoma in about 85% and hyperplasia in about 15%. Diagnosis of this condition can lead to appropriate treatment and prevention of dire complications.

Summary

Diseases of the thyroid and parathyroid glands may be elusive to detection since the symptomatology is often subtle and non-specific. Awareness of these problems by health professionals managing patients with these conditions is mandatory. The diagnosis is often made by a routine blood screen consisting of thyroid hormone estimations and serum calcium, as well as parathyroid hormone estimation. The benefits to the patient are incalculable.

21

Sleep and the elderly

Jaan Reitav and Jodi B Dickstein

The elderly person is confronted with a great number of challenges in life at a time when their capacity to manage those challenges, as well as their physical resilience, are gradually ebbing. Their bodies and their physiology are changing in ways that compromise their sleep patterns and reduce their daytime adaptability in meeting the challenges of life. These circumstances are progressive and irreversible, and therefore profound in their impact on many elderly persons.

In the face of these challenges, there is much that a well-informed and skilled health provider can do, yet many health-care providers have had little training in the specific challenges raised by patients with sleep problems. Questions abound: what would be considered a normal sleep pattern for older people? How is their sleep different from that of younger people? Is it true that they need less sleep? What emotional reactions are found among those who are most worried about their poor sleep? How would a clinician know whether their disrupted sleep pattern is negatively impacting their pain problem? How does this affect their family? What can a primary health-care provider do to help? And, finally, how can these perspectives be integrated into a clinical setting?

In 1990 the National Institutes of Health Consensus Development Conference on Sleep Disorders in Late Life[1] set a priority on preserving the integrity of sleep for as long as possible as a major public-health priority. However, meeting this goal requires that health-care providers attain an understanding of what needs to be done and what can be done, and develop clinical skills in accomplishing this goal with their patients. We hope that this chapter helps to accomplish these objectives. Although it has been written with chiropractors in mind, most of the discussion applies to any primary health-care provider.

The health-care provider who is able to help an elderly patient understand their sleep patterns, and make realistic adjustments in when and how they sleep, will be addressing these issues effectively and have a very appreciative patient. This chapter aims to provide all primary health-care providers with clinical knowledge, organized into five main sections: (i) description of the changes that happen to sleep with normal ageing; (ii) orientation to clinical evaluation of sleep problems; (iii) evaluation of specific conditions which must be screened for referral; (iv) clinical management strategies and interventions for the alternative health-care provider to improve the sleep of the elderly and (v) discussion of additional resources to turn to for more information.

This chapter is grounded in the scientific research into sleep which has occurred since the 1960s. However, its focus will be on managing the sleep complaints of elderly patients and providing a context in which to understand and treat their sleep problems.

Changes in sleep patterns with ageing

One way in which ageing changes the body's adaptability is by gradually, and persistently, restricting its ability to have a restorative night of sleep. Many older patients are aware of this, and increasing numbers begin to worry about their sleep. Sleep disruption causes wide-ranging impact on functioning, including physiological desynchronization, psychological distress, physical fatigue and cognitive distractibility. Sleep becomes more difficult to initiate and maintain with increasing age, and often results in a pattern of daytime napping as compensation. Understanding the nature of the sleep characteristics of these patients is fundamental to assisting them with the challenges that they face.

Ultradian rhythms of sleep stages

Sleep is a neurobehavioural state controlled by the central nervous system (CNS) acting in co-ordination with important organ systems. Sleep stages are therefore measured with all-night polysomnography of the electrical activity in the brain.[2] This consists of placing electroencephalogram (EEG) leads on the head, eyes and chin, and classifying the patterns into wakefulness, four stages of non-rapid eye movement (NREM) sleep, and stage REM (dreaming) sleep. Across the night brain waves shift back and forth through these sleep stages in the general manner indicated in Figure 21.1. Within these random shifts are ultradian rhythms lasting for 90–100 min, with each one usually being punctuated by a REM period.

On any given night the sequence of the stages, their duration and the total amount of time spent in each will vary. Nevertheless, the ultradian rhythms will tend to continue throughout the sleep period. Deep sleep or slow-wave sleep (SWS), which occurs in stages 3 and 4, will occur predominantly towards the beginning of the night. More of the REM sleep will occur at the end of the night. It is typical for all sleepers to awaken during the night. Young adult sleepers will wake up about twice a night. Good sleepers fall back to sleep within minutes, and will often not recall the night-time waking in the morning.

Age-related changes in sleep parameters suggest a flattening of the sleep–wake rhythm (as indicated in Figure 21.2). The amount of SWS (stages 3 and 4) declines from about 25% during the early adult years, to virtually disappearing by the mid-seventies.[3] This results in more of the sleep period being spent in very light (stage 1 or 2) sleep. This, in turn, means that the

elderly person is more easily awakened by noises and other environmental factors which previously had not disrupted sleep.[4] The average 65-year-old can wake up as many as five times a night, and frequently experiences problems getting back to sleep quickly. This results in a significant decrease in sleep efficiency from about 95% in the early adult years to under 80% by the seventies,[5] as well as more dissatisfaction with the quality of sleep.

These radical reductions in sleep efficiency are not due to a decrease in the need to sleep. In the face of decreasing night-time sleep efficiencies, most elderly people find themselves moving towards a pattern of daytime naps, to compensate for the poorer night-time sleep. In advanced age the ability to sleep, but not the necessity for sleep, is diminished.[6–8]

Reynolds et al.[9] noted that the REM sleep of older patients with major depression comorbid with Alzheimer's dementia showed no REM rebound (an increase in REM in the first night after a night of sleep deprivation), suggesting diminished physiological resilience and plasticity among this group. They concluded that successful adaptation in late life for healthy elderly people is most likely associated with stable preservation of REM sleep, rather than the number of wakenings, sleep efficiency or amount of delta sleep. Reynolds also noted the stability of REM sleep in elderly who can be described as ageing 'successfully' and proposed that REM sleep be considered the best marker, or correlate, of successful adaptation in late life.

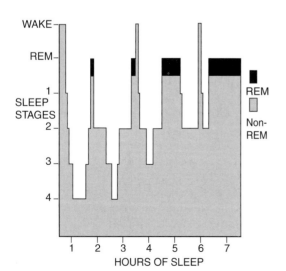

Figure 21.1 Sleep across a single night for young adults.

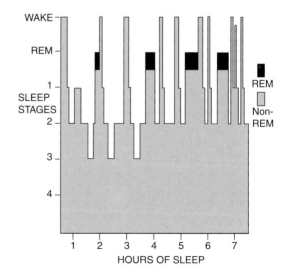

Figure 21.2 Sleep across a single night for the elderly.

Three stages of deterioration in sleep

A recent study by Van Cauter et al.[10] set out to determine the chronology of changes in sleep stages across late life. They found that there were two stages in the deterioration of sleep. The first stage, or midlife transition, occurs up the age of 50. There is a sharp reduction in the amount of stage 3 and 4 slow wave (SWS) sleep, from nearly 20% to under 5% of the total sleep time. The loss of SW delta sleep was compensated by an increase in light sleep (stages 1 and 2). Total sleep time did not change, nor was there any change in REM sleep.

The second stage, occurring from the patient's fifties to their eighties, was termed the late-life transition. It saw no further deterioration in SWS, but a fragmentation of sleep involving an increase in awake time of 27 min for every decade aged. Most of the lost sleep was at the expense of the light sleep (loss of 24 min per decade), but some was also due to reductions in REM sleep (loss of 10 min per decade). The resulting sleep profile of the average elderly person in late life is illustrated in Figure 21.2 The features of the sleep pattern include reduced or absent SWS, about five awakenings a night and a predominance of light sleep throughout most of the sleep period.

Results from an earlier study support the late-life transition stage in sleep continuity deterioration, but suggest that good sleep patterns can be maintained for longer. Hoch[11] followed subjective and polysomnographically defined sleep quality longitudinally for over 3 years among 50 elderly persons between 60 and 87 years of age. All subjects were carefully screened for medical and psychiatric status. In this cohort, subjective sleep quality, sleep continuity and SWS remained stable in subjects younger than 75, but diminished in the subjects 75 years and older.

The Van Cauter study has signalled a significant new development in understanding sleep in the elderly, namely, the highlighting of important substages within the overall gradual deterioration of sleep with ageing. To the two stages highlighted by Van Cauter a third must be considered: the transition back to a polycyclical, dysregulated sleep pattern, similar to patterns observed in infancy, which exhibit no effective circadian competency, or rhythmicity.[3,12]

Many demented patients experience extended sleep periods during the day and lengthy periods of wakefulness during the night.[13,14] Sleep patterns of these patients have lost their entrained circadian rhythms and have become totally disrupted, with nocturnal agitation occurring in the most serious cases. Causes for the latter can include loss of regular social interactions, anatomical deterioration of the suprachiasmatic nucleus (SCN), sleep apnoea, REM-related parasomnias, low ambient light and cold sensitivity.[3]

A recent study compared the sleep and wakefulness patterns of mild to moderately demented individuals with those of severely demented individuals.[14] The number of minutes spent asleep or awake for every hour across one 24 h period was measured. An hour was categorized as 'sleep' when greater than 90% of the time was spent asleep, and categorized as 'wakefulness' when greater than 90% of the time was spent awake. There were significant differences between the two groups in 13 of the 24 periods of 1 h, suggesting that progression of illness is paralleled by a progressive disruption of circadian rhythms. Both groups demonstrated wakefulness during the night, while the more severely demented showed a disproportionate amount of sleepiness during the day and night. There were differences between groups in total time sleeping, although the number of awakenings at night and number of naps during the day were not different for the two groups. The study concluded that with progression of dementia, both the capacity to maintain sleep at night and the capacity to maintain wakefulness during daytime are both impaired, and that this reflects changes in mental status rather than age per se.

What is not clear is the extent to which healthy older persons, even ones in their nineties and older, can maintain a relatively stable circadian sleep pattern, without the development of polycyclical characteristics. Future research will determine whether this third stage is entirely pathognomonic, or whether it comes to eventually define the sleep of all 'old old' elderly persons.

Circadian rhythms and endocrine functions

The circadian clock in humans is timed by the SCN, a group of cells within the hypothalamus.[15] Sensory information is obtained from the retina and passed on to the pineal gland, where melatonin is secreted. The SCN also triggers a neuroendocrine response in the hypothalamus, which then acts on the pituitary. This last pathway profoundly influences endocrine, immune, cardiovascular, and urinary systems.[15] Some of the hormones influenced by the circadian system include growth hormone (GH) and adrenocorticotropic hormone (ACTH). The latter causes the adrenal glands to release cortisol and aldosterone. With age, the body's ability to secrete adequate amounts of these substances is impaired.

The timings of the endocrine and immune systems are clearly intermeshed, as aldosterone and cortisol suppress the immune system, while melatonin appears to enhance it.[12] Sleep deprivation results in activation of the first line of host defence.[16] However, animal studies have shown that host defence fails during prolonged sleep deprivation. The existence of this link means that chronic disturbance in sleep processes can become critical to physical health concerns.[16] Researchers are just beginning to understand the ways in which sleep deprivation affects the immune system.

The circadian rhythm is also gradually disrupted by ageing, as underlying endogenous rhythms such as internal temperature, GH secretion and melatonin levels are attenuated, while insulin production increases.[12] Figure 21.3 shows the age-related changes in the circadian cycle of core body temperature. For young adults, sleep onset and continuity are facilitated by a marked decrease in temperature. Compared with young adults, the older person's temperature cycle is different in three ways: (i) the temperature begins to drop earlier in the night; (ii) the total decrease in temperature during the middle of the night is less than observed for younger sleepers; and (iii) the temperature begins to rise earlier in the morning. These changes are linked directly with corresponding changes in sleep. The older person will feel drowsy earlier in the evening, describe their sleep as much lighter than when they were young and have great difficulty sleeping in the morning.[17]

The Van Cauter[10] study also examined changes in the levels of endocrine activity, by tracking the release of GH and cortisol levels around the 24 h period. They observed a radical decrease in GH release: both in the total amount released across the 24 h period, as well as in the disappearance of the entrained circadian 'spike' occurring just after sleep onset (see Figure 21.4). The relative deficiency of GH among the elderly is associated with increased fatty tissue and abdominal obesity, reduced muscle mass and strength, and reduced exercise capacity.[18] Van Cauter et al.[10] found that reductions in secretion of GH paralleled the decreases in SWS, and postulated that both are governed by a common mechanism. Furthermore, in men it would appear that this mechanism, termed the somatotropic axis, is in decline as early as during the transition into midlife.

Rowe and Troen[19] stated that old age represented a hyperadrenergic state and noted that sympathetic overactivity resulted in changes in cardiovascular reflex, galvanic skin response and pupillary response. Furthermore, this overactive sympathetic nervous system (SNS) has also been thought to interfere with cognitive functions.

Van Cauter also noted that cortisol production is under the influence of another endocrine subsystem,

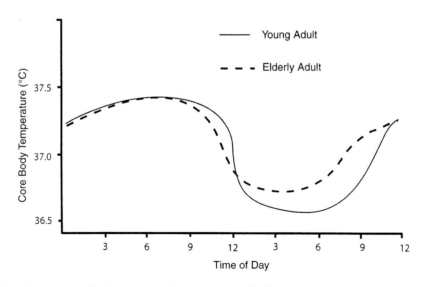

Figure 21.3 Circadian changes in body temperature for the young and old.

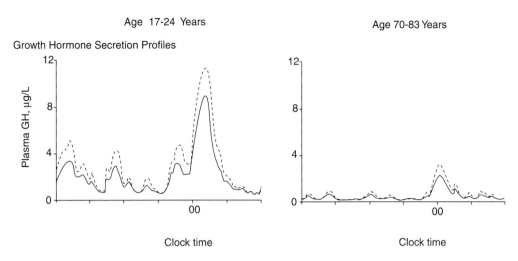

Figure 21.4 Sleep across a single night for young and elderly adults. Reprinted by permission of JAMA.[10]

called the corticotropic axis, which is tied in with circadian rhythmicity.[10] Circadian rhythmicity plays an important part in timing and consolidating sleep, and in the distribution of REM sleep. It is governed by the SCN. An evening elevation in cortisol is considered a hallmark of ageing and is thought to be implicated in the development of memory deficits associated with glucocorticoid excess, as well as in promoting further sleep fragmentation. Van Cauter *et al.* found that elevations in the levels of cortisol were noted in the transition from midlife (fifties) to late life (eighties), but not before, and were related to a progressive deterioration of sleep continuity.[10]

The above descriptions of developments in sleep patterns of the elderly are meant to provide an outline of recent discoveries in a still dimly understood area. For example, it must be remembered that the Van Cauter study was with men only, and the results for women could well differ in important ways.[20] Although the study investigated a cohort of 149 healthy men, only 12 were from the decade 71–80 years old and none was any older. Therefore, much further work needs to be done in clarifying the resilience of these physiological processes, and how it might be assisted.

Although the mechanism responsible for these changes is not entirely clear, some likely contributing processes have been identified. Regarding circadian rhythms it is thought that the SCN, which functions as the circadian pacemaker, shrinks as a function of age, possibly attenuating its effectiveness.[21] However, other factors related to use of these systems could also

be involved. Changes in behavioural patterns, such as activity levels and exposure to sunshine, could also moderate or exacerbate these age-related changes.[22] Although it is widely known that not everyone deteriorates at the same speed, what is not known is why some deteriorate slowly and others more rapidly; nor is it known how much these inevitable changes can be altered by lifestyle modifications such as increased social interaction and activity during the daytime.[23]

To summarize, there is ample evidence that circadian rhythms are dampened and advanced in older adults.[24] The most dramatic change is the flattening of the amplitude. This is evident in complaints of a reduction in night-time sleep quality, combined with complaints of reduced daytime alertness. In some elderly, an advance in sleep phase may be seen. This is evident from complaints of being very tired earlier at night, but if the person goes to sleep at this earlier time, they wake up much earlier, usually in the middle of the night. Still other elderly people may have a shortening of the circadian periodicity or a desynchronization of sleep rhythms; in both instances the patient will report a vacillating pattern of good and poor sleep.

The challenge of successful ageing

Within this environment of deterioration in the underlying physiological mechanisms that enable sleep, it is no surprise that correspondingly greater numbers of elderly people report clinically significant problems with sleep, daytime fatigue and, increasingly, physical illness and depressive affect. However, the inevitability of these changes does not imply that nothing can be done about these processes. Rowe and Kahn[25] make the distinction between 'normal' ageing and 'successful' ageing. This distinction is familiar to all chiropractors with a wellness-orientated practice. Rowe and Kahn emphasize the importance of making efforts to optimize the individual's adaptation to the inevitable physiological changes of ageing, which have been described. The central question of how to evaluate clinically the seriousness of a sleep problem is addressed in the next section.

Evaluation of sleep problems

Sleep complaints

Sleep problems among the elderly are ubiquitous and in many cases reflective of normal ageing. Every health-care provider will have to develop a plan for screening the seriousness of sleep problems, as well as determining their cause in the young and old alike. Many practitioners will also want to help the patient, either with education or by providing advice on improving sleep patterns. This section will acquaint the health-care provider with the assessment procedures necessary to meet the challenge of diagnosing the elderly patient's sleep problem.

How serious must a sleep problem be for one to consider it a clinical problem? The clinical criteria for insomnia generally can be considered to be longer than a 30 min sleep latency, total sleep of less than 6.5 h, or sleep efficiency of less than 85%. To diagnose insomnia these disruptions should occur on at least three nights out of seven. However, using only these sleep time criteria almost every elderly patient will be diagnosed with clinical insomnia. A better clinical rule of thumb for older patients is at least 2 h of sleep loss during the nightly bedtime period. Simon and VonKorff[26] have shown that about 10% of all adult patients presenting at a primary-care setting will meet this criterion, and that these patients usually have higher levels of functional impairment and medical utilization than do patients without insomnia.

There is evidence that self-reporting of sleep and wake times at night is different from the objective measures of sleep obtained by polysomnography, which are traditionally used to establish insomnia.[27] Only polysomnography was able to identify primary sleep disorders in their cohort (discussed in next section), even after subjects were screened for these disorders on the basis of questionnaires and interviews. The researchers recommended that more extensive use of polysomnography be incorporated into routine evaluations of the elderly.

Also interesting is a recent study by Lichstein et al.[28] which found that fatigue is very common among sleep-disordered patients, but that it is not the same thing as daytime sleepiness. The authors administered the Fatigue Severity Scale to over 200 adult patients of all ages attending at a sleep disorders clinic. Fatigue was present in a broad range of sleep disorders but was not related to daytime sleepiness, as measured by the multiple sleep latencies test. The authors identified a number of variables that predicted reports of fatigue, including being female, being a smoker, high body mass index (BMI), low sleep efficiency percentage and high ratings of psychological distress as measured by clinical elevations on the Minnesota Multiphasic Personality Inventory (MMPI).[28] Clinical evaluation of sleep should therefore explore sleep disruption, daytime sleepiness and fatigue independently.

A recent study by Ohayon et al.[29] found that as many as one-third of the general population meet the clinical criteria for insomnia, but as many as three-quarters of these report no sleep dissatisfaction. They concluded that sleep dissatisfaction is a necessary indicator of sleep pathology. The reports published by Ohayon[29–31] underline the puzzling fact that subjective and objective reports of sleep disturbance are not always consistent, and that often multiple lines of enquiry are necessary to understand the nature of the complaints being made by the patient. Polysomnographic study[32] of elderly insomniacs has suggested that sleep satisfaction was related to shorter sleep latency and increased stages 3 and 4 sleep, but not related to wake time after sleep onset or overall sleep efficiency.

Foley et al.[33] conducted a 3 year longitudinal study of almost 7000 elderly people over the age of 65, to determine the incidence rates (new cases) and remission rates of insomnia in a known study cohort. Nearly 15% of those who were normal sleepers at baseline had symptoms of insomnia 3 years later, suggesting an annual incidence rate of somewhere between 5 and 15%. In all but 7% of these new cases there was a precipitant for the insomnia, suggesting that the ageing process per se has little to do with sleep disturbances. This conclusion finds further support from the finding that half of the 2000 elderly who had initially reported insomnia no longer had these symptoms at follow-up and also reported improved self-perceived health.[33] With the remission rate exceeding the incident rate, there were fewer elderly in this cohort with an insomnia complaint 3 years later, again suggesting that insomnia is not inevitable with ageing.

Subjectively, as many as half of people over 65 years old express dissatisfaction with their quality of sleep, with as many as 25% reporting persistent problems with insomnia. The prevalence of insomnia detected among 2400 community-dwelling elderly people over 65 years of age averages from about one-third of elderly men to half of elderly women.[34] Chiu et al.[35] proposed that sleep disturbance and insomnia are two separate but overlapping constructs: among 1000 Chinese elderly over the age of 70 years, 75% reported occasional or persistent sleep disturbance, but only half of these complained of insomnia, that is subjectively inadequate or poor sleep. Among the institutionalized elderly the prevalence of insomnia has been reported to be as high as 80%, and is related to high levels of depression, pain problems, poor health and poor physical activity.[36] Nursing-home populations are therefore highly skewed, as the presence of serious illness is usually the reason for admission to such facilities in the first place.[36]

In all cases, the evaluator should be sure to ask the patient to identify how the sleep problem impacts on their daily functioning. A survey of a random sample of adults of all ages from across the USA showed that there were dramatic differences in reported quality of life measures for insomniacs, compared with those with no sleep disturbance.[37] These problems included impaired concentration, impaired memory, decreased ability to accomplish daily tasks and decreased enjoyment of interpersonal relationships. Most of these relationships were directly related to sleep disturbance; that is, as sleep disturbance worsened, the impact on waking quality of life increased. This result has been supported by a study with the SF-36, often taken as the gold standard for measuring quality of life. Insomniacs obtain lower mean scores on all subscales of the SF-36, suggesting broad-based impairments in all domains usually assessed in quality of life evaluation.[38]

One study investigated how sleep disruption affects cognitive performance of elderly insomniacs on a range of neuropsychological tests of cognitive functioning.[39] Results showed that subjective ratings of sleep disturbance were more related to poor performance than

were objective (polysomnograph) measures, although both indicated poor performance on cognitive functioning. Subjective ratings of disrupted sleep were related to poor performance on subtests of vigilance, psychomotor speed, recall memory and executive function. The objective measures were only related to performance on the word-list retention subtest. This suggests not only that subjective ratings are important in determining the quality of the night-time sleep of elderly patients, but also that they are important determinants of daytime performance, and related to impairment of cognitive functioning for this group of patients. A more recent study determined that cognitive functions are not impacted for elderly persons without insomnia, but are for insomniacs and would appear to be related to specific SWS deficiencies.[40]

The National Institute of Mental Health (NIMH) Consensus Conference[41] suggested classifying insomnia into three groups for the purpose of treatment decisions, with the distinction between groups based on duration. These are: (i) transient insomnia, which lasts for a few nights; (ii) short-term insomnia, which lasts for a few weeks; and (iii) chronic insomnia, which lasts for longer than a month. Most cases of transient and short-term insomnia are due to stress or disturbances in the sleep–wake routine, and can be resolved by providing the patient with appropriate support and assistance, to help them through the event that has precipitated the sleep problem. These occurrences are common and most health providers are accustomed to dealing with these events. However, the chronic sleep problem requires more systematic evaluation.

Clinical interviewing

Shochat et al.[42] recently posed the question: what factors would lead an elderly patient to discuss their sleep disturbance with their physician? The four primary predictors included how the patient felt physically, the number of years that they had struggled with their insomnia, their age and their income. What is interesting about this finding is that it confirms what is often found anecdotally, namely that patients do not ordinarily commence discussion of their sleep problems with their physicians readily, or in a timely way. It tends to be something that becomes apparent only after the condition has worsened, has physical concomitants and has become chronic. A more proactive approach to these issues by all primary-care physicians would be very helpful.

In all clinical evaluation with elderly patients a number of opposing principles must be balanced effectively, including: (i) the use of multiple methods of assessment, while being as brief and focused as possible; (ii) discriminating developmental change from pathological change, while also being mindful of comorbidity in symptom development; and (iii) incorporation of strengths and weaknesses into the final treatment plan.[43]

Clinical diagnosis of sleep disorders is made on the basis of a thorough clinical evaluation, mostly from the clinical interview. An in-depth sleep history can guide the health practitioner in patient management.[44] A complete sleep history should encompass the following elements:

- The specific sleep problem should be defined: With the elderly, it is important to differentiate between daytime fatigue, which results from insomnia at night, and excessive daytime somnolence, which can be associated with a primary sleep disorder.
- A complete assessment of the sleep–wakefulness pattern: This can be achieved by keeping a sleep diary or a sleep log in which the patient records activities, including each time they got into bed, each time they got out of bed, the time they began and ended a sleep period, use of the toilet during sleep time, each alcoholic drink, each caffeinated drink, every time they took a sleeping pill, meals, snacks and exercise periods. A variety of sleep log formats is available for clinical use.[45–47] This type of log will evaluate daily routine and sleep–wakefulness patterns, which is important in the elderly because the sleep cycle can become polycyclical. Frequent naps can alter the sleep–wake schedule and cause circadian rhythm disorder.
- An interview with the bed partner or care giver: This can give clues that will help in the further management of the patient. For example, excessively loud snoring, temporary cessation of breathing or restless movements in bed are important pointers to the diagnosis of obstructive sleep apnoea (OSA) or periodic limb movement syndrome (PLMS).
- A family history of a sleep disorder: Certain sleep disorders, e.g. narcolepsy, hypersomnia, sleep apnoea, and restless legs syndrome (RLS), may have a family history.
- A complete medical history: Elderly individuals with sleep problems often have a variety of medical disorders that may disrupt sleep. Particular attention should be paid to painful musculoskeletal conditions, urological problems, cardiopulmonary disease, thyroid dysfunction, neurological disorders, substance abuse, upper airway pathology and gastric disorders.
- A careful drug history: Many of the medications used to treat medical disorders can cause insomnia, including CNS stimulants, β-blockers and antihypertensives. Many CNS depressants, including hypnotics, sedative and antidepressants, may cause excessive daytime somnolence.
- A review of the patient's psychosocial life context. This leads to a psychiatric history, with particular emphasis placed on the evaluation of depression and anxiety. Psychophysiological arousal subsequent to life events and the recurrence of psychiatric disorders are among the most common causes of insomnia in the elderly.

A good outline for a clinical interview can be found in Morin's[46] text. The Insomnia Interview Schedule touches on the most important clinical issues in sleep assessment. This structured interview assesses the onset, course and current status of the sleep problem, as well as the environmental, psychosocial and psychiatric factors that can affect sleep. Morin also provides a Sleep Impairment Index that the patient can fill out, as well as a Beliefs and Attitudes Survey; these assess their perception of how much the sleep problem affects them, and their thoughts and beliefs about their sleep, respectively. Both instruments can be helpful in working with these patients. Other resources on sleep assessment include Espie[48] and Lichstein and Reidel.[49]

The clinical process by which the evaluator moves through collecting information in a systematic way and considering the evidence for each possible cause of the sleep problem can be described as formulating the clinical complaint. This process includes making a diagnosis, but is broader than just that. It involves thinking in more than one way about the sleep problem. As insomnia is the final common pathway for a broad range of underlying complaints, it means that each possible contributing cause must be considered seriously. Chronic insomnia has multiple causes, some intrinsic, some extrinsic and some circadian, and all of which can contribute to the final clinical complaint. The task is to identify all of these components and address all of them in the treatment plan. The strategic process of formulating the patient's sleep complaint is reviewed in the following section.

Clinical decision making in managing insomnia

After establishing that one is dealing with a chronic sleep problem, and determining its specific characteristics, the health-care provider will formulate what factors are contributing to the problem, to determine what exactly needs to be done. To accomplish this, the doctor conducts a reasoned enquiry into the specific features of the patient's clinical presentation, through a series of steps. There are two goals to this process:

(A) To screen for conditions requiring referral:
1. Establish the chronicity of the sleep complaint and its impact on daytime functioning.
2. Understand the clinical course, previous episodes and previous treatment.
3. Screen for primary sleep disorders.
4. Identify concurrent physical and psychiatric disorders, and drug involvement.
(B) To identify all contributing causes for primary intervention:
1. Identify the role of pain in the patient's sleep problems.
2. Identify psychosocial factors relevant to the current life context.
3. Identify other extrinsic factors impacting on sleep.
4. Consider multiple causes for insomnia and establish an integrated treatment plan.

The remainder of this chapter follows these two different clinical tasks systematically. The first is to conduct a careful screen for primary sleep disorders, as well as serious conditions and illnesses. These will require referral of the patient for consultation with a sleep disorders centre, sleep specialist or other health-care provider. The second is to do a thorough work-up of the patient's sleep complaint, to understand all factors that are contributing to the sleep disruption, in order to develop a treatment plan for the primary intervention that you will provide to your patient. This is the task of helping the patient to age 'successfully.'

Assessing for conditions requiring comanagement

Disrupted daytime functioning

Disrupted sleep will usually impact on the patient's daytime functioning. Indeed, this criterion is usually required to confirm that there is a clinical sleep disorder. For patients who report disrupted sleep but no impact on daytime functioning, a clinical diagnosis is rarely made. For example, the individual could be a person requiring less than 7 h of sleep per night.

The kinds of disruption usually reported by patients include unstable mood (irritability, depression, distress, etc.), poor concentration and daytime fatigue, sometimes with daytime naps. For example, it has been shown that elderly insomniacs, whether taking medications or not, perform worse on tests requiring attention or concentration than do good sleepers.[50] The researchers attributed this finding to a state of hyperarousal among elderly insomniacs.

Excessive daytime sleepiness can be due to sleep that has become excessively fragmented (owing to poor sleep habits, use of drugs or alcohol, or a primary sleep disorder), or due to excessive or inappropriate sleep intrusions (due to narcolepsy or another clinical condition). A good way of assessing the seriousness of the daytime sleepiness of the patient is with the Epworth Sleepiness Scale (ESS).[51] This measure has been shown to correlate with objective measures of daytime sleepiness obtained in the sleep laboratory. Any patient who reports falling asleep while driving should be sent to a sleep laboratory for evaluation.

Whitney et al.[52] reported on excessive daytime sleepiness among the elderly in the Cardiovascular Health Study. They found that about 20% of subjects complained of excessive daytime sleepiness, as measured by the ESS. Higher ESS scores were associated with non-white race, depression, loud snoring, frequent nocturnal awakenings, a sedentary lifestyle and limitation of activities of daily living (ADLs). The use of pills for congestive heart failure was positively associated, but the use of tricyclic antidepressants, benzodiazepines or alcohol to aid sleep was not associated with excessive daytime sleepiness.

Particularly important is the evaluation of the extent of daytime napping. Daytime sleepiness has been related strongly to poor health and limitations in ADLs, and correlated with age.[52] A multisite, multiyear prospective study of almost 4000 people over the age of 65 found that daytime nappers were more likely to be male, urban, more depressive, heavier, more limited in physical activity, and to have more functional impairments. The 4 year mortality rate was accelerated 1.73 times among older people who nap most of the time, and who also made two or more errors on a cognitive status examination.[53] For patients with such a clinical presentation, particular attention must be paid to the possibility of having a primary sleep disorder and to drug usage.

Assessing the course of a condition will give clues to the probable causes of the sleep disorder. In most cases of chronic insomnia, the sleep disturbance is multiply determined, meaning that there is usually more than one factor that contributes to the continuation of the sleep problem. Finding out whether the onset of the complaint was sudden or gradual, whether there are seasonal variations or variations in the sleep environment are all very important clinical issues that will suggest possible causes for the problem. At the least, it will suggest whether intrinsic, extrinsic or circadian factors could be involved. Previous treatment efforts will give a good indication of the patient's insight and motivation to change their behaviour, and therefore of the probability of successful intervention.

Primary sleep disorders and parasomnias

Sleep disorders are classified according to the American Sleep Disorders Association's International Classification of Sleep Disorders Diagnostic and Coding Manual.[54] This classifies sleep problems into dyssomnias, parasomnias and sleep disorders secondary to other medical or psychiatric conditions. Dyssomnias are defined as insufficient or inefficient sleep (in quality or quantity) or the opposite, excessive sleepiness. Dyssomnias therefore have two clusters of conditions: one with inadequate sleep to support daytime activity, referred to as the 'insomnias', and another characterized by having a persistent and excessive need for sleep that impairs daytime functioning, called 'hypersomnias'.[55] Further, the dyssomnias are subclassified into three groups, according to whether the cause of the sleep disturbance arises from within the body (intrinsic), from environmental factors (extrinsic) or from inappropriate timing of sleep within the 24 h day (circadian). Other diagnostic systems such as the World Health Organization's International Classification of Diseases (ICD-10) and the American Psychiatric Association's Diagnostic and Statistical Manual (DSM-IV) may differ in terms of terminology used, but not in any substantive way.[56]

The primary sleep disorders most common among the elderly include sleep apnoea and periodic limb movements. For all of these, the clinician will screen for the sleep disorder with a clinical interview. This section will provide the information to conduct such screenings efficiently. However, there is a questionnaire[57] available that will systematically review the essential features of the primary sleep disorders. The Sleep Disorders Questionnaire, developed by Stanford University, is a research questionnaire used to determine the likelihood of sleep apnoea, periodic limb movement, narcolepsy and insomnia secondary to psychiatric causes. It contains 175 questions and would probably take an elderly person a long time to complete. A shorter alternative, suitable for many uses in a primary health-care office, would be the Pittsburgh Sleep Quality Index, which is composed of 19 items and provides information on seven component scores.[58]

Snoring and sleep apnoea

Approximately 60% of men and 40% of women above the age of 60 years snore. These figures are almost twice the level of just 20 years earlier.[59] Snoring can be benign to the snorer,[60] but is always problematic for the bed partner. More importantly, it can be part of the syndrome of obstructive sleep apnoea (OSA).

OSA is more common in the elderly than in any other age group, and is an important cause of daytime sleepiness. Prevalence studies suggest that 24% of independently living elderly have at least a mild form of sleep apnoea,[61] defined as an apnoea index (AI) of greater than 5. The prevalence drops to 10% of the elderly population if one sets the criteria at the more usual cut-off for clinical apnoea, an AI of greater than 10. OSA can occur by itself or more typically, as part of a variety of other syndromes, such as chronic obstructive pulmonary disease, congestive heart failure, hypertension and renal disease.[62] It occurs more frequently among the obese, and has been found to be three times more common among the US Hispanic population.[63]

Bliwise[62] has been conducting a longitudinal study of 256 elderly individuals for the past two decades. Preliminary results indicate that increased sleep-disordered breathing is associated with progressive neuropsychological impairment, decreased vital capacity and increased risk for mortality. He concluded that several lines of evidence suggest that sleep apnoea, especially during REM sleep, could be the mechanism underlying 'natural' death during sleep. As such, early detection and treatment could extend the life of many such patients.

Another study[64] of over 400 elderly patients with sleep apnoea reported on a follow-up of clinical patients grouped into minimal, mild–moderate and severe apnoea. A follow-up of patients at 10 years showed that elderly people with severe sleep-disordered breathing were at a higher mortality risk, dying as much as 2 years earlier than those with less sleep-disordered breathing.

Not all researchers would agree that apnoea is routinely a risk factor. Bixler et al.[65] found a monotonic increase in the prevalence of sleep apnoea with age, but the severity of apnoea decreased with age, whether one looked at the number of events or the resultant oxygen desaturation. The authors suggested that the sleep laboratory criteria for diagnosing apnoea should be adjusted for age. However, Chokroverty[3] pointed out that the cerebral blood flow (CBF) in the elderly decreases with age and appears to be related to a decrease in cerebral metabolic rate. During SWS the decrease in CBF becomes excessive and interacts with the hypoxaemia related to the apnoea, creating a higher risk for sudden death or stroke.

OSA is characterized by periodic apnoeas and hypopneas during sleep that produce asphyxia and fragmented sleep. OSAs are caused by complete upper airway obstruction that occurs in the pharynx following sleep onset. Pharyngeal collapse causes airflow to stop despite continuing efforts to breathe against the obstructed airway. Both apnoeas and hypopneas result in progressive asphyxia which stimulates breathing efforts against the collapsed airway, typically until arousal from sleep occurs. Arousal is accompanied by a surge in activity of the upper airway muscles that restores upper airway potency and airflow. These sleep patients rapidly return to sleep, the pharynx collapses and the cycle begins again.

Symptoms of OSA include excessive daytime sleepiness, depression, headaches, memory loss and cognitive impairment. It is important to diagnose OSA early since it can usually be treated effectively, yet if left untreated, it can result in the development of hypertension and cardiovascular disease.[66] Questions that can be asked during the clinical interview to assess the possibility of sleep apnoea include the following:

• Are you a loud, habitual snorer?
• Do you usually feel tired and groggy on awakening?
• Do you struggle with fatigue throughout the day?
• Are you overweight?
• Do you wake out of sleep with the sensation that you are choking?
• Do you regularly wake up with a headache?

Where more than one answer is given affirmatively, follow-up evaluation in a sleep clinic would be advisable. Treatment for sleep apnoea[67] includes behavioural modifications to minimize sleeping on the back, weight loss and regular exercise, avoidance of alcohol and other respiratory depressants before bed, and the use of oral appliances that advance the mandible to enlarge the airway. Other options include the use of a nasal continuous positive airway pressure (CPAP) device, respiratory stimulants and surgery involving the upper airway. However, to date not a single controlled clinical trial has been conducted for sleep apnoea treatments at any age, let alone in the elderly.[62] A full discussion of the relationship between apnoea and ageing can be found in Levy et al.[68]

Periodic limb movements in sleep and restless legs syndrome

There is a prevalence in older adults for the development of two sleep-related neuromuscular dysfunctions: PLMS and RLS. PLMS, also called nocturnal myoclonus, occurs during sleep, is characterized by rapid stereotypic and periodic flexions of the leg and foot, and is associated with repeated awakenings throughout the night. These can last for 1 or 2 s and occur as often as hundreds of times a night. The number of limb movements often increases with age, resulting in increasing disruption of normal sleep patterns, especially of the descent into the deeper levels of stage 3 and 4 sleep. Prevalence rates for this condition are estimated at about 45% among the elderly.[69]

The condition does not appear to be associated with neurological dysfunction or other serious physical disease. It is usually non-progressive in any given individual patient. Caffeine and alcohol may exacerbate nocturnal myoclonus. PLMS can also be a complicating feature of other sleep disorders, such as OSA. The mechanisms controlling the appearance of these movements are not known with certainty, but dopamine depletion in the CNS may play a role in the pathogenesis.

Not all patients experiencing pronounced PLMS will have restless legs syndrome (RLS), but many do. Prevalence rates range from 5 to 15%. RLS is characterized by an aching, crawling sensation in the muscles which may also be described as a tingling, crawling or prickling sensation. The condition usually gets worse at night, resulting in repeated leg movements before bed. Correlations with iron deficiencies have been noted. Pathogenesis has been attributed to both CNS neurotransmitter deficits and peripheral axonal neuropathy.[70]

Questions that can be asked during the clinical interview to assess the possibility of PLMS and RLS include:

- Do you struggle with fatigue throughout the day?
- Does your bed partner report that you kick them during the night?
- Do your legs ache when you are inactive?
- Do the symptoms become worse in the evening and at night?
- Does movement improve the aching sensation?

PLMS can be reliably determined from an all-night polysomnograph, although more than one night's sleep in the sleep clinic may be required. Patients with this problem can be advised to get up and walk around when they feel the restless sensation, rub their legs, or take a hot bath or shower. For more severe presentations treatment with dopaminergic agents can be helpful,[71] but should be prescribed within specific guidelines. Some patients may benefit from iron replacement, or the use of opioid, benzodiazepine, anticonvulsant and adrenergic medications. The use of oestrogen, progesterone, or both, has also been shown to decrease the appearance of PLMS in women. Sleepiness and bed rest can exacerbate the symptoms of RLS.

Narcolepsy

Narcolepsy is a rare but incapacitating chronic disorder that affects the brain, where the regulation of sleep and wakefulness occurs. It is a benign neurological condition that consists essentially of the features off REM sleep disrupting the waking experience. The clinical features include the occurrence of 'sleep attacks', which can last from 1 to 30 min. These irresistible attacks may cause a person to fall asleep while driving a car or in the middle of talking to a friend. It can be dangerous because of the exposure to accident and injury. It is debilitating because it can make gainful employment difficult. Narcoleptics also report cataplectic episodes, which consist of limpness in muscles, paralysis on awakening and dream experiences as they are falling asleep (hypnogogic dreams).

Cataplectic phenomena are often triggered by emotions, but the condition is not a psychiatric or psychological disorder. The condition is not curable, but is managed with medications to reduce daytime sleepiness. Positive diagnosis is made with overnight polysomnography and a multiple sleep latencies test during the day. Many mild cases are not diagnosed until later in life.[72] The treatment of choice for this neurological condition is modafinil (Provigil).[73] It works so effectively in reducing sleepiness among this very difficult patient group that it is now also being tried with sleep apnoea.

Parasomnias

Parasomnias refer to sleep complaints that involve behaviours that do not normally belong in sleep, for example bruxism, sleepwalking or nightmares; they are not disorders of sleep–wake organization. These could arise because of autonomic nervous system activation, stress or other factors. They are a consideration among the elderly as onset can occur late in life. For example, β-blockers are well known to cause nightmares in some patients.

The most common are REM sleep behaviour disorder, sleepwalking and night terrors. REM sleep behaviour disorder is characterized by the intermittent loss of paralysis accompanying the REM state, with the result that motor activity associated with dream mentation appears. This can include punching, kicking or leaping from the bed. It typically appears at least 90 min after sleep onset. Violent episodes can occur, with variable frequency. REM sleep behaviour disorder can be suspected from the history given by the bed partner.

Parasomnias can not only lead to daytime fatigue but also result in injury during or after an episode. An acute transient form can accompany withdrawal from alcohol and medications. Drug-induced cases have been reported during treatment with tricyclics and biperiden. The frequency of the disorder is less than 1 in 100, but it is reported to have a good response to clonazepam.[74] Others have suggested that REM sleep behaviour disorder is an early feature in some patients who go on to develop Parkinson's disease,[75] or a consequence of cerebrovascular events,[7] and therefore such new presentations should prompt a more extensive neurological assessment.

Secondary sleep disorders

Sleep disorders can also be 'secondary' to somatic disease and psychiatric disorder. These can include pain conditions, use of drugs and a variety of illnesses. A recent prospective study of factors associated with sleep complaints in the elderly[76] concluded that the apparent association between sleep difficulties and age is primarily due to increased depressed mood and physical health problems among such patients, rather than advancing age per se.

Physical health problems

The elderly patient faces a much higher risk of various physical illnesses as the years pass, and this has been shown to increase reports of sleep disturbance correspondingly. However, one study[77] demonstrated that when somatic diseases are controlled statistically, some types of insomnia complaint showed no age-related increase at all. Therefore, taking the sleep complaint as an early associated symptom of somatic disease, or of a depressive disorder, is always the best strategy in the initial evaluation of sleep complaints of the elderly.

In all evaluation of sleep disorders, it is important to identify and treat any somatic conditions that could underlie the sleep disruption. A cross-section of physical conditions that could cause sleep disruption is presented in Table 21.1. In this regard, maintaining regular contact with the patient's medical doctor is an important part of managing these patients effectively. Where this is not possible, care of the patient will suffer.

Prevalence rates of sleep disorders among a number of neurological illnesses are very high.[7] For example, 90% of Parkinson's patients report sleep problems.[62] In Alzheimer's patients there is a strong relationship between daytime cognitive impairment and the amount of wakefulness at night.[78] For many patients with dementias there can be nocturnal confusional episodes, sometimes called 'sundowning', which are thought to be related to circadian rhythm dysregulation.[62]

Other neurological conditions should also be considered when an elderly patient presents with sleep disturbances. For example, sleep–wake cycle disturbance is an essential component of delirium, and cholinergic deficiency is thought to be the major pathogenic mechanism underlying the disorder. For other conditions, circadian factors may lead to nocturnal awakening episodes and can become associated with wandering.[13]

After consideration of the neurological disorders, one can consider a wide variety of other conditions. Among the most prominent are pain,[79] and cardiac, respiratory, urological, and gastrointestinal conditions.[80] Any physical disorder that has pain as a symptom can affect sleep patterns. As the evaluation of pain is such a core focus of assessment in chiropractic practice, this is discussed more fully in the next section. Among the other classes of diseases, respiratory and cardiac conditions[81] must be considered carefully, as must gastric conditions such as gastro-oesophageal reflux disorder and peptic ulcers. For example, lying down at night can worsen gastro-oesophageal reflux. Finally, numerous other conditions can be exacerbated by sleep. Nocturnal sleep cycles can affect headaches[82] and epileptic activity.

As an older person's sleep pattern is much lighter than that of younger persons, their sleep is easily interrupted by a variety of environmental and internal stimuli. The most common trigger in older people is frequent micturition or nocturia.[62] Prevalence data suggest that one in two elderly people awaken at least twice a night to urinate, and this is found more often among women than in men.[83] Nocturnal incontinence has been found in patients with congestive heart failure or nocturnal shortness of breath, and those who use sleep medications.[84] Bliwise speculates that data from sleep laboratory studies, in which nocturnal micturation was related to awakenings occurring after

Table 21.1 Physical illnesses associated with sleep disturbances

Neurological disorders	Other physical disorders	
Parkinson's disease	Congestive heart failure	Hypothyroidism
Alzheimer's disease	Cardiac arrhythmias	Diabetes mellitus
Dementias	Chronic pain and fibromyalgia	Chronic fatigue
Stroke	Degenerative joint disease	Renal disorders
Delirium	Gastrointestinal disorders	Prostatism
	Chronic obstructive pulmonary disease	

sleep apnoea episodes, could be taken as evidence that frequent nocturnal micturition is a proxy for the occurrence of episodes of sleep apnoea.[85]

Drug and alcohol use

As all drugs will impact on the architecture of sleep in some way, it is especially important to conduct a careful review of both prescription and non-prescription drugs. As many elderly do not easily remember the names of specific medications, it can be helpful to ask them to bring in all medications and sleep aids that they are currently taking. Alcohol usage also needs to be reviewed in detail, as it exacerbates most sleep disturbances and fragments sleep, making it less restorative.

Drugs that have been shown to be associated with disturbed sleep include lifestyle drugs such as caffeine, nicotine and alcohol, as well as medically prescribed drugs such as thyroid hormone, β-blockers, steroids, antihistamines, analgesics, non-steroidal anti-inflammatories and antiarrhythmic agents, and over-the-counter agents such as nasal decongestants.[62,86] Numerous other medications such as narcotic analgesics, antispasmodics, central α-agonists, tricyclic antidepressants and antihistamines taken during the day may have sleepiness as a side-effect.[86]

In addition to the known clinical effects of individual drugs, with the elderly one must be mindful of drug interactions and synergies from the ingestion of multiple drugs. The number of current medications taken by the elderly patient has been shown to correlate with the level of sleep disturbance reported.[87]

The evaluating clinician also needs to be mindful of the fact that drug pharmacokinetics are influenced by the physiological changes of ageing. Drug absorption, metabolism and elimination can all be altered by ageing. Perhaps for these reasons, the elderly can be more subject to adverse reactions to otherwise routine immunization procedures; for example, disrupted

sleep. The first author evaluated a retired man who began to have very bad insomnia after an immunization about 1 year previously. All other factors were reviewed carefully and excluded as precipitating and perpetuating factors. The immediate physical symptoms related to the immunization normalized quickly, but the sleep disruption continued for over a year and required 2 months of behavioural and cognitive treatment to normalize.

Psychiatric disorders

Many psychiatric disorders are accompanied by sleep disturbances, usually insomnia, and of short-term duration, but it can become chronic in some patients. The elderly have very little in the way of a buffer protecting sleep quality, and often any life crisis can precipitate an adjustment reaction with moderate anxiety or depression and cause an insomnia that thereafter becomes chronic. Often the original psychiatric disorder has resolved, but the sleep disturbance persists.

It has been estimated that up to half of chronic insomnia can be causally related to psychiatric illness, most of it clinical depression.[88] It has also been shown that the presence of anxiety and depression increases the subject's perception of disturbance in their sleep, well beyond that which objective sleep measures would support.[89] A recent study comparing anxious and depressed patients with associated sleep disturbances found that depressed patients experienced more repercussions than any other group,[90] making it especially important for primary-care physicians to be alert to these disorders. Table 21.2 lists some of the most common psychiatric disorders that can have sleep disturbance as a prominent feature of the presentation.

The natural course of insomnia often begins with anxiety resulting from stressful life events, proceeds through a phase in which the insomnia becomes chronic, and finally places the individual at risk for

Table 21.2 Psychiatric disorders associated with insomnia

Depressive conditions	Anxiety conditions	Other disorders
Major depression	Panic disorder	Personality disorder
Bipolar disorder	Post-traumatic stress disorder	Somatoform disorder
Dysthymic disorder	Generalized anxiety	Schizophrenia
Cyclothymic disorder	Obsessive–compulsive disorder	Eating disorders
Seasonal affective disorder	Adjustment disorder	Cognitive disorders

clinical depression.[89] Anxiety initially affects falling asleep more than it affects sleep maintenance. If the worrying and psychophysiological arousal have become chronic, then one finds a persistent disruption of all aspects of sleep. The extent of anxiety in a given patient can be evaluated with the use of the Beck Anxiety Inventory, for which norms for community-dwelling adults exist.[90] In general, because somatic symptoms are more generally prevalent in the elderly than in other age groups, diagnosis should rely more on the cognitive and behavioural dimensions of anxiety.

A detailed discussion of the issues involved in differential diagnosis of anxiety, insomnia, medication use and substances of abuse is presented in a monograph by Folks and Fuller.[91] Treatment of the disorder can involve relaxation training, biofeedback and other approaches that target the psychophysiological arousal of these patients. Learning to relax is like developing any other skill: it requires time and persistence. A review of the treatment of secondary insomnia has concluded that treatment focusing on the sleep component of insomnia secondary to medical or psychiatric conditions can be effective, with beneficial results persisting at 3 month follow-up.

The hallmark of depression is the early-morning awakening, but this is not pathognomonic for depression, nor is it the only feature typical of the sleep of depressed patients.[62] Such patients have a flattening of the sleep–wake rhythm, meaning that they have very little energy during the day, and feel alert and have trouble falling asleep at night. Depression is also likely to alter the architecture of sleep stages, particularly that of REM sleep.

Among depressed elderly it is estimated that 10–20% demonstrate cognitive impairment. When this is particularly severe, these patients can present as a 'pseudodementia' which is reversible when the depression is treated. In addition, it is estimated that 10% of the elderly population suffer cognitive decline of a pathological nature[7] which also compromises sleep and could provoke a secondary depression. These latter conditions are not reversible, but effective intervention can reduce the problematic symptomatology.

In a 2 year study of almost 1600 community-dwelling elderly people, respondents with persistent depressive symptoms across the study period tended to be older, report more sleep disturbances and experienced declining health, compared with those whose depressive symptoms remitted.[92] It would seem that depressive illness, once present, and especially once it has become persistent, can exacerbate predisposition to other illness, by impairing sleep and thereby probably compromising immune functioning.

Reynolds et al.[93] summarized how depression affects sleep by comparing groups of bereaved elderly who volunteered to participate in a sleep study. Those with a full depressive syndrome exhibited diminished sleep efficiency, shorter REM latency and reduced early SWS generation. The depressed widows and widowers also carried a heavier burden of medical illness, and reported poorer sleep quality and more early-morning awakening. More importantly, sleep among the non-depressed bereaved subjects was similar to that of healthy control subjects, suggesting that depression is not an eventuality, even when an elderly person has to deal with a major life event.

Reynolds and his colleagues went on to ask what factors among the non-depressed patients in this cohort provided a buffer against the threat of depressive symptomatology? They found that greater stability of psychosocial rhythms and higher levels of perceived social support among their subjects tended to be associated with less depression. This supported the view of George[94] that: 'high levels of social support are associated with decreased risk of psychiatric morbidity and that perceived support is the dimension most strongly related to mental health outcomes' (p. 215).

More interestingly, Reynolds went on to explore what it was about this factor that helped to buffer the impact of the death on the mood and sleep of the bereaved.[95] They found that the individual subject's sense of mastery, that is the feeling of a sense of competence in the face of calamity, predicted whether the depressive syndrome would or would not follow, and individuals with more social supports were more likely to feel that they were still in control of their life.

A recent broad-based prospective study of over 2000 elderly[96] confirmed that sleep disturbance and depression were related, and also highlighted other factors that were related to the occurrence of depression. Specific risk factors included being female, older age, social isolation, low education, financial strain and functional impairment. The study did not address whether any of these correlated factors were causes of depression, but the fact that they are related to the occurrence of this disruptive condition would make them very important factors to review in the clinical assessment of these patients.

Referral decisions

Where primary sleep disturbances are suspected, referral to a sleep disorders centre is required, to evaluate the presence of the sleep disorder and its seriousness. Sleep apnoea increases the risk of mortality. For all other sleep disorders referral is made to improve the patient's quality of life. Sleep clinics investigate the quality of sleep through polysomnography, the collection of physiological parameters during sleep. Brain-wave activity, chin muscle tone, eye movements, heart function, breathing patterns, blood oxygen saturation and leg muscle activity are monitored during a sleep study. This is achieved by attaching electrodes, small metal discs, on to the surface of the skin for the all-night study.

The overnight sleep study is used to help to diagnose primary sleep disorders such as sleep apnoea and RLS that can cause excessive daytime sleepiness. Having identified the problem, the sleep physician can choose the appropriate treatment. It should be noted that the one-night polysomnographic evaluation is not designed to understand the causes of insomnia, only to rule out specific sleep pathologies. It does the latter very well, but rarely has much of value to offer for the former.[97]

The Consensus Conference of Treatment of Sleep Disorders among the elderly concluded that 'hypnotic medication should not be the mainstay of management for most of the causes of disturbed sleep'.[1] The use of hypnotic medications among the elderly is usually restricted to short-term insomnia that is severe, disabling and subjecting the individual to extreme distress.[98] It is rarely endorsed beyond 3 weeks, and then with low-dose hypnotics, with regular and frequent assessments of side-effects, and a planned taper schedule.[99] In other words, treatment for chronic insomnia among the elderly must rely on treatment approaches other than hypnotic medication.

Hypnotics with short and intermediate half-lives are preferable over longer lasting drugs in the elderly because of the lower potential of hangover effects and accident risk.[100] Zaleplon, the newest benzodiazepine receptor agonist, is among the medications with the best profile of drug action for an elderly population.[101] In treating elderly patients with severe diseases and poor quality of life, sleep medication must sometimes continue for lengthy periods, but should be carefully monitored.[102]

Elderly patients who present with a pattern of habitual and prolonged use of hypnotics, in the absence of good clinical reason for such medication usage, will typically have a hypnotic-dependent insomnia that will require intervention by a sleep specialist.[103] Ohayan[30] estimated that as many as 10% of the elderly are currently on such medications. Discontinuation of medications for this group of patients is a complex process requiring attention to sleep parameters and the expectations of the patient, as well as attitudes and fears that the patient has about his or her sleep. The process involves a period of tapering from the medication that could be between 4 and 16 weeks in length, and is conducted under the close supervision of a physician.

Discontinuation from medications can also include stopping over-the-counter substances that an individual patient has been taking for a long time. A nation-wide survey conducted in the USA[104] suggested that 40% of insomniacs used alcohol and other over-the-counter remedies to help them to sleep. While many insomniacs believe that alcohol will promote sleep, it in fact exacerbates existing sleep problems. Over-the-counter medications have not been shown to be effective and withdrawal from them may present some clinical problems.[105]

There is widespread consensus that the development of effective non-pharmacological interventions is a necessity in helping elderly insomniacs.[106,107] These psychological treatments include both behavioural and cognitive strategies. A meta-analysis of studies employing non-pharmacological interventions[108] demonstrated the clinical utility of these approaches on improving disrupted sleep, and that these improvements persisted on follow-up. A recently published randomized controlled trial[107] of cognitive behaviour therapy (CBT) demonstrated its equal efficacy to pharmacological treatment, or CBT combined with pharmacological treatment. However, only the CBT groups maintained improvement over baseline at 2 year follow-up. There is also evidence that non-pharmacological treatment is rated as more acceptable and more suitable than drug treatment by olders people.[109]

For patients with significant psychological conflicts, who are struggling with bereavement issues, or have more complex or longstanding insomnia complaints, referral to a psychologist for more systematic behavioural treatment should be considered. Elements of a self-management programme could include relaxation training, a stimulus control approach to sleep, sleep restriction therapy, or a cognitive approach to their beliefs and attitudes about sleep.[46] Treatment focused on helping patients with insomnia secondary to medical or psychiatric disorders has generally been found to be effective.[86]

Clinical management of sleep problems

Having ruled out the conditions that could benefit from evaluation and treatment by other health-care professionals, the remaining and still complex clinical issue is to consider how the chiropractor can best improve the sleep pattern of that particular elderly patient. A more detailed review of clinical findings in a number of specific areas is central to accomplishing this goal.

Pain

Many patients seen in the chiropractor's office will be experiencing pain, either intermittent or chronic, and pain invariably disrupts sleep. Chronic pain conditions, whether involving headache,[79] musculoskeletal pain[82,110,111] or fibrositis,[112] and whether diffuse or localized in presentation, have a great impact on sleep functions and require evaluation by the practitioner. In addition, contemporary biopsychosocial models of pain emphasize the interrelationships between these biological factors and psychological and social processes.[113] For example, many pain patients will avoid movement and activity based on their fear of pain, and can become even further sensitized to pain.

Poor sleep also aggravates pain experiences. Sleep deprivation has been shown to give rise to pain complaints even in the sleep of healthy young adults. Specifically, deprivation of SWS resulted in increased muscle tenderness[114] and other complaints commonly reported by fibromyalgia patients. When SWS was systematically disrupted for three consecutive nights, subjects reported significant increases in tender point pain. The same result was not found when REM sleep was disrupted. Whether the increase in pain was directly related to the loss of the SWS or to the disruption of other processes associated with SWS, for example secretion of GH, is not known.

A recent study of healthy young adults during final examinations[115] also found significant decreases in musculoskeletal pain thresholds, but they were not correlated to any of the sleep parameters reported by subjects on their sleep logs. This study made no effort selectively to deprive SWS. Nevertheless, the increased sensitivity of these subjects to pain was strik-

ing. As these findings were obtained during final examinations, it was reasoned that the decreased pain thresholds were most likely to be the result of increased anxiety.

Anxiety involves stimulation of the SNS which results in the release of noradrenaline. Other studies have linked increased pain reports with a rise in plasma adrenaline levels,[116] and reported a positive correlation between the general level of life stress and pain intensity ratings among hospitalized patients.[117] It appears that anxiety, pain, sleep, and the biochemical and hormonal events associated with them, are interdependent phenomena, which can influence each other under certain circumstances. The dynamics between them have not yet been clearly elaborated and continue to require study.

The pain experience of chronic pain sufferers often impacts negatively on sleep experiences. Morin et al.[118] reported a study conducted with 105 chronic pain patients, most of whom were younger adults (average age 41.5 years). Subjects completed self-report measures of their sleep disturbance, as well as ratings of the intensity of their pain experience, and their level of anxiety and depression. Subjects were grouped into good sleepers and poor sleepers. Poor sleepers reported more difficulties in both initiating sleep and maintaining sleep, as well as higher levels of pain, than did the good sleepers. However, they did not have increased levels of anxiety or depression. These results indicate that sleep disturbance goes hand in hand with worsening of pain symptoms, but is not always accompanied by clinical anxiety or depression.

With time, the mood and self-esteem of chronic pain patients can also begin to be affected. Once this develops there is even greater sleep disturbance and the cycle intensifies further. The long-term course of this cycle will mean weight gain, from inactivity, and depression, both of which will negatively affect pain perception.

Active intervention in this cycle is required if the cycle is going to be reversed. Chiropractors, as drugless practitioners, are in an excellent position to take an educational and wellness-orientated approach with the pain patient. Most pain patients will complain of sleep problems, especially difficulties in falling asleep. With fewer other distractions from their pain at sleep onset, many pain patients will naturally focus on their pain at this time. If the elderly person has other stresses as well, such as depression precipitated by the loss of a loved one, then the downward spiral of increased pain, decreased sleep, and increased fear and hopelessness is all but certain.

Psychosocial factors

Many challenges come with old age; some of these are physical, others are social and emotional. Among treatment-seeking individuals with a primary complaint of insomnia, one-third displays a concurrent psychiatric condition, one-third exhibits psychological symptoms related to life stressors, but below the threshold for a psychiatric condition, and the final one-third presents with insomnia as a disorder unrelated to any psychological distress.[119] Another review of insomnia in relatively healthy elderly persons concluded that in this population insomnia is more closely associated with psychological factors than with lifestyle or health status.[120] Therefore, understanding which issues are troubling to a given patient, and how they try to cope with these, can be very helpful in understanding their sleep difficulties.

Lifestyle changes confront every elderly person who retires from their work responsibilities. Many elderly people do not have the financial resources to accommodate the lifestyle that they had been accustomed to. Just as important is whether the elderly person can make the adjustment to using their new-found spare time, and to putting energies into greater exercise and activity levels. Active elderly people will find that their sleep patterns are much more restorative and provide them with a buffer against the inevitable physiological changes that are taking place within them.

There are many ways in which a health professional can be helpful to the elderly patient. One is to help the patient to evaluate how well prepared they are for retirement, socially, emotionally and financially. How successfully they make the transition has a tremendous impact on physical and mental health, and sleep functions. Helping to establish regular activities, getting started in the morning and making other suggestions outlined later in this chapter would all be very important.

Probably the most important task of the elderly is to come to terms with death. Death will surround them increasingly as time passes. They must deal with the death of peers, loved ones and, most importantly, spouse. The death of the spouse often hits them psychologically in many ways. It takes away their life partner, with whom they have shared their triumphs and their tragedies. Now, when they have to deal with their greatest tragedy, they must learn to deal with it alone.

A spouse's death also takes away many activities that were done together, and places added burdens at the same time. For example, in a marriage where a wife coordinated social activities and the husband took care of banking, either partner would be left with having to learn new responsibilities at a time when just getting through the day was difficult enough. Making new friends is not easy when one has no interest in leaving the house or may be afraid to venture out. All of these effects are synergistic and the final impact on the elderly person is potentially devastating. Where children and other family members have moved away, the result can be loneliness, depression and despair.

An epidemiological study of insomnia in the general population found that being separated, divorced or widowed was highly associated with the presence of insomnia complaints for both men and women,[30] with a higher relationship than with the presence of physical illnesses. This result could be either because of depressed feelings due to the loss, or because of living alone, resulting in more anxieties or physical self-absorption. Whatever the reason, the association with sleep disturbance is highly significant and merits enquiry with individual elderly patients.

The health-care provider is in an excellent position to be empathic, to fuel the patient's efforts to rebuild his or her life, and to assist the elderly patient in building a sense of mastery, even in the face of catastrophic loss. Whatever improvement can be made in the patient's lifestyle is vital to offsetting the negative effects of the physiological changes of ageing. Although challenges from death and other changes are inevitable, they can be eased by a proactive approach to helping the older person to manage these changes in lifestyle more effectively. A wealth of information is available for patient or practitioner to explore at the website of the American Association of Retired Persons at http://www.aarp.org, including help with financial matters, assisting in independent living, finding health information, legal information, and a thousand other links and resources. Anyone who deals with older patients will find this a helpful place to start.

Finally, one needs to evaluate how the elderly person thinks about their sleep problem. Do they worry about their sleep? Their health? How much of a preoccupation is it? Some useful tools to help to understand these dimensions of their concerns include the

Self-Statement Test: 60+,[121] the Sleep Behaviors Scale: 60+,[122] and the Attitudes and Beliefs about Sleep Questionnaire.[123] In all cases where the patient is awake for longer than 30 min before sleeping, it is important to enquire into their thoughts during these periods. It is very common for many elderly to feel afraid, even frightened, of a range of different stressors, and these need to be identified and addressed.

Other extrinsic and circadian factors

This phase of the evaluation assesses a broad range of factors that can impact on sleep–wake patterns. First, one should attend to the environment in the bedroom itself, including noise, light and comfort. A systematic review is needed of the use of stimulants such as caffeine and nicotine, other substances such as alcohol and an assortment of over-the-counter sleep remedies, such as Nytol. Some form of sleep medication is taken by about 20% of subjects aged over 70.[124]

One survey of 176 ambulatory elderly persons aged 60–92 years found that half had used at least one therapy for their sleep problem in the past year.[125] About half of that half used non-prescription products, many of which were not marketed as sleep enhancing, but were perceived to be helpful by the subjects themselves. One-third of these elderly took these remedies daily, while the majority took them less often, but at least once a week. The same study found that subjects were taking an average of four concurrent medications, so the risk of drug interactions is very high.

Special attention needs to be paid to factors related to regularity of circadian patterns.[126] Irregular sleep–wake times, irregular meal times and daytime napping all contribute to the breakdown of entrained rhythms. Patients who can be considered at risk for poor circadian rhythm patterns are those who have histories of shift work or who report being a chronically light sleeper.

Integration of clinical findings

Before deciding which clinical interventions could be most effective for a given patient, one has to determine the range of possible contributory factors. This step is usually not a simple one for sleep disturbances. In most cases of chronic insomnia there are multiple factors that contribute to the final sleep patterns observed. For example, a multicentre study of diagnoses made for over 200 patients of all age ranges found that 77% of patients with a primary insomnia had a psychiatric disorder as an additional contributory factor.[127]

Even after one has identified all primary sleep disorders, as well as current physical and psychiatric conditions, one must still consider a variety of possible additional causes for sleep complaints. These include short sleepers, 'normal' sleep fragmentation due to ageing, psychophysiological insomnia, learned insomnia, and circadian disorders. Identification of all important contributing factors is essential to successful intervention. Furthermore, not all of these identified factors will have the same potency in affecting the sleep disturbance observed.

Reynolds et al.[128] proposed a biopsychosocial model of pathogenesis of sleep disorders, which identifies the most important predictors of poor sleep and circadian dysregulation in late life. The model proposes that changes in health status, cognitive status and negative life events (particularly bereavement) are hypothesized to lead to 'decay' in sleep and sleep quality.[129] The resultant net effect of these factors is determined by the presence of two primary mediating factors of either a negative shift in affect balance (onset of depression) or a worsening of sleep-disordered breathing. However, they propose that a range of moderating factors can provide a buffer against further sleep decay, including stability of social rhythms, social support, nutrition, physical fitness and gender.

The authors note that the model works synergistically in both directions: deterioration of sleep quality predisposes to problems with mood, and in time with other social and health functions. Conversely, improvements in depressed mood or OSA, from appropriate treatment, coupled with improved sleep hygiene, activity and social interaction, lead to much improved sleep overall. Improvement in each component adds weight to the overall sleep improvement obtained, so all factors must be addressed in the treatment plan.

Finally, it must be noted that the collection of research evidence to support the model has only begun. However, the model is consistent with clinical experience, and at least it provides a conceptual framework to guide clinical enquiries and direct interventions. There is also plenty of room for considering other factors which emerge from alternative health-care philosophies, such as chiropractic, as mediating variables in the improvement of the sleep of the elderly.

For the clinician with an elderly person with a sleep complaint, this model is helpful in that it guides clinical enquiry to three main triggering causes of deterioration: health, cognition and trauma. In this aspect of the model, chiropractic may have contributions to make to alternative more conservative ways of treating the health problems of the elderly, especially many pain conditions.

Most interestingly, while a health or trauma event can often not be reversed, cognition can be changed. Even in situations where health and trauma are involved, the way in which elderly people thinks about what is happening to them is a critical factor in how the other two factors impact on them. Cognitive factors as key to intervention strategies are discussed in the section on attitude and belief, later in the chapter.

In general, although depression and OSA can respond well to passive medical treatment, the chronic forms of insomnia seen in the elderly are *not* appropriate for traditional medical treatment with continuous medications.[1] The risks of falling or having a car accident are much higher.[130] Not only are medications riskier, but they are also unlikely to be effective without the clinician and patient addressing and making changes in a variety of exacerbating lifestyle factors. In this regard, management of sleep problems is like that of musculoskeletal injuries, which the chiropractor has a wealth of experience in treating. As Reynolds[131] recently commented, insomnia complaints among the elderly tend to be chronic and recurring, and therefore management strategies will generally occur in the primary-care setting, where new initiatives need to be devised and tested.

Interventions for successful ageing

Rapport building

Active involvement of the patient is necessary throughout the intervention process. The purpose of all effective sleep intervention is to: (i) create a sense of understanding about sleep; (ii) inspire a positive expectancy that efforts at making changes of different kinds will benefit sleep; (iii) use treatment strategies built on creating incremental improvement in many functions simultaneously; and (iv) focus on augmenting the patient's sense of mastery over their sleep problem.

Since sleep problems occur over time, chiropractors who plan to make some intervention with patients will be required to obtain ongoing information on the nature of the patient's sleep complaint. This will mean using a sleep log to evaluate the longitudinal pattern of the sleep disturbance, as well as the use of questionnaires which can help in determining the nature and severity of the sleep disturbance. A baseline of logging at least 2 weeks of sleep–wake patterns is necessary to assess sleep-onset latency problems, and at least 3 weeks for sleep-maintenance problems.[132]

Sleep logs are invaluable as a source of independent corroboration of the patient's descriptions. Although not as objective as polysomnographic study, they have good reliability and validity for the purposes of clinical intervention.[133] Often the simple task of tracking sleep night by night helps to clear up biases and misperceptions that the patient has about their own sleep. Even when this does not happen there is clinical value to seeing variations in the general patterns of sleep and understanding why such variations appear. This task is rarely redundant, even when patients are reluctant to comply with the task.

The clinical tasks required of the patient for improvement require a strong doctor–patient alliance,[134] changes in long-maintained behavioural patterns must usually be made to change the consequent sleep patterns successfully. Change in basic behavioural patterns, including simple lifestyle matters, can be effected within 2 months. However, when one is dealing with a long-term pattern of dependence on hypnotic medications, therapeutic success takes from 3 to 6 months.[46] For the practitioner to be effective in managing these problems, he or she must be effective at engaging the patient in a process of change.

Morin[46] advises that treatment should begin by examining the patient's expectations of treatment. It is very helpful, even essential, for treatment goals to be set early in the process. In all cases goals should be individualized, realistic and operational. The goal is often improving existing sleep patterns, setting realistic objectives for regular sleep patterns, and teaching skills for managing flare-ups and residual difficulties. In all cases, the patient should become knowledgeable enough to understand what is happening to him or her, and what to do to minimize the effects of the problem.

Sleep–wake behaviour

As a health professional the chiropractor can advise a sleepy patient on how to achieve a good night's sleep by modifying his or her sleep–wake habits. These habits, known as sleep hygiene, involve elements related to behaviour, diet, substance use and misuse, and managing light, noise and other environmental factors.

At the centre of this approach is the setting of sleep rituals and habits which provide a quiet, peaceful and predictable pattern for sleep. Setting a consistent sleep time is of importance, as is establishing the principle of only getting into bed when actually feeling sleepy. For many elderly, it is important to establish a consistent sleep ritual. Part of this ritual may be the exposure to bright light in the late evening period, when many elderly will feel prematurely tired and lethargic.[22,135] If people give in to this early drowsiness, they are likely to wake up, completely alert, in the middle of the night. A study of 16 insomniacs of at least 1 year showed improvements in sleep efficiency when subjected to bright-light exposure, a result comparable to that achieved with medications.[136] However, no follow-up data were provided to see whether the changes persisted beyond the treatment time.

Maintaining good sleep hygiene is an effective way of managing sleep disturbances by changing behaviours. Many of the lifestyle recommendations at the heart of sleep hygiene are principles very familiar to chiropractors who incorporate a good deal of wellness counselling into their practices. Among these are the recommendation to avoid foods, beverages and medications which may contain stimulants. The following guidelines can be recommended to patients to help to promote a good night's sleep:

- Maintain a regular schedule. Get up and go to sleep at the same time every day. Keep regular times for meals, medications and activities.
- Establish relaxing presleep rituals such as taking a warm bath, reading, listening to music and meditation.
- Exercise regularly. If you exercise vigorously, do so at least 5 h before bedtime. Mild exercise and stretching should be done at least 4 h before bedtime.
- If you nap, try to do so at the same time every day, before to 3 pm, and for less than an hour.
- Make the sleep environment comfortable by minimizing light, noise and extremes in temperature in the bedroom.
- Avoid eating or drinking anything containing caffeine within 6 hours of bedtime. Review prescription medications for the use of stimulants.
- Minimize all distractions from sleep, including TV and pets in the bedroom at night.
- Do not drink alcohol within 6 hours of bedtime.
- Avoid sleeping pills for anything but transient severe insomnia.
- Avoid smoking close to bedtime.

Activity is recommended, and suggestion is made to explore when this would be most advantageous to daily sleep–wake rhythms.[137] For an older person a pattern of going out for a walk after dinner may help to counteract the advanced sleep phase which becomes more pervasive with ageing. Vigorous exercise can improve the quality of nocturnal sleep and increase the percentage of SWS.[7] Production of GH can be stimulated, which can have an anabolic effect on protein metabolism, helping to restore muscle mass, accelerating cicatrization and enhancing the production of high-density lipoproteins.

Exercise has also been shown to be effective in helping elderly depressed patients.[138] A 10 week randomized control trial of weight training three times a week was compared with an attention control group. The subjects in the supervised weight-training programme improved both their subjective sleep quality and their depression. Depression measures were reduced by twice the amount seen in controls, and quality of life measures indicated significant broader improvement. Although the percentage increase in strength of these subjects predicted improvement in the Pittsburgh Sleep Quality Index, this improvement did not translate into increases in habitual activity of these patients.

Use of lifestyle stimulants such as caffeine, alcohol and tobacco should be limited for all patients with moderate or severe sleep disturbance. In every case, the use of such substances after midday can disrupt the next night's sleep. Naps in the afternoon can also interfere with the sleep pattern for the coming night. Few studies exist of the impact of these interventions, but preliminary results[139] suggest that sleep hygiene alone is as effective as more complex treatments in helping the elderly insomniac. A comprehensive discussion of sleep hygiene counselling for elderly patients can be found in Riedel's recent review.[140]

Attitudes and beliefs

There is a broad literature which demonstrates a relationship between neuroticism and sleep disturbance. Morin and his colleagues examined the beliefs, expectations and attributions relating to a number of sleep-related themes for elderly good sleepers and insomniacs.[123] They found that the insomniacs endorsed stronger beliefs about negative consequences of insomnia, and expressed more hopelessness about the fear of losing control of their sleep and more helplessness about its unpredictability. Clearly the person's beliefs and attitudes about sleep can be instrumental in perpetuating insomnia, and cognitive evaluation and intervention should be part of a systematic treatment programme for older insomniacs. Morin's Attitudes and Beliefs Questionnaire is helpful in understanding subjects' ideas about their sleep.[46]

Fichten et al.[97] provided an excellent review and summary of personality characteristics of elderly patients with insomnia. They note that in most cases of chronic insomnia, behavioural factors make a relatively small contribution to the sleep disturbance. Much more important are the multidimensional components of physiological activation, and psychological stimulation and facilitation. The key components include hyperarousal of the CNS, affective distress about sleep disruption and cognitive activity.

The types of cognitive activity that are particularly characteristic of the insomniac include cognitive hyperarousal, and distressing and intrusive thoughts. The Sleep Self-Statement Test (SST): 60+[121] was designed to capture the characteristics of night-time mentation of insomniacs. It gives two ratings of generalized positive and negative thinking of the elderly insomniac at night. Negative thoughts have been strongly and significantly related to sleep disturbance measures, as well as to complaints of daytime functioning.[97]

This work is an important extension of Morin's earlier work. While Morin's Attitudes and Beliefs Questionnaire asks subjects for their general views, the SST asks subjects for the specific thoughts that plague them and keep them awake at night. The SST also provides a way of evaluating the relative prevalence of negative thoughts, by calculating a ratio, or relative frequency of negative thoughts. Finally, once one has determined that there is an unhealthy prevalence, relative to positive thoughts, the SST identifies which particular negative thoughts are most salient for this particular elderly patient.

Fichten et al. propose a cognitive model of insomnia, in which cognitive factors play a critical role in the development of hyperarousal, and in the interpretation of the meaning of that hyperarousal for the individual elderly insomniac.[97] Specifically, negative cognitive activity (worrying and anxious thoughts and self-statements during periods of nocturnal wakefulness) is hypothesized to be the important mediator of insomnia complaints. Their data show that the patient's per-

ception of the severity of their sleep problem, and negative thoughts both make significant and independent contributions to the variability in distress about poor sleep.

Overall, their cognitive model identifies which aspects of the sleep and daytime experiences of the elderly insomniac to evaluate, provides tools to evaluate those processes, and identifies strategies to help the patient to change these patterns in a focused treatment process. It offers a comprehensive approach to treating the difficulties of elderly insomniacs, and should be reviewed in detail by anyone planning to provide intervention to these patients. Morin's review of cognitive therapy provides a context and closer description of the process of working with insomniacs within a cognitive behavioural model.[141]

Education

In addition to the above, it is often helpful to direct patients to read other sources to understand more about sleep and ways to improve their sleep patterns. Three of the best resources here are Charles Morin's Relief from Insomnia,[142] Hauri and Linde's No More Sleepless Nights[143] and Ancoli-Israel's All I Want is a Good Night's Sleep.[144] In many cases, the elderly may have to be encouraged to follow-up by making use of such resources.

Nevertheless, there is evidence that, with appropriately motivated patients, such a treatment approach can be very successful and very helpful for the patient. Mimeault and Morin[145] demonstrated that providing a general adult population of primary insomniacs with self-help treatment booklets every week for 6 weeks had a significant benefit on total wake time and sleep efficiency at post-treatment. Waiting list controls did not demonstrate such an improvement, and subjects also receiving a 15 min telephone contact from a sleep professional did not do any better. The authors concluded that cognitive–behavioural bibliotherapy, with or without professional guidance, is an effective approach for treating primary insomnia.

Other remedies

Several herbal and hormonal remedies have been touted as promoting good sleep. Recently, melatonin, valerian, camomile tea, Kava Kava and others have been suggested as being of help to the patient with insomnia. Woodward[146] has suggested that acupuncture may be helpful to some patients. To date there have been no controlled studies of these substances, but a review of clinical reports[147] concluded that valerian has not been shown to be effective in treating insomnia. In contrast, ginkgo biloba has been found effective in delaying the course of dementias.

Melatonin has received more attention than the others remedies. The issues involved in the debate over melatonin's effectiveness for insomnia are reviewed by Kryger[148] and Geoffriau et al.[149] A recent study of melatonin by Monti et al.[150] found clinically significant improvements in sleep for at least half of the 10 subjects in the study cohort.

An ongoing clinical trial of melatonin with insomniac, depressed and demented elderly people[151] reported improved sleep for all three groups, but improved next-day alertness only for the primary insomniacs. A follow-up study of 14 Alzheimer's patients receiving 9 mg of melatonin daily for 2–3 years found a significant improvement in the sundowning usually found in these patients, although no change in cognitive functioning was evident.

A pilot study with the use of melatonin in fibromyalgia patients found that in 1 month of treatment there were significant improvements in sleep, as well as reductions in both the number of tender points and the severity of pain reported at these sites.[152]

In our clinical work with the elderly, patients are not dissuaded from trying the herb or remedy that they wish to take, but not before a 3 week baseline measure of sleep patterns has been recorded. This is then followed by a trial of the active ingredient. In all cases, the person takes the remedy for at least a 3 week period and continues to keep a sleep log throughout this period. After a suitable length of time the patient and doctor can determine whether there is any sustained benefit from the remedy.

The one caveat here is where the elderly patient is already on prescription drugs of various kinds. In this situation there may be unknown interactions between the herbal remedy and the prescribed drugs. Caution is advised and consultation with the prescribing physician is suggested.

Additional sleep resources

This chapter is meant as an introduction to a broad and evolving literature. Contributions to sleep medicine come from physiologists, anatomists, the entire range of primary-health care practitioners and the sleep disorders centres. We hope that this chapter has created better awareness of the importance of taking the sleep complaints of the elderly seriously, and has helped in beginning to fashion the diagnostic and treatment skills needed to manage these problems more effectively.

Practitioners who would like to continue to develop skills in assessing and treating these problems are directed to a number of other sources. Two excellent volumes are available to expand the outline presented in this chapter. Understanding Sleep provides a comprehensive overview of topics including elaboration of the underpinnings of sleep and assessment methodology, and how sleep is impacted by a variety of specific medical conditions.[153] The recently published Treatment of Late-life Insomnia elaborates on many clinical issues involved in providing treatment to the elderly.[154] This book teaches the clinical procedures needed to treat late-life insomnia, in the style of a clinical handbook.

In addition, sleep specialists have two excellent organizations, the American Sleep Disorders Association and the Sleep Research Society. These organizations publish a journal of sleep and sleep disorders research entitled Sleep. They also hold an annual convention, usually in mid June. More information is available on the internet at http://www.asda.org. A highly recommended and very detailed source of research and clinical information is Principles and Practice of Sleep Medicine.[155]

Other websites worth visiting for updated information include the Mayo Clinic website on Sleep Disorders in the Elderly, at http://www.mayo.edu/geriatrics-rst/Sleep_ToC.html, the Website of the Canadian Sleep Society, at http://css.to/about/index.htm, and the Center for Biological Timing website, at http://www.cbt.virginian.edu/index.html. Additional sites and information can be searched for using the search engine at http://www.dogpile.com.

The authors welcome any feedback, suggestions or questions. If the reader is encountering sleep-related problems with elderly patients and this chapter has not addressed them directly, they may contact the primary author, Dr Jaan Reitav, at jreitav@cmcc.ca.

Acknowledgements

The authors wish to express their gratitude to their colleagues at the Canadian Memorial Chiropractic

College, and both the Sleep Disorders Centers of Metropolitan Toronto, and the Toronto Western Hospital, for their support and assistance in the writing of this chapter.

References

1 National Institutes of Health. Consensus development conference statement: the treatment of sleep disorders of older people. Sleep 1991; 14: 169–177. [Abstracted from NIH. Diagnosis and Treatment of Sleep Disorders in Late Life. Bethesda, MD: NIH, 1990.]

2 Hirshkowitz M, Moore CA, Hamilton CR et al. Polysomnography of adults and elderly: sleep architecture, respiration, and leg movements. J Clin Neurophysiol 1992; 9: 56–63.

3 Chokroverty S. Sleep disorders in elderly persons. In: Chokroverty S, ed. Sleep Disorders Medicine: Basic Science, Technical Considerations, and Clinical Aspects. London: Butterworth-Heinemann, 1994: 401–415.

4 Zepelin H, McDonald CS, Zammit GK. Effects of age on auditory awakening thresholds. J Gerontol 1984; 39: 294–300.

5 Bliwise DL. Normal aging. In: Kryger MH, Roth T, Dement WC, eds. Principles and Practice of Sleep Medicine, 2nd Edn. Philadelphia, PA: WB Saunders, 1994: 26–36.

6 Roffwarg HP, Muzio JN, Dement WC. Ontogenetic development of the human sleep–dream cycle. Science 1966; 152: 604–619.

7 Culebras A. Sleep in old age. In: Culebras A, ed. Clinical Handbook of Sleep Disorders. Boston, MA: Butterworth-Heinemann, 1996; 375–395.

8 Ancoli-Israel S. Sleep problems in older adults: putting myths to bed. Geriatrics 1997; 52(1): 20–30.

9 Reynolds CF, Hoch CC, Buysse DJ et al. Normal and abnormal REM sleep regulation: REM sleep in successful, usual, and pathological aging: the Pittsburgh experience 1980–93. J Sleep Res 1993; 2: 203–210.

10 Van Cauter E, Leproult R, Plat L. Age-related changes in slow wave sleep and REM sleep and relationship with growth hormone and cortisol levels in healthy men. JAMA 2000; 284: 861–868.

11 Hoch CC, Dew MA, Reynolds CF et al. Longitudinal changes in diary- and laboratory-based sleep measures in healthy 'old old' and 'young old' subjects: a three-year follow-up. Sleep 1997; 20: 192–202.

12 Touitou Y, Haus E. Biological rhythms and aging. In: Touitou Y, Haus E, eds. Biological Rhythms in Clinical and Laboratory Medicine Berlin: Springer, 1992: 188–207.

13 Evans LK. Sundown syndrome in institutionalized elderly. J Am Geriatr Soc 1997; 35: 101–109.

14 Pat-Horenczyk R, Klauber MR, Shochat T et al. Hourly profiles of sleep and wakefulness in severely versus mild–moderately demented nursing home patients. Aging 1998; 10: 308–315.

15 Moore-Ede M, Sulzman F, Fuller C. The Clocks that Time Us: Physiology of the Circadian Timing System. Cambridge, MA: Harvard University Press, 1982.

16 Everson CA. Sleep deprivation and the immune system. In: Pessman MR, Orr WC, eds. Understanding Sleep: The Evaluation and Treatment of Sleep Disorders. Washington, DC: American Psychological Association Press, 1997: 401–424.

17 Haimov I, Lavie P. Circadian characteristics of sleep propensity function in healthy elderly: a comparison with young adults. Sleep 1997; 20: 294–300.

18 Corpas E, Harman SM, Blackman MR. Human hormone and human ageing. Endocr Rev 1993; 14: 20–39.

19 Rowe JW, Troen BR. Sympathetic nervous system and aging in man. Endocr Rev 1980; 1: 167.

20 Rediehs MH, Reis JS, Creason NS. Sleep in old age: focus on gender differences. Sleep 1990; 13: 410–424.

21 Hoffman MA, Fliers E, Goudsmit E et al. Morphometric analysis of the suprachiasmatic and paraventricular nuclei in the human brain: sex differences and age-dependent changes. J Anat 1988; 160: 127–143.

22 Czeisler CA, Allan JS, Strogatz SH et al. Bright light resets the human circadian pacemaker independent of the timing of the sleep–wake cycle. Science 1986; 233: 667–671.

23 Monk TH, Reynolds CF, Machen MA et al. Daily social rhythms in the elderly and their relationship to objectively recorded sleep. Sleep 1992; 15: 322–329.

24 Myers BL, Badia P. Changes in circadian rhythms and sleep quality with aging: mechanisms and interventions. Neurosci Biobehav Rev 1995; 19: 553–571.

25 Rowe JW, Kahn R. Human aging: usual and successful. Science 1987; 237: 143–149.

26 Simon GE, VonKorff M. Prevalence, burden, and treatment of insomnia in primary care. Am J Psychiatry 1997; 154: 1417–1423.

27 Libman E, Creti L, Levy RD et al. A comparison of reported and recorded sleep in older poor sleepers. J Clin Geropsychol 1997; 3: 199–211.

28 Lichstein KL, Means MK, Noe SL et al. Fatigue and sleep disorders. Behav Res Ther 1997; 35: 733–740.

29 Ohayon MM, Caulet M, Guilleminault C. How a general population perceives its sleep and how this relates to the complaint of insomnia. Sleep 1997; 20: 715–723.

30 Ohayon MM. Epidemiological study of insomnia in the general population. Sleep 1996; 19(3): S7–S15.

31 Ohayon MM, Caulet M, Priest RG et al. DSM-IV and ICSD-90 insomnia symptoms and sleep dissatisfaction. Br J Psychiatry 1997; 171: 382–388.

32 Riedel BW, Lichstein KL. Objective sleep measures and subjective sleep satisfaction: how do older adults with insomnia define a good night's sleep? Psychol 1998; 13: 159–163.

33 Foley DJ, Monjan AA, Simonsick EM et al. Incidence and remission of insomnia among elderly adults: an epidemiological study of 6,800 persons over three years. Sleep 1999; 22 (Suppl 2): S366–S372.

34 Maggi S, Langlois JA, Minicuci N et al. Sleep complaints in community-dwelling older persons: prevalence, associated factors, and reported causes. J Am Geriatric Soc 1998; 46: 161–168.

35 Chiu HF, Leung T, Lam LC et al. Sleep problems in Chinese elderly in Hong Kong. Sleep 1999; 22: 717–726.

36 Zanocchi M, Ponsetto M, Spada S et al. Sleep disorders in the elderly. Minerva Med 1999; 90: 421–427.

37 Roth T, Ancoli-Israel S. Daytime consequences and correlates of insomnia in the United States: results of the 1991 National Sleep Foundation survey II. Sleep 1999; 22(Suppl 2): S354–S358.

38 Zammit GK, Weiner J, Damato N et al. Quality of life in people with insomnia. Sleep 1999; 22(Suppl 2): S379–S385.

39 Hart RP, Morin CM, Best AM. Relationship of sleep disturbance to cognitive functioning in insomniac elderly. Aging Cognition 1995; 2: 268–278.

40 Crenssaw MC, Edinger JD. Slow-wave sleep and working cognitive performance among older adults with and without insomnia complaints. Physiol Behav 1999; 66: 485–492.

41 Consensus Development Panel, Freedman, D, chair. Drugs and insomnia: the use of medications to promote sleep. JAMA 1984; 251: 2410–2414.

42 Shochat T, Umphress J, Israel AG, et al. Insomnia in primary care patients. Sleep 1999; 22(Suppl 2): S359–5365.

43 Lichtenberg PA. Introduction. In: Lichtenberg PA, ed. Handbook of Assessment in Clinical Gerontology. New York: John Wiley and Sons, 1999: 1–10.

44 Kales A, Kales JD. Evaluation and Treatment of Insomnia. New York: Oxford University Press, 1984.

45 Spielman AJ, Glovinsky PB. The diagnostic interview and differential diagnosis for complaints of insomnia. In: Pressman MR, Orr WC, eds. Understanding Sleep: The Evaluation and Treatment of Sleep Disorders. Washington, DC: American Psychological Association, 1997.

46 Morin CM. Insomnia: Psychological Assessment and Management. New York: Guilford Press, 1993.

47 Espie CA. Assessment and differential diagnosis. In: Lichstein KL, Morin CM, eds. Treatment of Late-life Insomnia. Thousand Oaks; AC: Sage, Publications, 2000: 81–108.

48 Espie CA. The Psychological Treatment of Insomnia. Chichester: John Wiley and Sons, 1991.

49 Lichstein KL, Reidel BW. Behavioral assessment and treatment of insomnia: a review with an emphasis on clinical application. Behav Ther 1994; 25: 659–688.

50 Vignola A, Lamoureux C, Bastien CH et al. Effects of chronic insomnia and use of benzodiazepines on daytime performance in older adults. J Gerontol Psychol Soc Sci 2000; 55: P54–P62.

51 Johns MW. A new method for measuring daytime sleepiness: the Epworth Sleepiness Scale. Sleep 1991; 14: 540–545.

52 Whitney CW, Enright PL, Newman AB et al. Correlates of daytime sleepiness in 4578 elderly persons – the Cardiovascular Health Study. Sleep 1998; 21: 27–36.

53 Hays JC, Blazer DG, Foley D et al. Risk of napping: excessive daytime sleepiness and mortality in an older community population. J Am Geriatr Soc 1996; 44: 693–698.

54 Diagnostic Classification Steering Committee, Thorpy MJ, Chair. International classification of sleep disorders. Rochester, MN: American Sleep Disorders Association, 1997.

55 Anders TF. Sleep disorders. In: Gabbard GO, Atkinson SD, eds. Synopsis of Treatments of Psychiatric Disorders. 2nd edn. Washington, DC: American Psychiatric Press, 1996: 167–176.

56 Morgan K. Sleep and aging. In: Lichstein KL, Morin CM, eds. Treatment of Late-life Insomnia. Thousand Oaks, CA: Sage, 2000: 3–36.

57 Douglass AB, Bormstein R, Nino-Murcia G et al. The Sleep Disorders Questionnaire I: creation and multivariate structure of the SDQ. Sleep 1994; 17: 160–167.

58 Buysse DJ, Reynolds CF, Monk TH et al. The Pittsburgh Sleep Quality Index: a new instrument for psychiatric practice and research. Psychiatry Res 1989; 28: 193–213.

59 Lugaresi E, Cirignotta F, Caccagna G et al. Some epidemiological data on snoring and cardiocirculatory disturbance. Sleep 1980; 3: 221–224.

60 Hoffstein V. Is snoring dangerous to your health? Sleep 1996; 19: 506–516.

61 Ancoli-Israel S, Kripke DF, Klauber MR et al. Sleep disordered breathing in community dwelling elderly. Sleep 1991; 14: 486–495.

62 Bliwise DL. Sleep and aging. In: Pressman MR, Orr WC, eds. Understanding Sleep: The Evaluation and Treatment of Sleep Disorders. Washington, DC: American Psychological Association Press, 1997: 441–464.

63 Kripke DF, Ancoli-Israel S, Klauber MR et al. Prevalence of sleep-disordered breathing in ages 40–64 years: a population-based survey. Sleep 1997; 20: 65–76.

64 Ancoli-Israel S, Kripke DF, Klauber MR et al. Morbidity, mortality and sleep-disordered breathing in community dwelling elderly. Sleep 1996; 19: 277–282.

65 Bixler EO, Vgontzas AN, Ten HT et al. Effects of age on sleep apnoea in men I: Prevalence and severity. Am J Respir Crit Care Med 1998 ;157: 144–148.

66 Coy TV, Dimsdale JE, Ancoli-Israel S et al. The role of sleep-disordered breathing in essential hypertension. Chest 1996; 109: 890–895.

67 Saskin P. Obstructive sleep apnoea: treatment options, efficacy, and effects. In: Pressman MR, Orr WC, eds. Understanding Sleep: The Evaluation and Treatment of Sleep Disorders. Washington, DC: American Psychological Association Press, 1997: 283–297.

68 Levy P, Pepin JL, Malauzat D et al. Is sleep apnoea syndrome in the elderly a specific entity? Sleep 1996; 19(3): S29–S38.

69 Ancoli-Israel S, Kripke DF, Klauber MR et al. Periodic limb movements in sleep in community dwelling elderly. Sleep 1991; 14: 496–500.

70 Mayo Clinic Website on Sleep Disorders in the Elderly at http://www.mayo.edu/geriatrics-rst/Sleep_ToC.html

71 Chesson AL, Wise M, Davila D et al. Practice parameters for the treatment of restless legs syndrome and periodic limb movement disorder. An American Academy of Sleep Medicine Report, Standards of Practice Committee. Sleep 1999; 22: 961–968.

72 Rye DB, Dihenia B, Weissman JD et al. Presentation of narcolepsy after 40. Neurology 1998; 50: 459–465.

73 Broughton RJ, Fleming JA, George CF et al. Randomized, double-blind, placebo-controlled crossover trial of modafinil in the treatment of excessive daytime sleepiness in narcolepsy. Neurology 1997; 49: 444–451.

74 Chiu HF, Wing YK, Chung DW et al. REM sleep behavior disorder in the elderly. Int J Geriatr Psychiatry 1997; 12: 888–891.

75 Tan A, Salgado M, Fahn S. REM sleep behavior disorder preceding Parkinson's disease with therapeutic response to levodopa. Mov Disord 1996; 11: 214–216.

76 Roberts RE, Sheema SJ, Kaplan GA. Prospective data on sleep complaints and associated risk factors in an older cohort. Psychosom Med 1999; 61: 188–196.

77 Gislason T, Almqvist M. Somatic diseases and sleep complaints. Acta Med Scand 1987; 221: 475–481.

78 Vitiello MV, Prinz PN, Williams DE et al. Sleep disturbances in patients with mild-stage Alzheimer's disease. J Gerontol Med Sci 1990; 45: M131–M138.

79 Wittig RM, Zorick FJ, Blumer D et al. Disturbed sleep in patients complaining of chronic pain. J Nerv Ment Disord 1982; 170: 424–431.

80 Mant A, Eyland EA. Sleep patterns and problems in elderly general practice attenders: an Australian survey. Community Health Stud 1988; 12: 192–199.

81 Hyyppa MT, Kronholm E. Quality of sleep and chronic illnesses. J Clin Epidemiol 1989; 42: 633–638.

82 Cook NR, Evans DA, Funkenstein H et al. Correlates of headache in a population based cohort of elderly. Arch Neurol 1989; 46: 1338–1344.

83 Brocklehurst JC, Fry J, Griffiths L et al. Dysuria in old age. J Am Geriatr Soc 1971; 19: 582–592.

84 Umlauf MG, Goode S, Burgio KL. Psychosocial issues in geriatric urology: Problems in treatment and treatment seeking. Urol Clin North Am 1996; 23: 127–136.

85 Kutner N, Schechtman KB Ory MG, et al. Older adults' perceptions of their health and functioning in relation to sleep disturbance, falling, and urinary incontinence. J Am Geriatr Soc 1984; 42: 757–762.

86 Lichstein KL. Secondary insomnia. In: Lichstein KL, Morin CM, eds. Treatment of Late-life Insomnia. Thousand Oaks, CA: Sage, 2000: 297–319.

87 Morgan K, Healey DW, Healey PJ. Factors influencing persistent subjective insomnia in old age: a follow-up study of good and poor sleepers aged 65–74. Age Ageing 1989; 18: 117–122.

88 Reite M, Ruddy J, Nagel K. Evaluation and Management of Sleep Disorders. 2nd edn. Washington, DC: American Psychiatric Press, 1997.

89 Ware JC, Morin CM. Sleep in depression and anxiety. In: Pressman MR, Orr WC, eds. Understanding Sleep: The Evaluation and Treatment of Sleep Disorders. Washington, DC: American Psychological Association Press, 1997: 483–503.

90 Ohayon MM, Caulet M, Lemoine P. Co-morbidity of mental and insomnia disorders in the general population. Compr Psychiatry 1998; 39: 185–197.

91 Folks DG, Fuller WC. Anxiety disorders and insomnia in geriatric patients. Psychiatr Clin of North Am 1997; 20: 137–164.

92 Kennedy GJ, Kelman HR, Thomas C. Persistence and remission of depressive symptoms in late life. Am J Psychiatry 1991; 148: 174–178

93 Reynolds CF, Hoch CC, Buysse DJ et al. EEG sleep in spousal bereavement and bereavement-related depression of late life. Biol Psychiatry 1992; 31: 69–82.

94 George LK. Social factors in geriatric psychiatry. In: Busse F, Blazer DG, eds. Social and Economic Factors in Geriatric Psychiatry. Washington, DC: American Psychiatric Press, 1989: 203–234.

95 Prigerson HG, Frank E, Reynolds CF et al. Protective psychosocial factors in depression among spousally bereaved elders. Am J Geriatr Psychiatry 1993; 1: 296–309.

96 Roberts RE, Shema SJ, Kaplan GA. Sleep complaints and depression in an aging cohort: a prospective perspective. Am J Psychiatry 2000; 157: 81–88.

97 Fichten CS, Libman E, Bailes S et al. Characteristics of older adults with insomnia. In: Lichstein KL, Morin CM, eds. Treatment of Late-life Insomnia. Thousand Oaks, CA: Sage, 2000: 37–79.

98 Morgan K. Managing sleep and insomnia. In: Woods RT, ed. Handbook of the Clinical Psychology of Ageing. New York: John Wiley and Sons, 1996: 303–316.

99 Shorr RI, Robin DW. Rational use of benzodiazepines in the elderly. Drugs Aging 1994; 4: 9–20.

100 Bandera R, Bollini P, Garattini S et al. Long-acting and short-acting benzodiazepines in the elderly: kinetic differences and clinical relevance. Curr Med Res Opin 1994; 8 (Suppl 4): 94–107.

101 Ancoli-Israel S. Insomnia in the elderly: a review for the primary care practitioner. Sleep 2000; 23 (Suppl 1): S23–S30; S36–S38.

102 Asplund R. Sleep disorders in the elderly. Drugs Aging 1999; 14(2): 91–103.

103 Morin CM, Baillargeon L, Bastien C. Discontinuation of sleep medications. In: Lichstein KL, Morin CM, eds. Treatment of Late-life Insomnia. Thousand Oaks, CA: Sage 2000: 271–296.

104 Gallup Organization. Sleep in America: a national survey of U.S. Adults. Princeton, NJ: National Sleep Foundation, 1991.

105 Roth T. Social and economic consequences of sleep disorders. Sleep 1996; 19(8): S46–S47.

106 Morin CM, Culbert JP, Schwartz SM. Nonpharmacological interventions for insomnia: a meta-analysis of treatment efficacy. Am J Psychiatry 1994; 151: 1172–1180.

107 Morin CM, Colecchi C, Stone J et al. Behavioral and pharmacological therapies for late-life insomnia: a randomized controlled trial. JAMA 1998; 281: 991–999.

108 Pallesen S, Nordhus IH, Kvale G. Nonpharmacological interventions for insomnia in older adults: a meta-analysis of treatment efficacy. Psychotherapy 1998; 35: 472–482.

109 Morin CM, Gaulier B, Barry T et al. Patients' acceptance of psychological and pharmacological therapies for insomnia. Sleep 1992; 15: 302–305.

110 Moldofsky H. Sleep influences on regional and diffuse pain syndromes associated with osteoarthritis. Semin in Arthritis Rheum 1989; 4 Suppl. (2): 18–21.

111 Moldofsky H. Sleep and musculoskeletal pain. In: Vaeroy H, Merskey H, eds. Progress in Fibromyalgia and Myofascial Pain. Amsterdam: Elsevier, 1993: 137–148.

112 Moldofsky H. Sleep and fibrositis syndrome. Rheum Dis Clin North Am 1989; 15: 90–103.

113 Reitav J, Hamovitch GN. Psychological aspects of head and neck pain. In: Vernon H, ed. The Cranio-Cervical Syndrome: Mechanisms, Assessment and Treatment. London: Butterworth Heinemann (2001).

114 Moldofsky H, Scarisbrick P. Induction of neurasthenic musculoskeletal pain syndrome by selective sleep stage deprivation. Psychosom Med 1976; 38 35–44.

115 Reitav J, McClean K, Cook T et al. Changes in sleep and muscular pain thresholds in college students during final examinations. 2000 (in press).

116 Janssen SA, Arntz A, Bouts S. Anxiety and pain: epinephrine-induced hyperalgesia and attentional influences. Pain 1998; 76: 309–316.

117 Volicer BJ. Hospital stress and patient reports of pain and physical status. J Hum Stress 1978; 4: 28–37.

118 Morin CM, Gibson D, Wade J. Self-reported sleep and mood disturbance in chronic pain patients. Clin J Pain 1998; 14: 311–314.

119 Morin CM, Ware JC. Sleep and psychopathology. Appl Prevent Psychol 1996; 5: 211–224.

120 Beullens J. Determinants of insomnia in relatively healthy elderly: a literature review. Tijdschr Gerontol Geriatr 1999; 30: 31–38.

121 Fichten CS, Libman E, Creti L et al. Thoughts during awake times in older good and poor sleepers: the Self-Statement Test: 60+. Cognitive Ther Res 1998; 22: 1–20.

122 Libman E, Creti L, Amsel R et al. What do older good and poor sleepers do during periods of nocturnal wakefulness? The Sleep Behaviours Scale: 60+. Psychol Aging 1997; 12: 170–182.

123 Morin CM, Stone J, Tinkle D et al. Dysfunctional beliefs and attitudes about sleep among older adults with and without insomnia complaints. Psychol Aging 1993; 8: 463–467.

124 Englert S, Linden M. Differences in self-reported sleep complaints in elderly persons living in the community who do or do not take sleep medications. J Clin Psychiatry 1998; 59: 137–144.

125 Sproule BA, Busto UE, Buckle C et al. The use of non-prescription sleep products in the elderly. Intl J Geriatr Psychiatry 1999; 14: 851–85

126 Neubauer DN. Sleep problems in the elderly. Am Fam Physician 1999; 5: 2551–2560.

127 Nowell PD, Buysse DJ, Reynolds CF et al. Clinical factors contributing to the differential diagnosis of primary insomnia and insomnia related to mental disorders. Am J Psychiatry 1997; 154: 1412–1416.

128 Reynolds CF, Dew MA, Monk TH et al. Sleep disorders in late life: a biopsychosocial model for understanding pathogenesis and intervention. In: Coffey CE, Cummings JL, eds Textbook of Geriatric Neuropsychiatry. Washington, DC: American Psychiatric Association, 1996: 323–331.

129 Nowell PD, Hoch CC, Reynolds CF. Sleep disorders. In: Coffey CE, Cummings JL, eds. Textbook of Geriatric Neuropsychiatry Washington, DC: American Psychiatric Press, 2000: 401–413.

130 Hemmelgarn B, Suissa S, Huang A et al. Benzodiazepine use and the risk of motor vehicle crash in the elderly. JAMA 1997; 278: 27–31.

131 Reynolds CF, Buysse DJ, Kuupfer DJ *et al.* Treating insomnia in older adults: taking a long-term view. JAMA 1999; 281: 1034–1035.

132 Wohlgemuth WK, Edinger JD, Fins AI *et al.* How many nights are enough? The short- term stability of sleep parameters in elderly insomniacs and normal sleepers. Psychophysiology 1999; 36: 233–244.

133 Rogers AE, Caruso CC, Aldrich M. Reliability of sleep diaries for assessment of sleep/wake patterns. Nurs Res 1993; 42; 368–372.

134 Buysse DJ, Morin CM,. Reynolds CF III. Sleep disorders. In: Gabbard GO, Atkinson SD, eds. Synopsis of Treatments of Psychiatric Disorders 2nd edn. Washington, DC: American Psychiatric Press, 1996: 1013–1041.

135 Campbell SS, Terman M, Lewy AJ *et al.* Light treatment for sleep disorders: consensus report; V. Age-related disturbances. J Biol Rhythms 1995; 10: 151–154.

136 Campbell SS. Bright light treatment of sleep maintenance insomnia and behavioral disturbance. In: Lam RW *et al.*, eds. Seasonal Affective Disorder and Beyond: Light Treatment for SAD and non-SAD Condition. Washington, DC: American Psychiatric Press, 1998: 289–304.

137 King AC, Oman RF, Brassington G *et al.* Moderate-intensity exercise and self-rated quality of sleep in older adults. JAMA 1997; 277: 32–37.

138 Singh NA, Clements KM, Fiatarone MA. A randomized controlled trial of the effect of exercise on sleep. Sleep 1997; 20: 95–101.

139 Friedman L, Benson K, Noda A *et al.* An actigraphic comparison of sleep restriction and sleep hygiene treatments for insomnia in older adults. J Geriatr Psychiatry Neurol 2000; 13: 17–27.

140 Riedel BW. Sleep hygiene. In: Lichstein KL, Morin CM, eds. Treatment of Late-life Insomnia. Thousand Oaks, CA: Sage, 2000: 125–146.

141 Morin CM, Savard J, Blais FC. Cognitive therapy. In: Lichstein KL, Morin CM, eds. Treatment of Late-life Insomnia. Thousand Oaks, CA: Sage, 2000: 207–230.

142 Morin CM. Relief from Insomnia: Getting the Sleep of Your Dreams. New York: Doubleday, 1996.

143 Hauri P, Linde S. No More Sleepless Nights. New York: John Wiley and Sons, 1990.

144 Ancoli-Israel S. All I Want is a Good Night's Sleep. St Louis: Mosby Books, 1996.

145 Mimeault V, Morin CM. Self-help treatment for insomnia: bibliotherapy with and without professional guidance. J Consuit Clin Psychol 1999; 67: 511–519.

146 Woodward M. Insomnia in the elderly. Aust Fam Physician 1999; 28: 653–658.

147 Ernst E. Herbal medications for common ailments in the elderly. Drugs Aging 1999; 15: 423–428.

148 Kryger MH. Controversies in sleep medicine – melatonin. Sleep 1997; 20: 898.

149 Geoffriau M, Brun J, Chazot G *et al.* The physiology and pharmacology of melatonin in humans. Horm Res 1998; 49: 136–141.

150 Monti JM, Alvarino F, Cardinali D *et al.* Polysomnographic study of the effect of melatonin on sleep in elderly patients with chronic primary insomnia. Arch Gerontol Geriatr 1999; 28: 85–98.

151 Brusco LI, Fainstein I, Marquez M *et al.* Effect of melatonin in selected populations of sleep-disturbed patients. Biol Signals Recept 1999; 8: 126–131.

152 Citera G, Arias MA, Maldonado-Cocco JA *et al.* The effect of melatonin in patients with fibromyalgia: a pilot study. Clin Rheumatol 2000; 19: 9–13.

153 Pressman MR, Orr WC. Understanding Sleep: The Evaluation of Sleep Disorders. Washington, DC: American Psychological Association, 1997.

154 Lichstein KL, Morin CM. Treatment of Late-life Insomnia. Thousand Oaks, CA: Sage, 2000.

155 Kryger MH, Roth T, Dement WC. Principles and Practice of Sleep Medicine 3rd Edn. Philadelphia, PA: Saunders, 2000.

22

Iatrogenic drug reactions

Brian J Gleberzon

Despite differences in principles and philosophy, a common feature of chiropractic care is the preference for a non-pharmacological solution to a patient's clinical condition whenever possible. Clearly, there are instances when allopathic intervention is essential for the survival of a patient or the successful management of a particular clinical condition. Type I diabetes, coronary heart disease, infective processes such as pneumonia and tuberculosis, neoplasms requiring aggressive chemotherapies and emergency procedures all dictate a medical approach. Very few chiropractors or other complementary and alternative medicine (CAM) providers would dispute this general principle. However, it is equally true that exclusive reliance on drug therapies can be inherently dangerous and often unnecessary. In many cases, a drugless approach can and should be the initial treatment of choice. The importance of this concept is nowhere more compelling than with the prescription of medications for older adults.

Definitions

The study of ageing and pharmacology in humans has been termed geriatric clinical pharmacology, which is a subdiscipline within the broad field of clinical pharmacology.[1] To understand the issues of geriatric clinical pharmacology, several terms must be defined. These include: polymedicine, polypharmacy, adverse drug reaction (ADR), iatrogenic drug reaction and the prescription cascade.

Polymedicine describes the use of medications in an older patient for the treatment of multiple comorbid conditions.[2] Polypharmacy represents a less than desirable state of multiple drug consumption with duplicative medications, interactions between drugs, and inadequate attention to pharmacokinetic and pharmacodynamic principles.[2,3]

According to the World Health Organization, an ADR is defined as any noxious, unintended or undesired effect of a drug, which occurs at doses used in humans for prophylaxis, diagnosis or therapy.[4] This definition excludes therapeutic failures, intentional and accidental poisoning (drug overdoses), errors in administration or non-compliance on the part of the patient.[4]*

Iatrogenic drug reactions refer to those ADRs that occur as the result of treatment by a physician, either in private practice or during hospitalization.[3]

The prescription cascade is a specific category of ADRs. It is not uncommon for the undesired side-effects of a prescription medication to be either misinterpreted as a new clinical complaint, or recognized as a consequence of the drug but considered insignificant. In either case, the original drug dose is continued and a new prescription drug is provided to the patient to combat the symptoms of the first drug. This new drug may, either because of its own physiological effects or by interacting with the first drug, cause the development of a new symptom pattern, which is often treated with yet another medication.

Age-related changes, pharmacokinetics and pharmacodynamics

It is imperative for those health-care providers who make use of medications, whether prescription or over-the-counter, to be aware of the normal physiological changes that occur in older patients which result in an increased likelihood of ADRs. Even those health-care providers who recommend botanical medicines or other supplements and remedies must be cognizant of these physiological changes, since such changes may necessitate a modification to recommended dosage levels and/or frequency of use.

As a person ages, there is a decline in both hepatic and renal function.[5–7] By the age of 80, there is a 30%

(or more) decline in glomerular filtration rate, renal mass and blood flow, and also a decline in hepatic mass, enzymatic activity and blood flow.[6,7] This causes a concomitant decline in drug clearance, which results in an increase in the bioavailability of a drug. The recommended dose of a drug is partially determined by its expected rate of clearance from the body. If the organs responsible for this clearance (liver and kidneys) are not functioning optimally, a drug may be present in a patient's body for a longer period than might otherwise be expected. In older patients, the effect that drug concentrations have at the site of action (pharmacokinetics) and the responsiveness to the drug by end-organs may be concomitantly and simultaneously altered.[7]

Moreover, there are changes to a person's body composition with age that may alter the physiological effects of medications. Muscle mass and body-water content decline by 30% and 15%, respectively, as a person ages, although total body weight may not change or may increase.[6] Even in thin people, the ratio of body fat to body muscle increases, resulting in a greater pharmacokinetic effect of fat-soluble drugs.[6]

As in any patient, problems of tolerance (the need to increase the size of subsequent doses in order to achieve the same effect obtained previously), withdrawal (unpleasant physiological changes that occur when drug use is abruptly discontinued) and dependence (the psychological or physiological need to repeat or continue administration of a drug to achieve a desired effect, produce pleasure or avoid discomfort) may occur with many prescribed medications.[8]

Medical statistics of drug use in older patients

Thirty per cent of all prescription drugs and 40% of all over-the-counter drugs, are purchased by adults over the age of 65 years.[9,10] Two-thirds of Americans over the age of 65 use at least one drug a day, with 45% of the elderly taking several prescriptions concurrently.[5,10] This translates to an annual cost to the American Health Care system of $10 billion.[5] It has been estimated that almost 25% of older outpatients receive inappropriate medications.[14] Two-thirds of all physician visits lead to a drug prescription and 40% of visits result in the prescription of two or more medications.[5]

The most commonly misused prescription medications are antibiotics.[5] It has been estimated that over 60% of antibiotic use in hospitalized patients is either unnecessary or inappropriately dosed.[5] Furthermore, three-quarters of ADRs are dose dependent, with many occurring at the manufacturer's recommended dose.[10] Although statistics vary, non-steroidal anti-inflammatory drugs (NSAIDs) are thought to result in between 8000 and 16000 deaths and more than 100000 hospitalizations annually in the USA.[10]

Estimates of drug utilization among older persons

There is considerable variation in the estimates of the number of prescription and over-the-counter drugs, homoeopathic or naturopathic remedies, vitamins, minerals and other supplements that older patients consume on a daily basis. This variation is primarily a reflection of the setting in which the person is residing. In general, most experts agree that patients living in long-term institutions are prescribed many more drugs than those living in the community.[5,10] The estimate of the number of prescription medications taken daily by older community-dwelling seniors is three to eight, with seven being the number most frequently cited.[5,6,10] It is further estimated that these seven drugs can be divided into three to four prescription and three to four non-prescription medications.[5,6] However, these numbers may not include supplements or self-prescribed remedies. The geriatric 'Model Curriculum' developed at the Palmer College of Chiropractic estimates that the total number of preparations that an older person consumes daily for a desired clinical effect is 12.[11] Among community-dwelling seniors, the most common types of prescribed medications used are analgesics, diuretics, cardiovascular drugs and sedatives.[7]

The estimate for the number of drugs provided to elderly inpatients ranges from eight to 10 medications daily.[5,6] For nursing-home residents, the most commonly prescribed medications are antipsychotics, sedative–hypnotics, diuretics, antihypertensives, analgesics, cardiac drugs and antibiotics.[7]

The human cost of adverse drug reactions in the USA

The annual national cost of drug-related morbidity and mortality in the USA has recently been estimated at $76.6 billion, with the majority ($47 billion) related to hospital admissions.[12] Several studies have calculated the incidence of ADRs in hospitalized patients.[13–17] The Boston Collaborative Drug Surveillance Project estimated that approximately 30% of hospitalized patients experience adverse events attributable to drugs, and that 3–28% of all hospital admissions are related to ADRs.[13,17] Similarly, ADRs were the most common type of adverse event experienced by patients in the Harvard Medical Practice Study, a study of over 30 000 hospitalized patients.[14,15] The Harvard study documented that at least 3.7% of all hospitalized patients developed serious, disabling and clinically important adverse events during their hospitalizations, of which 20% were ADRs.[14,15,17] Other studies have estimated the rate of ADRs to be 6.5 per 100 hospital admissions, of which 28% were judged to be preventable.[16]

Several recent studies have sought to measure the economic cost and increase in length of stay at hospitals as the result of ADRs.[16,17] In a study by Bates *et al.*,[16] who examined 4108 admissions to 11 medical and surgical units and two tertiary-care units over a 6 month period, the postevent costs attributable to an adverse drug event (ADE) were $2595 for all ADEs and $4685 for the 28% of ADEs judged to be preventable. Of all ADEs, 57% were judged to be significant, 30% serious, 12% life-threatening and 1% fatal. Analgesics (30%) and antibiotics (30%) accounted for the largest percentage of non-preventable ADEs. Preventable ADEs were most often caused by analgesics, sedatives, antibiotics and antipsychotics.[16] The organ systems most commonly affected were the central nervous system (18%), gastrointestinal system (18%) and cardiovascular system (16%), and allergic/cutaneous complications occur in 16%.[16] This study estimated that the annual costs attributable to all ADEs and preventable ADEs for a 700-bed hospital to be $5.6 million and $2.8 million, respectively.[16]

A similar study conducted by Clemen *et al.*[17] concluded that ADEs complicated 2.43 per 100 admissions to the LDS hospital that they studied, resulting in increased hospital stays of 1.91 days at a cost of $2282. The increased risk of death among hospitalized patients experiencing ADEs was 1.88. The authors commented that if these numbers were to be extrapolated to the USA as a whole, 770 000 hospitalized patients may experience ADEs annually.[17]

A prospective meta-analysis conducted by Lazarou *et al.* sought to estimate the number and incidence of serious and fatal ADRs in hospitalized patients in the USA.[4] The researchers reviewed prospective data obtained over a 32 year period on two different groups: those admitted to hospitals due to ADRs, and those experiencing an ADR while in the hospital. Their study indicated the overall incidence of serious ADRs to be 6.7% with a fatality rate of 0.32% among hospitalized patients. The authors estimated that, in 1994, 2 216 000 patients in the two groups studied had serious ADRs, and 106 000 had fatal ADRs, making these reactions between the fourth and sixth leading causes of death, a ranking higher than either pneumonia or diabetes.[4] The authors of the study concluded that serious ADRs are more frequent than generally recognized and that the incidence of ADRs has remained constant since the 1970s.[4]

Adverse drug reactions in older persons

About one half of all deaths attributable to ADRs occur in persons aged 60 and older.[10] Between 10 and 17% of all hospital admissions in the elderly are the result of inappropriately used medications.[5,6,10] Another study investigating nursing home-eligible, homebound seniors revealed that the number of drugs taken daily was 5.3 ± 2.9.[18] Forty per cent of the group under review had received one inappropriate prescription, with 10% having received two or more inappropriate prescriptions.[18]

The incidence of ADRs is dramatically increased in older patients residing in long-term institutions, such as nursing homes.[5,6,19] A recent study by Cooper revealed that, over a 4 year period, ADRs may affect as many as one in seven residents of nursing facilities.[20] It was his opinion that the high incidence of ADRs was related to polypharmacy (estimated at 7.9 ± 2.6 drugs used daily) as well as inattention to patient history for contraindications and previous ADRs.[20] Another study by Williams *et al.* concluded that the prescription of drugs was related more to symptom resolution than to documented medical evidence.[21] Although this group of researchers discovered that the average number of daily medications per resident was five, the investigators found that a general lack of recorded diagnoses limited their ability to evaluate the drug therapy.[21] The authors suggested that improvements in record keeping, periodic medication reviews, and resident, staff and prescriber education are necessary to ensure appropriate drug utilization in such settings.[21]

An intriguing statistic was reported from a study investigating morbidity and mortality in nursing facilities.[22] The investigators calculated that, for every one dollar spent on drugs in nursing facilities, $1.33 in health-care resources was consumed in the treatment of drug-related problems.[22]

Andrews et al. reported that, in a study of over 1000 patient hospital files, 18% were identified as having at least one serious adverse event while under hospital care, and the likelihood of experiencing an adverse event increased by 6% for each day spent in the hospital.[23]

The human cost of adverse drug reaction around the world: a demographic review

Many epidemiological studies have investigated the incidence of ADRs around the world. In general, studies reveal that ADRs in older patients are a very common occurrence, and ADRs are a leading cause of morbidity and mortality in elderly persons worldwide. Studies conducted in Italy,[24,25] Denmark,[26–28] south Wales,[29] France,[30–34] Spain,[35] Portugal[36] and Australia[37,38] all reveal that many older patients are consuming more than one prescription medication daily. Percentages range from 13% in one Italian study[25] to 48% in a Danish study.[28] Reported international rates of ADRs range from 5.7% elderly persons in Denmark[26] to 13.6% of Spanish seniors.[35]

A Portuguese study reported that 44% of elderly hospitalized patients had one or more iatrogenic illness.[36] Of the reported iatrogenic disorders, 18% were due to diagnostic tests and 59% due to therapeutic interventions (32% were directly attributed to drug therapy).[36]

A study conducted in Australia reviewing patient files in general practice revealed that ADRs may be even more prevalent in private practice than in hospital settings.[37] Specifically, problems with therapeutic use occurred in 26% of cases in private practice, compared with 8% in hospitals. The prescribing of contraindicated medications occurred in 15% of patients in private practice, compared with 5% in hospitals. Such contraindications included prescription of a drug to which the patient was known to be allergic (4%), prescription of medications for which there was a recognized potential for a drug interaction (4%) and contraindication due to pathophysiological factors (4%).[37] Another Australian study estimated that

80 000 medication-related hospitalizations occur in Australia each year, and that between 32 and 69% of these hospitalizations were avoidable.[38]

Several different French studies have calculated that 10% of patient admissions to an intensive care unit were for iatrogenic diseases, with ADRs being the most common cause.[30–34] One group of researchers referred to the 'geriatric paradox', which consists of an overprescribing of drugs despite the fact that side-effects are more frequent in older patients.[32] Another group of French researchers concluded that the incidence of iatrogenic disease resulting in hospitalization remained unchanged between 1975 and 1999, despite 25 years of experience with high-technology medicine.[30]

Examples of iatrogenic and adverse drug reactions

Many commonly prescribed medications result in a plethora of adverse reactions and physiological, behavioural and cognitive impairments (Table 22.1). Established ADRs range from cognitive compromise, depression and behavioural changes to urinary incon-

Table 22.1 Example of drug-induced clinical impairments as the result of commonly prescribed medications[5,6]

Drug	Clinical impairment or significance
Corticosteroids	Hyperglycaemia, insomnia, depression, osteoporosis, arthralgia, myopathies.
Non-steroidal anti-inflammatory drugs	Inhibition of platelet aggregation, headache, tinnitus, vertigo, confusion, gastrointestinal distress.
Tylenol	Hepatotoxicity
Anticholinergics	Urinary incontinence, delirium, insomnia, sedation, agitation, irritability, psychosis
β-blockers	Hyperglycaemia, hypotension
Diuretics	Electrolyte imbalance, orthostatic hypotension, hyperglycaemia, hepatitis
Benzodiazepines	Hypotension, psychomotor retardation, incontinence
Antihistamines	Urinary incontinence, psychomotor retardation
Cimetidine (Tagamet)	Central nervous system depression

Table 22.2 Common adverse drug reactions in older persons[7,8]

Adverse reaction	Clinical presentation	Common causes
Anticholinergic effects	Confusion, nervousness, drowsiness, dry mouth, urinary incontinence	Antihistamines, antidepressants, antipsychotics
Confusion	Disorientation, delirium	Antidepressants, narcoanalgesics, anticholinergics
Depression	Intensive sadness, apathy	Alcohol, antihypertensives, antipsychotics, barbituates, β-blockers, corticosteroids
Dementia	Increased confusion, delirium	Antiepileptics, antidepressants, anticholinergics
Dizziness	Loss of balance, falling	Sedatives, antipsychotics, narcoanalgesics, antihistamines
Fatigue and weakness	Loss of strength and inability to perform activities of daily living	Muscle relaxants, diuretics
Hypertension	Increase in blood pressure	Non-steroidal anti-inflammatory drugs
Orthostatic hypotension	Dizziness, loss of balance, increased risk of falling	Antihypertensives, antianginal agents, tricyclic antidepressants
Osteopenia	Bone fragility and fracture	Corticosteroids
Sedation	Drowsiness and sleepiness	Antipsychotics, narcoanalgesics, sedative–hypnotics

tinence, orthostatic hypotension and extrapyramidal symptoms (Table 22.2).

NSAIDs deserve special discussion. These drugs are among the most commonly prescribed medications, especially for patients experiencing spinal pain. However, the risks of NSAID use include serious gastrointestinal complications such as gastritis, ulcers, perforation and bleeding.[39] Complications from NSAID use have been calculated at a fatality rate of 0.04%, accounting for 3200 deaths annually,[40] and a 2.74% rate of serious gastrointestinal events.[41] Other studies estimate 2600 deaths and 20 000 hospitalizations annually are attributable to NSAID use, with an incidence rate of 390–3200 serious gastrointestinal events per million.[42,43] As mentioned in Chapter 10, NSAIDs have other side-effects such as hypertension, they may interfere with hypertensive therapy and NSAID use is associated with an increased risk of renal insufficiency, especially if combined with medications such as diuretics and certain cardiac drugs.[39]

Botanical medicines

The herbal market in the USA is experiencing unprecedented growth.[44] Many patients are presenting to naturopaths, homoeopaths and other CAM providers (Chapter 27) who primarily use botanical and herbal medicinals. The use of herbal medicines increased by 57% in 1997, with an estimated 60 million Americans accounting for $3.14 billion in sales.[44] It is important to note that studies estimate that 70% of patients do not reveal their herbal use to their allopathic physician.[44] A study by Eisenberg *et al.* estimated that 15 million adults in 1997 took prescription medications concurrently with herbal remedies and/or high-dose vitamins (18.4% of all prescription drug users).[45] Although they provide some benefit for a variety of clinical conditions including dizziness (ginger, gingko), headache (feverfew), dementia (ginkgo), sleep disorders (chamomile) and benign prostatic hypertrophy (saw palmetto), many botanical medicines can also result in adverse reactions and are contraindicated in certain clinical conditions[44,46] (see Table 22.3).

Recent studies have sought to measure the efficacy and side-effects of some of the more commonly used botanical medicines.[44–49] For example, Gaster and Holroyd analysed the results of eight randomized controlled studies examining the use of St John's wort for depression.[47] The authors concluded that the response rate with the use of St John's wort ranged from 23 to 55% or higher than with a placebo, but

Table 22.3 Examples of adverse reactions and contraindications to some commonly utilized botanical medicines[44,46]

Botanical medicine	Adverse reactions	Contraindications
Aloe vera	Severe abdominal cramping, nephritis, gastritis, vomiting, bloody diarrhoea	Pregnancy and menstruation
Echinacea	None known	Autoimmune disorders, e.g. diabetes, lupus, rheumatoid arthritis; progressive systemic diseases, e.g. multiple sclerosis, tuberculosis
Gingko	Gastrointestinal disorders, headache, spontaneous bleeding (very rare)	Pregnancy and lactation (?)
Ginseng	Insomnia (Asian ginseng), hypertension, vomiting, headache, epistaxis	Hypertension, acute illness, premenopausal women, diabetes; pregnancy and lactation (?)
St John's wort	Photosensitivity, dizziness, gastrointestinal upset, sedation	Pregnancy and lactation
Valerian	Sedation	Driving or operating hazardous machinery; pregnancy and lactation

ranged from 6 to 18% lower compared with tricyclic antidepressants, although the rate of side-effects was found to be low.[47]

Houpt *et al.* recently reported on a randomized controlled trial (RCT) investigating the efficacy of glucosamine hydrochloride.[48] Their study followed 118 patients with osteoarthritis of the knee over a 21 week period. The investigators concluded that there was no significant difference in pain reduction between glucosamine hydrochloride and the placebo group, as measured by the Western Ontario and McMaster University Osteoarthritis Index (WOMAC).[48] However, the authors noted that, for some patients, there was a cumulative pain reduction as measured by a daily dairy and improvements in knee examination finding (range of motion). About 12% of both the placebo and glucosamine groups reported mild gastrointestinal symptoms.[48] A systematic review of all RCTs investigating glucosamine concluded that the literature supports the efficacy and safety of glucosamine for patients with osteoarthritis.[49]

Adverse drug–herb interactions

The ever-increasing use of botanical medicines and herbs comes with the increased potential for cross-reactions between these medicinals and prescribed drugs. A recent study by Miller[44] explored the potential interactions between prescribed drugs and the more commonly used botanical medicines. These potential interactions are summarized in Table 22.4.

Final recommendations

Given the narrow margin of safety among older patients with respect to medications, a medical physician should always be wary of prescribing a drug unnecessarily and a non-pharmacological treatment should be considered first whenever possible. A prudent clinician is therefore always vigilant to the possibility that any presenting chief complaint may be the consequence of an ADR involving prescription medications, botanical medicines or a combination of both.

If a patient presents with an extensive list of prescription medications, over-the-counter drugs and other remedies, the chiropractor must ask the patient whether they have informed their medical provider(s) of their complete drug profile: this includes all substances that the patient is 'putting in their mouth' for a physiological effect. The patient's medical doctor, and perhaps their pharmacist, can then better advise them and take charge of their drug and drug dosage schedule. Moreover, as many as 70% of older patients use self-selected medications, often obtaining both prescriptions and advice from friends, usually without discussion with their physicians (45). It is not uncommon for one of a patient's medical specialists to be unaware of the prescription drug(s) provided by another medical specialist. The chiropractor can therefore provide an important role in facilitating the sharing of this information by bringing this situation to the patient's attention. If the chiropractor deduces that a clinical symptom or condition may be

Table 22.4 Potential drug–herb interactions[44]

Botanical medicine/herb	Cross-reacting drugs	Potential consequences
Echinacea	Anabolic steroids, amidarone, methotrexate, ketoconazole	Hepatoxic effects
Feverfew	Non-steroidal anti-inflammatory drugs	Negation of effect on migraine headaches
Feverfew, garlic, gingko, ginger, ginseng	Warfanin	Alter bleeding time
Ginseng	Phenelzine sulfate	Headache, manic episodes, tremulousness
Ginseng	Oestrogens, corticosteroids	Possible addictive effects
St John's wort	Monoamine oxidase inhibitors, selective serotonin uptake inhibitors	Unknown mechanism of St John's wort; may cause headache, sweating, agitation
St John's wort	Piroxicam, tetracycline hydorchloride	Photosensitivity
Valerian	Barbiturates	Excessive sedation
Evening primrose oil, borage	Anticonvulsants	Lower seizure threshold
Hawthorn, Siberian ginseng, kyushin, liquorice	Digoxin	Cardiac dysfunction
Chamomile	Anticoagulants (?)	Changes in coagulation (?)

the result of an ADR or polypharmacy, the chiropractor can advise the patient to seek further consultation with their medical provider. Directly informing a patient to discontinue taking a prescribed medication is beyond the scope of chiropractic practice.

References

1 Vestal RE. Aging and pharmacology. Cancer 1997; 80: 1302–1310.
2 Monane M, Monane S, Semla T. Optimal medication use in elders. Key to successful aging. West J Med 1997; 167: 233–237.
3 Elliot M. Dorland's Illustrated Medical Dictionary. 28th edn. Philadelphia, PA: WB Saunders, 1994.
4 Lazarou J, Pomeranz B, Corey P. Incidence of adverse drug reactions in hospitalized patients. JAMA 1998; 279: 1200–1205.
5 Ferri F, Fretwell M, Wachtel T. Practical Guide to the Care of the Elderly Patient. 2nd edn. St Louis: Mosby-Year Book, 1997.
6 Lonergan E. Geriatrics. A Lange Clinical Manual. 1st edn. Stamford, CT: Appleton & Lange, 1996.
7 Abrams W. The Merck Manual for Geriatric Patients. 2nd edn. Whitehouse Station, NJ: Merck & Co., 1997.
8 Abrams W, Beers M, Berkow R. The Merck Manual. 2nd edn. Whitehouse Station, NJ: Merck & Co., 1995.
9 Salom I, Davis K. Prescribing for older patients: how to avoid toxic drug reactions. Geriatrics 1995; 50(10): 37–43.
10 Cohen J. Avoiding adverse reactions. Effective lower-dose drug therapies for older patients. Geriatrics 2000; 55(2): 54–64.
11 Killinger L, Azad A. Chiropractic Geriatric Education: An Interdisciplinary Resource Guide and Teaching Strategy for Health Educators. US Health Resources and Services Administration Contract, 1997.

12 Johnson JA, Bootman JL. Drug-related morbidity and mortality: a cost-of-illness model. Arch Inter Med 1995; 155: 1949–1956.
13 Jicks H. Drugs – Remarkably non-toxic. N Engl J Med 1974; 291: 824–828.
14 Brennan TA, Leape LL, Laird N et al. Incidence of adverse events and negligence in hospitalized patients: results from the Harvard Medical Practice Study. N Engl J Med 1991; 324: 370–376.
15 Leape LL, Brennan TA, Laird N et al. The nature of adverse events in hospitalized patients: results from the Harvard Medical Practice Study II. N Engl J Med 1991; 324: 377–384.
16 Bates DW, Spell N, Cullen DJ et al. The cost of adverse drug events in hospitalized patients. JAMA 1997; 277: 307–311.
17 Classen DC, Pestotnik SL, Evans S et al. Adverse drug events in hospitalized patients: excess length of stay, extra costs, and attributable mortality. JAMA 1997; 277: 301–306.
18 Golden AG, Preston RA, Barnett SD et al. Inappropriate medication prescribing in homebound older adults. J Am Geriatr Soc 1999; 47: 948–953.
19 Broderick E. Prescribing patterns for nursing home residents in the U.S. The reality and the vision. Drugs Aging 1997; 11: 255–260.
20 Cooper JW. Adverse drug reaction-related hospitalizations of nursing facility patients: a 4-year study. South Med J 1999; 92: 485–490.
21 Williams BR, Nichol MB, Lowe B et al. Medication use in residential care facilities for the elderly. Ann Pharmacol 1999; 33: 149–155.
22 Bootman JL, Harrison DL, Cox E. The health care cost of drug-related morbidity and mortality in nursing facilities. Arch Intern Med 1997; 157: 2089–2096.
23 Andrews LB, Stocking C, Krizek T et al. An alternative strategy for studying adverse events in medical care. Lancet 1997; 349: 309–313.
24 Nobili A, Tettamanti M, Frattura L et al. Drug use in the elderly in Italy. Ann Pharmacother 1997; 31: 16–22.

25 Zanocchi M, Ponzetto M, Spada S *et al.* Polypharmacy in the ambulatory care of aged patients. Rec Prog Med 1999; 90: 455–461.

26 Veehof LJ, Stewart R, Haaijer-Ruskamp FM, Meyboom-de Jong B. Adverse drug reactions and polypharmacy in the elderly in general practice. Eur J Clin Pharmacol 1999; 55: 533–536.

27 Bjerrum L, Sogaard J, Hallas J, Kragstrup J. Polypharmacy in general practice: differences between practitioners. Br J Gen Pract 1999; 49: 195–198.

28 Rosholm JU, Bjerrum L, Hallas J *et al.* Polypharmacy and the risk of drug–drug interactions among Danish elderly. Dan Med Bull 1998; 45: 210–213.

29 Thomas HF, Sweetnam PM, Janchawee B, Luscombe DK. Polypharmacy among older men in South Wales. Eur J Clin Pharmacol 1999; 55: 411–415.

30 Sternon J, Gilles C. Polymedicine and drug interaction in geriatrics. Rev Med Brux 1996; 17: 389–396.

31 Imbs JL, Pouyanne P, Haramburu F *et al.* Iatrogenic medications: estimation of its prevalence in French public hospitals. Therapie 1999; 54: 21–27.

32 Darchy B, Le Miere E, Figueredo B *et al.* Iatrogenic diseases as a reason for admission to the intensive care unit: incidence, causes and consequences. Arch Intern Med 1999; 159: 71–78.

33 Darchy B, Le Miere E, Figueredo B *et al.* Patients admitted to the intensive care unit for iatrogenic diseases. Risk factors and consequences. Rev Med Intern 1998; 19: 470–478.

34 Queneau P, Grandmottet P. Prevention of avoidable iatrogenic effects; the obligation for vigilance. Press Med 1998; 27: 1280–1282.

35 Recalde JM, Zunzunegui MV, Beland F. Interaction of prescribed drugs in a population over 65 years of age. Aten Primaria 1998; 22: 434–439.

36 Carvalho-Filho ET, Saporetti L, Souza MA *et al.* Iatrogeny in hospitalized elderly patients. Rev Saude Publica 1998; 32: 36–42.

37 Steven ID, Malpass A, Moller J *et al.* Towards safer drug use in general practice. J Qual Clin Pract 1999; 19: 47–50.

38 Roughead EE. The nature and extent of drug-related hospitalization in Australia. J Qual Clin Pract 1999; 19: 19–22.

39 Simon LS. Risk factors and current NSAID use (Editorial). J Rheumatol 1999; 26: 1429–1431.

40 Fries JF. Assessing and understanding patient risk. Scand J Rheumatol 1992; 29 (Suppl): 21–24.

41 Gabriel SE, Jaakkimainen L, Bombardier C. Risk of serious gastrointestinal complications related to use of nonsteroidal anti-inflammatory drugs. A meta-analysis. Ann Intern Med 1991; 115: 787–796.

42 Roth SH, Tindall EA, Jain AK *et al.* A controlled study comparing the effects of nabumetone, ibuprofen, and ibuprofen plus misoprostol on the upper gastrointestinal tract mucosa. Arch Intern Med 1996; 153: 565–571.

43 Tamblyn R. Medication use in seniors: challenges and solutions. Therapie 1996; 51: 269–282.

44 Miller LG. Herbal medicines. Selected clinical considerations focusing on known or potential drug–herb interactions. Arch Intern Med 1998; 158: 2200–2211.

45 Eisenberg D, Davis R, Ettner S *et al.* Trends in alternative medicine use in the United States, 1990–1997. JAMA 1998; 280: 1569–1575.

46 Boon H, Smith M. The Botanical Pharmacy. The Pharmacology of 47 Common Herbs. Kingston: Quarry Press, 1999.

47 Gaster B, Holroyd J. St John's wort for depression: a systematic review. Arch Intern Med 2000; 160: 152–156.

48 Houpt JB, McMillan R, Wein C, Paget-Dellio SD. Effects of glucosamine hydrochloride in the treatment of pain and osteoarthritis of the knee. J Rheumatol 1999; 26: 2423–2430.

49 Towheed TE, Anastassiades TP. Glucosamine therapy for osteoarthritis. J Rheumatol 1999; 26: 2294–2297.

50 McCarthy KA. Management consideration in the geriatric patient. Top Clin Chiropractic 1996; 3(2): 66–75.

23

Chronic illnesses and care of the terminally ill patient

Brian J Gleberzon

This textbook has explored many clinical disorders that successfully respond to pharmacological, botanical and/or chiropractic treatments. Such disorders include diabetes the degenerative arthritides, cardiovascular diseases, and many neurological conditions, as well as acute and chronic spinal pain. Regrettably, however, there are certain diseases that preferentially affect older persons that result in severe morbidity and respond poorly to many different therapeutic approaches. This chapter will review these severe chronic illnesses, as well as many issues surrounding the care of the terminally ill patient.

Chronic obstructive lung disease

Chronic obstructive lung diseases (COLDs) are a group of conditions frequently encountered in the elderly.[1] Affecting more than 15 million Americans, COLDs are the fifth leading cause of death among older persons, and the prevalence of these conditions is increasing.[1–3] Epidemiological evidence also indicates that the incidence of COLD has risen more rapidly than any of the 10 other most common causes of death in persons over the age of 65 years during the 1980s and 1990s.[3] COLDs are characterized by chronic airway obstruction which is either reversible (asthma), associated with mucus hypersecretion (chronic bronchitis) or associated with destruction of alveolar tissue (emphysema).[1] Other associated symptoms include dyspnoea, cough and impaired gas exchange.

A combination of genetic predisposition and environmental exposure leads to COLD.[3] Cigarette smoking is the most common environmental risk factor, and is believed to contribute to over 80% of all cases of COLD.[3] It is unfortunately not uncommon for patients to present with indolent symptoms of COLD in their seventies or eighties even after having discontinued tobacco use up to two decades earlier.[1] Cigarette smoke leads to inflammatory changes in the lungs, invariably leading to an increased ratio of mucous glands to bronchial wall thickness (the Reid index).[3] Other histological changes to lung tissue include increased peribronchial muscle, fibrosis, goblet cell metaphasia and increased intraluminal mucus.[3]

Presenting signs and symptoms of COLD include productive cough, increased sputum production, dyspnoea and wheezing.[3] The cough may be mild, or it may be disabling, causing episodes of syncope, vomiting or stress incontinence.[3] Among persons with osteoporosis, the cough may result in spinal or costal fracture.[3] Pursed lip breathing is a characteristic sign often observed.[3] Patients may also find it easier to breathe in a seated position with their elbows resting on their thighs.[3] Bacteria such as *Haemophilus influenzae* or *Streptococcus pneumoniae* may exacerbate symptoms, especially among patients with bronchitis.[3]

There are two stereotypical patients with severe COLD: pink puffers and blue bloaters. Pink puffers are typically asthenic, barrel-chested emphysematous patients who exhibit pursed lip breathing with no evidence of cyanosis or oedema.[3] These patients usually use extrathoracic muscles to breathe, produce minimal sputum and experience little fluctuation in day-to-day levels of dyspnoea.[3] Diaphragmatic breathing is reduced, and breath and heart sounds are distant.[3] Arterial blood gas studies reveal only mild to moderate hypoxaemia. In contrast, the blue bloater is usually overweight, cyanotic and oedematous, exhibiting a chronic productive cough.[3] Arterial blood gases demonstrate hypoxaemia and hypercapnia, and nocturnal hypoxaemia is often profound.[3]

In addition to physical examination findings, a diagnosis of COLD may be confirmed by various laboratory findings, including plain-film chest radiographs, spirometry and arterial blood gas levels.[3] Airflow obstruction is confirmed if there is a less than expected ratio (less than 80%) of forced expiratory volume in 1 s to the forced vital capacity (FEV_1/FVC).[2,3]

Medical management

The therapeutic goals of geriatric patients with COLD are to maintain functional independence and to avoid repeated hospitalizations.[3] Medical treatment primarily consists of bronchodilator therapy.[1] In general, inhaled drugs are preferred over systemic medications.[1] Anticholinergic inhalers are often the drugs of choice, owing to their record of fewer systemic side-effects. Many older patients often require more than the typically recommended two puffs four times a day to achieve maximal results.[1] Some medical practitioners maintain that the use of oral corticosteroids should be instituted in all asthmatic patients requiring daily bronchodilator therapy to control their symptoms.[1] Medications are considered to be therapeutically beneficial if they achieve a 15% improvement in FEV_1 as measured by spirometry.[1] Lastly, because of the patient's vulnerability to pulmonary disease, a patient must be ever vigilant as to the potential risk of possible infection. Influenza vaccination and pneumococcal immunizations are often suggested as prophylactic measures.[1,3]

In cases of severe hypoxia, in which the partial pressure of oxygen is measured at less than 55 mmHg, many patients benefit from oxygen therapy.[1–3] The goal of oxygen therapy is to achieve oxygen saturation in excess of 90%. Oxygen therapy has been shown to improve sleep quality, reduce nocturnal arrhythmias, improve daytime activities, alleviate the signs and symptoms associated with COLD, and prolong life.[1–3]

Non-pharmacological management

Exercise conditioning is essential to improve maximal oxygen consumption and reduce ventilation rate and heart rate.[2] It is the cornerstone of non-pharmacological therapies for COLD. A patient who smokes should be encouraged to quit. Support groups such as the Better Breathers, a course offered through the American Lung Association, can guide a patient to conserve his or her energy, avoid panic attacks and improve bronchial hygiene, and instruct patients in breathing retraining exercises to help them to cope with chronic breathlessness.[1] Educational initiatives may help a patient with other activities as well. For example, sexual function often improves if the person is rested, uses a bronchodilator 20–30 min beforehand and avoids consuming large amounts of food or alcohol, and if sexual activity is scheduled during the 'better breathing' parts of a person's day, being mindful of those positions that put less pressure on the person's chest or abdomen.[3]

Asthma

Asthma in particular warrants special discussion. It affects 10% of elderly Americans, and one-half of all elderly patients with asthma have an onset of symptoms after the age of 65.[1,2] Mortality due to asthma has been increasing over the past decades, and adults over the age of 45 have a 20-fold higher mortality rate than children under the age of 15.[2,4] The annual cost of asthma care in the USA is estimated to be more than $6 billion.[4]

Clinically, patients with asthma present with recurrent episodes of wheezing, shortness of breath, chest tightness, non-productive cough and persistence of upper respiratory disease.[5] In addition, older asthmatic patients may demonstrate weight loss and fatigue.[6] In cases of acute, severe asthma, patients are often agitated and somnolent, display interrupted speech and need to sit in an upright position to breathe.[5,6]

An article by Smyrnios[4] lists the six key strategies for the medical management of asthma among older persons. These are: patient education, objective measurements of lung function, environmental control, pharmacological therapy for chronic asthma, pharmacological therapy for acute asthma and regular follow-up care.[4] Since up to 75% of asthmatic patients demonstrate allergies to environmental triggers, such as house dust mites,[2] avoidance or reduction of household allergens has been recommended by others as an effective strategy for asthma prevention.[7,8] Methods to achieve allergen control or avoidance include:[7]

- covering mattresses and pillows with plastic or vapour-permeable fabric covers
- damp wiping the mattress every 2 weeks
- washing all bedding weekly in hot water
- replacing feather pillows
- avoiding basement bedrooms
- removing carpeting in bedrooms

- covering air ducts into bedrooms with filters
- maintaining a smoke-free environment
- vacuuming any carpets weekly
- maintaining a humidity of 30–50%
- washing pets regularly
- avoiding upholstered furniture
- increasing ventilation with air conditioning.

If allergen avoidance is not possible, immunotherapy may be necessary. β-Blockers have been shown to be very effective in the management of patients with asthma, but only if a patient is given clear instructions on how to utilize his or her 'puffer'.

Some recent studies have examined the effects of spinal manipulative therapy (SMT) on patients with asthma.[9–11] Although these studies failed to demonstrate changes in objective lung function of the asthmatic patient receiving SMT as measured by spirometry, it is noteworthy that these patients reported many subjective benefits such as decreased symptoms, decreased medication usage and increased quality of life.[9–11] A recent review by Hondras et al. for the Cochrane Library concluded that there is currently insufficient evidence to support or refute the use of manual therapies for patients with asthma.[9] SMT for this condition is traditionally delivered to the upper cervical and mid-thoracic segments.[12,13] Adjunctive therapies that may be used by chiropractors for their asthmatic patients include thoracic percussion, relaxation techniques, and soft-tissue therapies such as trigger point therapy directed at thoracic, intercostal and paraspinal muscles.[14,15]

Cancer

The American Cancer Society, the National Cancer Institute and the Centers for Disease Control and Prevention have all reported that, in general, cancer incidence rates decreased on average 0.7% per year between 1990 and 1995.[16] Death rates from the four most common types of cancer, lung, breast, prostate and colorectal, also decreased significantly during the same period.[16] That said, some authorities still predict that the likelihood that an American would develop cancer over his or her lifetime is about 40%.[17] Moreover, cancer is primarily a disease of the elderly, and the approach to it, in terms of both treatment and palliative care, is becoming a major component of geriatric care and, with the ageing of the population, foreshadows impending concerns within the health-care delivery system.[1,3,18] Indeed, age is the major

determinant of cancer risk, with most life-threatening cancers occurring in patients over the age of 65 years.[1,3] In addition, nearly one-third of all cancers occur in persons over the age of 70 years,[1] with the incidence of lung, breast and prostatic cancers all having risen dramatically over the past 20 years in that age group.[3] Before the age of 50 years, the incidence of cancer is higher among women than men; however, after the age of 60, there is a remarkable rise in the incidence of cancers among men.[3]

It is not known whether the increased incidence of cancer in the elderly is the result of biological changes associated with the ageing process or the result of prolonged exposure to carcinogens.[3] There is evidence to support both theories. For example, observed age-dependent declines in mitochondrial activity may lead to an impaired cellular repair ability,[3] and changes in the immune system (often called immune senescence) include a decline in interleukin-2 levels, decreased T-cell function and impaired mitogen responsiveness which, in turn, are thought to result in a decreased ability to recognize and destroy neoplastic mutations.[3] In addition, prolonged lifetime exposure to known carcinogens increases the incidence of many cancers (lung, gastric, skin, etc.).[3]

Regrettably, many diagnostic and treatment decisions are often based solely on a person's age.[3] Because many health-care providers may associate chronological age with poor prognosis, cognitive impairment, decreased quality of life, limited life expectancy and decreased social worth, compared with younger people older persons may receive less thorough screening for cancers, less staging of diagnosed cancer, less aggressive therapy, and often no treatment at all.[3] For example, mammography, breast self-examination, prostatic examinations and guaiac testing are commonly performed less often than recommended for older persons.[3] In addition, Cleary and Carbone[18] report that older patients are less likely than younger persons to receive proper pain management for cancer, thus imposing a barrier to their palliative care.

Often the attitudes or belief systems of an older person may interfere with administrative efforts for cancer management.[3,16] Attitudes that create barriers to treatment include the patient declining a diagnostic or therapeutic procedure because they do not understand or appreciate the advances made in medicine, or the patient may believe that there is no hope for the successful treatment of his or her cancer.[3,18]

Clearly, cancer diagnosis and treatment is predominantly within the realm of conventional medicine, typically involving aggressive pharmacological or surgical interventions. Thus, an in-depth and detailed description of cancer diagnosis and management would go beyond the scope of this textbook. However, a chiropractor or other CAM provider can play an important role in health care by being aware of the presenting signs and symptoms of various cancers, and referring a patient to the appropriate medical physician as circumstances dictate. The chiropractor may also be an important educational resource for patients. This section therefore discusses those cancers most commonly encountered in the older population. Cancers reviewed include: lung cancer, breast cancer, prostatic cancer, endometrial, cervical and ovarian cancers, colorectal and pancreatic cancers, and myeloproliferative disorders.

Lung cancer

The World Health Organization (WHO) has estimated that each year 3 million people die of lung cancer worldwide,[19] with the highest rate of lung cancer among North Americans.[2,3] It is estimated that there were 178 000 new cases of lung cancer in the USA in 1997.[19] Lung cancer is the most common cause of cancer deaths among American men and women, accounting for 160 000 deaths annually.[2,3,19] Although the incidence of lung cancer has dropped among men since the 1980s, lung cancer surpassed breast cancer as the most common cause of cancer death among American women during that same period.[19]

Demographic studies reveal that, since the 1940s, the increase in lung cancer mortality in both genders has followed the pattern of an increase in cigarette smoking, with a 20 year time lag.[3] About 90% of lung cancer in men and 80% of lung cancer in women is directly attributable to cigarette smoking.[3,19] The overall risk associated with smoking and lung cancer is proportional to both the number of cigarettes a person smokes each day and the total number of years the person has smoked.[19] However, it is noteworthy that smoking cessation reduces the risk of lung cancer mortality at any age, and even an older, lifelong smoker can lower his or her lung cancer risk by quitting. Moreover, the earlier a person quits smoking, the greater the impact on lung cancer risk.[3] Currently, the 5 year survival rate is only 10–15% for persons with lung cancer.[1] It is also estimated that 3000 non-smokers die annually from

secondhand smoke.[19] Other causes of lung cancer include exposure to certain radioactive or mineral dusts such as uranium, asbestos, arsenic and nickel.[19]

Signs and symptoms

Unfortunately, most cases of lung cancer are untreatable at the time they are diagnosed.[19] This is because lung cancer tends to be clinically silent as it develops over many years.[19] The signs and symptoms that should alert a clinician to the possibility of lung cancer include unexplained weight loss, dyspnoea, chest pain, bone pain, haemoptysis, wheezing or stridor, signs of brain metastasis (seizure, headache), and recurrent or unresolving pneumonia and other pneumonic symptoms such as fever and productive cough.[2,3,19] If the tumour has invaded other associated regions of the chest, signs and symptoms may include hoarseness, hemidiaphragm elevation, pleural effusion and cardiac symptoms.[3] Lung cancer may also be detected incidentally on thoracic or chest X-rays. In particular, patients over the age of 50 years who are either current or former smokers and present with community-acquired pneumonia should be aggressively investigated.[3] Currently, however, there are no screening protocols for asymptomatic persons.[3]

Metastatic tumours can produce a wide variety of symptoms, depending on the site of invasion. The four most common sites for lung cancer metastases are bone, brain, liver and the adrenal glands.[19] Bone metastases may cause insidious, progressive pain, especially in the spine and pelvis.[19] Chiropractors must therefore include this alternative in their differential diagnoses for those patients who present with spinal pain and a suspicious history (primarily a history of smoking) who do not respond well to treatment.[19] Lastly, metastases to the brain may result in seizures or various neurological dysfunctions.[19]

Staging and types

Lung cancers are classified using the TNM staging system. This system describes tumour size (T), nodal involvement (N) and the presence or absence of metastasis (M).[3] Histologically, lung cancers may be squamous cell, large-cell, small or oat-cell, or adenocarcinoma.[3] Adenocarcinoma has recently over-taken squamous cell carcinoma (SCC) as the most common type of lung cancer,[19] accounting for 30–35% of all cases.[19] Adenocarcinoma is the most common type of lung cancer among women and non-smokers, and it generally has a worse prognosis than SCC.[3,19] SCC is the second most common type of cancer, but it is the most common lung cancer among the elderly, accounting for 45% of all lung cancers in that group of persons.[3] SCC is strongly linked to cigarette smoking, and these types of tumour are typically the most slow growing.[3,19]

Treatment

Treatments for lung cancer include surgery, radiotherapy, chemotherapy and a combination of each of these. The treatment approach is often dictated by the stage of the tumour.[1–3] There is a growing interest in alternative or unconventional treatments for cancers of all types. Examples of unconventional treatments include Essiac (a herbal mixture that has been used in Canada since the 1920s), Iscator (trade name of European mistletoe), vitamins A, C and E, and 714-X, an agent available in Canada, Mexico and some European countries.[19–21]

Prognosis

The prognosis for patients with lung cancer tends to be poor. Overall, 87% of all people with lung cancer will die from it within 5 years of diagnosis.[19]

Breast cancer

Demographics

Breast cancer is the most commonly diagnosed cancer among American and Canadian women, and is second only to lung cancer in terms of cancer deaths among women in these two countries, affecting one in nine adult women.[1,2,21] In 1990, for example, 150 000 new cases of breast cancer were diagnosed in the USA.[1] Breast cancer represents 29% of all cancers among American women and accounts for 18% of all cancer deaths in that group.[1] In the USA, 44 000 women die from breast cancer annually.[1,2] Among women from 15 to 54 years of age, breast cancer is the leading cause of cancer death. However, breast cancer is of concern to older women as well, with 45% of all breast cancer cases occurring in women over the age of 65 years and 170 000 new cases diagnosed in the USA annually in this age group.[1,3] Seventy per cent of all breast cancers are diagnosed after the age of 50 years.[1,21] Moreover, the likelihood of developing breast cancer increases for a woman every decade beyond the age of 40 years.[1] Since the 1970s, the incidence of breast cancer has risen more rapidly among black women than among white women.[3] Some authorities attribute these increases in the incidence of breast cancer to increased awareness and education, as many breast cancers are detected in the early stages of development during screening mammograms.[21] Early detection is important as breast cancer is one of the most treatable of all types of cancer, with a good overall prognosis, although one-third of women who develop breast cancer will die from it.[21]

Breast cancer relapses are common, typically developing within the first 2–6 years following the initial diagnosis and treatment.[21] It is important for the chiropractic clinician to be aware of this fact as 50% of breast cancer survivors will develop metastases.[21] Of these cases of metastases, 40–60% will appear in bone and 7–15% in soft tissue.[21] This has obvious implications for clinical practice, particularly with respect to methods of treatment.

Risk factors

Currently, the causes of breast cancer are only partially understood. However, many factors have been identified as contributing to the risk of developing breast cancer. These include; gender (99% of all breast cancers occur in women), age (over 50 years), exposure to oestrogen, diet, genetic factors, socioeconomic status (breast cancer is more common in women of higher socioeconomic status), radiation exposure, personal history of endometrial or ovarian cancer, and history of benign breast disease[1–3,21] (Table 23.1).

Exposure to oestrogen has been identified as the major factor affecting breast cancer development.[1] There is a correlation between a woman's menstrual

Table 23.1 Breast cancer development: major and minor risk factors[3,21]

Major risk factors	Minor risk factors
Female gender	Never having breast fed
Increased age	Heavy alcohol consumption
Family history	High dietary fat
Personal history of cancer	Obesity
Onset of menarche before the age of 12 years	Adult weight gain
Onset of menopause after the age of 55 years	Oral contraceptive use
First pregnancy after the age of 30 years/nulliparity	Hormone-replacement therapy
Genetic alterations (*BRCA1, BRCA2, p53*)	Smoking
Exposure to radiation	Socioeconomic status

history and the development of breast cancer.[1,21] In general, the longer a women is exposed to oestrogen, the greater her chance of developing breast cancer. This is not because oestrogen is mutagenic, but because oestrogen may promote the growth of established cancer cells.[21] For example, women who have had early menarche (defined as before the age of 12 years) are at increased risk for breast cancer, and those women who experience menopause after the age of 55 years are at twice the risk of developing breast cancer.[1,21] Women who experience menopause by the age of 45 years have half the incidence of breast cancer of those women who enter menopause after the age of 55 years.[21] There is also an association between the establishment of a regular menstrual cycle and the risk of breast cancer. Evidence suggests that those women who establish regular menstrual periods during their first year of menstruation have a risk three times greater than those who do not.[21]

Pregnancy appears to convey some protection from breast cancer development. This is thought to be related to the increase in circulating prolactin, which imparts a protective effect.[21] This effect is enhanced with each subsequent pregnancy.[21] A first pregnancy after the age of 30 years is associated with a four- to five-fold increase in breast cancer risk, and nulliparity is also associated with an increased risk of breast cancer.[1,21] The relationship between breast cancer risk and the use of oral contraceptives is still controversial, although prolonged (greater than 5 years) use of oestrogen replacement therapy for postmenopausal symptoms slightly increases the risk of breast cancer.[1,21] Artificial or premature menopause as the result of surgery, drugs or radiation provides some protection from breast cancer development.

A large body mass and android (abdominal) obesity are associated with an increased risk of breast cancer.[1-3,21] This increased risk is attributed to the increase in oestrogen levels associated with an increase in adipose tissue.[21] Some evidence also suggests that dietary fat and total caloric intake may be the promoting factors, and that these dietary factors may explain the increased risk of breast cancer among women who immigrate from countries with a low breast cancer prevalence (such as Japan) to countries with a higher prevalence (such as the USA).[1] Some authorities also link tobacco and alcohol use with an increase in breast cancer risk.[1,21]

Familial clustering of breast cancer has long been observed and is thought to be a major risk factor for its development.[1] The risk is higher if the family member with breast cancer is a first-degree relative (mother, sister, daughter).[21] The number of first-degree relatives with breast cancer augments the risk of breast cancer development, as well as whether the cancer was diagnosed in the family member premenopausally or in both breasts.[21] A family history of colon and endometrial cancer is also associated with an increased risk of breast cancer.[2,3]

Other genetic factors associated with an increased risk of breast cancer include mutations to the gene *BRCA1*, located on chromosome 17. Mutations of this allele increase the carrier's lifetime risk of breast cancer development by 85%, and the chance of developing a second primary breast tumour is 65%.[21] Women with this genetic allele also have a 40–60% chance of developing ovarian cancer.[21] Other genes linked to an increased risk of breast cancer include the inactivation of *p53*, a tumour suppressor gene also located on chromosome 17.[21] The alteration of *BRCA2* (on chromosome 13) also increases the risk of breast cancer in both men and women.[21]

Exposure to high levels of radiation has been associated with an increased risk of breast cancer.[1] However, radiation exposure after the age of 40 years does not seem to increase this risk and, most importantly, mammography and chest radiography pose a negligible risk for breast cancer development.[1] Lastly, there is an increase in breast cancer risk among women found to have hyperplasial ductal changes with cellular atypia upon biopsy.[1]

Screening for breast cancer

Along with recommendations to perform monthly breast self-examinations (1 week after menstruation) and to have a breast examination performed every 3 years until the age of 40 and yearly thereafter, the American Cancer Society has endorsed screening for breast cancer as part of routine health maintenance for women.[1,2,21] As a guideline, the American College of Physicians recommends obtaining an initial baseline mammogram between the ages of 35 and 40 (the American Cancer Society recommends that this should begin at 40), every 2 years from 40 to 50 years of age, and yearly thereafter.[2,3,21] The Canadian Cancer Society has recommended a screening mammogram every 2 years for women between the ages of 50 and 69 years.[21] It is estimated that appropriate screening can reduce breast cancer-related mortality among women between the ages of 50 and 75 years by 20% to 25%.[3] Unfortunately, less than half of the women over the age of 65 have undergone mammography.[3]

Signs and symptoms

The most common clinical presentation of breast cancer is a palpable mass.[1,3] Lesions are typically firm nodules within the breast which are usually not painful, but they may be tender.[1,21] Ulcerations may occur, and lesions within or near the nipple may produce discharge.[3] The presentation of deep, boring bone pain may indicate metastasis to bone, which is a very common occurrence.[21] A mass clustering of microcalcifications seen on mammography is suggestive of carcinoma. In suspicious cases, fine-needle biopsy is performed to establish a diagnosis. This procedure is both safe and effective, with 94% sensitivity.[2,3]

Histological classifications and staging

There are four types of breast cancers: Paget's disease of the breast, inflammatory carcinoma, ductal carcinoma *in situ* and lobular carcinoma *in situ*.[3] Breast cancers are staged using the TNM system.[1,3] Breast cancers are designated as stage I, II, III or IV, depending on tumour size, the site and number of lymph nodes, and the presence or absence of metastasis. Stage IV breast cancer is the most serious. The average survival time is only 3–6 months if the patient has liver or lymphangitic lung metastasis, 24 months if the patient has nodular lung metastases, and greater than 5 years if metastases are confined to only bone.[3] With this in mind, involvement of axillary lymph nodes must be determined. In general, approximately 40–50% of all breast tumours are associated with axillary lymph-node involvement at diagnosis.[1] The assessment of lymph-node involvement must involve biopsy as physical examination of the axilla is imprecise, since 25% of palpable lymph nodes are proven to be histologically negative and 30% of non-palpable lymph nodes are found to contain breast cancer cells.[1] The presence or absence of axillary lymph nodes is inversely related to patient survival rates, and lymph-node involvement determines patient prognosis.[1,3]

Treatment

Treatment options for patients with breast cancer are determined by the stage of the disease. In general, treatment for stage I and II breast cancers may involve partial (lumpectomy) or total mastectomy and lymph-

Table 23.2 Breast cancer development: preventive strategies[21]

Primary revention	Exercise
	Balanced diet, including antioxidants such as vitamins A, C and E
	Increased linolenic acid
	Decreased use of oral contraceptives
	Prophylactic mastectomy (only for women at very high risk level)
Secondary prevention	Breast self-examination
	Clinical breast examination
	Mammography
Tertiary prevention	Postoperative care
	Follow-up visits
	Patient education

node dissection.[1,3] Absolute contraindications for breast-conserving surgery include large tumour size (greater than 5 cm), prior breast irradiation, male breast cancer, recurrence after previous breast-conserving surgery, existent carcinoma *in situ*, synchronous breast tumours, inflammatory breast cancer and the inability to achieve clear surgical margins.[1]

Radiation therapy following breast-conserving surgery is an integral component of breast cancer therapy.[1] For patients with metastatic disease, radiation therapy is an important palliative modality, and is effective in controlling symptoms caused by tumour compression, obstruction or lysis.[1] Other therapeutic options include hormone therapy, chemotherapy or both.[1,3] The following factors are associated with a favourable prognosis: older age, postmenopausal status, small tumour size, absence of axillary lymph-node involvement, high steroid hormone receptor content, good tissue differentiation, the absence of intratumour lymphatic invasion and the absence of metastases.[2] Unconventional therapies for breast cancer include vitamins A, C and E, Essiac, Iscador, green tea, hydrazine sulfate and 714-X.[21] Most experts agree that the best treatment for any disease is its prevention. Table 23.2 provides some preventive strategies to reduce a woman's risk of breast cancer.

Prostatic cancer

More than 50% of men over the age of 70 years have histological evidence of prostatic cancer.[3] It is the second most common cause of cancer death in men.[3] Current estimates predict that 244 000 American men will be diagnosed with this cancer in any given year, and over 40 000 men are predicted to die from this disease annually.[1] Cancer of the prostate accounts for 32% of all cancers occurring in men.[1] African-American men in the USA have the highest incidence of prostate cancer in the world (approximately one in every nine men).[2]

As discussed in Chapter 5, benign prostatic hypertrophy (BPH) is now thought to be related to an increase risk of prostatic cancer. The signs, symptoms, investigation strategies and treatment options for cases of BPH were reviewed in Chapters 5 and 18. Unlike BPH, however, prostatic cancer is typically asymptomatic;[3] therefore, 50% of prostatic cancers are clinically advanced at the time of discovery.[3] Early presenting signs and symptoms may include acute retention and haematuria and, very often include symptoms of distant metastases (pain, weight loss and lymphadenopathy).[3] Prostatic cancer typically metastasizes to bone, leading to bone pain and anaemia.[3]

Screening tests for the presence of prostatic cancer include annual digital rectal examination (which is beyond the scope of chiropractic practice in many jurisdictions) and the prostate-specific antigen (PSA) test.[3] Unfortunately, the PSA test misses about one-third of clinically important cancers and is falsely positive in about 60% of cases, which may in turn lead to unnecessary and costly diagnostic evaluations.[3] It may also cause a great deal of needless anxiety in the patient. Transrectal prostatic ultrasonography is regarded as more sensitive than digital rectal examination and it is useful to guide a biopsy; however, its use as a primary screening tool is limited by the high cost and low availability of the test.[2] A bone scan is often used to determine the presence and extent of metastases.[2] Prostate tumours are staged using the TNM classification model previously described. The prognosis is poorer if the cancer has invaded tissue beyond the prostate and if the lymph nodes are involved.[2]

Treatment options for clinically localized prostatic cancer include radical surgery, radiation and watchful waiting. In cases of locally invasive prostatic cancer, radiation therapy is the most common medical intervention. It is important to reassure a patient with prostatic cancer that a large percentage of men with this cancer will not die of it, in part because this type of cancer progresses slowly.[3]

Endometrial, cervical and ovarian cancer

Endometrial cancer is the most common gynaecological malignancy in the USA, predominantly affecting post-menopausal women.[3] Endometrial cancer accounts for one-half of all gynaecological cancers in the USA.[1] The aetiology of endometrial cancer is poorly understood, although contributing factors are obesity, late menopause, use of exogenous oestrogen, hypertension, nulliparity, diabetes and ovarian disease.[1] Post-menopausal bleeding is the harbinger of endometrial cancer, and any patient reporting postmenopausal bleeding must be referred to the appropriate health-care provider and aggressively assessed.[1,3] Treatment is primarily surgical, and endometrial cancers are generally associated with a better prognoses than other gynaecological cancers.[3] Radiotherapy and chemotherapy may also be required for tumours in advanced stages.[3]

Cervical cancer is the second most common gynaecological cancer, and its peak incidence occurs in the fifth and sixth decades. The median age of presentation for cases of cervical cancer is 52 years.[1] Several human papillomaviruses, as well as herpes simplex virus type 2, have been implicated in the development of cervical cancer, and the rise of this disease has been attributed to more promiscuous sexual behaviours.[1,3]

Although ovarian cancer is less common than either endometrial or cervical cancer, it is much more deadly.[3] Ovarian cancer is the leading cause of death from gynaecological cancers in the USA and the incidence of this cancer is greatest in the 65–85-year-old age group.[1] The aetiology of ovarian cancer is unknown, although established risk factors include increased age, nationality (more common in the USA, Israel and Scandinavian countries), familial syndromes, the presence of other cancers (breast, colon) and race (more common in Caucasians), and it is also associated with exposure to known carcinogens (such as asbestos).[1] The symptoms develop late and are usually non-specific, often presenting as only a vague abdominal or gastrointestinal discomfort.[3] Unfortunately, elderly patients tend to present with more advanced stage ovarian cancers.[1] There are many subtypes of ovarian cancer, although most (85–95%) are epithelial in origin.[1] Surgery is the treatment of choice and the prognosis depends on proper surgical staging.[1]

Colorectal and pancreatic cancer

Colorectal and pancreatic cancers are highly prevalent among older persons in the USA, and these cancers are second only to lung cancer as the most common malignancies among both men and women.[1,3] Colorectal cancers are the second most common cause of cancer-related deaths in the USA.[1,3] In the USA, 90% of all cases of colorectal cancers occur in persons over the age of 50 years,[1] with 150 000 new cases reported each year.[2] As such, colorectal cancers represent the leading cause of mortality and morbidity in the elderly.[1] The incidence of colorectal cancers begins to rise at the age of 40 and doubles every 5 years thereafter.[3] Adenocarcinoma constitutes 95% of all cases of colorectal cancers. Whereas rectal cancer occurs more frequently among men, colon cancer occurs equally among men and women.[3]

Demographics

The incidence rates of colorectal cancinoma are highest in North America, Australia and New Zealand, intermediate in areas of Europe, and less common in Asia, South America and sub-Saharan Africa.[1] Colorectal cancers are more common in upper socioeconomic classes.[1,3] These demographic differences in the incidence of colorectal cancer are attributable to differences in dietary factors. Epidemiological evidence suggests that colorectal cancers are associated with diets comprised of high animal fat, refined sugar and char-grilled meat intake. Conversely, a diet of restricted refined sugar, lower animal fat and high fibre is associated with a lower incidence of colorectal cancers.[1,3]

Risk factors

Risk factors associated with an increased incidence of colorectal cancers include age, family history, diet (see above), presence of inflammatory bowel disease (ulcerative colitis more so than Crohn's disease), adenomatous polyps and incidence of other colon tumours.[2]

Signs and symptoms and diagnostic testing

Colorectal cancers are typically asymptomatic and are only discovered by screening examinations.[2] However, the presence of colorectal cancer should be suspected if occult faecal blood is discovered for any reason, if a person over the age of 40 years develops iron-deficiency anaemia, or if a large abdominal mass is detected during routine abdominal examination.[2] Anorexia and unexplained weight loss are often associated with colon cancer.[2]

Because most cases of colorectal cancer are asymptomatic, many authorities suggest a yearly digital rectal examination for patients over the age of 40 years, a yearly stool test for occult blood after the age of 50

in low-risk persons and after the age of 40 in high-risk persons, a flexible sigmoidoscopy at the age of 50 and every 5 years thereafter, and a colonoscopy or double air-contrast barium enema every 3 years for high-risk persons after the age of 40, although these last two suggestions are controversial.[2,3]

Colorectal cancers are graded using the TNM system following the Duke's stage (A–D).[2,3] In general, colorectal cancers that have not spread to the lymph nodes are 70–90% curable.[2] Tumours that have spread to four or more lymph nodes are 50% and 30% curable if located in the colon and rectum, respectively.[2] Those tumours that exhibit distant metastases (Duke's stage D) are generally not curable.[2]

Treatment

The treatment of colorectal cancer typically requires surgery and adjuvant chemotherapy. Some patients may require a combination of palliative chemotherapy and radiation therapy, although these procedures often provide only limited benefits.[2]

Pancreatic cancer

Pancreatic cancer is the fourth most common cancer in the USA, with over 25 000 cases reported annually.[1] Tumours are classified as either ductal adenocarcinomas or cystadenocarcinomas.[1]

Risk factors

The cause of pancreatic cancer is not fully known, but many authorities believe that environmental factors probably contribute to its development.[1] Environmental factors thought to contribute to pancreatic cancer include cigarette smoking, diabetes mellitus and other glucose-intolerance disorders, history of chronic cholecystitis or gastrectomy, dietary factors such as alcohol use, high saturated fat and consumption of coffee, and exposure to industrial carcinogens.[1]

Signs and symptoms

The most common presenting signs and symptoms in patients with pancreatic cancer are progressive unexplained weight loss, jaundice and abdominal pain.[1]

Treatment and prognosis

Because cigarette smoking has been linked to the development of pancreatic cancer, smoking cessation is an important prevent measure.[1] Treatment options include surgery, chemotherapy and radiation therapy.

Regrettably, the 5 year survival rate for persons with unresectable pancreatic cancer is about only 10%, and patients with unresectable cancer rarely survive beyond 2 years.[1]

Myeloproliferative disorders

The leukaemias

Leukaemias are categorized as either acute or chronic. Acute leukaemia is primarily a disease of the elderly. Fortunately, current treatment has greatly improved survival rates for leukaemia patients, but the most dramatic results are usually observed in the young.[3] Acute leukaemias include acute lymphocytic leukaemia (ALL) and acute non-lymphocytic leukaemia [also known as acute myelogenous leukaemia (AML)], according to the morphological characteristics of cells in peripheral blood and bone-marrow smears.[3] About 80% of adults with acute leukaemia have the AML type, whereas 80% of children with acute leukaemia have ALL.[3]

ALL is a cancer of primitive lymphoid cells.[1] The cause of ALL is largely unknown, although transfer of genetic material from chromosome 9 to 22 (the 'Philadelphia' chromosome) is often associated with ALL, especially among older persons, and other chromosomal rearrangements have been associated with AML as well.[1] Other causes of acute leukaemia include exposure to radiation or viruses. The development of leukaemia has been associated with certain oncogenes.[3]

In general, the presenting signs and symptoms of acute leukaemias are constitutional (fatigue, weakness, pallor, weight loss), a history of infections, easy bruising and bleeding, lymphadenopathy and hepatosplenomegaly.[1–3] Diagnosis is confirmed by laboratory investigations of the blood and bone marrow.[1–3] Treatment consists of chemotherapy and, in cases of AML, bone-marrow transplantation.[1–3] As mentioned earlier, prognosis among older persons with acute leukaemia is generally poorer than that in children with acute leukaemia, with infections being the most common cause of morbidity and mortality.[3]

Chronic leukaemias are similarly classified as being either chronic lymphocytic leukaemia (CLL) or chronic myelogenous leukaemia (CML). CLL is the most common leukaemia in the elderly, with 80% of all cases of CLL occurring in persons over the age of 50 years, and nearly two-thirds of cases occurring in persons over 60 years.[1,2] Genetic components appear to be involved in the development of chronic

leukaemias, although certain viruses [notably the Epstein–Barr virus (EBV)] have also been suggested as a possible cause.[3] Chronic leukaemias tend to be asymptomatic and are often incidental findings during routine laboratory testing, although the patient may present with constitutional signs.[1–3] The diagnosis is confirmed by laboratory studies. If the leukaemias are detected early, treatment is often not rendered, as the complication of chemotherapy may be more deleterious to the patient than the original condition.[3] However, for late-stage chronic leukaemias, chemotherapy, radiation therapy and bone-marrow transplantation may be required.[1–3] Prognosis is typically fair to poor, with reported 5 year survival rates of only about 50%.[1,3]

Another common form of leukaemia is hairy cell leukaemia (HCL). The mean age of diagnosis of this disease is 50 years, and HCL occurs almost exclusively among men.[2] HCL is a malignant B-cell proliferation of unknown cause, which is often asymptomatic.[1,2] Treatment options range from no treatment, to splenectomy (less common today than in the past) or chemotherapy in advanced cases.[2] Prognosis is usually very good, with remission rates approaching 85%, and patient survival rates may return to those of the general population.[1,2]

Multiple myeloma

Multiple myeloma is a neoplastic disorder resulting from the proliferation and accumulation of immature plasma cells in the bone marrow.[3] These cells synthesize abnormal amounts of monoclonal immunoglobulins (IgG, IgA, IgD or IgE).[3] The consequences of abnormal plasma cell growth are plasma cell tumours, osteolysis, haematopoeitic suppression, paraproteinaemia and renal disease.[3]

Multiple myeloma is more common among African-Americans than Caucasians, it occurs equally among men and women, and it usually occurs in persons over the age of 50 years.[3] Causes linked to the development of multiple myeloma include genetic factors, exposure to high levels of radiation (as shown in survivors of the Hiroshima and Nagasaki atomic bombs), osteomyelitis, cholecystitis, repeated exposure to allergen injections, exposure to known toxins (asbestos, heavy metals, pesticides, benzene, etc.) and viral illnesses.[3]

Bone pain is the most common symptom of multiple myeloma, occurring in over two-thirds of patients.[1,3] Pain most often occurs in the lower thoracic region or the ribs, and the pain often gradually increases in intensity over time.[3] The sudden onset of pain may indicate a compression fracture of a vertebra, or a pathological fracture in such bones as the pelvis, rib or clavicle.[3] Other signs and symptoms include pallor, weakness, fatigue, dyspnoea and palpitations, cord or nerve root compression signs, and renal failure or infection.[1,3] Diagnosis is confirmed by serum electrophoresis, bone-marrow aspiration and X-ray[3] (see Chapter 8).

Treatment includes chemotherapy and radiation therapy if lytic pathological fractures are identified.[1–3] The mainstay of the chemotherapeutic regimen is monthly therapy with oral melphalan and prednisone.[1–3] Patients should be encouraged to stay active to prevent further bone demineralization, infections must be treated promptly, and patients should drink sufficient fluids to increase urine excretion of light-chain immunoglobulins, uric acid and other metabolites.[3] The prognosis for patients with multiple myeloma is variable.

Lymphoma

Lymphomas are primary malignancies of the lymph nodes. They are categorized as Hodgkin's disease or non-Hodgkin's disease. In general, Hodgkin's lymphoma is histologically differentiated from non-Hodgkin's lymphoma by the presence of Reed–Sternberg cells.[3] Hodgkin's lymphoma has a bimodal distribution, with an initial peak incidence between the ages of 15 and 35 years, and a second peak between 50 and 80 years.[1,3]

The cause of these lymphomas is unknown, although viruses have been implicated in both diseases, with EBV associated with Hodgkin's lymphoma and the human immunodeficiency virus (HIV) associated with non-Hodgkin's lymphoma.[3]

Persons with Hodgkin's lymphoma often present with enlarged lymph nodes, especially those located in the central or axial regions.[3] Symptoms range from asymptomatic to fever, night sweats, loss of body weight and pruritus.[2,3] Lymph-node biopsy, X-ray, bone-marrow examination and computed tomographic (CT) scans are often used to confirm the disease.[2,3] These tests are especially important in lymphoma as clinical staging determines the course of treatment.[3] Treatment consists of chemotherapy and radiation therapy.[2,3] With treatment, almost 70% of

patients with Hodgkin's lymphoma are long-term survivors and cure rates are over 75%, regardless of histological findings.[3] In cases of non-Hodgkin's lymphoma, combined chemotherapy can result in a cure rate of 80%, even in cases with unfavourable biopsy types.[2]

Chronic pain

Chronic pain must be included in any discussion of conditions leading to chronic morbidity in any patient population, but this topic is especially relevant when discussing the elderly. Many of the clinical conditions described throughout this textbook often present with, or result in, chronic pain. Neck pain among older patients has been discussed in Chapter 16, and considerations for the chiropractic management of many painful clinical conditions affecting older persons are discussed in detail in Chapter 25. Therefore, only a brief description of this topic is provided here.

It is estimated that 80–85% of all people experience a significant health problem that predisposes them to pain at some time after the age of 65 years.[22] Among this group, 25–50% will experience significant pain, and the percentage rises to 45–80% among those living in nursing homes.[22] Moreover, the age-specific morbidity rates for persistent pain increase with age for most conditions, and 36–83% of older persons report that some degree of pain that interferes with daily activities and quality of life.[22] Clinical conditions associated with a high incidence of pain in older persons include rheumatoid arthritis, temporal arteritis, polymyalgia rheumatica, osteoporosis, osteomalacia, angina, herpes zoster and various neuropathies (as in diabetes).[22]

The Iowa 65+ study reported on the prevalence of pain among 3693 community-dwelling seniors living in the rural midwest of the USA.[23] In this study, 86% of the respondents reported some type of pain in the past year and 59% of those with pain (51% of the sample) reported multiple painful complaints.[23] Other studies have concluded that women are more likely to report musculoskeletal pain and multiple pain sites than men.[22] This is significant when one considers that women comprise 60% of the population over the age of 65 years, and are predicted to comprise 73% of the population aged 85 years and older by 2020.[22]

Paradoxically, most epidemiological studies report that the overall prevalence of pain complaints, as well as migraines and low back pain, peaks in middle age, and steadily declines thereafter.[23] For example, in the Iowa 65+ study previously cited,[23] persons over the age of 85 years reported a significantly lower prevalence of pain than those in other age groups. Other studies have found similar results: among community-dwelling seniors, the prevalence of pain peaks or plateaus by the age of 65 years, after which it steadily declines. Gallagher et al. posit that there may be several reasons for this phenomenon:[22] (i) age-related changes in nociception pathways may reduce the intensity of pain; (ii) older persons may be more reluctant to report painful symptoms than younger persons; and (iii) the decline in pain-reporting with age may be an artefact of higher mortality rates or an increased likelihood of institutionalization for the more seriously ill.[22]

Chronic pain in and of itself does not always diminish a person's quality of life. Quality of life is often compromised by such pain-associated problems as sleeplessness, impaired physical and social functioning, depression and an increased need to use health services.[22,24] Indeed, symptoms of pain and depression are often associated with each other, and each may intensify the severity of the other.[22] As reported by Gallagher et al.,[22] health-related quality-of-life indices of people with chronic non-malignant pain are among the lowest observed for any medical condition.

Many authorities in the area of pain management maintain that the intensity or character of the pain does not necessarily impact a person's life as much as the person's perception of his or her pain. In a recent article, Hoffman[24] reviewed the issues confronting practitioners who were treating patients with low back pain. Hoffman expanded on the biopsychosocial model first popularized by Waddell in the late 1980s.[24] In this biopsychosocial model, disease is defined as any source of tissue damage and irritation that causes pain sensation. Illness, or illness behaviour, is the patient's interpretation and reaction to the pain sensation. Illness behaviour by a patient is modulated by several biobehavioural factors, such as the degree of pain sensation and psychological and social factors. These social, psychological, environmental and psychophysiological factors may attenuate or exacerbate the discrepancy between pathology, pain, impairment, functional limitation and disability.[24]

Certain factors have been identified as predictive of whether a patient with acute low back pain will develop a chronic pain profile. Patients who demonstrated such factors as greater self-reported pain and disability, psychological distress on the Minnesota Multiphasic Personality Inventory, and worker's compensation or personal injury status were 90% more likely to have chronic symptoms.[24]

Hoffman advocates that the patient should be an active participant in his or her health care.[24] Studies indicate that patients who perceive themselves to be actively involved in their health care tend to have better relationships with their physicians, an increased sense of self-control and ability to tolerate pain, and overall better clinical outcomes. As might be expected, studies also indicate that physician-dominated consultations lead to poorer patient satisfaction and outcomes. Hoffman also suggests that clinicians orientate the patient away from the exclusive goal of pain relief and instead emphasize the importance of restoring functional abilities. In his words, 'patients should be made to understand that as function returns pain will decrease, rather than as pain decreases function will resume'.[24] Waddell echoes this sentiment by stating that 'treatment often fails when relying on too narrow a conceptual model of pain'.[24] This shift away from a pain-based model to a function-based model is nowhere more important than in the care of older patients, whose painful symptoms are often the result of degenerative, irreversible conditions. Nevertheless, functional gains are often obtainable under chiropractic care.

Chiropractic considerations in the care of the terminally ill patient

Breaking bad news

Breaking bad news to a patient is one of the most difficult and stressful, and least enjoyable aspects of doctoring.[25,26] The key to conveying bad news to a patient is to do so in such a manner as to facilitate acceptance and understanding, while minimizing the risk of patient denial, ambivalence, unrealistic expectation, overwhelming distress or collusion.[25]

But, what is bad news? According to Bor et al., it is those 'situations where there is either a feeling of no hope, a threat to a person's mental or physical well-being, a risk of upsetting an established lifestyle, or where a message is given which conveys to an individual fewer choices in his or her life'.[27] Or, put more simply, it is any information that will change a person's life for the worse, or alter dramatically a patient's view of his or her future.[25] However, it is clear that the interpretation of this news is dependent upon both subjective and objective variables, and what exactly constitutes 'bad news' may be different for either the doctor or patient.[25] What is unclear is which personal, interpersonal, news-specific, situation-specific and transmission-specific variables are important predictors of the receiver's (and giver's) reaction to this news.[25,26] It is also important to remember that the news may be expected, and the doctor may only be confirming a patient's pre-existing suspicion.

Bowers[25] posits that the ability to convey bad news compassionately with a patient is crucial from several different perspectives. First, this task is not optional and it cannot be delegated to a surrogate. Secondly, jurisprudence dictates that a patient be informed about the nature, extent and implications of his or her illness. Lastly, if this is handled tactfully, the rapport between the patient and the doctor may be fortified. Conversely, bad news delivered insensitively is emotionally damaging to both the doctor and the patient. Furthermore, it may impede the patient's long-term adjustment to the news.[25]

Authorities agree that the key to conveying bad news successfully to a patient is strong communication skills.[25,26] Indeed, poor communication is among the most common causes of patient complaints lodged against physicians, and it is a major factor in medicolegal actions.[25] There are several strategies that can enhance these communication skills when they are most urgently needed:[22,23]

- Give the news in person.
- Ensure a quiet location with no interruptions.
- Set aside extra time for the patient.
- Sit close to the patient, with no physical barriers between you.
- Avoid technical jargon.
- Give the patient a warning shot ('I've got some bad news …').
- Avoid euphemisms.
- Treat the patient with respect.
- Have a supportive person present.
- Give some measure of hope.
- Maintain eye contact.
- Provide reassurance by physical touch (hand-holding).
- Invite questions by periodically asking the patient whether you are making sense.
- Provide documentation.

- Be honest, compassionate, caring, hopeful and informative.
- Bad news should be delivered at the patient's pace.

The physical and social setting

The news should be delivered in a quiet, comfortable setting that offers the patient privacy, and can accommodate a friend or family member, if their presence is desired by the patient. The time should be convenient for the patient, and the clinician's schedule should be arranged to allow for whatever extra time the patient may require.[25,26] Several studies have indicated that physicians may delay breaking bad news to the patient because the physician is anxious or uncomfortable, or because the physician may wish to avoid a discussion of a patient's poor prognosis, even though most (but not all) patients want to hear it.[26] Therefore, to break bad news to a patient effectively, the practitioner must do so when he or she is most comfortable. It is likely that the patient's perceptions will be clouded if the practitioner is perceived to be anxious, depressed, irritated or pressured for time.[25]

Experts agree that the news should be given in person. The clinician should sit close to the patient, with no physical barriers (desk, chairs, tables) separating them.[25,26] The doctor and patient should not face each other, but rather sit at about 90 degrees to each other. In this manner, the physician can more effectively respond to emotional cues from the patient. Again, most experts emphasize the benefits of touch while conveying bad news.[25] Eye contact is crucial and interruptions must be avoided.

The message

The clinician must be certain of the information before he or she gives it to the patient. As Bowers opined: 'Giving a patient bad news one day and then retracting it later is unconscionable and inexcusable'.[25] That said, Berwin[28] describes three ways to deliver bad news. The first is bluntly and insensitively, which leaves the patient feeling isolated and angry. The second is kindly and sadly, which may deprive the patient of any hope or sense of optimism. The third approach is to be understanding and positive, to be flexible, reassuring and empathetic, helping the patient to plan for the immediate future. Complete disclosure is imperative, as is delivering the news at the receiver's pace.[25,26] In this manner, the physician may ensure that the patient comprehends the information being conveyed.

Authorities agree that the delivery of the message should begin with a warning shot, such as 'I have some bad news'.[26] This tactic is thought to reduce the element of shock. Moreover, it is important for the clinician to be aware that the first thing the patient hears is often remembered best, and all the information that follows may be nothing but a blur.[26] Therefore, it is important to convey hope in the opening remarks. This does not mean that the physician should be less than completely truthful, nor does this imply that the doctor should promise an impossible cure, but rather he or she should offer the patient sincere, controlled optimism.[25] It may also be helpful periodically to ask the patient: 'Am I making sense'. This may allow the patient to ask a question, which he or she may be reluctant to do during a conversation that he or she may not completely understand.[25]

Because the patient may remember little of what is said after the crux of the message is delivered, the practitioner may want to give the patient a written summary of the news, or the physician or patient may want to audiotape the conversation.[26] This allows the patient to read or listen to the discussion at a later time, when they are more relaxed and less shocked.[26]

There is some disagreement about whether specific medical terminology should be used.[26] While it is important to avoid technical information that the patient may not be able to understand, the use of specific terminology will enable the patient to gather additional information on his or her own (from such sources as the internet).[26] The majority of authorities also agree that euphemisms should be avoided, as the ambiguities that may arise from their use may block effective understanding and impair subsequent discussions or decisions.[25] If the patient has cancer, the physician should say so, rather than describing the illness as a 'growth' or 'tumor'.

A few studies have investigated the issue of receiving bad news from the perspective of the patient. A study conducted by Girgis and Sanson-Fischer[29] reported that patients believed that it was better if the bad news was given in private in a quiet location, free of jargon, with some measure of hope and with documentation. Other studies indicated that the patient wanted their physician to be honest, compassionate, caring, hopeful and informative.[26] Patients wanted the information to be told to them in person, in a private setting, as soon as possible, at their own pace with time for discussion, and with a support person present.[26]

The manner in which a patient will respond to the news varies. While some patients may not be surprised by the news, others may respond with anger, stunned silence, acute distress or guilt.[26] Some patients may have an unspoken fear that the clinician will abandon them. The patient should therefore be assured that the doctor will be available for support or consultation, even if he or she will not be actively involved in the patient's treatment.[26]

While breaking bad news is clearly stressful to the patient, some research has demonstrated that this process also places a great strain on the clinician.[25,26] There are many possible contributory factors that may add to a physician's fear or anxiety while breaking bad news to his or her patients. These factors include being blamed for the illness, fear of the unknown, fear of unleashing an emotional response, discomfort of not knowing the answers to all of the patient's questions, and personal fear of the unknown and death.[25] Signs that a clinician may be experiencing professional 'burnout' include feelings of anxiety, feelings of being unable to cope with work or family, dreading going to work, depression, sleeplessness or substance abuse.[25]

Chiropractic care

Little has been written on the topic of chiropractic management of terminally ill patients. This may reflect the fact that chiropractic care is more geared towards treating the secondary symptoms that may arise from morbific diseases (pain, loss of motion) rather than the diseases themselves, although there is an intriguing case in the literature that describes the remission of hepatocellular carcinoma in a patient receiving only upper cervical care.[30] Several articles describe cases of spinal pain in adults later attributed to prostatic metastasis,[31,32] bronchial carcinoma,[33] abdominal aortic aneurysms[34,35] and other serious pathologies.[36–38] Thus, a clinician must always include such pathologies in any differential diagnosis, particularly when assessing an older patient presenting with spinal pain.

There are various cancer prevention strategies that a chiropractor can suggest to his or her patient. These include recommendations to quit smoking, avoid excessive alcohol use, minimize exposure to sunlight (unprotected), and take exercise and proper nutrition (see also Chapters 27 and 30). Jamison[39] suggested five mechanisms by which nutrients may block the access of genotoxic compounds and tumour promoters. These include: (i) adsorption of carcinogens; (ii) dilution of carcinogen concentration; (iii) modification of microbial intestinal metabolism; (iv) induction of enzymatic activities; and (v) modification of gene expression.[39] Dietary components thought to have a cancer-preventive effect include β-carotene, fibre, vitamins A, C, D and E, folic acid and calcium.[39] In addition, various herbal products are likewise thought to exert a cancer-preventive effect.[40] For example, cartilage extract, genistein and mistletoe are thought to have an antiangiogenetic effect (prevent tumour growth), whereas astragalus, ginseng, bromelain and green tea are thought to exert a chemopreventive effect, possibly by stimulation of the immune system.[40]

End-of-life issues

Palliative care can be defined as 'a special kind of health care for individuals and families who are living with a life-threatening illness that is usually at an advanced stage'.[41] There are several goals of palliative care. These include providing comfort and dignity to the person living with the illness, as well as providing the best quality of life possible to both the individual and his or her family. An important objective of palliative care is relief of pain and other symptoms. Palliative care should provide not only for the individual's physical needs, but also for his or her psychological, social, cultural, emotional and spiritual needs[41] (Table 23.3). Thus, a 'good death' may be achieved if the person is pain free, is operating at the highest possible level of functioning, has resolved long-standing conflicts, and has satisfied any final wishes.[41]

Health-care providers can help the patient to attain these important goals by encouraging opportunities for the individual to reminisce, and to express feelings of anger, fear, desire and so on. At such times, it is important for the practitioner to be a good listener and attempt to empower the dying person whenever possible. This sense of empowerment may be achieved by involving the individual in all health-care decisions and respecting whatever choices he or she may select.

Towards that end, it is important to suggest to a terminally ill patient that they prepare those legal documents that will provide health-care practitioners with clear instructions. For example, a 'living will' can indicate which treatments a patient may or may not want performed in the event that they are incapacitated or otherwise unable to make their wishes known to an emergency-care doctor or nurse. This may include the desire not to be given food or water intravenously or

Table 23.3 Determinants of health associated with goals of end-of-life care [adapted from Ref. 41]

Determinant of health	End-of-life goal
Health service	Control pain and other symptoms
	Optimize physical functioning
Personal health practices and coping skills	Foster a sense of control by the patient
	Eliminate fear and anxiety
	Allow the patient to 'die well', according to his or her choices
Social environment	Provide a supportive environment
	Provide opportunities for social contact with family, friends and peers
Culture	Provide care that is consistent with the patient's cultural and religious values, beliefs and practices
Income and social status	Encourage the use of legal documents for planning end-of-life issues

by tube. Patients can also indicate that they do not wish 'heroic means' be used if they are near death ('do-not-resuscitate' orders). Moreover, a patient can clearly express his or her decision regarding organ donation. This issue has recently become very contentious in Ontario, where the provincial government is attempting to make organ donation more common by asking the next-of-kin for their consent in the event that the patient's wishes are unclear or undocumented. Other contentious end-of-life issues include euthanasia, hospice versus at-home care, and ethics of pharmacological pain control versus the desire of the patient to avoid sedation. Several important resources for both clinicians and patients are provided at the end of this chapter.

Death is an inevitable aspect of life. A person's death need not be a time of unnecessary angst, confusion or suffering for either the individual or his or her family or friends. If prepared for, it is possible for a person to have a 'good death'.

References

1 Lonergan E. Geriatrics: A Lange Clinical Manual. 1st edn. Stamford, CT: Appleton & Lange, 1996.
2 Ferri F, Fretwall M, Wachtel A. The Care of the Geriatric Patient. 2nd edn. St Louis, MO: Mosby-Year Book, 1997.

3 Abrams M. Merck Manual of Geriatrics. 2nd edn. Whitehouse Station, NJ: Merck and Co., 1995.

4 Symrnios NA. Asthma: a six-part strategy for managing older patients. Geriatrics 1997; 52(2): 36–44.

5 Wilkins RL, Dexter JR, eds. Respiratory Disease: A Case Study Approach to Patient Care. 2nd edn. Philadelphia, PA: FA Davis Co., 1998.

6 Sherman CB. Late-onset asthma: making the diagnosis, choosing drug therapy. Geriatrics 1995; 50: 24–33.

7 Jones AP. Asthma and the home environment. J Asthma 2000; 37: 103–124.

8 Lewitt GT, Watkins AD. Unconventional therapies in asthma – an overview. Allergy 1996; 51: 761–769.

9 Hondras MA, Linde K, Jones AP. Manual Therapy for Asthma. The Cochrane Library, Issue 2. Oxford: Update Software, 2000: 17.

10 Balon J, Aker P, Crowther ER *et al*. A comparison of active and simulated chiropractic manipulation as adjunctive treatment for childhood asthma. N Engl J Med 1998; 339: 1013–1020.

11 Nielson NH, Bronfort G, Bendix T *et al*. Chronic asthma and chiropractic spinal manipulation: a randomized clinical trial. Clin Exp Allergy 1995; 25: 80–88.

12 Jamison JR, McEwen AP, Thomas SJ. Chiropractic adjustments in the management of visceral conditions: a critical appraisal. J Manipulative Physiol Ther 1992; 15: 171–180.

13 Wiles MR, Diakow P. Chiropractic and visceral disease: a brief survey. J Can Chiropractic Assoc 1982; 26: 65–68.

14 Frischer AA, Mootz RD, Adams AH. Evaluation and management of the adult patient presenting with a cough. Top Clin Chiropractic 1995; 2: 13–23.

15 Lines DH. A holistic approach to the treatment of bronchial asthma in a chiropractic practice. Chiropractic J Aust 1993; 23: 4–8.

16 Jamison J. Nutritional prevention of cancer: current status, future possibilities. Top Clin Chiropractic 1999; 6(1): 45–53.

17 Hinck G. The role of herbal products in the prevention of cancer. Top Clin Chiropractic 1999; 6(1): 54–62.

18 Cleary JF, Carbone PP. Palliative medicine in the elderly. Cancer 1997; 80(7): 1335–1347.

19 Elkington W. An overview of lung cancer for the chiropractor. Top Clin Chiropractic 1999; 6(1): 18–24.

20 Kaegi E. Unconventional therapies for cancer. Can Med Assoc J 1998; 158: 897–902.

21 Berestiansky L. Breast cancer: a current summary. Top Clin Chiropractic 1999; 6(1): 9–17.

22 Gallagher RM, Verma S, Mossay J. Sources of late-life pain and risk factors for disability. Geriatrics 2000; 55(9): 40–47.

23 Mobily PR, Herr KA, Clark MK, Wallace RB. An epidemiological analysis of pain in the elderly: the Iowa 65+ study. J Aging Health 1994; 6: 139–154.

24 Hoffman B. Confronting psychosocial issues in patients with low back pain. Top Clin Chiropractic 1999; 6(2): 1–7.

25 Bowers L. 'I've got some bad news …' Top Clin Chiropractic 1999; 6(1): 1–8.

26 Ptacek JT, Eberhardt TL. Breaking bad news. A review of the literature. JAMA 1996; 276: 496–502.

27 Bor R, Miller R, Goldman E, Scher I. The meaning of bad news in HIV disease; counseling about dreaded issues revisited. Counsel Psychol Q 1993; 6: 69–80.

28 Berwin TB. Three ways of giving bad news. Lancet 1991; 337: 1207–1209.

29 Girgis A, Sanson-Fischer RW. Breaking bad news: consensus guidelines for medical practitioners. J Clin Oncol 1995; 13: 2449–2456.

30 Lee G, Jenson CD. Remission of hepatocellular carcinoma in a patient under chiropractic care: a case report. J Vertebral Subluxation Res 1998; 2: 125–130.

31 Johnson T Jr. Diagnosis of low back pain, secondary to prostate metastasis to the lumbar spine, by digital rectal examination and serum prostate-specific antigen. J Manipulative Physiol Ther 1994; 17: 107–112.

32 Rodgers R. Prostatic metastases confirmatory diagnostic procedures: a case study. J Neuromusculoskeletal System. 1994; 2: 79–82.

33 Lemire J, Mierau D, Yong-Hing K. Metastatic bone disease presenting as low back pain: a case study. J Neuromusculoskeletal System 1994; 2: 131–139.

34 Hadida C, Rajwani M. Abdominal aortic aneurysms: case report. J Can Chiropractic Assoc 1998; 42: 216–21.

35 Van der Velde GM. Abdominal aortic aneurysms. Two case reports and a brief review of its clinical characteristics and ramifications. J Can Chiropractic Assoc 1998; 6: 76–83.

36 Diamond M. Ominous lower-back pain – a case report. J Chiropractic 1994; 31(2): 25–27.

37 Yurkiw D. Pancreatic cancer and chronic thoracic back pain – a case report. J Can Chiropractic Assoc 1995; 39(1): 18–21.

38 Demetrious J. Metastatic renal cell carcinoma of the sternum and spine that mimicked costochondritis: a case report. J Neuromusculoskeletal System 1995; 3: 16–19.

39 Jamison J. Nutritional prevention of cancer: current status, future possibilities. Top Clin Chiropractic 1999; 6(1): 45–53.

40 Hinck G. The role of herbal products in the prevention of cancer. Top Clin Chiropractic 1999; 6(1): 54–62.

41 Fisher R, Ross MM, MacLean MJ. A guide to end-of-life care for seniors. University of Toronto and University of Ottawa, with funding by Population Health Directorate, Health Canada, 2000.

Further reading

Byock I. Dying Well: The Prospect for Growth at the End of Life. New York: Riverhead Books, 1997.

Remen RN. Kitchen Table Wisdom: Stories that Heal. New York: Riverhead Books, 1996.

Additional resources

American Academy of Hospice and Palliative Medicine. PO Box 14288 Gainesville, FL, 32604-2288, USA. Tel. +1-352-377-8900; e-mail aahpm@aahpm.org

American Pain Society. Tel. +1-847-375-4715; e-mail aps@amctec.com

Association of Death Education and Counseling. 638 Prospect Ave., Hartford, CT 06105-4298, USA. Tel. +1-860-586-7503; website http//www.adec.org

Catholic Health Association of the United States. Tel. +1-314-427-2500.

Choice in Dying, Inc. Tel. +1-212-366-5540; e-mail cid@choices.org

National Hospice Foundation. Tel. +1-703-516-4928; e-mail www.nho.org

National Hospice Organization. Tel. +1-800-658-8898; website http://www.nho.org

Section IV: Treatment and management considerations for the older person

24

Different health-care strategies for the older person

Brian J Gleberzon and Robert Mootz

Since its early days, the chiropractic profession has emphasized its connection with the health of the entire person. This sentiment, which embraces the concept of holism, is considered to be a basic tenet of chiropractic principles.[1] Along with other principles such as conservatism, rationalism, humanism, naturalism and vitalism, holism is a concept that is also intimate with complementary and alternative medicine (CAM) approaches such as naturopathy and homoeopathy. Approaches utilized by CAM disciplines such as herbalism, bone-setting and acupuncture have roots extending back centuries, yet these tenets are surprisingly congruent with the emerging contemporary focus on prevention, health promotion and wellness.[2]

The dominant Western approach to medicine, based in great measure on allopathic traditions, has sometimes been characterized as viewing a patient as no more than the sum of his or her parts.[3] Black has termed this a 'molecular approach'.[4] Coulter describes a paradigm shift in health care away from this compartmental, disease-based approach (the germ theory) towards an approach that considers the entire person, their body, mind and spirit, as the issue at hand to be addressed. Health is considered the natural end-product of normal processes of living, not just as the absence of disease. The role of the CAM practitioner, in turn, helps to marshal the patient's natural (or innate) recuperative abilities.[3] This approach has also been called the 'contextual approach'.[4–6] Health-care disciplines frequently included under the CAM umbrella traditionally prefer an equalitarian relationship between the practitioner and the patient, as opposed to what Hawk has called a patriarchal medical model.[2] As Gerin *et al.* emphasize, 'Attention is focused on patients themselves, as human beings, and not just on their illness'.[7]

Exploring molecular and contextual paradigms

The concepts of contextual and molecular medicine are neither extreme opposites nor mutually exclusive. Rather, they represent complementary viewpoints. Table 24.1 contrasts some underlying characteristics that may be representative of each approach. The adjective 'contextual' emphasizes that disease may simply be a predictable 'reaction' to a variety of environmental, psychosocial, genetic and other factors (the belief systems of the patient and the doctor, the surroundings and accoutrements of a healing encounter, and so on). A contextual viewpoint considers disease as a process rather than a discrete entity and that trying to separate such a process from the circumstance that produced it is rather arbitrary.[5]

In contrast, interventions that primarily deal with physiological reactions to circumstances (disease processes) might be termed 'molecular' medicine to emphasize a focus on 'specific causation' at the physiological level. A molecular viewpoint recognizes that a myriad of contributing factors play a role in disease, and the role is often viewed as a background constant of sorts. However, the molecularists' contributing factor might be considered the pivotal focus of intervention by a CAM practitioner.

To illustrate what is meant by the concept of 'contextual', consider a droplet of water. The same water molecule may exist as a gas, liquid or solid depending on its environmental context. Temperature, air circulation and various other factors make the difference between rain, steam, snow or hail. A molecularist might try to manipulate hydrogen bonds by adding salt to the water in order to change its state for a useful purpose.

Table 24.1 Characteristics of molecular and contextual healing

Molecular approaches	Contextual approaches
Emphasize 'specific causation' as primary contributors to disease (e.g. germ theory)	Emphasize multivariate causation of disease. Consider disease to be a natural and normal response to 'contextual' circumstances (e.g. theory of holism)
Emphasize reductionist approaches to scientific enquiry of biochemical and molecular processes (e.g. respiratory distress in tuberculosis from caseating granulomas in the lung)	Favour qualitative approaches to scientific enquiry that emphasize interactions between many variables (e.g. clinical focus on host resistance in relationship to virulence of environmental pathogens)
Emphasize *in vitro* studies and tight controls (internal validity) in scientific design	Emphasize in vivo studies and generalizability to practical settings (external validity) in scientific design
Require certain assumptions regarding interplay of components in order to generalize to complexities of healing processes	Require certain (different) assumptions regarding interplay of components in order to generalize to complexities of healing processes

A contextualist might suggest moving it to a warmer environment to accomplish the same thing. Which approach is better depends on a number of factors. In winter, the contextualist would win to make a glass of drinking water, but the molecularist would win to increase traction on an icy road.[6]

Similarly, there are no absolute rights or wrongs in terms of molecular or contextual healing approaches. In fact, both CAM and conventional medical approaches are made up from elements of both. Perhaps the greatest differences lie in what the circumstances are when an intervention is performed. Although contextual prevention and lifestyle approaches may be valuable in managing and preventing cardiovascular disease, when an acute myocardial infarct occurs, molecular-orientated intervention may make more sense. In contrast, in a disease such as cancer, contextual methods may have a more meaningful yield in terms of quality of life.

Just like water droplets, human cells function within variable contexts that determine their physiological expression, albeit with far greater complexity. Diet, environmental factors (air, climate), social and psychological factors (work, family) and an organism's activity level will all affect how cells behave. Even though a relatively finite number of molecules make up living beings, a combinatorial explosion occurs when one considers all the behaviours possible. Thus, physicians and scientists are confronted with huge challenges in trying to operationalize strategies for clinical interventions. Complexities may arise simply from the existence of more variables. In addition, simple systems may interact in ways that lead to complex and unpredictable behaviours. The process of crystalliza-

tion in physics, geological formations or weather patterns in nature, and Mandelbrot equations in mathematics represent examples of where a theoretically finite number of variables can combine in ways that exhibit complex behaviours.[6] While the system remains essentially the same, its context impacts on its expression and behaviour.

Pros and cons of molecular approaches

Molecular approaches help physicians and scientists to focus on what is practically manageable at a given point in time under a given set of circumstances. By breaking problems down into manageable components, confusion and uncertainty can be reduced when looking at real life events. Molecular approaches are very systematic and allow sequential experimentation (or therapeutic trials) to produce a manageable accumulation of knowledge. Rigorous and quantitative description is possible, which helps to contribute to predictability, a hallmark of desirability in health-care interventions in modern society. Thus, molecular medicine has provided tangible breakthroughs that excel in emergent situations (myocardial infarct), can dramatically counter environmental virulence (antibiotics) and can induce hosts to develop defences against known environmental agents (immunization).

However, molecular approaches may oversimplify problems and fail to account for the unpredictability of complex systems (or simple ones that behave in a complex manner). Molecular approaches may often exhibit a robustness that can be misleading. It is easy for doctors or scientists to ignore phenomena that are not explained by their models by simply avoiding their study. Reducing complex systems to component parts may fragment things artificially. Modern medicine is full of experiences where something appeared to work in the laboratory and the theory notebooks, but when brought to market was ineffective or even harmful (e.g. many drugs, routine spinal fusion surgery). The temptation for molecularists to assume generalization from simplified reductionistic models to real-world phenomena is great and occurs frequently. Combinatorial explosion is not uncommon, leading to complexity and chaos. The highly successful novel and movie Jurassic Park popularized this very premise a few years ago.

Pros and cons of contextual approaches

Contextual approaches are often intuitively attractive. Chiropractors have experienced this kind of acceptance from patients with low back pain. The medical doctor hears the patient explain how they bent over and lifted something to initiate the problem, and then he or she prescribes a chemical remedy applied to through the gastrointestinal system. The chiropractor, on hearing the same history, looks at the back and posits a mechanical remedy applied to where the patient perceives the problem is coming from. Contextual approaches often deal with the richness of human experience and readily attain cultural acceptance. They may be easier to communicate and may even prevail despite disapproval from orthodoxy. The survival and growth of CAM methods within Western cultures illustrate this.

Yet, despite their intuitive clarity and tangibility, contextual approaches offer abundant room for error. History is also rich with examples of intuitively attractive beliefs and feelings becoming institutionalized, then turning out to be wrong. The need for rigor and critical appraisal in contextual methods is just as great as it is with molecular approaches. Contextual approaches may lack the quantifiability that permits others to learn readily to reproduce them. Often it is difficult to build a common knowledge base around contextual approaches. This can be seen in the proliferation and high variability of techniques within chiropractic, for example. It is obvious that contextual methods have an outsider status within the scientific and health-care mainstream. Contextual medicine has not really demonstrated tangible and pivotal clinical breakthroughs that rapidly impact the evolution of health care beyond its current status. Such subtle contributions are easily overlooked.

Chiropractic's context within classic health-care philosophies

Chiropractic's emphasis on structure and function and how that relates to overall health resonates well with traditional naturalist or naturopathic philosophies that disease is really a result of diminished host resistance, not necessarily related to any specific environmental pathogen. Naturopathic interventions are frequently concerned with general strengthening of the patient in order cope with the environment, regardless of which environmental factors may be wreaking havoc. Diet, exercise, fresh air, mental outlook and other large-scale issues are among the highest priorities for intervention, rather than agents of specific diseases. Chiropractic and osteopathic models gravitate toward this paradigm as well, emphasizing the role that somatic structure plays in the host's ability to function within diverse environments.[6] In contrast, classic allopathic perspectives view the virulence of environmental pathogens as being central in disease processes. Thus, allopathic remedies are based on determining specific causation in order to determine how to counter whatever environmental intrusions occurred. By recognizing such 'root' causes of disease, better strategies can be developed to counter the responsible environmental agents or their effects. Thus, much of contemporary biomedical model building and belief systems regarding health and disease focuses on the microscopic and molecular levels of physiologic processes because it leads to identification of specific causation.

Homoeopathic approaches have elements of specific causation from allopathic traditions and host resistance from the naturalists' viewpoints. Homoeopathy recognizes specific environmental causes of disease, but seeks specific (rather than general) means to harness the body's intrinsic defence mechanisms. Such remedies aim to trigger inherent host responses (rebound) to environmental pathogens by seeking a remedy that stresses the body in a similar, but less virulent fashion, to that of the pathogen. Today, all health professions use interventions that could be categorized in all three philosophies; and many interventions might fall into more than one, or really belong somewhere other than the paradigm from which it has been popularized. For example, symptom suppression as a goal or outcome of killing a bacterial infection may have allopathic overtones, but symptom suppression to allow a good night's sleep so that the body can fight off the infestation might be naturopathic.

Chiropractic, the profession

Chiropractic is a health-care profession, not a treatment modality. Consideration of its attributes as a profession and discipline requires sociological, historical, economic and health services research methods. Spinal manipulation or adjusting are interventions commonly used by chiropractors. The study of manipulation requires epidemiological and physiological methods of exploration. Chiropractic is the third largest learned health-care profession behind medicine and dentistry, with some 60 000 practitioners in the USA. There 19 accredited doctoral level training institutions in North America alone and nearly as many others world-wide.[8] Studies suggest that 10–15% of the US population has utilized chiropractic services, with upwards of 35% of all low back pain patients using it. Chiropractors' caseloads comprise roughly 90% musculoskeletal pain condition complaints.[9] As a profession, chiropractic has made the greatest advances in social acceptance and utilization of any CAM discipline, with accredited training, licensure in all states and provinces in the USA and Canada, and substantive insurance reimbursement. The profession is often viewed as a mainstream discipline by other CAM professions, yet it is still considered alternative within mainstream circles.

Case management used by chiropractors reflects approaches standard to all health-care disciplines, including diagnostic evaluation, care planning and case management.[8] Interventions commonly include spinal manipulation and manual therapies, exercise and rehabilitation methods, physiotherapeutic modalities, advice on lifestyle, nutrition, ergonomics, hygiene and health promotion, as well as assorted complementary/alternative procedures.[9]

Chiropractic does not represent a unified clinical approach, although nearly all practitioners share the intervention of spinal adjusting or manipulation as a central focus of therapy. Like conventional medicine, chiropractic also represents a spectrum of perspectives towards intervention, even within what are often considered common philosophies.

For example, Owens has characterized four distinct practice objectives that chiropractors might have, ranging from a monocausal subluxation-only emphasis to that of a musculoskeletal condition-based specialty.[10] Some chiropractors may approach patient care in as reductionist a fashion as does any conventional medical provider. Others emphasize a 'non-therapeutic' approach that proponents believe to be of value for sustaining health. Whatever the belief, or practice, research on CAM methods in general and chiropractic interventions in particular has focused on what transpires when they are used with people that have some kind of measurable clinical condition. Among the many challenges ahead for CAM models is operationalizing attributes of contextual perspectives that can be rigorously quantified. For the time being, science can help us to assess utility in the care of people with various clinical conditions.

Spinal manipulation

A variety of manual therapies may be used by a variety of practitioners. Different definitions and categorization schemes exist but no definitive accepted taxonomy has been adopted by all professions providing the service. In the USA, chiropractors perform some 95% of manipulation provided to patients.[9] Therefore, terminology used here will be based on chiropractic taxonomies.[10,11] A glossary of common terms and brief definitions is given in Table 24.2. Many theoretical models regarding the mechanisms associated with manipulation have also been proposed and described, and they may fall into generic descriptions of physiological models or appear using syntax unique to a given profession or discipline.[13]

Safety issues and side-effects with spinal manipulation

Manipulation may have side-effects. Case reports, usually of severe consequences, predominate in the literature. One systematic study from Scandinavia collected self-report data from more than 1000 patients in order to inventory side-effects.[14] Two comprehensive literature reviews have been conducted to inventory published reports of complications of manipulation.[15,16] Nearly half of all patients experience side-effects, usually involving local discomfort, headache or tiredness with onset within 4 hours of the procedure.[14] Some 15% describe effects as 'severe' in intensity; however, most disappear within 24 h. Serious complications are extremely rare, but can occur. None has ever been reported among some 2500 subjects in over 50 randomized clinical trials published to date.

A literature review performed by RAND identified 118 cases of serious complications from cervical spinal

Table 24.2 Glossary of common terminology related to manipulation

Mobilization	'Passive' movement within physiological joint range of motion (range typically performed by intrinsic musculature)
Manipulation	'Passive' movement into paraphysiological range (range typically requires application of external force) but not exceeding anatomical range of motion
Spinal manipulative therapy	Generic umbrella term used for various procedures that may include chiropractic adjustment.
Chiropractic adjustment	Term typically favoured by chiropractors which characterizes neurological and segmental specificity in application (as opposed to mechanical and directional articular specificity typical of manipulation descriptions)
Manipulable spinal lesion models	Generic: biomechanical, neurophysiological, trophic, psychosocial, combination models Profession-derived: e.g. chiropractic vertebral subluxation, osteopathic somatic dysfunction, manual medicine joint block or fixation
Active care	Manual movement performed by the patient
Passive care	Manual movement performed by or with assistance from a clinician
Manipulation technique categories	Generic: mechanical/clinical descriptions, e.g. specific contact thrust, or manual force mechanically assisted Developer-named: e.g. Gonstead, Cox, Diversified, Logan-basic, craniosacral

manipulation reported in the English literature, including 21 fatalities, 51 major impairments and 42 that resolved favourably.[17] Hurwitz *et al.*[15] and Haldeman *et al.*[16] performed an extremely comprehensive search of literature for reports of vertebrobasilar artery dissection, the most serious complication that has been associated with a type of cervical spine manipulation. Of 367 case reports from all causes, 160 cases occurred due to spontaneous onset, 115 cases were found with onset after spinal manipulation, 58 cases associated were associated with trivial trauma and 37 cases were caused by major trauma (three cases were classified in two categories). Unfortunately, the nature of the precipitating trauma, neck movement or type of manipulation that was performed was poorly defined in the literature, and it was not possible to identify a specific neck movement or trauma that could be considered the offending activity in the majority of cases (see also Chapters 16 and 25). Table 24.3 provides an overview of the research findings on spinal manipulation.

Complications from lumbar manipulation are much rarer, with only 29 reported since 1911. Serious complications include vertebrobasilar and cerebral reactions, disc herniation and cauda equina syndrome.[18] Side-effects do not appear to have an age dependency, although a slightly higher incidence may exist among women.[14,19]

Overall, RAND estimated the rates of serious complications as 5–10 in 10 million for vertebrobasilar reactions, 3–6 in 10 million for major impairment, fewer than 3 fatalities per 10 million manipulations, and about 1 per 100 million complications involving cauda equina.[15] At the high end, occurrences have been estimated to be 1 in 400 000–500 000.[20–22] Other estimates indicate 1 per 1.3–2 million manipulations.[9,23] Serious complication from manipulation should be placed in perspective.[24,25] The most common medical treatment for musculoskeletal conditions (routinely cared for by chiropractors) is the prescription of non-steroidal anti-inflammatory drugs (NSAIDs). Complications from NSAIDs have been documented at 0.04% fatality rate (accounting for 3200 deaths annually)[26] and a 2.74% rate of serious gastrointestinal events.[27] Other reports estimate 2600 deaths and 20 000 hospitalizations annually from NSAIDs with between 390 and 3200 serious gastrointestinal events per million.[28] NSAID use can be of greater concern in older populations. Strategies to minimize risk have been developed and are standard within chiropractic, including the identification of appropriate clinical indications, appropriate patient selection and appropriate expertise, yet their value is limited.[11,16,29,30] Other concerns over iatrogenic drug reactions are discussed in further detail in Chapter 22.

Comparing spinal manipulation to alternative interventions and placebo

Spinal manipulation has become a well-studied intervention. Its evidentiary basis includes long-term clinical experience, observational studies, randomized

Table 24.3 Brief overview of research findings on spinal manipulation

Acute lower back pain: 14 RCTs	7 favoured manipulation
	4 found significance in subgroups
	3 found no difference
Subacute and chronic lower back pain: 11 RCTs	7 favoured manipulation over other treatments
	3 reported no significant differences
	1 made no conclusions from the data
Mixed lower back pain: 13 RCTs	9 favoured manipulation
	1 significant in subgroup only
	3 reported no difference
Manipulation vs placebo: 11 RCTs	8 favoured manipulation (including 4 of the 5 best-designed
(4 sham manipulation, 7 detuned modalities)	studies)
Acute and chronic neck pain: 10 RCTs	4 favoured manipulation
	6 found no statistical difference
	Statistical pooling of five better studies yielded a 0.06 effect size favouring
	manipulation (a change of 16 on a 100 point scale)
Headache: 8 RCTs	5 favoured manipulation (muscle tension/cervicogenic)
	3 equivocal (migraine, chronic muscle tension)
Chiropractic literature in older populations:	15 case studies
40 articles	1 retrospective case series
	1 diagnostic technology assessment
	18 clinical overviews
	19 commentaries

clinical trials, meta-analyses and systematic literature reviews, formal expert consensus panels, and government reports and guidelines.[9] Manipulation has been compared with placebos, exercise and advice, no treatment (natural progression), back school, analgesics and NSAIDs, infrared, shortwave diathermy, ultrasound, flexion exercises, massage, electrical stimulation and various combinations of these. In general, 39 randomized clinical trials have evaluated spinal manipulation for low back pain. At least 26 of them favoured manipulation (including eight of the 10 best-designed studies) and 13 found outcomes from manipulation comparable to other treatments.[31,32] A recent review by Bronfort[33] suggests that there is moderate evidence of benefit from manipulation for acute, subacute and chronic low back pain, but inadequate data for making any conclusions regarding radiculopathy. There have been at least 18 randomized trials for manipulation with head and neck pain complaints. Nine favoured manipulation and eight found manipulation equal to other treatments.[15,34] In 1995, Assendelft *et al.* reported that 34 of 51 reviews favoured manipulation.[35] No studies have found any other comparable treatments to work better than manipulation for the musculoskeletal complaints studied. Several meta-analyses have been performed, all of which reiterate the effectiveness of manipulation. One

of the best-designed analyses considered acute lower back pain studies and concluded benefit from spinal manipulation.[31] Some examples of published trials and reviews we listed in the appendix.

Non-spine-related disorders

Far less literature has considered manipulation for non-musculoskeletal disorders, and among the studies that have, evidence favouring benefit has been much less robust. Case studies predominate along with a few well-designed pilot studies. Few conclusions can be drawn from these. Among the better-designed reported are comparisons of manipulation with usual care for primary dysmenorrhoea, chronic pelvic pain, childhood asthma and hypertension.[36–38] The primary outcomes of all studies have been essentially equivocal to non-treatment or random treatment groups thus far. Some benefit with reduced medication use was reported in the asthma study.

Research issues for spinal manipulation, chiropractic and other complementary and alternative medicine models

As with any field with limited resources for research, much remains to be done. There are quality and methodology issues for all of the published manipulation studies to date. Among issues warranting improvement are the heterogeneity of study patients, and blinding of patients, clinicians and outcomes assessors. In addition, theory development issues and a generally poor understanding of pain syndromes represent areas for further investigation. Among the most complex of research issues confronting methodology for spinal manipulation trials are challenges associated with placebo effects and other confounders including doctor–patient interactions, the nature of physical touch, and doctor and patient expectations. The entire area of prevention, wellness and non-therapeutic interventions will require much more work in the area of methodologies and measurement. This holds true for all of the CAM disciplines, but also is of interest in preventive medicine. Capturing subtle effects requires large populations and long-term follow-up. This can be roughly translated into one word: 'expensive'.

Developing the research infrastructure for chiropractic including personnel, facilities, expertise and funding also remains challenging.[39] The Consortial Center for Chiropractic Research has been established and is currently funded as a National Institutes of Health, National Center for Complementary and Alternative Medicine (NIH-NCCAM) Research Center. In Europe, Canada, the USA and Australia, a small but significant chiropractic research enterprise has been established and the quality and productivity of chiropractic research activity have become laudable. Still, much more financial and economic support will be required for more and better research to be sustained. A fundamental social priority issue is likely to plague initiatives to explore contextual methods and questions of interest in greater depth: what near-term benefits will accrue to society that can justify diversion of resources from cancer, heart disease, retro-viruses and other accepted health-care needs?

Chiropractic management considerations with the elderly

Older patients may make up approximately 15% of chiropractic patient populations.[40] Of patients between 65 and 75 years of age, 14% report using chiropractic services but that drops off to 6% among those over the age of 75.[41] However, access issues may account for these numbers. There is great regional variation, and one study examining two rural midwestern communities found that two-thirds of individuals over

the age of 65 used chiropractic care.[42] The number increases substantially among men over 70 years old. Overall, chiropractic utilization by the elderly mirrors that of the general population, with the notable exception that ready access to chiropractic in medically underserved areas dramatically increases utilization. Those that do use chiropractic services tend to be in good health, less likely to use nursing-home or hospital services, and use fewer prescription drugs, but more over-the-counter medications.[40]

Effectiveness studies of manipulation on geriatric populations per se have not been conducted. To date, most studies have recruited otherwise healthy adult patients in the 18–65 age range. Thus, the applicability of such findings to an older population must be made with caution. It would be reasonable to expect the same sorts of challenges in implementation of manipulation studies on older populations that exist in other care settings (e.g. ambulation issues, compliance with care, access). The elderly may often take multiple medications that can be a source of masked treatment effects. Common issues concerning an ageing population will also impact on study designs. For example, physiological healing times prolong with age, access to study locations may be challenging, and connective tissue and joint pliability changes may require modification of interventions on a case-by-case basis, hindering the ability to standardize manipulative interventions.

Reliance on clinical experience in the care of elderly patients is the norm within chiropractic, and a great deal of qualitative attention to geriatric care issues can be found in chiropractic training and clinical literature.[43–45] Manipulation techniques are frequently modified to suit the exigencies and tolerances of patients and specific considerations have been reported in chiropractic literature.[46] Age-appropriate modifications to chiropractic evaluation protocols may also be warranted and have been described as well.[47, 48] Chiropractors also report providing an eclectic host of interventions beyond manipulation for elderly patients, including exercise, nutrition, relaxation and physical therapy.[49]

Contextual approaches in geriatric chiropractic care

There is a growing trend permeating throughout health care that focuses on how well an individual can carry out his or her activities of daily living (ADLs), as opposed to the definitive resolution of a disease process.[50] Recent chiropractic literature emphasizes approaches that consider the entire person's health in terms of physiological abilities, psychosocial interactions and emotional well-being.[2,3,43,44,47,51–53] Thus, it may be concluded that there is a shift away from molecular medicine to contextual medicine, especially in the area of chiropractic geriatric care.

Some authors refer to such changes in function synonymously with changes in quality of life or health-related quality of life (HRQOL).[7,51,54] In the parlance of chiropractic, these factors are often grouped together under the umbrella term of 'wellness' or global well-being. The literature describing the assessment and management of an older patient emphasizes this holistic, functionally based approach.[2,3,43,44,47,51–53] The recommended assessment of an older patient is termed a comprehensive geriatric assessment (CGA), which has been defined previously.

According to Bowers, a functional assessment is the cornerstone of a geriatric assessment.[47] The assessment of an older patient, therefore, is not only in quantitative terms (degrees of range of motion, responsive to provocational tests and so on), but must also be in qualitative terms that assesses quality of life improvements. Combining a patient's functional abilities with their quality of life status serves as a guide to his or her overall well-being.[7,51,54]

For older patients the preservation (or increase) of the patient's quality of life is necessary for 'successful' or 'optimal ageing', which is defined as the optimalization of a person's health while minimizing any physiological declines as the result of the ageing process.[43,47] In contrast to successful ageing, a person who succumbs to the ravages of time and manifests degenerative changes in health status due to genetic predispositions and poor lifestyle choices (smoking, excessive alcohol consumption, obesity, sedentary lifest) is said to exhibit 'normal' or 'usual' ageing.[43,47]

It is not the intent of this discussion either to diminish the importance of conventional medicine in caring for conditions that arise with age, or to portray any of medicine's misanthropic features. Holism does have its champions in modern medicine. Wilson and Cleary describe the importance of linking clinical variables with HRQOL measurements in a recent article published in the Journal of the American Medical Association.[54] In the article, the authors state that there is increasing evidence that HRQOLs are valid and reliable, are responsive to clinical changes and are a useful and important supplement to traditional physiological and psychological outcome measures.[54]

This sentiment was echoed by Gerin et al., who emphasized that because 'an individual's personal experience is the only realistic reference for use in the subjective quality of life assessment … it is the person himself who is best qualified to make the assessment'.[7] The authors go on to state that 'in therapeutic trials, the effects of a treatment on both the objective and subjective quality of life should be simultaneously but independently assessed'.[7]

Measuring wellness

There are many different evaluation instruments available to measure a patient's quality of life. These include the Global Well-Being Scale (GWBS), the Self-Related Health/Wellness Survey (SRHW) and the SF-36. The SF-36 is by far the most commonly used evaluation instrument to measure quality of life.

Dr Cheryl Hawk of Palmer College of Chiropractic developed the Global Well-Being Scale (GWBS).[55] The GWBS is a visual analogue scale on a horizontal 10 cm line that has at one end the statement 'The Best I've Ever Felt' and at the other end 'The Worst I've Ever Felt' (Figure 24.1). The patient is asked to mark a line on the scale that best matches how they feel on that day.

The reliability and validity of the GWBS as an outcome instrument have been studied and documented.[56] A pilot study using the GWBS as a measure of change in patient's health under a form of chiropractic care (bioenergetic synchronicity technique or BEST) was conducted in 1995.[56] Statistically significant

---

Global Well-Being Scale

Date:

Patient ID#:

Please think about how you are feeling right now – your general sense of health and well-being. On the line below, make a straight vertical (up and down) mark on the line to show how you feel right now:

Worst you	Best you
could possible	could possibly
feel _____	feel

Figure 24.1 Global well-being scale.

improvements in wellness were observed.[56] An important finding of this pilot study was that patients reported being more well after treatment, despite the re-emergence of their physical pain and symptoms.[56] The GWBS was also used as an outcome measure in a 1999 study comparing improvements in patient's wellness receiving either an actual or a sham (activator set to zero) adjustment.[57]

Similar research has been conducted by a joint Sherman College–Life University study.[58–60] In that study, the investigators found that GWBS and SF-36 scores improved in patients receiving only upper cervical chiropractic treatments.[58–60] Interestingly, pain symptoms (measured as body pain by the SF-36) did not improve to the level of the general population after completion of chiropractic care.[58–60] Had an individual examined this study only for changes in objective measures such as pain, the reader would have had to conclude that upper cervical care was ineffective for pain resolution. However, such an examination of this study may have been inappropriate because practitioners utilizing upper cervical techniques do not have as their intent or goal of treatment symptom resolution. Instead, many chiropractors utilizing upper cervical techniques have as their intent the attainment of wellness.

A recently published longitudinal study conducted at the New Zealand School of Chiropractic assessed patient self-related health wellness and quality of life while under chiropractic care at a training clinic.[61] The Self-Related Health/Wellness Survey (SRHW) was used to evaluate health status of patients. The SRHW was developed and first used by Blanks *et al.* in a retrospective study of patients receiving Network Care.[62] The New Zealand school reported significant positive perceived changes in Physical State, Mental/Emotional State and Combined Wellness in patients under chiropractic care.[61]

The most commonly used and most extensively tested instrument to measure changes in quality of life is the Medical Outcomes Study Short Form-36 Health Survey, Rand modification 1.0 Rand SF-36.[63] The SF-36 is a self-administered, generic (meaning the measures are relevant to individuals generally and not to a specific condition) measure of quality of life. In a study conducted by Beaton *et al.* that compared five different generic health status measures in a group of patients, the SF-36 was the most appropriate questionnaire to measure health changes.[51] According to

Ware, the SF-36 can be administered in 5–10 min with a high degree of acceptability and data quality to the general population and to young and elderly patients.[64] Normative values exist for the general populations.[64] Specifically, the SF-36 gathers information in eight different health domains: (i) physical functioning; (ii) role limitations due to physical health (role–physical); (iii) role limitations due to emotional problems (role–emotion); (iv) energy/fatigue; (v) emotional well-being (mental health); (vi) social functioning; (vii) body pain; and (viii) general health.[64] The SF-36 can used to compare conditions and treatments.[65] According to Wilson, the SF-36 has been used in more than 400 clinical trials in the USA, and its use in that country (including number of projects and organizations using the survey) exceeds 4500.[66]

Challenges to promoting wellness

There are many intellectual challenges to the development of a preventive and wellness approach for CAMs.[2] The most important of these challenges is the lack of knowledge and established evidence that preventive or maintenance care can result in a higher level of patient health or wellness, in spite of the fact that both patients and practitioners place a high value on these outcomes.[2,49,67] This is further hampered by the requirement of third-party payers, such as Medicare, for evidence indicating the 'therapeutic necessity' of a service being submitted for compensation (see below). From a methodological perspective, how can prevention be measured? How can a study objectively demonstrate that a patient is healthier ('more well') if he or she receives periodic spinal adjustments that are supposed to prevent illness, as opposed to a symptom-based approach, which has demonstrable changes in 'quantitative' measures such as pain perception, range of motion and diminished response to orthopaedic tests?

The promotion of a wellness paradigm is further hampered by pedagogical gaps in health-care training, during which public-health strategies and epidemiology are not traditionally emphasized.[2] Moreover, training at many CAM colleges has not, by and large, prepared its students to form alliances with public-health departments and government agencies.[2]

There are some fundamental challenges to the financing of CAM services under contemporary reimbursement methods, particularly those focused on prevention and wellness care.[68] Fortunately, the dilemma permeates preventive conventional medicine service as well. The crux of the matter revolves around the very nature of indemnity insurance. The idea is for many people in society who do not require a product or service in everyday life to contribute a small amount of money, via insurance premiums or taxation, to pay for something that would be beyond the individual's normal resources to afford. Coverage for automobile accidents exemplifies this concept. Individuals pay an affordable premium. In the event of an accident, the necessary financial resources are available to deal with any damage to the car or injury to the driver or passengers. The system would fall apart if all insured persons either were required to remit expensive collision coverage premiums every month, or required large reimbursements on a regular basis.

The same principles apply to health-care coverage. Many individuals contribute an affordable amount to cover an expensive situation in the event of a crisis. If all insured persons needed expensive medical services simultaneously, the system would collapse. Health insurance, by its very nature, is condition orientated. Many CAM interventions that focus on wellness care or prevention, therefore, have a dilemma. While many healthful activities such as eating vegetables has been shown to prevent some diseases, it is unlikely that an insurance company would ever pay a person's grocery bill.

The same thought process must apply to chiropractic care. Even assuming that chiropractic maintenance care may prevent certain diseases in some percentage of the population, unless the direct cost of the diseases prevented exceeded the cost of compensating for universal chiropractic care, insurance carriers would not reimburse the chiropractic users. It is more cost efficient for individuals to pay directly for such services with community subsides for the needy. It seems more likely that should evidence eventually support the use of chiropractic care for general wellness, and further provided that the patient can document each appointment, a person may then qualify for a 'wellness' discount. Certain regular medical interventions, such as mammograms, pap-smears and immunizations, along with some lifestyle behaviours (e.g. not smoking) are examples of procedures that currently justify this approach.

A key challenge for CAM providers and proponents of wellness or preventive services is econometric documentation. Such research takes years and is costly. In the meantime, reimbursement for CAM services will have to struggle to fit into existing condition-based reimbursement requirements.[68]

The challenge of developing evidence-based medicine for complementary and alternative medicine

Sackett describes evidence-based medicine as the 'conscientious, explicit and judicious use of the current best evidence in making decisions about the care of individual patients'.[69] This implies that procedures and behaviours have been subjected to rigorous standards of scientific observations, experimentations and documentation.[70] Many CAM providers are faced with the duel need and frustration of having to develop and promote evidence-based medicine. Third-party payers (health-insurance plans, government agencies) are demanding that CAM practitioners provide evidence as to the efficacy of their therapeutic interventions. The frustration, however, is that many features of CAM are difficult both to define and to measure.[70] In chiropractic, for example, no clear definition exists for 'subluxation', which is for some the anchor-term of chiropractic, and minimal research has been performed to identify the extent to which a subluxation compromises a person's health.[70] Moreover, with hundreds of different system techniques described, many of which advocate a different model of care (structural, postural, vitalistic, etc), it is difficult to determine how best to allocate the limited research resources. Perhaps the most daunting challenge is the inability of chiropractors to agree on the intent of provided care. Is chiropractic a portal of entry into the health system (not unlike dentistry), or is it primary care?[71] Is the primary goal of care the removal of subluxations only? Is it the restoration of homoeostasis within a patient? Should CAMs be preferentially concerned with the alleviation of pain and symptoms? If the latter, how can a practitioner justify the importance of 'maintenance care', which is the provision of care as a prophylactic measure, often in the absence of symptoms, for reimbursement by third-party payers? Operational definitions for terms such as 'health' and the chiropractic 'adjustment' are similarly difficult to develop.[70]

In a recent article, Meeker identified concepts germane to the application of evidence-based medicine to chiropractic theory.[70] He reminded the reader that many of the approaches used by all health-care providers, including medical physicians, lack strong supportive evidence. As Meeker describes, scientific induction begins with empirical observations, from which hypotheses, theories and laws are ultimately developed.[70] The importance of incorporating clinical observations in the development of evidence-based medicine is further emphasized by Sackett, who wrote 'the practice of evidence-based medicine means integrating individual clinical expertise with the best available external clinical evidence from systematic research'.[69]

Although randomized clinical trials (RCTs) are considered to be at the pinnacle of evidence-based medicine, evidence of the effectiveness of chiropractic treatments also comes from clinical experience, case studies and observational cohort studies.[29] Moreover, there are several limitations to RCTs.[72] For example, RCTs are usually of short or moderate duration, most do not include a true placebo group, and they may not truly represent clinical practice because some patients (typically those at higher risk) may be excluded from the trials.[72] More importantly, RCTs focus primarily on a priori end-points, and do not necessary monitor other benefits of therapy, such as prevention of the progression of the disease, reduced impact of comorbid conditions and improved quality of life.[72] Additional barriers to RCTs are their cost, the time required to perform them and the scarcity of skilled researchers to conduct them. The alternative of large-scale, longitudinal, population-based, observational studies, which may overcome some of the limitations of RCTs, is also exorbitantly resource intensive.

Notwithstanding these barriers, chiropractic and other CAMs have taken the challenges of evidence-based medicine seriously. The CAM professions have encouraged individuals to develop the necessary research skills, they continue to promote the agenda of evidence-based medicine, and CAM organizations are allocating the resources required to test their health models. The evidence base for manipulation and rationale applications to use in geriatric populations that have appeared in the chiropractic literature make a reasonable case for the use of these services.[73]

Coverage and effectiveness decisions being made by both public- and private-sector health policy are under ever-increasing scrutiny.[74] Competition for a limited pool of revenue resources is increasing owing to higher costs for health care, greater demands of an increasing older population, and consumer and accountability pressures from the public. Policy makers are under pressure to pay only for procedures that are effective. When procedures are of equivalent effectiveness, cost can become the determining factor. The challenge of evidence-based medicine is not simply 'does it work?' Paying customers are posing legitimate questions such as: 'Is this kind of care really effective? What evidence is it based on? Is it merely based on theory or with treatment philosophy? Does this kind of care improve quality of life? Is this kind of care better (superior, faster, or less expensive clinical and social outcomes) than the care received from the traditional allopathic approaches or from those of other alternative health-care disciplines?'[75]

CAM providers are not being singled out. Such tough questions are being asked of everyone, including traditional conventional generalists and specialists, hospital systems, rehabilitation centres, long-term care centres, dentists and most allied health-providers. These realities have helped to inform the future chiropractic research agenda.[75] However, the best available evidence, and the nature of health-care reimbursement itself, will probably focus the discussion on condition care. The province of wellness care seems likely to be elective or limited in terms of third-party pay for some time.

Technology assessment

Among the newer buzzwords in the field of evidence-based medicine is technology assessment.[74] Technology assessment can be defined as a form of policy research that attempts to evaluate technology for the purpose of providing decision makers with information on different policy options.[74] It is required by many different stakeholders, including insurance companies, government agencies, the public and health-care providers (to name just a few) to determine the impact of a particular technology on issues such as safety, efficacy, effectiveness, cost–benefit, quality of life changes and cost-effectiveness.[74]

The need for technology assessment is nowhere more striking than in the field of chiropractic care. This is because many technique system entrepreneurs have an unfair advantage over chiropractic colleges, because the former are able to make virtually any unsubstantiated claim without fear of professional censure and they need only ensure that they stay out of the criminal system and avoid being seen as fringe enough to have practitioners barred from practising the given technique.[76] In contrast, the chiropractic colleges are accountable to public-health agencies, the scientific community, student loan-granting agencies, alumni, students and their own faculty.[76] Therefore, it may be argued that it is the responsibility of chiropractic colleges to provide students with the necessary information to prevent the more outlandish producers from exploiting them because of their inexperience.[76,77]

Technology assessment is at the centre of many of the decisions made by managed care administrators.[76] As Mootz *et al.* wrote: 'No one (especially an insurance company) wants to pay for clinical procedures that are ineffective, overpriced, or unnecessary ... The advent of better technologies to synthesize research, establish professional consensus, and determine appropriateness has offered a reasonable alternative to the arbitrary and proprietary methods of the past'.[78]

It is important for practitioners not be afraid of the results that may come out of research projects, and they must be prepared to modify or reject current behaviours, attitudes or therapeutic approaches, regardless of their historical appeal, if they are proven to be ineffective at best, or harmful at worst. The authors have heard the dangers of research described as the slaying of a beautiful idea by an ugly fact. As Cooperstein and Schneider recounted, '... [negative] results are never encouraging ones to bring back to students or alumni who wonder aloud why the colleges would undermine confidence in their own core curricula'.[76] However, Coulter and Adams remind us that 'what is clear is that if chiropractors do not develop [guidelines] for themselves, outside parties (such as third-party payers) will do it for them'.[79] All of this becomes necessary given the wide fluctuations in chiropractic utilization that occur geographically, the large variation in the number of office visits and the diverse number of methods in common use.[76]

Irrespective of its importance, no health-care approach can rely exclusively on an evidence-based approach. As O'Malley observed, many practitioners can relate anecdotal examples of a seemingly capricious patient's body responding to treatment at variance with textbook expected outcomes of predefined syndromes.[80] Because of this, while evidence-based medicine may be the preferred treatment method of choice, it is not necessarily the most beneficial at all times for all patients, and a trial-based therapeutic approach, specifically structured for the special needs of a particular patient, must continue to be the cornerstone of both allopathic and CAM use.

This approach has recently been echoed by Goodwin who opined:

Evidence-based medicine is not kind to the elderly. This movement trusts only the products of randomized, controlled trials or, preferably, meta-analyses of those trials. But subjects over the age of 75 years are rarely found in such trials, thus rendering this population invisible to scientific medicine. If we teach only what we know, and if we know only what we can measure in clinical trials, then we can say little of importance about the care of the elderly. The most important resources required in caring for the very old – sufficient time and empathy – are not included in the critical pathways of managed care.[80]

The future of complementary and alternative medicine

In Chapter 2 (Geriatric demographics), possible future trends in health-care were discussed in general terms. These included the development of an integrated health-care system, which has as one goal health cost containment. However, Dillard has recently described the drawbacks facing CAMs to being 'integrated' or 'mainstreamed' into allopathic health care, in a process that he termed 'medicinization.[82] Dillard warns of the risks of emulating what he calls a (medical) reductionist approach, the tyranny of managed care, and that an integration into medicine may result in the sacrifice of a discipline's diversity and robust heterogeneity.[82] Notwithstanding Dillard's cautions, it seems inevitable that CAM will become mainstream, for the ultimate benefit of the practitioners, professions and patients alike.

In a recent conference, Coulter has suggested that there are two possible futures specific to CAM.[83] In the first scenario, Coulter opined that CAM may act as a type of health care 'Trojan Horse', whose members will attempt to change the traditional reductionist allopathic model to a holistic paradigm from within. This would be achieved by establishing strong interprofessional working relationships and rapports.

The second of Coulter's scenarios, simultaneously more troubling and yet seemingly more plausible, is that allopathic medicine will agree with the concept of an holistic approach to such an extent that medicine will simply assimilate the CAM foundational tenets and therapeutic methods, not unlike the co-optation of osteopathy.[83] Coulter suggested that leaders in medical pedagogy may come to accept the efficacy of spinal manipulative therapy, botanical medicines and acupuncture. Educators may simply insert training in these modes of therapy into the core curriculum of a medical college. With an established infrastructure for third-party payers already in place, along with the legislative privileges to prescribe medications and perform spinal manipulative therapy, this scenario could prove to be the most formidable challenge facing the CAM disciplines. Indeed, a recent survey of 117 of the 125 medical schools in the USA revealed that 64% offer some type of CAM instruction.[84] Moreover, a survey of medical doctors seemed to indicate a growing acceptance or chiropractic care, with 39% of respondents describing it as a 'legitimate medical practice'.[84] Lastly, Meeker notes that many prestigious medical journals, such as the New England Journal of Medicine, Annals of Internal Medicine and Journal of the American Medical Association, have devoted more and more space to the issues surrounding CAM.[84]

Strategic planning by the chiropractic profession, and CAM providers in general, is urgently needed. Otherwise, CAM practitioners could find themselves left out of key discussions on health-care delivery system and perhaps future systems themselves. A recent futures forecasting issue from the journal Topics in Clinical Chiropractic was devoted to assessing near-term trends that are likely to impact the profession. The editors offered three defining issues for the chiropractic profession in confronting the future: (i) no one cares about our internal disputes and agendas except for us; (ii) how we define our interface between condition-based care and wellness-based care determines where we fit in to reimbursement systems; and (iii) adaptability to the information age (where our patients and competition increasingly know the same things that we do) will determine how well we survive.[85]

Chiropractic has grown to the third largest learned health profession within a century, an accomplishment in which we can take great pride. However, consider how conventional medicine ascended from the days of medical protest movements, with Flexner taking the medical profession to task for its medieval allopathy of lances, leaches, tinctures and quinine, to its contemporary position of predominance. Obstacles still exist for CAM practices:[83]

- lack of research on efficacy
- economic consideration/costs
- ignorance about CAM by both the public and medical field
- provider competition and division

- lack of standards of practice and licensing
- fear of change by the medical establishment
- cultural bias and prejudice
- lack of usage data on CAM
- lack of consumer or employer demand for CAM
- lack of insurance reimbursement for CAM
- lack of provider networks including CAM
- resistance to methods of the medical establishment.

However, for those who doubt the possibility of medical acceptance and the eventual envelopment (displacement?) of CAM, consider the following commentary by Dr Albert Abrams:

> Others, less scientific but more astute, have determined empirically that manipulation of the spine does sometimes cure conditions which have failed of cure in the hands of experienced physicians ... Neither the fury of tongue nor the truculence of pen can gainsay the confidence that these systems of practice have inspired in the community.[86]

What is sobering about this statement is that Dr Abrams, a medical physician considered to be a heretic in his time, wrote this opinion in 1912. The methods promoted by CAM are not new, and their popularity has risen and fallen over the centuries and across cultures. For health disciplines to flourish, not only must their paradigms resonate within the culture, but also their proponents must astutely and seamlessly position themselves among the resources and problem-solvers of the community.

References

1 Gatterman M. Chiropractic Management of Spinal Related Disorders. Baltimore, MD: Williams & Wilkins, 1990.
2 Hawk C. Should chiropractic be a 'wellness', profession? Top Clin Chiropractic 2000; 7(1): 23–26.
3 Coulter I. Alternative Philosophical and investigatory paradigms in chiropractic. J Manipulative Physiol Ther 1993; 16: 419–425.
4 Black D. Inner Wisdom: The Challenge of Contextual Healing. Springville, UT: Tapestry Press, 1990.
5 Black D. Fine Tuning: The Promise of Contextual Healing. Springville, UT: Tapestry Press, 1991.
6 Mootz RD. The contextual nature of manual methods: challenges of the paradigm. J Chiropractic Humanities 1995; 5(1): 28–40.
7 Gerin P, Dazord A, Boissel J, Chifflet R. Quality of life assessment in therapeutic trials: rationale for and presentation of a more appropriate instrument. Fundam Clin Pharmacol 1992; 6: 263–276.
8 Chapman-Smith DA. The Chiropractic Profession. West DesMoines, IA: NCMIC Group, 2000.
9 Cherkin DC, Mootz RD, eds. Chiropractic in the United States: Training, Practice, and Research. AHCPR Pub. No. 98-N002. Rockville, MD: Agency for Health Care Policy and Research, 1997.

10 Owens EF. Theoretical constructs of vertebral subluxation as applied by chiropractic practitioners and researchers. Top Clin Chiropractic 2000; 7(1): 74–79.

11 Haldeman S, Chapman Smith D, Petersen D, eds. Guidelines for Chiropractic Quality Assurance and Practice Parameters. Gaithersberg, MD: Aspen, 1993.

12 Bartol KM. A model for categorization of chiropractic treatment procedures. J Chiropractic Technique 1991; 3(2): 78–80.

13 Gatterman MI, ed. Foundations of Chiropractic: Subluxation. St Louis, MO: Mosby 1995.

14 Senstad O, Leboeuf-Yde C, Borchgrevink C. Frequency and characteristics of side effects of spinal manipulative therapy. Spine 1997; 22: 435–440.

15 Hurwitz EL, Aker PD, Adams AH *et al.* Manipulation and mobilzation of the cervical spine. A systematic review of the literature. Spine 1996; 21: 1746–1759.

16 Haldeman S, Kohlbeck FJ, McGregor M. Risk factors and precipitating neck movements causing vertebrobasilar artery dissection after cervical trauma and spinal manipulation. Spine 1999; 24: 785–794.

17 RAND.

18 Assendelft WJ, Bouter LM, Knipschild PG. Complications of spinal manipulation: a comprehensive review of the literature. J Fam Pract 1996; 42: 475–480.

19 Leboeuf-Y de C, Hennius B, Rudberg E *et al.* Side effects of chiropractic treatment: a prospective study. J Manipulative Physiol Ther 1997; 20: 511–515.

20 Dvorak J, vOrelli F. How dangerous is manipulation to the cervical spine? Case report and results of a survey. J Manual Med 1985; 2: 1–4.

21 Patjin J. Complications in manual medicine: a review of the literature. J Manual Med 1991; 6(3): 89–92.

22 Lee KP, Carlini WG, McCormick GF, Albers GW. Neurologic complications following chiropractic manipulation: a survey of California neurologists. Neurology 1995; 45: 123–1215.

23 Klougart N, Leboeuf-Yde C. Rasmussen LR. Saftey in chiropractic practice, Part I: The occurrence of cerebrovascular accidents after manipulation to the neck in Denmark from 1978–1988. J Manipulative Physiol Ther 1996; 19: 371–377.

24 Terrett AGJ. Misuse of the literature by medical authors in discussing spinal manipulative therapy injury. J Manipulative Physiol Ther 1995; 18: 203–210.

25 Fries JF. Assessing and understanding patient risk. Scand J Rheumotol Suppl 1992; 92: 21–24.

26 Gabriel SE, Jaakkimainen L, Bombardier C. Risk for serious gastrointestinal complications related to use of nonsteroidal anti-inflammatory drugs. A meta-analysis. Ann Intern Med 1991; 115: 787–796.

27 Roth SH, Tindall EA, Jain AK et al. A controlled study comparing the effects of nabumetone, ibuprofen, and ibuprofen plus misoprostol on the upper gastrointestinal tract mucosa. Arch Intern Med 1996; 153: 565–571.

28 Tamblyn R. Medication use in seniors: challenges and solutions. Therapie 1996; 51: 269–282.

29 McGregor M, Haldeman S, Kohlbeck F. Vertebrobasilar compromise associated with cervical manipulation. Topics Clin Chiropractic 1995; 2: 63–73.

30 Senstad O, Leboef-Yde C, Borchgrevink C. Predictors of side effects to spinal manipulative therapy. J Manipulative Physiol Ther 1996; 19: 441–445.

31 Shekelle PG, Adams AH, Chassin MR *et al.* Spinal manipulation for low-back pain. Ann Intern Med 1992; 117: 590–598.

32 Van Tulder MW, Koes BW, Bouter LM. Conservative treatment of acute and chronic nonspecific low back pain. A systematic review of randomized controlled trials of the most common interventions. Spine 1997; 22: 2128–2156.

33 Bronfort G. Spinal manipulation: current state of research and its indications. Neurol Clin 1999; 17: 91–111.

34 Vernon H, McDermaid CS, Hagino C. Systematic review of randomized clinical trials of complementary/alternative therapies in the treatment of tension-type and cervicogenic headache. Complementary Med Ther 1999; 7: 142–155

35 Assendelft WJ, Koes BW, Knipschild PG, Bouter LM. The relationship between methodological quality and conclusions in reviews of spinal manipulation. JAMA 1995; 274: 1942–1948.

36 Goertz CM, Mootz RD. A review of chiropractic management strategies in the care of hypertensive patients. J Neuromusculoskeletal Syst 1993; 1: 91–108.

37 Balon J, Aker PD, Crowther ER *et al.* A comparison of active and simulated chiropractic manipulation as adjunctive treatment for childhood asthma. N Engl J Med 1998; 339: 1013–1020.

38 Hondras MA, Long CR, Brennan PC. Spinal manipulative therapy versus a low force mimic maneuver for women with primary dysmenorrhea: a randomized, observer-blinded, clinical trial. Pain 1999; 81: 105–114.

39 Marchiori DM, Meeker W, Hawk C, Long CR. Research productivity of chiropractic college faculty. J Manipulative Physiol Ther 1998; 21: 8–13.

40 Coulter ID, Hurwitz EL, Aronow HU *et al.* Chiropractic patients in a comprehensive home-based geriatric assessment, follow-up and health promotion program. Topics Clin Chiropractic 1996; 3(2): 46–55.

41 National Center for Health Statistics (NCHS). Public Use Data Tape Documentation Part 1, National Interview Survey 1989. Hyattville, MD: National Technical Information Service, US Department of Commerce, NA-22161, 1990.

42 Lavsky-Shulan M, Wallace RB, Kohout FJ *et al.* Prevalence and functional correlates of low back pain in the elderly: the Iowa 65+ Rural Health Study. J Am Geriatr Soc 1985, 33(1): 23–28.

43 Killinger LZ, Azad A, Zapotocky B, Morschauser E. Development of a model curriculum in chiropractic geriatric education:process and content. J Neuromusculoskeletal Syst 1998; 6: 146–155.

44 McCarthy K. Management consideration in the geriatric patient. Topics Clin Chiropractic 1996; 3(2): 66–75.

45 Mootz RD, Bowers LJ, eds. Chiropractic Care of Special Populations. Gaithersburg, MD: Aspen, 1999.

46 Bergman TF, Larson L. Manipulative care and older persons. Topics Clin Chiropractic 1996; 3(2): 56–65.

47 Bowers LJ. Clinical assessment of geriatric patients: unique challenges. Topics Clin Chiropractic 1996; 3(2): 10–22.

48 Taylor J, Hoffman E. The geriatric patient: diagostic imaging considerations of common musculoskeletal disorders. Topics Clin Chiropractic 1996; 3(2): 23–35.

49 Rubert RL, Manello D, Sandefur R. Maintenance care: health promotion services administered to US chiropractic patients aged 65 and older, Part II. J Manipulative Physiol Ther 2000; 23: 10–19.

50 Bulpitt CJ. Quality of life as an outcome measure. Med Care 1997; 35: 613–617.

51 Beaton D, Hogg-Johnson S, Bombardier C. Evaluating changes in health status; reliability and responsiveness of five generic health status measures in workers with musculoskeletal disorders. Clin Epidemiol 1997; 50: 79–93.

52 Hawk C, Killinger LZ, Zapotocky B. Chiropractic training in the care of the geriatric patient: an assessment. J Neuromusculoskeletal Syst 1997; 5: 15–25.

53 Killinger LZ, Azad A. Chiropractic Geriatric Education. An Interdisciplinary Resource Guide and Teaching Strategy for Health Providers. Chicago, IL: Palmer College, Center for Chiropractic Research, 1998.

54 Wilson I, Cleary P. Linking clinical variables with health-related quality of life. JAMA 1995; 273: 59–65.

55 Hawk C, Dusio M, Wallace H et al. A study of the reliability, validity and responsiveness of a self-administered instrument to measure global well-being. Palmer J Res 1995; 2(1): 15–22.

56 Hawk C, Morter M. The use of measures of general well health status in chiropractic patients: a pilot study. Palmer J Res 1995; 2(2): 39–45.

57 Hawk C, Azad A, Phongphua C, Long C. Preliminary study of the effects of a placebo chiropractic treatment with sham adjustments. J Manipulative Physiol Ther 1999; 22: 436–443.

58 Hoiriis K, Brud D, Owens E. Changes in general health status during upper cervical chiropractic care. Presented at the Proceedings of the World Federation of Chiropractic, 5th Biennial Congress, Auckland, May 17–22, 1999.

59 Hoiriis K, Owens E, Pfleger B. Changes in general health status during upper cervical chiropractic care: a practice based research project. www.life-research.edu/crj/outcome.html

60 Owens E, Hoiriis K. Changes in the general health status during upper cervical chiropractic care: PBR Progress Report. Chiropractic Res J 1998; 5(1): 1.

61 Marino M, Langrell P. A longitudinal assessment of chiropractic care using a survey of self-related health wellness and quality of life: a preliminary study. J Vertebral Subluxation Res 1999; 3(2): 65–73.

62 Blanks R, Schuster T, Dobson M. A retrospective assessment of network care using a survey of self-related health, wellness and quality of life. J Vertebral Subluxation Res 1997; 1(4): 15–31.

63 RAND Health Sciences Program. RAND 36-Item Health Survey 1.0. RAND, 1982.

64 Ware J. The SF-36 Health Survey. www.sf-36.com/general/sf36.html.

65 Sanders C, Egger M, Donovan J et al. Reporting on quality of life in randomised controlled trials: bibliographic study. BMJ 1998; 317: 1191–1194.

66 Wilson T. Applications of the SF-36 health status. J Rehabilitation Outcomes Measure 1997; 1: 26–34.

67 Rupert R, Manello D, Sandefur R. Maintenance care: health promotion services administered to US chiropractic patients aged 65 and older, Part I. J Manipulative Physiol Ther 2000; 23: 1–9.

68 Bielinski LL, Mootz RD, eds. Issues in Coverage for Complementary and Alternative Medicine Services: Report of the Clinician Workgroup on the Integration of Complementary and Alternative Medicine. Olympia, WA: State of Washington Office of the Insurance Commissioner, 2000.

69 Sackett DL. Evidence-based medicine (Editorial). Spine 1999; 23: 1085–1086.

70 Meeker WC. Concepts germane to an evidence-based application of chiropractic theory. Topics Clin Chiropractic 2000; 7(1): 67–73.

71 Nelson C. Chiropractic scope of practice. J Manipulative Physiol Ther 1993; 16: 488–497.

72 JNC VI – The Sixth Report of the Joint National Committee on Prevention, Detection, Evaluation, and Treatment of High Blood Pressure. Arch Intern Med 1997; 157: 2413–2446.

73 Mootz Rd, Meeker WC. An evidence-based update on spinal manipulation with considerations for an aging population. 1st National Symposium on Complementary and Alternative Geriatric Health Care, Logan College of Chiropractic, April 30, 2000.

74 Hansen DT, Mootz RD. Formal processes in technology assessment: a primer for the chiropractic profession. Top Clin Chiropractic 1996; 3(1): 71–83.

75 Mootz RD, Coulter ID, Hansen DT. Health services research related to chiropractic: review and recommendations for research prioritization by the chiropractic profession. J Manipulative Physiol Ther 1997; 20: 201–217.

76 Cooperstein R, Schneider MS. Assessment of chiropractic techniques and procedures. Top Clin Chiropractic 1996; 3(1): 44–51.

77 Gleberzon BJ. Name technique in Canada: current trends in utilization rates and recommendations for their recommendations at the Canadian Chiropractic Memorial College. J Can Chiropractic Assoc 2000; 4(3): 55–69.

78 Mootz RD, Shekelle PG, Hansen DT. The politics of policy and research. Top Clin Chiropractic 1995; 2(2): 56–70.

79 Coulter I, Adams A. Consensus methods, clinical guidelines, and the RAND study of chiropractic. Am Chiropractic Assoc, J Chiropractic 1992; 29: 50–61.

80 O'Malley J. Toward a reconstruction of the philosophy of chiropractic. J Manipulative Physiol Ther 1995; 18: 285–292.

81 Goodwin JS. Geriatrics and the limits of modern medicine (commentary). New Engl J Med 1999; 340(16): 1283–1285.

82 Dillard J. Chiropractic as a mainstream health benefit versus an alternative/complementary benefit. Top Clin Chiropractic 2000; 7(1): 57–60.

83 Coulter I. Closing keynote address. 1st National Symposium on Complementary and Alternative Geriatric Health Care, Logan College of Chiropractic, April 30, 2000.

84 Meeker WC. Public demand and the integration of complementary and alternative medicine in the US health care system. J Manipulative Physiol Ther 2000; 23: 123–126.

85 Mootz RD, Hansen DT. Way back in the 1990s. Top Clin Chiropractic 2000; 7(1): iv–v.

86 Abrams A. Spondylotherapy: Physiotherapy of the Spine Based on a Study of Clinical Physiology. 3rd edn. San Francisco, CA: Philopolis Press, 1912: 673.

Appendix: Clinical trials on manipulation

Andersson GB, Lucente T, Davis AM et al. A comparison of osteopathic spinal manipulation with standard care for patients with low back pain. N Engl J Med 1999; 341: 1426–1431.

Anderson R, Meeker WC, Wirick B et al. A meta-analysis of clinical trials of spinal manipulation. J Manipulative Physiol Ther 1992; 15: 181–194.

Arkuszewski Z. The efficacy of manual treatment in low-back pain: a clinical trial. Manual Med 1986; 2: 68–71.

Balon J, Aker PD, Crowther ER et al. A comparison of active and simulated chiropractic manipulation as adjunctive treatment for childhood asthma. N Engl J Med 1998; 339: 1013–1020.

Bergquist-Ullman M, Larsson U. Acute low back pain in industry. A controlled prospective study with special reference to therapy and confounding factors. Acta Orthop Scand 1977; Suppl 170: 11–117.

Blomberg S, Hallin G, Grann K et al. Manual therapy with steroid injections in low-back pain. Spine 1994; 19: 569–577.

Boline PD, Kassak K, Bronfort G et al. Spinal manipulation versus amitriptyline for the treatment of chronic tension-type headaches: randomized clinical trial. J Manipulative Physiol Ther 1995; 18: 148–154.

Bove G, Nilsson N. Spinal manipulation in the treatment of episodic tension-type headache, a randomized controlled trial. JAMA 1998; 280: 1576–1579.

Brodin H. Cervical pain and mobilization. Manual Med 1982; 20: 90–94.

Bronfort G. Chiropractic versus general medical treatment of low-back pain: a small-scale controlled clinical trial. Am J Chiropract Med 1989; 2: 145–150.

Browning JE. Chiropractic distractive decompression in treating pelvic pain and multiple system pelvic organic dysfunction. J Manipulative Physiol Ther 1989; 12: 265–274.

Carey TS, Evans AT, Hadler NM et al. Acute severe low back pain. A population-based study of prevalence and care-seeking. Spine 1996; 21: 339–344.

Carey TS, Garrett J, Jackman A et al. The outcomes and costs of care for acute low back pain among patients seen by primary care practitioners, chiropractors, and orthopedic surgeons. N Engl J Med 1995; 333: 913–917.

Cassidy JD, Lopes AA, Yong-Hing K. The immediate effect of manipulation versus mobilization on pain and range of motion in the cervical spine: a randomized controlled trial. J Manipulation Physiol Ther 1992; 15: 570–575.

Cherkin DC, Deyo RA, Battie M et al. A comparison of physical therapy, chiropractic manipulation, and provision of an educational booklet for the treatment of patients with low back pain. N Engl J Med 1998; 339: 1021–1029.

Cherkin DC, MacCornack FA. Patient evaluations of low back pain care from family physicians and chiropractors. West J Med 1989; 150: 351–355.

Christian GH, Stanton GJ, Sissons D et al. Immunoreactive ACTH, beta-endorphin, and cortisol levels in plasma following spinal manipulative therapy. Spine 1988; 13: 1411–1417.

Coxhead CE, Meade TM, Inskip H et al. Multicentre trial of physiotherapy in the management of sciatic symptoms. Lancet 1981; i: 1065–1068.

Delitto A, Cibulka MT, Erhard RE et al. Evidence for use of an extension-mobilization category in acute low-back syndrome. A prescriptive validation pilot study. Phys Ther 1992; 73: 216–223.

Doran DM, Newell DJ. Manipulation in treatment of low back pain. A multicentre study. BMJ 1975; ii: 161–164.

Evans DP, Burke MS, Lloyd KN et al. Lumbar spinal manipulation on trial. Rheumatol Rehabil 1978; 17: 46–53.

Farrell JP, Twomey LT. Acute low back pain. Comparison of two conservative treatment approaches. Med J Aust 1982; 1: 160–164.

Gibson T, Harkness J, Blackgrave P et al. Controlled comparison of short-wave diathermy treatment with osteopathic treatment in non-specific low back pain. Lancet 1985; i: 1258–1261.

Glover JR, Morris JG, Khosla T. Back pain: a randomized trial of rotational manipulation to the trunk. Br J Ind Med 1974; 31: 59–64.

Godfrey CM, Morgan PP, Schatzker J. A randomized trial of manipulation for low back pain in a medical setting. Spine 1984; 9: 301–304.

Hadler NM, Curtis P, Gillings DB, Stinnett S. A benefit of spinal manipulation as adjunctive therapy for acute low-back pain: a stratified control trial. Spine 1987; 12: 702–706.

Hawk CK, Long C, Azad A. Chiropractic care for chronic pelvic pain: a prospective single-group intervention study. J Manipulative Physiol Ther 1997; 20: 73–79.

Herzog W, Conway PJ, Willcox BJ. Effects of different treatment modalities on gait symmetry and clinical measures for sacroiliac joint patients. J Manipulative Physiol Ther 1991; 14: 104–109.

Hoehler FK, Tobis JS, Buerger AA. Spinal manipulation for low back pain. JAMA 1981; 245: 1835–1838.

Howe DH, Newcombe RG, Wade MT. Manipulation of the cervical spine. A pilot study. J R Coll Gen Pract 1983; 574–579.

Hoyt WH, Shaffer F, Bard DA et al. Osteopathic manipulation in the treatment of muscle-contraction headache. J Am Osteopath Assoc 1979; 78: 322–325.

Hurwitz EL, Aker PD, Adams AH et al. Manipulation and mobilization of the cervical spine. A systematic review of the literature. Spine 1996; 21: 1746–1759, Discussion 1759–1760.

Hviid CS. A comparison of the effect of chiropractic treatment on respiratory function in patients with respiratory distress symptoms and patients without. Bull Eur Chiropractic Union 1978; 26: 17–34.

Jensen OK, Nielsen FF, Vosmar L. An open study comparing manual therapy with the use of cold packs in the treatment of post-traumatic headache. Cephalalgia 1990; 10: 241–250.

Jordan A, Bendix T, Nielsen H et al. Intensive training, physiotherapy, or manipulation for patients with chronic neck pain. A prospective single-blind randomized clinical trial. Spine 1998; 23: 311–319.

Kinalski R, Kuwik W, Pietrzak. The comparison of the results of manual therapy versus physiotherapy methods used in treatment of patients with low back syndromes. Manual Med 1989; 4: 44–46.

Koes BW, Bouter LM, Mameren HV et al. A randomized clinical trial of manual therapy and physiotherapy for persistent back and neck complaints: subgroup analysis and relationship between outcome measures. J Manipulative Physiol Ther 1993; 16: 211–219.

Koes BW, Bouter LM, Van Mameren H et al. The effectiveness of manual therapy, physiotherapy, and treatment by the general practitioner for nonspecific back and neck complaints: a randomized clinical trial. Spine 1992; 17: 28–35.

Kokjohn K Schmid DM, Triano JJ, Brennan PC. The effect of spinal manipulation on pain and prostaglandin levels in women with primary dysmenorrhea. J Manipulative Physiol Ther 1992; 15:79–285.

MacDonald RS, Bell CMJ. An open controlled assessment of osteopathic manipulation in nonspecific low back pain. Spine 1990; 15: 364–370.

Mathews JA, Mills SB, Jenkins VM et al. Back pain and sciatica: controlled trials of manipulation, traction, sclerosant and epidural injections. Br J Rheumatol 1987; 26: 416–423.

Mckinney LA. Early mobilisation and outcome in acute sprains of the neck. BMJ 1989; 299: 1006–1008.

Meade TW, Dyer S, Browne W, Frank AO. Randomised comparison of chiropractic and outpatient management for low back pain: results from extended follow up. BMJ 1995; 311: 349–351.

Meade TW, Dyer S, Browne W et al. Low back pain of mechanical origin: randomized comparison of chiropractic and hospital outpatient treatment. BMJ 1990; 300: 1431–1437.

Mealy K, Brennan H, Fenelon GC. Early mobilisation and outcome in acute sprains of the neck. BMJ (Clin Res Edn) 1986; 292: 656–657.

Nelson CF, Bronfort G, Evans R et al. The efficacy of spinal manipulation, amitriptyline and the combination of both therapies for the prophylaxis of migraine headache. J Manipulative Physiol Ther 1998; 21: 511–519.

Nilsson N. A randomized controlled trial of the effect of spinal manipulation in the treatment of cervicogenic headache. J Manipulative Physiol Ther 1995; 18: 435–440.

Nilsson N, Christensen HW, Hartvigsen J. The effect of spinal manipulation in the treatment of cervicogenic headache. J Manipulative Physiol Ther 1997; 20: 326–330.

Nordemar R, Thorner C. Treatment of acute cervical pain: a comparative group study. Pain 1981; 10: 93–101.

Nwuga VCB. Relative therapeutic efficacy of vertebral manipulation and conventional treatment in back pain management. Am J Phys Med 1982; 2: 143–146.

Nyiendo J, Haas M, Goodwin P. Patient characteristics, practice activities, and one-month outcomes for chronic, recurrent low-back pain treated by chiropractors and family medicine physicians: a practice-based feasibility study. J Manipulative Physiol Ther 2000; 23: 239–245.

Parker GB, Tupling H, Pryor DS. A controlled trial of cervical manipulation for migraine. Aust N Z Med 1978; 8: 589–593.

Pope MH, Phillips RB, Haugh LD et al. A prospective randomized three-week trial of spinal manipulation, transcutaneous muscle stimulation, massage and corset in the treatment of subacute low back pain. Spine 1994; 19: 2571–2577.

Postacchini F, Facchini M, Palieri P. Efficacy of various forms of conservative treatment in low back pain. A comparative study. Neuro-Orthopedics 1988; 6: 28–35.

Rasmussen GG. Manipulation in treatment of low back pain. A randomized clinical trial. Manual Med 1979; 1: 8–10.

Rupert RL, Wagnon R, Thompson P, Ezzeldin MT. Chiropractic adjustments: results of a controlled clinical trial in Egypt. ICA Int Rev Chiropractic 1985; Winter: 58–60.

Sanders GE, Reinert O, Tepe R, Maloney P. Chiropractic adjustive manipulation on subjects with acute low back pain: visual analog pain scores and plasma B-endorphin levels. J Manipulative Physiol Ther 1990; 13: 391–395.

Shekelle PG, Adams AH, Chassin MR et al. Spinal manipulation for low-back pain. Ann Intern Med 1992; 117: 590–598.

Siehl D, Olson DR, Ross HE , Rockwood EE. Manipulation of the lumbar spine with the patient under general anesthesia: an evaluation by EMG and clinical neurologic examination of its use for lumbar nerve root compression. J Am Osteopath Assoc 1971; 70: 433–441.

Sims-Williams H, Jayson M, Young SM, Baddeley H. Controlled trial of mobilization and manipulation for patients with low back pain in general practice. BMJ 1978; ii: 1338–1340.

Sims-Williams H, Jayson MIV, Young SMS et al. Controlled trial of mobilization and manipulation for low back pain: hospital patients. BMJ 1979; ii: 1318–1320.

Skargren EI, Oberg B, Carlsson P, Gade M. Cost and effectiveness analysis of chiropractic and physiotherapy treatment for low-back and neck pain: 6 month follow-up. Spine 1997; 22: 2167–2177.

Skargren EI, Carlsson PG, Oberg BE. One-year follow-up comparison of the cost and effectiveness of chiropractic and physiotherapy as primary management for back pain. Spine 1998; 23: 1875–1884.

Sloop PR, Smith DS, Goldenberg EVA, Dore C. Manipulation for chronic neck pain. A double-blind controlled study. Spine 1982; 7: 532–535.

Triano JJ, McGregor M, Hondras MA, Brennan PC. Manipulative therapy versus education programs in chronic low back pain. Spine 1995; 20: 948–955.

Vernon HT, Dhami MS, Howley TP, Annett R. Spinal manipulation and beta-endorphin: a controlled study of the effect of a spinal manipulation on plasma beta-endorphin levels in normal males. J Manipulative Physiol Ther 1986; 9: 115–123.

Vernon HT, Peter A, Burns S et al. Pressure pain threshold evaluation of the effect of spinal manipulation in the treatment of chronic neck pain: a pilot study. J Manipulative Physiol Ther 1990; 13: 13–16.

Waagen GN, Haldeman S, Cook G et al. Short term trial of chiropractic adjustments for the relief of chronic low-back pain. Manual Med 1986; 2: 63–67.

Zylbergold RS, Piper MC. Lumbar disc disease: comparative analysis of physical therapy treatments. Arch Phys Med Rehabil 1981; 62: 176–179.

25

Chiropractic techniques in the care of the geriatric patient

Robert Cooperstein and Lisa Killinger

When I was a student, there seemed to be developing in the profession a feeling of increased reluctance to use manipulative treatment in the elderly because of the physiologic changes in their spine. Reference was made to the presence of osteoporosis, making the bone structure easy to fracture. Comments were made to the effect that by treating with manipulation one might break off the spurs of the ever-present degenerative arthritis and that the subsequent reactions of the body would make the patient feel worse. Various other reasons were advanced for not employing manipulative techniques in the elderly and the critically ill.

Unfortunately, this tendency has increased since I graduated. Such an attitude is deleterious to the profession and results in the shortchanging of our patients. They are deprived of the full benefit of our education and skills in the treatment of their problems and illnesses. [Nonetheless] All treatment is dose-related. The type and amount of treatment depend on the problems your evaluation elicits; the anatomic, physiologic, and psychologic condition of the patient; and your own skill in the use of a variety of techniques.[1]

D. Dodson

Introduction

Dodson poignantly told of his experience (or lack thereof) in providing care for older patients in his osteopathic education and practice experience. Although by 'manipulation' he sometimes refers to low force manual interventions, not the thrusting techniques chiropractors often use, they experience many of the same care issues as osteopathic providers. The essence of the message above is that we must make a full range of chiropractic care available, albeit cautiously, to the ageing population. The elderly patient is most deserving of, and perhaps most in need of, alternatives to the traditional pharmaceutical and surgical options offered through allopathic providers.

Most of the elderly patients seen in chiropractic practice are in the 'young old' category, less than 75 years old. The National Board of Chiropractic Examiners Job Analysis of Chiropractic 2000 states that approximately one-third of chiropractic patients are aged 50 and older. In this category, 21% of chiropractic patients are 51–64 years of age, while nearly 13% are over 65. They tend to be ambulatory and are fit enough to perform successfully most of the activities of daily living (ADLs) without assistance. There are many issues to consider when providing care for the older patient, with the safety and comfort of the patient of special significance. The chiropractor's choice of adjusting techniques and ancillary procedures should be made with due consideration of the entire clinical picture. Each geriatric patient brings to the chiropractic practice a lengthy health history and frequently a complex health status. Thus, geriatric patients afford the chiropractor numerous and special challenges and opportunities.

There are two relevant trends in today's health-care setting that should be noted at the outset: the rapid growth of the geriatric population, and the increase in society's use of complementary and alternative medicine (CAM) health-care services.[2] Chiropractic, with a century-plus tradition of providing effective, conservative heath care, is particularly well positioned to take on an important role in providing health care to the rapidly growing numbers of older patients.

Why geriatric technique?

In principle, chiropractic technique includes both examination and adjustment procedures, we have chosen to emphasize the latter in preparing this chapter. This is because the examination of the geriatric patient does not differ nearly as much in the protocols that would be used in a younger person as do the treatment protocols, where there are many age-related variables to take into account. That stated, the PARTS acronym, described by Bergmann and Larson,[3] is quite applicable to the geriatric setting; patient assessment includes:

- Pain/tenderness in articular structures and soft tissues
- Asymmetry of joint alignment and motion
- Range of motion findings
- Tissue tone, texture and temperature abnormalities
- Special testing procedures that are mostly unique within specific technique systems.

There is no hard and fast dividing line that separates chiropractic technique for the geriatric patient from chiropractic technique for any other patient, although there are several considerations that deserve special emphasis in this select patient population. There are, after all, special considerations in managing typical geriatric cases: greater difficulty in obtaining a history and a greater amount of history that needs to be obtained, the likelihood of multiple pathologies confounding the differential diagnosis, the complications that accrue to prescriptions for possibly numerous pharmaceutical agents, and age-specific contraindications for certain types of chiropractic adjustive care.[4]

Even the notion of age-specific care requires qualification,[5] since a patient who is geriatric in the chronological sense may be in better musculoskeletal and general health than many younger patients, and thus amenable to being treated no differently from them.[6] Rollis argues that geriatric chiropractic care is not fundamentally different, but adds, 'it has more depth; more is required of the chiropractor'.[7] Although it is certainly true that adjustive techniques need to be modified to some extent for geriatric patients, the uniqueness of this patient population has as much to do with 'expectations and practicality',[6] establishing an appropriate level of expectations,[8] as it does with physical matters. A 10% improvement that a younger patient would judge a treatment failure could mark a dramatic improvement in the life of an elderly patient trying to avoid a wheelchair or confinement to a nursing facility.[6]

The importance of gaining information about the patient through a competently administered health history and examination has been addressed in previous chapters of this text. Once such health status information has been gathered, the chiropractor will need to make the important decisions about the core of chiropractic practice, the adjustive strategy. Beyond that, it will be necessary to design an overall management plan that effectively addresses the physical needs of the patient, while considering financial, ethical and practical issues. One should avoid the introduction of counterproductive psychological attitudes through the indiscriminate use of negative suggestive terms ('degeneration', 'bone loss', etc.[9]).

Safety of chiropractic adjustive care in the geriatric setting

There are very few age-stratified data on the frequency of adverse reactions to spinal manipulation. In a Norwegian study, the incidence of side-effects to spinal manipulative therapy (including thrusting adjustive methods) was 49% among patients 47–64 years of age and 60% among those 27–46 years of age.[10] LeBoeuf-Yde, on the other hand, failed to find a comparable age association in a similar Swedish study.[11] Given that the Norwegian study involved 1058 patients, whereas the Swedish study only involved 625 patients, it is reasonable to conclude that older patients may not suffer more adverse responses to spinal manipulation than younger patients, and may even suffer fewer. Were that to be the case, one would not be able to tell from these studies whether the comparative safety of chiropractic adjustive care in the elderly results from a patient-related variable (e.g. perhaps their greater joint stiffness protects them from injuries related to poorly directed or excessive force), a doctor-related variable (perhaps their greater reliance on low force techniques and more prudence), or both patient and doctor-related variables. In either case, these are encouraging numbers that should dispel the most obvious type of scepticism concerning the value of chiropractic adjustive care in this select population.

Clinical value of geriatric chiropractic care

Most clinical studies on chiropractic adjustive care exclude by design geriatric patients, so the evidence base by necessity is heavily based on personal experience, supplemented by the small amount of practice-based research that exists. Hawk et al.[12] gathered data from 96 practices in 32 states and two Canadian provinces on 805 eligible patients aged 55 and over during a 12 week study period, in 1997–1998. Since practice-based research is conducted using volunteers, the characteristics of the care rendered and the results obtained cannot be extrapolated to the population of chiropractors and their patients in general. Nonetheless, it is certainly encouraging that in this study, in which 72.3% of the patients had pain as their chief complaint, improvement was noted in the Pain Disability Index instrument, and patient use of pain medications declined. The most commonly used adjustive method was Activator at 56.6%, followed by Diversified at 23.5%. This choice of adjustive methods should not be considered representative of chiropractic practice patterns in general, since the Activator technique organization was the only one of six organizations contacted that elected to participate and recruit doctors for the study. Their efforts in that regard appear to date as far back as 1991, when what amounts to a feasibility study and case report was published.[13]

Rupert et al.[14,15] investigated the impact of maintenance care (services intended to prevent illness and promote health) on chiropractic patients in people aged 65 and above, who had received at least four visits per year for at least 5 years. These patients mostly received a variety of ancillary procedures in addition to manipulation. The most frequently applied chiropractic adjustive technique was Diversified, which probably included high-velocity, low-amplitude (HVLA) thrusting, at 70.4%, followed by Activator at 28.3%, Thompson technique at 21.9%, and Nimmo/other soft-tissue techniques at 20.6%. Most of the patients (68.2%) were advised to perform exercises. Compared with individuals over 65 not receiving chiropractic maintenance care, the patients in this study tended to exhibit an improved health status. The authors suggest caution in interpreting the study for a number of reasons: many of the contacted chiropractors declined to participate in the study, the patients differed in some respects from the population of geriatrics in general, the study design does not allow a causal relation to be inferred between maintenance care and improved health status; and various other problems arose in the conduct of the study.[14,15]

General goals of care in the geriatric setting

Various perceived patient care goals exist in chiropractic, each of which should be acknowledged in constructing a care plan. It is important that the goals be realistic.[16] These might include:

- promoting wellness, actual and potential[17,18]
- removing nerve interference (i.e. neurological dysfunction) through adjusting subluxations
- reducing pain, and thereby the dangers of drug dependence and the iatrogenic complications of drug therapy[19]
- increasing joint mobility
- compressing morbidity[17]
- increasing the patient's overall quality of life
- maintaining a positive patient attitude[8]
- avoiding surgery.[5]

Most clinicians find that among patients in general, acute conditions respond more favourably that chronic conditions. Deshpande et al.[20] found as much in their experience rehabilitating acute and subacute geriatric patients for a variety of ailments, including stroke and hip fractures. This observation naturally should bear on the expectations imparted to the geriatric patient.

Only a few adjustive procedures are illustrated in this chapter. The illustrations and descriptions available in many of the chiropractic profession's excellent chiropractic technique textbooks, such as Chiropractic Technique by Bergmann et al.,[21] are more detailed and very useful. These techniques may be safely applied in the geriatric setting in accordance with some of the stipulations and modifications in this chapter. The reader should consult Grieve's works[22,23] and Hammer's work,[24] especially for their excellent illustrations and descriptions of mobilization and soft-tissue methods, of particular relevance in a geriatric context. Since contraindications are condition specific, not age specific, existing guidelines for the population at large, such as are found in the Guidelines for Chiropractic Quality Assurance and Practice Parameters,[25] are entirely amenable to being extrapolated to geriatric patients. Since there is very little literature available on the manual treatment of geriatric patients, the authors by necessity draw heavily on their own experience.

Geriatric chiropractic technique: relevant terminology

Before going further, some of the relevant terminology is discussed, in order to avoid misinterpretation.

Manipulation and mobilization

The biggest problem concerns the term manipulation. In some fields, such as osteopathy, 'manipulation' may refer to a variety of treatment methods by hand: massage, ischaemic compression, low-force joint movements, vigorous thrusting, reflex techniques, etc. Chiropractors generally (but not always) use 'manipulation' to refer to an HVLA thrust, of the type intended to produce cavitation. Obviously, in dealing with a geriatric population, one would not want to be misunderstood while recommending or warning against the use of manipulation: it could make the difference between assisting the patient and breaking a bone. 'Mobilization', as used in this chapter, refers to the application of low forces to bones, joints and other soft tissues so as to increase joint range of motion, perhaps through stretching soft tissues, reducing the severity of adhesions or some combination thereof. 'By taking the joint to its barrier and repetitively moving along or beside it, it is thought that the barrier will be encouraged to recede'.[3] Although some believe that several types of mobilization include what is defined here as manipulation (high-velocity thrusting), for the sake of clarity, the term is not used in that way herein. As an example, much (but not all) of what Nwuga[26] calls 'manipulation' is actually about mobilization (as used in chiropractic terminology), a distinction that has at times been neglected by some who cite his work. In yet another example, Dodson's excellent article entitled Manipulative therapy for the geriatric patient[1] is not about high velocity, low amplitude thrusting at all; rather, it describes manual treatment with low-force methods.

Subluxation and adjustment

Much ink has been spilled defining terms such as 'adjustment' and 'subluxation', much of it having to do with the specificity of the target of intervention, and the examination or treatment methods used. However, many of the distinctions and refinements that some have brought to bear on these terms seem less relevant in a geriatric patient population. In this chapter, the term 'adjustment' is used to refer to the chiropractic armamentarium of treatment methods, mostly but not exclusively manual, aimed at improving neuromusculoskeletal structure and function. These methods include:

- application of forces using both short and long leverage;
- addressing bone position, joint motion, or both
- addressing conditions in which neuropathology ('nerve interference') is obvious and/or prominent, and others in which it is not

- using manual, mechanically assisted and instrument-assisted adjustive procedures[27]
- addressing segmental and regional targets of intervention[28]
- using high (e.g. HVLA)[27] and low-force manoeuvres.[27]

'Subluxations' in the present usage are abnormal states of components of the neuromusculoskeletal system, which are addressed by the adjustive methods described. Whatever the benefits of being very specific about what one is treating in a young population, in geriatrics, the entity under care is frequently if not usually a regional matter, or a kinetic chain of events that must be addressed globally, as a syndrome with a whole web of connections. For an opposing view, emphasizing the traditional importance of specificity in this select population, see Markham[29] and Clemen.[30]

Technique or technique?

Another term prone to much misinterpretation is 'technique', as in 'chiropractic technique'. First, although the term should rightfully include both chiropractic examination and adjustive procedures, it is frequently understood to pertain largely or exclusively to treatment alone. It is in that sense that this chapter understands the term. Secondly, there is a big difference between 'technique' with a lower case t, and 'Technique' with an upper case t.[31] During its century-plus of existence, chiropractors have devised hundreds of different named Technique systems, such as the Gonstead Technique, the Palmer Method and Sacro-occipital Technique. Most of these brand-name (or proprietary) techniques claim to be superior to the others, and to treat a great variety of (if not all) health problems without needing treatment methods that would be found in other technique systems. There is also a huge assortment of chiropractic adjustive methods whose rationale and mechanical style belong to the chiropractic common domain, and the totality of these generic treatment methods is what is meant by 'chiropractic technique' in this chapter. Therefore, the reader should not expect to find in this chapter any ringing endorsements for any particular system Techniques for geriatric patients in general or for specific conditions, although several types of technique manoeuvre are recommended.

Geriatric chiropractic technique: general considerations

Sound clinical judgement should provide patient benefit while avoiding stroke, postadjustment discomfort, spinal or rib fractures, intervertebral disc injury, and soft-tissue injuries (strains, sprains and bruising). Before exploring specific adjustive strategies, a few global observations are offered bearing on geriatric chiropractic care, including but not limited to the question of patient safety. The final section of this chapter considers the particulars of safely adjusting the geriatric population.

Level of force

The most obvious consideration in addressing the geriatric patient is determining the safe and effective level of force that can be used. Depending on the body structure that is contacted, the issue may be less one of force and more one of pressure. That is, a relatively ample force may be nonetheless safely used if it is applied to a broad enough area, even more safely than a lesser force applied to a small area. The 40.9 N generated by one kind of hand-held percussive instrument,[32] therefore, may be more threatening to an osteoporotic transverse process than the 117.6 N generated by a hand contact[32] spread out over a broad area, depending on the doctor's style.

Leverage must also be taken into account, in that a bony contact that is locally safe may produce a substantial mechanical impact on distant tissues. Although the authors are not aware of case reports, one could well imagine how achieving preadjustive tension through leverage in the knee area could fracture the neck of the femur, or how pressure on a rib could produce a fracture in a quite removed location. Fernandez remarks, however exaggeratedly: 'The doctor must pay particular attention not to put pressure upon the rib heads, because they surely will break. Any doctor who has heard the thud of a rib breaking knows about this'.[33] One doctor, while recommending reducing adjustive force in osteoporotic patients, comments: 'You, the doctor, understand that the vertebral subluxation complex is much more life threatening than a cracked rib sustained in the attempt to correct it ... [but] a patient won't stay with a doctor who increases his or her symptoms'.[30] The reader may draw his or her own conclusions from these comments, but reducing pressure and respecting leverage mini-

mizes the risk of fractures. Specific thrusts directed at very focal locations may not be as safe as more regional targets of intervention.

Spinal degenerative changes

During ageing, the spine undergoes degenerative changes that are likely to contribute to the overall clinical picture, including back pain. There may be predisposing curvature in the frontal plane (scoliosis) and also alterations in the sagittal curves, such as upper dorsal hyperkyphosis. The altered stress associated with abnormal weight bearing results in degenerative disc disease and osteophytosis. In the absence of any definitive evidence that such changes are reversible (see, however, refs 34–37 and assuming that a geriatric patient population is among the least likely to show reversibility of degenerative changes, the goal of care must remain largely palliative. If chiropractic adjustive care is not likely to reverse arthritic changes, it may at least slow progression. This is especially likely given that experimental joint immobilization hastens arthritic development,[38–40] lending credence to the hypothesis that increased flexibility through chiropractic adjustive care would retard osteoarthritic changes. Conversely, such changes may have a stabilizing impact that protect the patient to some extent, as noted by Kirkaldy-Willis in his well-known three-phase model of spinal degenerative disease: the stages of dysfunction, instability and stabilization.[41,42] Age-related degenerative changes reduce the risk of disc herniation in the elderly.[43] Markham's cautionary comments should be well heeded:

> The issue of destabilizing the patient through vigorous joint manipulation is ignored. We recognize that spinal intersegmental mobility, in the elderly, with a stable spine, there may be a little movement but there is often little pain and discomfort. [sic] When a doctor undertakes to remobilize the joints they need to recognize and inform the patient of the possibility of increased symptomatology for a period of time as the adjustments may create instability. Such instability will usually create more pain and may not be quickly abated.[29]

Posture and the trophostatic syndrome[9]

There is a long tradition in chiropractic, most closely associated with Carver[44] in the early days, of emphasizing the patient's posture as an important or even primary target of care. Rosenthal describes this as the structural approach,[45] an approach that remains well represented today.[46–48] In a similar vein, Sandoz describes a 'trophostatic syndrome'[9] characterized by an increase in the sagittal lordoses and kyphoses, associated with forward head syndrome and a series of local degenerative changes. He emphasizes that a 'global disturbance in spinal mechanics will first have regional static consequences; these in turn will modify the local mechanical condition and favour or hasten the development of local degenerative pathology'.[9] It follows that intervention should not be limited to the local hot spots, even under the assumption that they are the primary pain generators, but rather should address the global circumstances that favour their development.

Abnormal changes in the sagittal curves are codetermining and, according to Sandoz,[9] the dorsal hyperkyphosis is the primary offender, resulting in the cervical and lumbar hyperlordoses. Therefore, adjustive care emphasizes an attempt to reduce the dorsal hyperkyphosis, which has a remote impact upon the range of motion of the lumbar and cervical spines; like Sandoz, the authors have seen satisfying increases in cervical range of motion following some degree of upper dorsal flattening. Simply lying on the floor at home in the supine position (with a measured pillow under the head, if the patient cannot tolerate very much cervical extension) amounts to an exercise for many geriatric patients, and is buttressed in the chiropractic office by the doctor applying sustained and diffuse pressure to the dorsal spine of the prone patient.

As every chiropractor knows, improving a patient's posture is not as simple as suggesting that he or she 'stand up straighter'. Patients attempting to do so, prior to having received adjustive and rehabilitative care, assume the most awkward postures imaginable, constrained by musculotendinous and ligamentous contracture and joint rigidity. Once care has been initiated and initial benefits have been obtained, the patient is at the very least given a postural choice. Patients who want to walk around as though they bear the weight of the world on their shoulders will, but the chiropractor can at least provide other options. Although the resumption of poor posture is also possible, the patient may elect to assume a more normal carriage, a choice at first conscious but ultimately unconscious, as it becomes habitual.

Soft-tissue contractures

Understanding the special needs of the geriatric patient, from a manual technique point of view, is all about acknowledging that soft tissues have degenerated and undergone shortening. It follows that they will need to be stretched. Increasing the elasticity of soft tissues increases the pain-free range of motion of joints, allows strengthening exercises in ranges not formerly accessible, reduces the likelihood that such tissues will fail (tear) when subjected to the stresses of daily life, increases the safety of manual treatments (including manipulation), improves the likelihood of postural improvement and increases access to the normal activities of daily life.[49] Indeed, as so many have stated, in movement there is life, and especially in a geriatric population.

It is sometimes useful, prior to the application of manipulative and other adjustive procedures, to preposition (prestress) the patient so as to stretch abnormally contractured tissues. Troyanovich, at the year 2000's Research Agenda Conference,[50] attributed this seminal methodology to Dr Winterstein's 'stress reversal analysis/adjusting' of the 1960s at the National Chiropractic College. In the sagittal plane, this generally amounts to reducing the degree of exaggerated thoracic kyphosis, and (to patient tolerance, given the difficulty many geriatrics have with spinal extension) prestressing hypolordotic cervical and lumbar curves into extension prior to force application. In the frontal plane, this involves prestressing scoliotic curves into an opposite configuration (see Figure 25.1). For example, a person with left lateral curvature in the thoracic spine would be moved towards the right side of the table, and have the shoulder and pelvic girdles deflected towards the left side of the table, placing the spine in a doctor-created right lateral curvature during the application of prone adjustive procedures.

Of course, one should not realistically expect a spine which has undergone decades of bony remodelling into abnormal curves and curvatures to be fully 'corrected' by such manoeuvres, but these methods should improve the outcome of manual treatment procedures, thanks to having stretching contractured tissues.[17] Historically, chiropractors have tended to view abnormal alterations in anteroposterior or lateral disc angles as a matter of 'open wedges', whereas it is clear, especially in a geriatric population that has undergone spinal degenerative changes, that it is more a question of 'closed

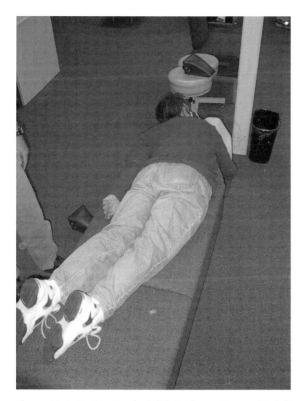

Figure 25.1 Prestressing for left lateral curvature and/or left lateral flexion restriction.

wedges' on the concave side of curvatures. After all, spinal curvature leads to decreased, not increased intervertebral disc height. The goal of care is thus to open closed wedges, not to close open wedges. Prepositioning the patient in an appropriate manner more directly impacts spinal curvature than 'torquing down the spine to close the wedge', as traditionalists might put it.

Flexibility and strength training

Although it is beyond the purview of this chapter, the chiropractic case management of the geriatric patient should include education in basic mechanics: how best to sit, walk, sleep and exercise.[51,52] Although dramatic postural changes are not expected, even incremental improvements can effect significant changes in the intensity of symptoms, apart from slowing the progression of degenerative changes. For any given level of musculoskeletal degeneration, more flexibility is usually preferred to less (barring instability), in addition to potentiating the value of specific interventions.

One must always keep in mind, as obvious as the point may seem, that what determines posture is the net additive result of a multitude of vectors, including both muscle tone and soft tissue (i.e. ligamentous) resistance, in addition to gravitational forces. The key to postural improvement may be more a question of increasing the elasticity of soft tissues than bulking up muscles and, at the least, muscles are more safely strengthened when they are exercised against diminished soft-tissue resistance. Certainly, flexibility and strengthening are additive in their benefits.[53] It is also true that a general exercise programme may increase the joint range of motion in the elderly.[54,55]

Although it will be necessary at some point for the elderly patient to undertake strength training, in order to secure the benefits of the adjustive care, it would be a mistake to increase strength before initiating stretching exercises, including instructions on warming up, improving agility, etc.[56] It is counterproductive, and even dangerous, to embark upon strengthening weak muscles before stretched contractured antagonistic muscles. It is also dangerous to undertake manipulative (even mobilization procedures, to a lesser extent) before having achieved some degree of greater tissue elasticity. After all, geriatric tissues may, in a word, be 'brittle'.[17] Since adhesions and scar tissue are fabricated from about the same collagen as ligaments and tendons, it is not always easy to design and introduce forces that are likely to stretch the 'bad' collagen without endangering to an unacceptable degree the 'good' collagen.

Fixation and misalignment among the elderly

Chiropractors often ascribe many of the patient's complaint to bones being out of alignment, and no doubt in some cases this is true. However, whatever the intrinsic merits of such a concept in relatively young patients, it is less applicable in an older patient population. Long-term segmental misalignment and abnormal regional spinal configurations (frontal plane lateral curvature and sagittal plane curve alterations) result in bone and soft-tissue remodelling, thus locking in the altered spinal structure. The goal of care and the prognosis, therefore, is unlikely to be restitution of normal structure; the results of chiropractic care among the elderly are subject to the 'limits of matter'.[57] Although there may be some postural improvement, the benefits of care are centred mostly around improving joint mobility, soft-tissue elasticity, nervous system functioning and vascular supply.

It follows from these considerations that the traditional chiropractic emphasis on 'specificity' (addressing a specific segment, with a specific line of drive, using short levers such as a spinous or transverse process) would benefit from reinterpretation in its application to a geriatric patient population, and perhaps other patients as well. If the neuromusculoskeletal problems of the elderly patient are largely regional (multisegmental), and if in addition the clinical substrate frequently involves kinetic chains, then the adjustive strategy should be commensurate: multisegmental (regional) in emphasis, and aimed at improved global range of motion and body posture. Apart from the direct clinical value in this approach, there is the added benefit that forces that are more broadly applied exert less focal pressure on the spinal contacts, and are thus safer in patients with osteoporosis. The Carver bridge (bilateral knife-edge) or bilateral thenar contact[21] (Figure 25.2), spanning several vertebrae is less likely to injure the patient than a single-hand contact on a spinous or transverse process, whether the doctor believes the patient to suffer from a segmental or more regional fault.

Similar considerations enter into the consideration of joint movement dysfunction. In a patient with left–right lateral bending in the cervical spine limited to 20 degrees, not at all uncommon among the elderly, there can be no question of identifying 'the' segment which is 'fixated' or 'misaligned', as though it alone, directly or indirectly, could somehow account for such a stiff neck. Subluxation among the elderly is best considered a regional condition; there may be a segmental, focal point of the pathology, but the adjustive approach is safest and most effective when regional considerations are taken into account. Whatever happens to be the most fixed and/or misaligned segment is the tip of the iceberg in such a patient, even if it were the focus of symptomatology: it is the iceberg that must be addressed.

Preadjustive tension

There are differences in manipulative approaches among chiropractic technicians. Some typically remove as much joint slack as possible prior to thrusting, whereas others do not, preferring to back off maximum preadjustive tension before adjusting. Whatever the merits of the two approaches in general, in a geriatric population it is safer to achieve maximum premanipulative tension, as this is the easiest way to assess the type and amount of resistance likely to be attained. In other words, it would not be prudent to thrust from a distance, as it were, since this could result in a sprain or strain injury to the patient. Sandoz speaks of a rule amounting to thrusting in the 'painless and free direction'.[9] Again, whatever the merits of such a rule in a general population, in a geriatric population, this should be observed and exceptions should be weighed carefully.

In a geriatric patient, one must take into account that a hard joint end-feel is obtained relatively quickly as preadjustive pressure is applied. The palpable 'fixation' at this point is likely to be due to osteophytic and other degenerative joint changes, compared with the fixation in a younger patient that is more likely to be due to muscle hypertonus or swelling. Therefore, it would be prudent not to try to overcome this 'bony fixation' forcibly in an elderly patient, as restriction in joint movement in this case is determined by the 'limits of matter', once again as the Palmers may have put it.[57]

In applying either supine or prone manipulative or mobilization procedures, the patient is prepositioned taking into account any lateral flexion restrictions that they may have. If bending the seated patient to the left and the right reveals, for example, that several segments in the mid-thoracic spine do not participate in left lateral bending, the patient would be prestressed on the table as indicated in Figure 25.1. If the patient happened to be 'saucered' (i.e. hypokyphotic) in this region, the prestressing would be identical, but the procedure would be anterior thoracic manipulation or mobilization, as seen in Figure 25.3.

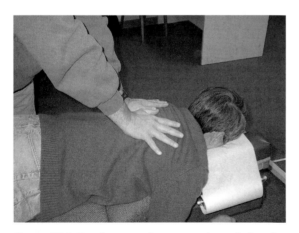

Figure 25.2 Broad contact increases safety of thrusting manoeuvres.

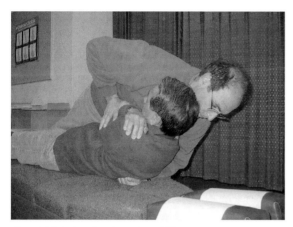

Figure 25.3 Anterior thoracic mobilization.

Geriatric chiropractic technique: regional considerations

Neck–shoulder–scapula complex

The neck–shoulder–scapula complex is an ideal example of what was described above as a kinetic chain, a set of regional connections that may give rise to related complaints. Nothing prevents a neck problem from arising in a patient with normal shoulder function, or a shoulder problem in a patient without a cervical problem, but the anatomical relations of muscles such as the trapezii, scalenes, sternocleidomastoids and levator scapuli often result in associated dysfunction. Although this is true for patients in general, it is particularly common among geriatric patients[58,59] because age-related changes tend to result in an anterior carriage of the head and neck in relation to the rib cage ['forward head syndrome' in medicine or 'anterior weight bearing'[60] in chiropractic], with round shoulders.[61] Menopausal females are at the most risk,[62] but men often come in with this problem. Typical complaints include cervicogenic headache; neck pain, shoulder and interscapular pain; tingling, pain and sometimes numbness in the arms; and difficulty working with the arms raised.

Wyke adds that the ageing cervical spine contributes to reflexogenic alterations in posture, balance and gait through the agency of cervical mechanoreceptors, which are functionally more important than the vestibular apparatus in humans.[63] Thoracic outlet syndrome (usually related to pectoralis minor tightness) is a common accompaniment, as is scapulocostal syndrome (restriction of scapular movements). The patient is invariably aware of the neck stiffness and

pain, but very frequently has failed to note the gradual loss of range of motion of the arm(s), especially abduction, and is quite surprised to have this limitation demonstrated immediately after the history of the chief complaint is taken. The shoulder range of motion into abduction dramatically improves if the upper thoracic hyperkyphosis is flattened to some extent, because the scapula then lies in a more vertical plane.

Neck complaints are unlikely to improve much until the shoulder and scapulocostal issues have been at least partially ameliorated. Active and passive stretching of contracted soft tissues works well in restoring scapular glide and humeral abduction. Ischaemic compression (trigger-point work) tends to provide less benefit if for no other reason than geriatric patients bruise so easily. The relationship of the cervical and shoulder–scapular problem is so intimate that humeral abduction almost serves as a marker for the level of cervical dysfunction and oft-related cervicogenic headache. Far less frequently, in the authors' experience, does addressing cervical complaints provide a direct benefit to shoulder and scapulocostal complaints.

Lumbothoracic junctional region manipulation

One of the most characteristic features of the geriatric gait is that the pelvis is carried very stiffly, with the legs swung from the hips and the torso failing to participate in ambulation. In more efficient walking, the pelvic and shudder girdles rotate around the y-axis in opposed directions, so that the angular momentum generated by swinging a leg forwards is conserved by swinging the opposite arm forwards simultaneously.[64] The geriatric patient usually exhibits a hypomobile lumbothoracic junctional area (loosely defined), rendering it difficult for the lumbothoracic spine to participate in the gait mechanism. This can be seen in the stiff, shuffling gait of an elderly person. What is particularly insidious about this, from the standpoint of addressing the patient's presenting complaints, is that the inability to walk in an efficient, comfortable manner without doubt negatively impacts on the value of whatever care is given. Proper walking is necessary for overall biomechanical and psychosocial fitness, and increases the short-and long-term benefits of adjustive care.

It is important to remember that one goal of geriatric care is to assist in maintaining the patient's independence

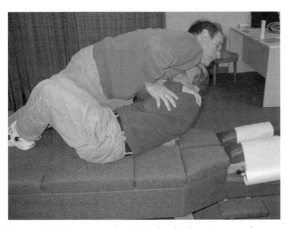

Figure 25.4 Prestressed anterior lumbothoracic procedure.

and functional status. Maintaining the integrity of gait and mobility is an essential component of functional status.

Therefore, the treatment of the geriatric patient, whatever the presenting complaints, should include increasing lumbothoracic mobility. When not contraindicated, the authors' favoured manipulative procedure is the 'anterior lumbothoracic', modelled after the well-known anterior dorsal manoeuvre but applied near or below the level of the floating ribs (see Figure 25.4). Where an HVLA thrust cannot be safely applied, the patient may be gently rocked in the same general position, while the doctor varies the application of the hand behind the spine to mobilize the spinal joints at the various levels. Patients who cannot tolerate being supported in the supine position can have their lumbothoracic articulations mobilized in the prone position, but this is not as effective, since this area is built more for flexion than extension, and therefore is best mobilized in flexion. If it must be done prone, a dorsal roll can be placed under the patient's midsection to introduce flexion, or a table that allows lumbopelvic flexion during treatment can be used.

Selected extremity considerations

Degenerative joint disease of the hip
There is a high incidence of degenerative joint disease of the hips among the elderly. The crippling effect on walking, and the huge negative impact on the patient's physical and emotional fitness, are obvious. It is therefore very important to find a way to improve hip-function. Frequently, there is no acceptable solution short of hip-replacement surgery, but mobilization procedures for the hip can prove very valuable. As

stated above, proper walking increases the short- and long-term benefits of adjustive care; hence the rationale for carefully examining the hip joints and addressing them in every geriatric case.

Our favoured manoeuvre involves placing the supine patient's lower leg between the standing doctor's legs, while the doctor leans back to apply significant traction to the hip. In this position, the doctor then uses his or her arms to circumduct the legs, in alternating directions, for a few minutes. The treatment concludes with a distractive pull, which often produces an audible release as the femoral head withdraws from the acetabulum. It can be amazing at how much motion can be introduced into the hip joint of a patient who experienced exquisite pain during Patrick–Fabere testing. This confirms that the application of traction during mobilization procedures increases the amount of motion that can be introduced for any given level of discomfort that the patient is able and willing to tolerate. (Although the present discussion concerns the hip, the same rationale can be applied to the glenohumeral, knee and elbow joints). This protocol should be applied to each hip, and not merely the symptomatic one. Not infrequently, the patient has a knee problem that precludes applying traction from the lower leg, in which case the protocol can be applied (although not as easily) through grasping the patient's thigh, just above the knee. One case report describes a situation in which a doctor produced a knee injury by applying a distractive thrust similar to what we describe above,[65] so the reader is forewarned to examine the knee carefully and ask about its current and historical status prior to applying such a thrust. Furthermore, the practitioner must be careful not to stress unduly the neck of the femur in particular, lest it be fractured.[26]

Wrist and fingers
Patients sometimes complain of often marked limitation in the range of motion of the wrist and/or finger, with associated pain. Some have signs of De Quervain's stenosing synovitis, others not. They have generally been to other providers (including chiropractors), who assured them that they had 'arthritis' and nothing could be done other than the daily administration of non-steroidal anti-inflammatory drugs (NSAIDs). This is true in some such cases, but some of these patients, if examined carefully enough, will be found to have contractures in the wrist flexors, extensors or both. This can be immediately demon-

strated to the patient by flexing and extending the wrist with the elbow held straight, then repeating the manoeuvre while the doctor applies a distractive force to the flexor or extensors by 'milking' the forearm musculature distally using the thumb and index finger: the 'arthritic' wrist or finger will now have a near-normal, pain-free range of motion.

Foot–knee–hip–pelvis kinetic chain

The vast literature on the interconnectedness of mechanical foot, knee, hip and pelvic problems need not be reviewed here, since others address it.[66] Suffice it to say that amelioration of a knee complaint may well depend on proper attention being paid to a (possibly asymptomatic) foot problem, as in the case of knee pain related to hyperpronation.[67,68] Likewise, functional and/or structural leg length inequality[69–72] can lead to sacroiliac and other complaints and dysfunction. Nothing particularly changes in this in looking at a geriatric population, except perhaps that they have the hardest time of all finding a pair of shoes that fits. Sometimes this is due to ankle oedema, but not always. Age-related hyperpronation whittles away at the shock-absorptive role of the arches of the foot during ambulation, communicating more stress to cephalad structures. Part of managing the geriatric case almost always will involve taking heed of lower extremity issues and complaints.

Geriatric chiropractic technique: adjustive approaches

Manipulation

Among the various adjustive techniques, it is manipulation that the public and many chiropractors equate with uniquely chiropractic care; and it is manipulation, the application of HVLA forces, that garners the greatest share of controversy when the topic of geriatric chiropractic technique comes up. Critics who are sceptical about the value of manipulation for patients in general become more outspoken when their concerns about the efficacy of spinal manipulation are amplified by their fear of adverse consequences. In addition to the bad press that chiropractic adjustive thrusting routinely receives from the mass media and other health professions, sadly, some chiropractic techniques have added to the furore by branding methods other than their own low-force and/or reflex methods dangerous, at least for certain regions of the axial skeleton.

All of this notwithstanding, manipulation in the geriatric setting can be very helpful and can be applied very safely, provided the clinician respects the relative and absolute contraindications that this chapter (and virtually every textbook of chiropractic) describes below. There are prone, supine and side-lying techniques, for all areas of the body, too numerous to describe beyond referencing the work of Bergmann et al.[21] The best direct evidence is that while side-effects are common, they are rarely serious;[10,11] and there is indirect evidence, based on the relative infrequency of published accounts of severe complications, that spinal manipulation is quite safe,[73] certainly in comparison with pharmacological alternatives.[74] Not one of the several dozen randomized clinical trials of spinal manipulation has ever reported an experimental subject to have been injured, which they would have been required to do had that been the case. Bergmann and Larson, in their article on manipulative care and older persons, write: 'Consideration can be given to the use of specific, high-velocity low amplitude thrust technique in the care of older patients'.[3] Winterstein comments: "Manipulative management of the geriatric patient is rarely contraindicated, but use of any adjustive procedure must be tempered by age-related factors, such as the presence of compression fracture, use of anti-coagulant medication, osteopenia and other modifiers'.[8] Fernandez suggests that the clinician applying rotational manipulation to the lumbar spine in side posture be careful not to involve the thoracic spine, so as to avoid fracturing a rib.[33] In addition side-posture low-back manipulative procedures should avoid extension (see Figure 25.5).

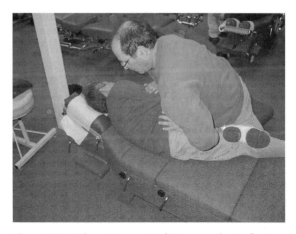

Figure 25.5 Side-posture manipulative procedure in flexion.

The safety of manipulation probably has more to do with pressure (force per unit area) than force per se. Thus, the chiropractor may favour relatively broad, diffuse contacts. Although this reduces the degree of specificity, it is consistent with the fact that geriatrics have less specific (more regional) complaints, and we are less concerned with segmental alignment and movement than with overall posture and flexibility.

Spinal extension can be quite uncomfortable for the geriatric patient, so that thrusting techniques should be applied accordingly: often, with the patient in flexion or at least neutrally positioned, and with caution not to hyperextend the spine. Chiropractors have been exceedingly creative in devising methods to thrust in flexion, including:

- pillow placed under prone patient
- segmented table arranged in flexion
- anterior thoracic adjustment, patient supine and flexed
- anterior thoracic adjustment, patient standing and slumped
- line of drive very inferior to superior, patient prone.

Through a combination of flexion and reduced force, manipulation can be rendered quite safe for the geriatric patient.

There is a variety of 'drop-assisted' thrust techniques.[75–79] J Clay Thompson pioneered the use of the drop table, an adjusting table with one or more sections capable of dropping a short distance when the doctor applies a thrust to the body section resting on that portion of the table. Although drop-table adjusting is commonly viewed as more conservative than other forms of manipulation, such as side-posture manipulation of the low back, it is not because low force is applied (although it can be). Rather, the short distance through which the table section moves when it is actuated limits the mutual displacement of body parts, compared with these other methods. Compare, for example, the potential extension of the lumbothoracic transitional area when a thrust is applied to a prone patient on a drop table, with that of a patient crouched on a knee–chest table. The authors are aware of no data confirming that drop-table adjusting provides an extra measure of safety, but it is not unreasonable to suppose this to be true. (As always, a careful clinician applying an adjustive method more capable of abuse is preferred to a less careful clinician using a 'safer' method unsafely.)

Whatever the mechanical safety factors involved, one wonders whether the impact on the patient when the table section abruptly bottoms out is capable of creating some problems. In other words, the relatively rapid deceleration of the contact body part, compared with that in other adjustive methods, may increase the force involved. Could the relatively inelastic collision of the dropping table section and its substrate produce a shock wave with hazardous effects on atherosclerotic plaque or aneurysms with potentially catastrophic consequences? Although the authors are aware of no data in regard to this, not having been able to locate even one case report of a vascular event (or a fracture, for that matter) following a drop-table thrust, it would be prudent to use lighter force when using this equipment with a geriatric patient than in a younger patient.

Some tables, with or without drop pieces (e.g. the Leander table), are designed with sections that can drop out or fall away, so that a posterior to anterior thrust on the spine does not exert excessive pressure on the ribs. The knee–chest table affords a similar benefit, provided the doctor is careful not to overextend the lumbothoracic transitional area.

Mobilization

The indications for mobilization are not really different from manipulation; it is just a question of force (although some clinicians feel that only high-velocity thrusting can reduce intra-articular adhesions). There is some evidence that manipulation obtains a better outcome than mobilization,[80] but also evidence that the two methods achieve equal outcomes.[81,82] Since geriatric patients and patients with severe age-related complaints are often excluded from clinical studies, it is unclear which approach is likely to achieve the best outcome in this select population. As is always the case with insufficient data, this means that one would expect greater variation in practice patterns as clinicians base more of their decisions on their own clinical experience. Common sense dictates that whatever a clinician's preference between the two in a younger population, the relative usage of mobilization should increase in a geriatric population. There is more potential harm inherent in a manipulative thrust that is too extreme for an elderly patient, than in using a mobilization procedure where a thrusting technique would have been well tolerated.

Mechanized equipment for mobilization

The Leander table is a segmented table with a motor-driven caudal section capable of cycling back and forth through flexion and extension at different stroke amplitudes and rates of movement. The caudal section is also capable of lateral flexion. The doctor's hands are at work at all times on the patient, serving as fulcrums adding to or subtracting from the motion effected by the table mechanism. Although this may be thought of as intermittent motorized traction, it may be more appropriate to regard the procedure as mechanically assisted, manual mobilization, in that it is used to take the patient's joints through an ample range of passive motion, in multiple and varying degrees of freedom, mostly in observance of the physiological coupling patterns described for those joints.

Stair-stepping and figure-of-8 manoeuvres

These procedures, borrowed from Sacro-occipital Technique,[83,84] involve lifting the head and neck of the supine patient from the table, and introducing a relatively light compressive force that winds up gliding the cervical joints. In effect, the head lifts from the table while the cervical vertebrae glide anteriorly. At any point in the process where restriction manifests, the doctor takes the head and neck through a figure-of-8 type of motion, after which it is generally found that the movement of the head and neck is improved.

Flexion manoeuvres

As stated above in the discussion of manipulation, extension is often eschewed; degenerative spinal changes often result in the geriatric patient being unable to extend very well, whether out of central canal stenosis or posterior joint arthrosis. That means that mobilization procedures are frequently done in flexion. This might entail something as obvious as a pillow under the supine patient's head while the neck is being mobilized, or a pillow under the chest while the prone patient's posterior thoracic joints are being mobilized. Many chiropractic tables are segmented so as to allow flexion of the prone patient, and the judicious use of pillows always helps if the table is not very versatile.

Anterior thoracic mobilization

Chiropractic clinicians are mostly familiar with the anterior thoracic manipulative procedure. This same procedure, minus the thrust, is very useful for gently mobilizing the lumbar and thoracic joints. The supine, sitting patient is lowered to the table, as though the spine were being unrolled on to the table (see Figure 25.3). In the meantime, the doctor's hand

underneath the patient sequentially establishes the segment that is being mobilized, starting with the most caudal segment of the region being treated. The doctor rocks each contacted segment in a variety of directions, back and forth, to the patient's tolerance. Patients with severe low-back pain cannot be held for very long in the supine position, and some patients are too heavy (depending on the doctor's size) to be controlled for long in this manner, but for most patients this is an easily executed and well tolerated treatment procedure.

Blocking

Although other classifications are possible, 'blocking' – in which the prone or supine patient lies across a pair of padded wedges in various combinations and orientations[84] – may be considered a form of mobilization, akin to some forms of traction. This allows gravitational forces to produce gentle, sustained joint mobilizations, in directions that are intended to effect improvements in posture and range of motion. It is possible to apply manual forces to the patient on the blocks, in which case the blocking procedure would have to be classified as mechanically assisted mobilization. The chiropractic clinicians most likely to use blocking procedures, Sacro-occipital Technique practitioners,[84] believe that these procedures may remotely impact upon cranial structures and the circulation of the cerebrospinal fluid but, more simply, blocks may be used in the region-specific manners described below.

Pelvic blocking

Figure 25.6 illustrates a pair of wedges positioned under a prone patient so as to correct pelvic torsion via pelvic blocking, and Figure 25.7 illustrates supine blocking. Supine blocking tends to approximate the sacroiliac joints, whereas prone blocking distracts the sacroiliac joints. Since the geriatric patient is more likely to be fixated than hypermobile, prone blocking is more effective. Since many geriatric patients, especially those suffering from diagnosed spinal stenosis, benefit from mobilization manoeuvres that flex the spine, it is sometimes useful to insert both padded wedges high, under the anterosuperior iliac spine (ASIS) area. In cases of discogenic back pain, with pain peripheralization into the lower extremities, a pair of low blocks may be inserted under the greater trochanteric area (provided contraindications to extension are noted and

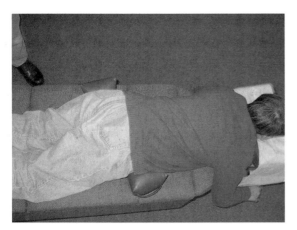

Figure 25.6 Prone blocking with padded wedges.

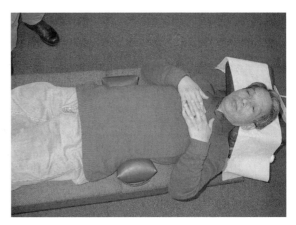

Figure 25.8 Lumbar blocking with padded wedges.

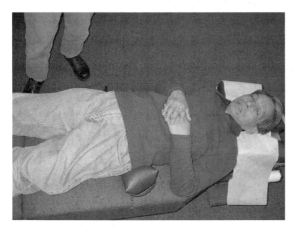

Figure 25.7 Supine blocking with padded wedges.

observed), in accordance with the McKenzie protocols.[85] This may result in increased low back pain, but is indicated under the proviso that leg pain and/or neurological symptoms are made less distal. Care must be taken to ensure that the geriatric patient who has been on the blocks for several minutes rises slowly, lest potential dizziness result in a fall.

Lumbar blocking

Again, in the event that a patient suffers from lumbar discogenic pain referral into the lower extremities, a pair of blocks may be applied under the mid-lumbar spine of the supine patient, provided contraindications to extension are noted and observed (see Figure 25.8). The mechanical effect is similar to that afforded by bilateral greater trochanteric blocking under a prone patient, except that it creates more extension and is less likely to be tolerated. Nonetheless, since a treat-

ment success always involves a lot of trial and error, supine lumbar blocking should be considered as a possibility for low back pain with lower extremity referred pain. Supine lumbar blocking amounts to a supine version of the McKenzie extension protocol for managing low back pain.[85,86]

Thoracic blocking

In essence, almost all people, if they live long enough, develop mid-to upper dorsal hyperkyphosis, a change accelerated by osteoporotic changes in postmenopausal women. It may be an element of the spondylosis syndrome, involving upper extremity paraesthesias, headaches and discogenic arthritic changes. It is useful to place a padded wedge under the upper dorsal spine of the patient, so as to hyperextend the area, with care being taken to provide an adequately sized pillow or other support for the head. The patient who is hyperkyphotic in this area generally cannot tolerate very much cervical extension. The patient's arms are abducted over the side of the table, to add to the stretching of the pectoral girdle and the anterior tissues in general; this would be done only to patient tolerance if he or she complained of thoracic outlet syndrome-related tingling in the fingers. A broad contact is taken bilaterally, with the doctors's fingers maximally spread, involving the clavicles, sternum, pectoral muscles and the tip of the shoulder if the doctor's fingers can reach it. The treatment either ends here, or if the doctor deems it safe to do so, a careful but focused thrust is delivered to the patient's chest area after the patient has been stretching on the blocks for a couple of minutes. It must be noted that many patients would not be able to tolerate the thrust, or would have enough osteoporosis to contraindicate the move. The prognosis for postural change is far from dramatic, but the introduction of even mild postural improvement, and improvement in upper dorsal extension capability, make a great difference in the patient's symptoms.

Traction manoeuvres

Although there is nothing distinctly chiropractic about traction, which is more properly thought of as a physical therapy modality, a small number of traction techniques may liberally be classified as forms of mobilization. In addition to the use of padded wedges, which may be considered as a means of using gravity to exert traction across asymmetrically placed fulcrums, other devices may be used to provide distraction (stretching) of contracted soft tissues in the geriatric patient. Again, the objective is not only to stretch as an end in itself, but to render manipulative and other hand treatments safer and more effective.

Some chiropractic tables feature mechanisms to stretch contractures on a prone patient. For example, some allow flexion of the lower extremities on the pelvis, and others feature a drop away section that allows the abdominal area to sag, thus extending a thoracic hyperkyphosis. Still others can raise the head relative to the rib cage to reverse a forward head posture coupled to increased upper thoracic kyphosis. In addition, a great variety of pillows is available from chiropractic equipment vendors that allow the various body regions to be supported in appropriate preadjustive and even postadjustive positions. As already noted, adequate time must be allowed for viscoelastic creep to have occurred prior to applying thrusts, in order not to tear brittle soft tissues.

In the special case of distraction technique,[87] a specially designed table allows the patient to be stretched and (usually) flexed simultaneously, while the doctor's hand makes a specific contact on the appropriate lumbar vertebra. This may thought of as manually assisted, segmentally specific traction.[88] Distractive procedures (traction) are thought to relax muscles, reduce the pressure on weight-bearing joints, promote the influx of nourishing fluids into discal spaces, relieve (at least temporarily) pressure on nerve roots where there is stenosis of the intervertebral foramen and ameliorate pain. There is a considerable body of evidence that the method is clinically valuable, including for geriatric patients.[89]

Similarly to the table used by distraction-technique practitioners, the Leander table also allows the patient to be moved in and out of flexion, differing in that it features a motor that allows cycling back and forth between flexion and extension. Some chiropractic clinicians apply a manual thrust at carefully chosen phases of the cycle, usually in flexion, considered to be of special benefit for the geriatric patient. Similarly but oppositely, the Reinert table (non-motorized) allows a thrust to be delivered in a precisely arranged attitude of patient extension.[90] The authors, not having used this table, are not certain of its value in treating elderly patients, especially since these person's are beyond the age where the disc herniation that the table is designed to help treat are most likely to occur.

Instrument-assisted adjusting

Many mechanical devices are available for delivering thrusts to patients, some hand-held and others mounted on a table or the floor. Many of these devices can be set at different force levels. Practitioners believe these devices to be particularly safe for geriatric patients, which is a reasonable assertion so long as one notes that tools such as these are capable of generating around 60 N at their maximum force levels, which is comparable to some types of hand adjusting.[32] Moreover, the percussive stylus could, under some circumstances, apply more pressure than hand adjusting which might be more forceful, but employs a broader contact with the patient.

Current research on chiropractic practice patterns indicates that a percussive instrument may be found in approximately one-half of chiropractic offices.[12,91] It is beyond the scope of this work to discuss the analytical systems commonly associated with instrument-assisted adjusting techniques, the most used of which is Activator Methods Chiropractic Technique,[92] which is heavily dependent on leg checking and reflex procedures. Nevertheless, there are several advantages of instrument adjusting: variable force application, highly accelerated thrust (believed by some practitioners to obviate the need to overpower the patient's muscle tension), very specific contact, physical ease for doctors, and the ability to adjust easily those patients who cannot lie in the side posture.

Miscellaneous low-force and soft-tissue techniques

The comment was made earlier that perhaps the most basic consideration in chiropractic geriatric care has to do with the level of force. Common sense suggests that lower levels of force would be indicated, although the authors are aware of no data suggesting that traditional manipulative techniques are less safe or contraindicated, if modified in accordance with the preventive strategies discussed earlier in this chapter. Therefore, a clinician need not be tempted to use a low-force method of dubious value simply because it is less likely to do harm, minus any reasonable expectation that they would achieve a good outcome beyond simply not injuring the patient. This exposes the elderly patient to the risk of substandard treatment or no treatment benefit beyond placebo. Many of the most outlandish, unscientific, and truly strange techniques in the history of chiropractic have been 'low force'; there is no excuse for emphasizing techniques such as these among the elderly, who deserve the same quality of treatment as younger patients. As Dodson so eloquently explained: 'All treatment is dose-related. The type and amount of treatment depend on the problems your evaluation elicits; the anatomic, physiologic, and psychologic condition of the patient; and your own skill in the use of a variety of techniques...I do not wish to leave anyone with the impression that high-velocity thrust techniques are not a viable option in manipulative treatment of the elderly'.[1]

These points having been made, it remains true that there are several low-force technique methods in chiropractic, although less clinically validated than manipulation, that have stood the test of time and have served generations of chiropractors and their patients. To invoke Dodson yet again, this time discussing osteopathic craniopathic procedures, 'I would simply caution you not to fall into the mental trap commonly referred to as "being down on what you are not

up on"'.[1] Nevertheless, no blanket endorsement of any of these named technique systems is given here, for geriatrics or any other select patient population, since many feature a mix of reasonable and questionable methods in their rationale and application. Table 25.1 provides a list of some of these common low-force and mostly reflex techniques. A reflex technique is thought to work in ways not currently described in mainstream physiology and anatomy books, often through remote effects on tissues distant to where the intervention is physically applied.[93] The table identifies a representative core adjustive procedure, which the authors endorse, and a brief, reasonable physiological rationale for the method, of lesser certainty. The methods described in the table may also be used by clinicians who do not profess to use the technique system in which it figures prominently, or may consider themselves practitioners of a different technique system altogether.

Table 25.2 lists several soft-tissue methods commonly used by chiropractors, many but not all of which have been recruited from allied health professions (e.g. osteopathy, physical therapy, oriental medicine). A soft-tissue technique may be thought of as a treatment method intended to improve the functioning of articular tissues, through its impact on related non-osseous tissues. It is with some reticence that the Receptor-Tonus technique of Nimmo is included in this list, since this chiropractor considered his methods adjustive in the strict sense of the term, and possibly with some justification. However, this indigenous chiropractic method may be considered so similar to Travell's trigger point therapy, commonly regarded as therapeutic rather than adjustive, that it would be more instructive to include Receptor-Tonus technique in the table than to exclude it.

Table 25.1 Low-force adjustive techniques commonly used in chiropractic

Low-force adjustive techniques commonly used in chiropractic	Representative core adjustive procedure	Physiological rationale
Sacro-Occipital Technique	Pelvic blocking with padded wedges	Vectored stretching of soft tissues
Logan Basic Technique	Cephalad tug on sacrotuberous ligament	Gentle mobilization of sacroiliac joints
Upper Cervical Technique	Adjustment of atlas (may be high or low force)	Remote effect on remote body locations
Activator Method Chiropractic Technique	Instrument-assisted application of force	Force may be carefully controlled in level and point of application
Distraction Technique	Axial traction of specialized tables designed for that purpose	Reduce muscle hypertonus, increase tissue elasticity and joint excursion, improve vascular supply, reduce disc bulge(?)

Table 25.2 Soft-tissue techniques commonly used in chiropractic

Sofe-tissue techniques commonly used in chiropractic	Representative examples	Physiological rationale
Massage (traditional)	Effleurage, petrissage, tapotement	Relax muscle, improve vascular supply to tissues
Massage (therapeutic)	Transverse frictional	Reduce contractures, including adhesion related
Nimmo Receptor-Tonus	Trigger point ischaemic pressure	Relax muscle and diminish pain
Reflex methods	Neurolymphatic reflexes of Chapman, neurovascular reflexes of Bennett, acupressure	Normalize muscle and organ function
Osteopathic contributions	Strain–counterstrain method of Jones, muscle energy technique	Normalize muscle function
Stretching, passive	Stretching connective tissues	Elongate contractures
Stretching, active	Proprioceptive neurofacillitation technique, actively resisted stretching of connective tissues	Improve neurological function, elongate contractures

Special note on upper cervical techniques

Various upper cervical techniques exist, many of which may be appropriately used in the chiropractic care of geriatric patients. Upper cervical chiropractic care is based on the belief that correction of atlas subluxation normalizes the structure and function of the entire body. A great variety of analytical procedures and adjustive equipment is used in the upper cervical setting. In some geriatric patients, frailty, thoracic spine compression fractures or hyperkyphosis, advanced lumbar or pelvic osseous degeneration or arthritides, or disc disease may contraindicate direct adjustments in these areas. In such cases, there still may be some advantage to caring for the upper cervical spine.

Despite the unique position of upper cervical care in the history of chiropractic, it may be regarded under the more general category heading of 'extraregional care': intervention in a given body location that is designed to have a remote impact on another body region. This is especially useful when the symptom-generating body region is more capable of being iatrogenically injured by adjustive care. In addition to upper cervical care, heel lifts, foot orthotics and lower extremity manipulation may be thought of as extraregional care of an ailing low back (or even head–neck region).

Ancillary modalities and treatments

Although ancillary treatments for the musculoskeletal problems of geriatric patients have been described and in some cases found to be effective, it is beyond the scope of this chapter to go into them. These treatments include physical therapy,[94,95] nutrition,[16,32,96–98] exercise (stretching and strengthening),[17,49,51,96,99,100] psychological intervention[8,28,101] and quality sleep.

Condition-based and subluxation-based care

At the Research Agenda Conference V in 2000, Reikeman distinguished condition-based chiropractic care, aimed at treating diagnosed conditions (e.g., back pain, gastric ulcers), from subluxation-based chiropractic care, aimed at reducing the severity of biomechanical derangements of the spine (vertebral subluxation), arguing that both have a role to play in the contemporary chiropractic setting. Spinal problems no doubt originate well before the emergence of spine-related symptoms, representing the tips of the icebergs. Therefore, it is important that chiropractic clinicians attempt to identify and proactively treat such biomechanical derangements before they become symptomatic. Nothing in all this changes in moving from a younger to a geriatric population, except perhaps for a reduced likelihood of spinal biomechanical derangements being asymptomatic. Therefore, one would expect to see more condition-based chiropractic care among the elderly; not because it is more important for them per se, but because almost the entire iceberg can be seen.

Geriatric preventive and maintenance care

Although the dividing line is not hard and fast, maintenance care intends to preserve the current health status of the patient, which may be normal or subnormal to some degree, whereas preventive care aims to reduce the risk of deterioration. Koch has coined the term 'meta-therapeusis' to embrace the continuum of preventive and maintenance care.[102] Given the prevalence of an age-related decline in health, the geriatric segment of the population should be encouraged to receive meta-therapeutic chiropractic care. Although there are few clinical data in support of this proportion, a recent study by Rupert *et al.* was consistent with the proposition that maintenance care in a geriatric population can improve their status compared with individuals not receiving chiropractic care.[14,15] Sprovieri makes a similar case for osteopathic care[103] and Lambert for medical care.[96]

Geriatric chiropractic technique: safety and risk management

Changes occur in patients as they age, many of which are considered to be 'normal' age-related changes. That is not to say that the patient is powerless to slow or reverse some of these changes, but the chiropractor must consider how such changes can and should affect their clinical decision making. Some of the consequences of normal ageing that may affect the choices of chiropractic techniques and procedures are listed below.[43] The reader should carefully consider this list, lending thought to preventing iatrogenic injuries. More general health changes are listed first, followed by specific spinal health changes:

- vision and hearing loss
- vascular plaque/stroke risk
- increased capillary, skin and bone fragility
- orthostatic hypotension
- decreased muscle mass
- decreased bone density
- decreased elasticity of ligaments and tendons
- loss of nucleus pulposis
- flattening of uncinate processes
- increased rigidity of dural root sleeves
- hypertrophy of the ligamentum flavum and some osteophytic changes.

Absolute and relative contraindications for manipulative care

Other chapters in this book pertain to the process of obtaining a history, performing an examination, conducting elective diagnostic procedures (laboratory, X-ray, advance imaging, etc.), deriving a clinical impression, devising a care plan and managing the geriatric case. Clearly, diagnoses such as acute fracture, osteomyelitis and malignancy require referral to the medical system prior to there being any question of concurrent care, let alone uniquely chiropractic care. Other less dramatic and life-threatening clinical scenarios, such as osteoporosis and degenerative joint disease, simply need be acknowledged in devising a safe and effective care plan. It usually comes down to common sense: the more severe the condition, the less aggressive the treatment should be.

Table 25.3 indicates absolute and relative contraindications for manipulative care.[3,21,104] An absolute contraindication precludes manipulative care, whereas a relative contraindication supports manipulation provided there are appropriate modifications. Non-manipulative forms of chiropractic adjustive care may be safely applied in many situations where higher force thrusting may not.

The controversy that surrounds the question of chiropractic care for the elderly really pertains to one issue and one issue alone: to manipulate, or not to manipulate. No one to our knowledge believes mobilization and other light force procedures risky, except perhaps when the patient has suffered a sprain that requires immobilization (at least in the acute phase). Unfortunately, when it comes to the safety of manipulation, each case must be evaluated on its own merits. The more osteoporotic, osteoarthritic, feeble and mentally challenged the geriatric patient, the less likely manipulation has a role to play, and even at that, the adjustive thrust should be gentle. One thing is certain: it requires more skill and experience to safely and effectively adjust the geriatric patient, for which reason it is all the important that chiropractic students need to obtain a broader exposure to this patient population.[105] What follows is a general discussion of selected safety issues in the chiropractic treatment of elderly patients.

The clinical context of geriatric chiropractic care

Vision and hearing loss

Since greater than half of all patients will have some level of hearing and vision loss in their later years[17] the chi-

Table 25.3 Absolute and relative contraindications to manipulative care [with permission from Bergmann *et al.*[21]]

	Conditions		Complication
	Absolute contraindications	Relative contraindications	
Vascular	Vertebrobasilar insufficiency		Infarction in brainstem
	Aneurysm		Haemorrhage
		Atherosclerosis	thrombus formation, haemorrhage
		Anticoagulant therapy	Haemorrhage
Articular		Advanced osteoarthritis	Increased instability, neurological compromise, increased pain
		Inflammatory arthritis (rheumatoid, psoriasis)	Transverse ligament rupture, increased inflammation
		Ankylosing spondylitis	Increased inflammation
		Joint instability, hypermobility	Increased instability, movement beyond physiological limits
	Disc prolapse with neurological deficit		Cauda equina syndrome, permanent neurological loss
Trauma	Fracture		Delayed or improper healing, increased instability
	Dislocation		Increased instability, permanent soft-tissue damage
		Severe sprains and strains	Increased instability, inflammation, pain
Bone-weakening disorders	Bone tumours		Pathological fracture
	Bone infections (tuberculosis)	Osteomyelitis	Pathological fracture
		Osteoporosis, osteomalacia	Pathological fracture
Neurological		Severe sacral nerve root compression	Cauda equina syndrome. permanent neurological loss
		Vertigo	Stroke, paralysis
		Severe pain, patient intolerance	Unnecessary or increased pain
		Space-occupying lesion	Permanent neurological loss
Psychological		Malingering	Secondary gain syndrome
		Hysteria	Prolonged treatment
		Hypochondriasis	Dependency on treatment

ropractor must learn to be a good communicator, sensitive to the needs of the elderly patient. If a patient has been unable to read the forms that they filled out before care, misinformation and missing information threaten to leave the chiropractor poorly informed about potentially important health information.

Preventive strategies

- Large print forms should be available to patients with visual impairments.
- In performing the health history and physical examination, the doctor should also be aware that if a patient does not hear well, the examination will take

extra time, and again misinformation is a possibility when the patient cannot hear the questions being asked.
- Doctors should position themselves close to the older patient, speak clearly and face the patient whenever possible to facilitate effective communication. Some patients will be embarrassed about, or unaware of their deficits, so the clinician should again be sensitive to the patient's special communication needs.
- It is essential to remove background noise, such as music, to assist a hearing-impaired patient in hearing the interviewer's questions and instructions.

Orthostatic hypotension

Orthostatic hypotension is a drop in blood pressure when patient moves from a sitting or lying position to standing. Orthostatic hypotension may be caused by compromised blood flow to the brain due to atherosclerosis, a side-effect of blood pressure or other medications, general low blood pressure, etc. Whatever the cause, the result is a patient in need of special consideration. Many older patients are prone to orthostatic hypotension, which in turn makes them susceptible to falls, which can be devastating.[6] Many factors contribute to the development of orthostatic hypotension and should be recognized by the clinician in order to develop appropriate procedures to prevent a fall in the chiropractic office during the patient's office visit.

Preventive strategies

- The patient should be told to hyperoxygenate with some deep breaths before and as they are brought up on the table from lying to standing or sitting.
- The doctor should support the patient with two hands when they are brought up on a Hi-Lo type of table, with one hand positioned firmly over the patient's thoracic spine (to prevent posterior or anterior falls). The doctor should hold the patient's arm or hand gently, to allow the patient temporary support of weight and balance assistance, as they step off the foot-plate. The doctor should continue to support the patient as the transition is made from the foot-plate to walking on other textured flooring, such as carpeting.
- The patient is given counselling regarding the importance of regular exercise[99] to increase balance, strength and bone mass, to prevent the catastrophic results of falls.
- The patient's medication use should be assessed regularly for potential drug interactions that lead to balance disorders, dizziness, orthostatic hypotension, etc.

Decreased muscle mass (sarcopenia)

Studies show that until people are approximately 69 years old, age-related changes in muscle are relatively small.[106] After the age of 70, however, these changes accelerate considerably. Changes in the distribution and size of muscle fibres are accompanied by an overall decrease in muscle mass. Since normal ageing-related changes in muscle mass do not result in an inability to gain strength with exercise,[43,107] exercise

programmes to maintain muscle mass and strength can be recommended,[99] thereby increasing the patient's ability to tolerate chiropractic adjustments and ancillary procedures.

Changes in muscle mass impact the manner in which practitioners apply chiropractic procedures in older patients, since muscles provide stability to spinal and other articulations, just like ligaments. Degenerative changes, despite their overall negative impact, tend to reduce spinal mobility, protecting the patient to some extent from the risk associated with sarcopenia in the context of manual adjustive procedures. Since older patients often have a decreased muscle mass, palpation of the osseous structures is often easier to perform, and can be done with a lighter touch. Adjustments and other manual procedures can also be accomplished with a lighter thrust, since there will be less muscle to adjust through, less resistance from the patient's existing muscle and a greater chance of straining the patient's muscles if the thrust is unnecessarily hard. The issue of muscle strain is related to the general increase in muscle rigidity often clinically manifested as a decreased tolerance for passive movement, and increased susceptibility to trauma.[108] The accompanying decrease in ligament elasticity and increase in capillary fragility in the older patient add to this concern over injury of the older patient.

Preventive strategies

- Palpation can be done with a lighter touch.
- Adjustments and other manual procedures should be administered with a lighter thrust.
- Lower settings should be used with physiotherapy modalities.
- Caution should be exerted in applying using heat and ice or cooling packs.

Osteoporosis

Osteoporosis, abnormal rarefaction of bone tissue, is one of the primary risk–benefit concerns that the chiropractor must address when caring for a geriatric patient. There is an increased risk of causing pathological fractures in a patient population more likely to exhibit bone malignancy, osteomyelitis and osteoporosis; and the patient's pain is more likely to be attributable to an osteoporosis-related fracture.[33] Causing a hip fracture, perhaps by using a side-posture technique that involves creating leverage by using the patient's leg, would clearly be a catastrophic adverse response,[26] given how frequently hip fracture represents a life-altering or even fatal event for the geriatric patient.[109,110] Particularly sobering in this regard is a case series of six nursing-home residents who sustained long-bone fractures without evidence of trauma or abuse.[111]

Although Sandoz wrote in 1989[9] 'I have yet to see a compression fracture produced by an adjustment!', Haldeman in 1992 presented a case series of four patients who alleged that they had undergone compression fractures during spinal manipulation,[110] although it is not certain that any of these patients were correct. One severely osteoporotic female, treated by a doctor using 'manual adjustments of specific vertebrae to correct aberrant spinal dynamics', was found to have compression fractures of T10, T12, L1, L2, L4, and L5 after 23 office visits over a span of 6 weeks.[110] (The only review of premanipulative and postmanipulation X-rays was performed by the defendant, who said there was no evidence of change.) Another of the patients, a severely osteoporotic woman who had been on prednisone for 9 years, the most likely among the four cases to have shown a cause and effect relationship between the manipulation and the fracture, was found to have three fractures following what was reported to be forceful manipulation. Haldeman stresses the importance of obtaining diagnostic X-rays in cases such as these, all of which involved trauma, and furthermore concludes that manipulation of a spinal area that has already undergone a compression fracture is likely to make the patient worse.[110]

It must also be remembered that spinal manipulation may induce a vertebral fracture in patients with malignancy, as in the two cases reported by Austin.[112] There is also some evidence[113] and opinion[114] that spinal manipulation can produce other than vertebral body fractures.

The following types of patients are at increased risk for osteoporosis (a more extensive discussion of this topic can be found in Chapter 30, Prevention and health promotion):

- fair-skinned, Caucasian or Asian
- female
- postmenopausal/early menopause
- small-framed, thin
- family history of osteoporosis
- allergy or aversion to dairy products

- hysterectomy at early age
- consumer of pop, coffee, alcohol or cigarettes
- high-protein diet

Preventive strategies

- The above risk factors must be considered carefully.
- An X-ray may assess the degree of bone loss, and rule out conditions predisposing towards iatrogenic fractures (malignancy, osteomyelitis, osteoporosis, etc.).[115]
- Adjustments and other manual procedures should be administered with a lighter thrust.

Vascular plaque/stroke risk

The single most controversial issue pertaining to the safety of manipulative care is concern over the possibility of postmanipulative vertebral artery injuries, which are thought to occur in about 1 in 1 million cervical manipulative adjustments.[116] Risk factors for strokes from all causes include:

- Plaqued arteries
- Orthostatic hypotension
- Smoking
- High cholesterol
- Previous strokes?
- familial history of strokes?
- High blood pressure
- Sedentary lifestyle
- Presence of bruits on auscultation of vessels

The majority of these adverse consequences occur in patients below the age of 65, even though the elderly are at greater risk of stroke from all causes.

It is tempting to speculate that the diminished range of motion of the geriatric neck exerts a protective effect, reducing the risk of stroke by preventing vertebra from mutually displacing enough to endanger the vertebral artery. After all, compared with the younger neck the geriatric neck has 12% less flexion, 32% less extension, 22% less lateral flexion and 25% less rotation.[62] In this light, one is hard pressed to interpret remarks such as 'Restricted range of motion of the cervical spine and so on may predispose the patient to injury to the arteries that supply blood to the brain'.[33] In any case, it is likely that clinicians exert more caution when manipulating geriatric cervical spines, because of fear of vascular or sprain/strain types of injury.

Although some investigators have suggested that rotational manipulation poses more of a threat than less rotatory manoeuvres, Haldeman *et al.* find no particular manipulative style to pose more risk than any other: 'The literature does not assist in the identification of the offending mechanical trauma, neck movement, or type of manipulation precipitating vertebrobasilar artery dissection or the identification of the patient at risk'.[117] The literature dealing with this issue is too vast to consider in this chapter, but many excellent reviews can be consulted[74,116–118] Some common signs of stroke are:

- Focally intense headaches of sudden onset
- Unexplained weakness, paraesthesia, tingling, numbness (especially one-sided)
- Unexplained or sudden onset difficulties with speech, etc.

Although it is always difficult to determine risk factors for rare events such as postmanipulative vascular accidents, pending the development of better data, it would be prudent to avoid excessive rotation in the patient set-up and thrust, although it is not easy to cite a definite number that would be safe. The available literature has been interpreted in a variety of ways, as is typically the case when an event is too rare to draw definitive conclusions. Pending the development of better and more data, it is comforting to note that whatever risk the chiropractic clinician believes attends manipulative care of the neck in general, there is no reason to think the risk greater among geriatric patients, certainly if the clinician displays an appropriate level of caution. When we handle an exceedingly stiff neck we are not generally tempted to thrust vigorously into it. In the case of a patient (geriatric or otherwise) who has already experienced a cervical vascular injury, manipulation should be avoided.

Preventive strategies

- X-rays are taken to visualize the presence and extent of plaque in vessels.
- One should listen for bruits and obtain bilateral carotid pulse and blood pressure readings.
- George's test or an equivalent protocol may be used; despite a lack of evidence that it predicts vascular accidents,[119,120] there is little harm in excessive, even if irrelevant, prudence.
- Care should be taken in applying adjustments to cervical spine, especially with excessive rotation.[116,118]

- Care in using the knee–chest table may be contraindicated in plaqued patients.
- Caution may be indicated in applying deep thrusts to lumbar spine if plaquing is present.

Degenerative joint disease

As the intervertebral discs thin, the posterior joints become more prone to subluxation and degenerative changes. This eventually leads to altered weight-bearing stresses, bony remodelling, hypertrophic changes and compromise of neural structures. It is plausible that chiropractic care can retard the progressive changes, especially if it embraces preventive components. Some patient are at increased risk for such changes, especially those with congenitally defective cartilage and collagen.

Preventive strategies

- One should avoid hyperextending osteophytic spines.
- Excessive force leading to sprains or strains should be avoided.
- The goal of care must be realistic. 'Normal ageing' involves a reduced range of motion and curve alterations; there should be no attempt at 'restoring' normal spinal structure and function, at least not age adjusted.
- Caution should be applied in addressing asymptomatic or slightly symptomatic spinal areas.
- Gradual and gentle stretch should be applied to body regions before manipulation.
- All interventions must be within the bounds of the patient's tolerance.

Summary

The elderly patient has had many years to develop adequate compensations for a whole host of musculoskeletal indiscretions. In some cases, it may be prudent to leave good enough alone, rather than risk destabilizing an effective, if not pretty, solution achieved by innate intelligence: the 'wisdom of the body', as physiologist Walter Cannon put it. However, an elderly patient seeking chiropractic care either fears experiencing or has already sustained a failure of the compensation mechanisms that result from age-related breakdown.

The ageing of the population in the USA and other countries means that chiropractors should increase their proficiency in treating elderly patients. This chapter described the hands-on part, the principles and practices that are likely to increase the safety and effectiveness of chiropractic care in the geriatric setting. In a way, it all comes down to using the same methods used for a younger patient, with mostly obvious modifications that take into account age-related changes. Almost always this means lower force, broader manual contacts, staying within the bounds of patient tolerance and being realistic about the goal of care. We urge our fellow chiropractors not to disdain the judicious administration of adjustive thrusts in favour of low-force methods that seem irrational, or even border on abject quackery, solely because these latter are less likely to fracture a bone.

Chiropractors should not simply refer very symptomatic patients into the medical system, if that means out of chiropractic care. Dr Kent's eloquent statement is an appropriate means of concluding this chapter:

> Some conditions may require interdisciplinary cooperative care. Some may require the chiropractor to modify adjusting techniques to maintain patient safety. It must be emphasized that the primary responsibility of the doctor of chiropractic is the detection and correction of vertebral subluxations. The presence of a pathology which contra-indicates certain techniques does not obviate this responsibility. Furthermore, a decision to seek medical treatment does not mean that a patient should remain subluxated. The geriatric challenge is for each chiropractor to develop a repertoire of techniques so that any subluxated patient may be safely adjusted.[115]

References

1 Dodson D. Manipulative therapy for the geriatric patient. Osteopathic Annals 1979; 7(3): 114–119.
2 Eisenberg DM, Kessler RC, Foster C et al. Unconventional medicine in the United States. Prevalence, costs, and patterns of use. N Engl J Med 1993; 328: 246–252.
3 Bergmann TF, Larson L. Manipulative care and older persons. Top Clin Chiropractic 1996; 3(1): 56–65.
4 Gleberzon BJ. Chiropractic geriatrics: the challenges of assessing the older patient. J Am Chiropractic Assoc 2000; Apr: 36–37.
5 Quincy C. Evaluation of the geriatric patient. Osteopathic Annals 1983; 11(5): 14–15, 18–19.
6 Argoe RT. Analyzing the special needs of the elderly patient. Today's Chiropractic 1989; 18(6): 16–19.
7 Rollis CM. Chiropractic and the elderly patient. Am Chiropractor 1980 May/June: 36, 83.
8 Winterstein J. Perspectives on clinical practice: practical management of the geriatric patient. J Aust Chiropractors Assoc 1990; 20(2): 62–65.
9 Sandoz R. Chiropractic care of the aged patient. Ann Swiss Chiropractic Assoc 1985; 8: 167–191.
10 Senstad O, Leboeuf-Yde C, Borchgrevink C. Predictors of side effects to spinal manipulative therapy. J Manipulative Physiol Ther 1996; 19: 441–445.
11 LeBoeuf-Yde C, Hennius B, Rudberg E et al. Side effects of chiropractic treatment: a prospective study. J Manipulative Physiol Ther 1997; 20:511–515.
12 Hawk C, Long CR, Boulanger KT et al. Chiropractic care for patients aged 55 years and older: report from a practice-based research program. J Am Geriatr Soc 2000; 48: 534–545.
13 Osterbauer PJ, DeVita T, Fuhr AW. Chiropractic treatment of chronic mechanical low back pain in a geriatric population: a practitioner-scientist protocol. In: Proceedings of the Foundation for Chiropractic Education and Research, 3rd Annual International Conference on Spinal Manipulation, Washington, DC, April 12–13, 1991: 230–231.
14 Rupert RL, Manello D, Sandefur R. Health promotion services administered to US chiropractic patients aged 65 and older. Maintenance care: part II. J Manipulative Physiol Ther 2000; 23: 10–19.
15 Rupert RL. A survey of practice patterns and the health promotion and prevention attitudes of US chiropractors. Maintenance care: part I. J Manipulative Physiol Ther 2000; 23: 1–9.
16 Schuman J. Can your elderly patient be rehabilitated? Can J Diagnosis 1996; 13: 129–138.
17 McCarthy K. Management considerations in the geriatric patient. Top Clin Chiropractic 1996; 3(2): 66–75.
18 Cox JM. Patient benefits of attending a chiropractic low back wellness clinic. J Manipulative Physiol Ther 1994; 17: 25–28.
19 Gregg JR. Chiropractic and our nation's aging population. ICA Int Rev Chiropractic 1994; 9(Sept/Oct): 9.
20 Deshpande S, Macneill S, Lichtenberg P et al. Functional outcome differences in acute versus subacute geriatric rehabilitation. Top Geriatr Rehabil 13(4): 30–38.
21 Bergmann T, Peterson DH, Lawrence DJ. Chiropractic Technique. New York: Churchill Livingstone, 1994.
22 Grieve G. Modern Manual Therapy of the Vertebral Column. Edinburgh: Churchill Livingstone, 1986.
23 Grieve G. Common Vertebral Joint Problems. 1st edn. Edinburgh: Churchill Livingstone, 1981.
24 Hammer W. Functional Soft Tissue Examination and Treatment by Manual Methods: New Perspectives. Gaithersburg, MD: Aspen, 1999.
25 Haldeman S, Chapman-Smith D, Petersen DM, eds. Guidelines for Chiropractic Quality Assurance and Practice Parameters. Gaithersburg, MD: Aspen, 1993.
26 Nwuga V. Manipulation of the Spine. Baltimore, MD: Williams & Wilkins, 1976.
27 Bartol KM. Algorithm for the categorization of chiropractic technique procedures. Chiropractic Technique 1992; 4(1): 8–14.
28 Cooperstein R. Chiropraxis. Oakland, CA: Self-published, 1994.
29 Markham JF. Ethical considerations and case management of geriatric patients. ICA Int Rev Chiropractic 1994; 9(Sept/Oct): 45–48.
30 Clemen MJ. Delivering effective force adjustments on patients with degenerative spinal conditions. ICA Int Rev Chiropractic 1988; Sept/Oct: 27–35.
31 Gardner S, ed. Chiropractic Secrets. Philadelphia, PA: Hanley & Belfus.
32 Kawchuk GN, Herzog W. Biomechanical characterization (fingerprinting) of five novel methods of cervical spine manipulation. J Manipulative Physiol Ther 1993; 16(9): 573-537.
33 Fernandez PG. Care of the geriatric patient. Today's Chiropractic 1989; 18(6): 13–15.

34 Gaby AR. Natural treatments for osteoarthritis. Altern Med Rev 1999; 4: 330–341.

35 van Roon JA, van Roy JL, Gmelig-Meyling FH *et al*. Prevention and reversal of cartilage degradation in rheumatoid arthritis by interleukin-10 and interleukin-4. Arthritis Rheum 1996; 39: 829–835.

36 Berkson DL. Osteoarthritis, chiropractic, and nutrition: osteoarthritis considered as a natural part of a three stage subluxation complex: its reversibility: its relevance and treatability by chiropractic and nutritional correlates. Med Hypotheses 1991; 36: 356–367.

37 Bland JH. The reversibility of osteoarthritis: a review. Am J Med 1983; 74(6A): 16–26.

38 Kallio PE, Michelsson JE, Bjorkenheim JM. Immobilization leads to early changes in hydrostatic pressure of bone and joint. A study on experimental osteoarthritis in rabbits. Scand J Rheumatol 1988; 17: 27–32.

39 Troyer H. Experimental models of osteoarthritis: a review. Semin Arthritis Rheum 1982; 11: 362–374.

40 Langenskiold A, Michelsson JE, Videman T. Osteoarthritis of the knee in the rabbit produced by immobilization. Attempts to achieve a reproducible model for studies on pathogenesis and therapy. Acta Orthop Scand 1979; 50:1–14.

41 Kirkaldy-Willis WH. Managing Low Back Pain. 1st edn. New York: Churchill Livingstone, 1983.

42 Pipher WL. Clinical instability of the lumbar spine. J Manipulative Physiol Ther 1990; 13: 482–485.

43 Souza T, Soliman S. Back to basics: normal aging. Top Clin Chiropractic 1996; 3(2): 1–9.

44 Carver W. Carver's Chiropractic Analysis of Chiropractic Principles as Applied to Pathology, Relatology, Symptomology and Diagnosis. 1st edn. Oklahoma City, OK 1921.

45 Rosenthal MJ. The structural approach to chiropractic: from Willard Carver to present practice. Chiropractic Hist 1981; 1(1): 25–29.

46 Troyanovich SJ, Harrison DD. Chiropractic biophysics (CBP) technique. Chiropractic Technique 1996; 8(1): 30–35.

47 Cooperstein R. Technique system overview: Chiropractic Biophysics Technique (CBP). Chiropractic Technique 1995; 7(4): 141–146.

48 Pettibon B. Introduction to Spinal Bio-Mechanics. Tacoma, WA: Pettibon Spinal Biomechanics Institute, 1989.

49 Kligman EW, Pepin E. Prescribing physical activity for older patients. Geriatrics 1992; 47(8): 33–34, 37–44, 47.

50 Troyanovich SJ. Modeling chiropractic concepts: displacements of resting posture as the chiropractic lesion. In: Research PCfC, ed. RAC V: Integrating Chiropractic Theory, Evidence, and Practice; 2000. Chicago, IL: Palmer Center for Chiropractic Research, 2000: 16–17.

51 Shephard RJ. Exercise and aging: extending independence in older adults. Geriatrics 1993; 48(5): 61–64.

52 McDonald JC. Geriatrics: Exercise and the chiropractic lifestyle. ICA Int Rev Chiropractic 1994; 9(Sept/Oct): 26–35.

53 Lazowski DA, Ecclestone NA, Myers AM *et al*. A randomized outcome evaluation of group exercise programs in long-term care institutions. J Gerontol A Biol Sci Med Sci 1999; 54: M621–M628.

54 Hubley-Kozey C, Wall J, Hogan D. Effects of a general exercise program on passive hip, knee, and ankle range of motion of older women. Top Geriatr Rehabil 1995; 10(3): 33–44.

55 Hubley-Kozey C, Wall J, Hogan D. Effects of a general exercise program on plantarflexor and dorsiflexor strength and power of older women. Top Geriatr Rehabil 1995; 10(3): 45–60.

56 Kallinen M, Markku A. Aging, physical activity and sports injuries. An overview of common sports injuries in the elderly. Sports Med 1995; 20: 41–52.

57 Stephenson RW. Chiropractic Textbook. Davenport, IA: Palmer School of Chiropractic, 1927.

58 Chakravarty K, Webley M. Shoulder joint movement and its relationship to disability in the elderly. J Rheumatol 1993; 20: 1359–1361.

59 Chakravarty KK, Webley M. Disorders of the shoulder: an often unrecognised cause of disability in elderly people. BMJ 1990; 300: 848–849.

60 Harrison DD. Chiropractic: The Physics of Spinal Correction. CBP Technique, 1994.

61 Lovett RW. Lateral Curvature of the Spine. 4 edn. Philadelphia, PA: P. Blakiston's Son & Co.; 1922.

62 Kuhlman KA. Cervical range of motion in the elderly. Arch Phys Med Rehabil 1993; 74: 1071–1079.

63 Wyke B. Cervical articular contributions to posture and gait: their relation to senile disequilibrium. Age Ageing 1979; 8: 251–257.

64 Gracovetsky S. An hypothesis for the role of the spine in human locomotion: a challenge to current thinking. J Biomed Eng 1985; 7: 205–216.

65 Haldeman S, Rubenstein SM. The precipitation or aggravation of musculoskeletal pain in patients receiving spinal manipulative therapy. J Manipulative Physiol Ther 1993; 16: 47–50.

66 Scott K. Closed kinetic chain assessment rehabilitation for improved function in the older patient. Top Geriatr Rehabil 1995; 11(1): 1–5.

67 Hintermann B, Nigg BM. [Pronation from the viewpoint of the transfer of movement between the calcaneus and the tibia]. Schweiz Z Sportmed 1993; 41: 151–156.

68 Sommer C, Hintermann B, Nigg BM, van den Bogert AJ. Influence of ankle ligaments on tibial rotation: an *in vitro* study. Foot Ankle Int 1996; 17(2): 79–84.

69 Friberg O. Leg length inequality and low back pain. Clin Biomech 1987; 2: 211–219.

70 McCaw ST, Bates BT. Biomechanical implications of mild leg length inequality [published erratum appears in Br J Sports Med 1991 25: 190]. Br J Sports Med 1991; 25: 10–13.

71 Baylis WJ, Rzonca EC. Functional and structural limb length discrepancies: evaluation and treatment. Clin Podiatr Med Surg 1988; 5: 509–520.

72 Rothbart BA, Estabrook L. Excessive pronation: a major biomechanical determinant in the development of chondromalacia and pelvic lists. J Manipulative Physiol Ther 1988; 11: 373–379.

73 Shekelle P. The appropriateness of spinal manipulation for low back pain. Chiropractic Technique 1992; 4: 5–7.

74 Dabbs V, Lauretti WJ. A risk assessment of cervical manipulation vs. NSAIDs for the treatment of neck pain. J Manipulative Physiol Ther 1995; 18: 530–536.

75 Stillwagon G, Stillwagon KL. The Pierce–Stillwagon technique. American Chiropractor 1983; July/Aug: 20–23, 28–31, 65.

76 Cooperstein R. Technique system overview: Thompson Technique. Chiropractic Technique 1995; 7(2): 60–63.

77 Hyman RC. The Thompson Chiropractic Technique. Publisher unknown, 1991.

78 Zemelka WH. The Thompson Technique. Bettendorf, IA: Victoria Press, 1992.

79 Thompson C. Thompson Technique Reference Manual. Elgin, ILL: Thompson Educational Workshops, Williams Manufacturing, 1984.

80 Cassidy JD, Lopes AA, Yong-Hing K. The immediate effect of manipulation versus mobilization on pain and range of motion in the cervical spine: a randomized controlled trial. J Manipulative Physiol Ther 1992; 15: 570–575.

81 Cherkin D, Deyo R, Battie M *et al*. A randomized trial comparing chiropractic manipulation, McKenzie therapy, and an educa-

tional booklet for low back pain. In: FCER, ed. 1996 International Conference on Spinal Manipulation. Bournemouth, Foundation for Chiropractic Research and Education, 1996: 103–104.

82 Cherkin DC, Deyo RA, Battie M *et al*. A comparison of physical therapy, chiropractic manipulation, and provision of an educational booklet for the treatment of patients with low back pain. N Engl J Med 1998; 339: 1021–1029.

83 DeJarnette B. Sacro-Occipital Technique. Today's Chiropractic 1986; May–June: 97–98, 115.

84 Cooperstein R. Technique system overview: Sacro Occipital Technique. Chiropractic Technique 1996; 8: 125–131.

85 McKenzie RA. The lumbar spine: mechanical diagnosis and therapy. Waikanae, New Zealand: Spinal Publications, 1981.

86 Sullivan MS, Kues JM, Mayhew TP. Treatment categories for low back pain: a methodological approach. J Orthop Sports Phys Ther 1996; 24: 359–364.

87 Cox JM, Feller J, Cox-Cid J. Distraction chiropractic adjusting. In: Top Clin Chiropractic 1996: 45–57.

88 Gatterman MJ, Cooperstein R, Lantz C *et al*. Rating chiropractic technique procedures for specific low back conditions: a process for guidelines development. In: WFC, ed. World Federation of Chiropractic, 5th Biennial Congress, 1999. Auckland, New Zealand: World Federation of Chiropractic, 1999: 159.

89 Cox J, Fromelt K, Shreiner S. Chiropractic statistical survey of 100 consecutive low back pain patients. J Manipulative Physiol Ther; 1983: 117–128.

90 Barrale R, Filson R. A study of chiropractic adjusting utilizing a novel passive extension table position. In: Conference Proceedings of the Chiropractic Centennial Foundation, 1995: 355.

91 Christensen MG. Job analysis of chiropractic. Greeley, COL: National Board of Chiropractic Examiners, 1993.

92 Cooperstein R. Technique system overview: Activator Methods Technique. Chiropractic Technique 1997; 9: 108–114.

93 Cooperstein R. Chiropractic technique. In: Gardner S, Mosby JS, ed. Chiropractic Secrets. Philadelphia, PA: Hanley & Belfus, 1999: 325.

94 Chiodo LK, Gerety MB, Mulrow CD *et al*. The impact of physical therapy on nursing home patient outcomes. Phys Ther 1992; 72:168–173, Discussion 173–175.

95 Janse J, Houser R. Chiropractic Principles and Technic. Lombard, ILL: National College of Chiropractic, 1947.

96 Gambert SR, Gupta KL. Preventive care: what it's worth in geriatrics. Geriatrics 1989; 44(8): 61–66, 71.

97 Bruno G. Musculoskeletal rehabilitation and correct nutritional supplementation. Today's Chiropractic 1989; 18(6): 24–26.

98 Epstein MC. Aging and the role of chiropractic. Digest Chiropractic Econ 1986; (Nov/Dec): 132, 134–138.

99 Simpson WM Jr. Exercise: prescriptions for the elderly. Geriatrics 1986; 41(1): 95–100.

100 Lowenthal D. Conversation with . . . David Lowenthal, MD, PhD: practical approaches to geriatric exercise [interview by Richard L. Peck]. Geriatrics 1990; 45(8): 76, 81–82.

101 Thomas AG. Psychological considerations in the care of the geriatric patient. ICA Int Rev Chiropractic 1994; 9(Sept/Oct): 42–44.

102 Koch D. Chiropractic maintenance and wellness care: a clinical research challenge. In: Research PCfC, ed. RAC V: Integrating Chiropractic Theory, Evidence, and Practice. Chicago, IL: Palmer Center for Chiropractic Research, 2000: 19–20.

103 Sprovieri J. Geriatric programs emphasize wellness. DO 1989; Jan: 112–113.

104 Gatterman MI. Chiropractic management of spine-related disorders. Baltimore, MD: Williams & Wilkins, 1990.

105 Cassata DM. The aging American. An interview with Donald M. Cassata, D.C., Ph.D. on chiropractic care of the elderly. ACA J Chiropractic 1991; Oct: 22–24.

106 Carmeli E, Reznick AZ. The physiology and biochemistry of skeletal muscle atrophy as a function of age. Proc Soc Exp Biol Med 1994; 206: 103–113.

107 Jette AM, Lachman M, Giorgetti MM *et al*. Exercise – it's never too late: the strong-for-life program. Am J Public Health 1999; 89: 66–72.

108 Villareal DT, Morley JE. Trophic factors in aging. Should older people receive hormonal replacement therapy? Drugs Aging 1994; 4: 492–509.

109 Zuckerman JD, Fabian DR, Aharanoff G *et al*. Enhancing independence in the older hip fracture patient. Geriatrics 1993; 48(5): 76–78, 81.

110 Haldeman S, Rubinstein SM. Compression fractures in patients undergoing spinal manipulative therapy. J Manipulative Physiol Ther 1992; 15: 450–454.

111 Kane RS, Goodwin JS. Spontaneous fractures of the long bones in nursing home patients. Am J Med 1991; 90: 263–266.

112 Austin RT. Pathological vertebral fractures after spinal manipulation. BMJ (Clin Res Ed) 1985; 291: 1114–1115.

113 Dan NG, Saccasan PA. Serious complications of lumbar spinal manipulation. Med J Aust 1983; 2: 672–673.

114 Plaugher G. Compression fractures in patients undergoing spinal manipulative therapy (Letter; Comment). J Manipulative Physiol Ther 1993; 16: 193–195.

115 Kent C. The imposters: imaging findings in selected conditions of the geriatric patient which may mimic the vertebral subluxation complex. ICA Int Rev Chiropractic 1994; 9(Sept/Oct): 36–41.

116 Klougart N, Leboeuf-Yde C, Rasmussen LR. Safety in chiropractic practice, Part I; The occurrence of cerebrovascular accidents after manipulation to the neck in Denmark from 1978–1988. J Manipulative Physiol Ther 1996; 19: 371–377.

117 Haldeman S, Kohlbeck FJ, McGregor M. Risk factors and precipitating neck movements causing vertebrobasilar artery dissection after cervical trauma and spinal manipulation. Spine 1999; 24: 785–794.

118 Klougart N, Leboeuf-Yde C, Rasmussen LR. Safety in chiropractic practice. Part II: Treatment to the upper neck and the rate of cerebrovascular incidents. J Manipulative Physiol Ther 1996; 19: 563–569.

119 Licht PB, Christensen HW, Hoilund-Carlsen PF. Is there a role for premanipulative testing before cervical manipulation? J Manipulative Physiol Ther 2000; 23: 175–179.

120 Cote P, Kreitz BG, Cassidy JD, Thiel H. The validity of the extension–rotation test as a clinical screening procedure before neck manipulation: a secondary analysis. J Manipulative Physiol Ther 1996; 19: 159–164.

26

Clinical nutrition for the geriatric patient

Susan St. Clair

'Successful ageing' lengthens the time to mortality while decreasing the years of morbidity.[1] Humans now have longer life expectancy (although some argue that it is still shorter than possible), but with it come years of pathology. The aged population in Western societies today faces a plethora of chronic degenerative diseases, each with its proposed cause and intervention. The current mitochondrial theory of ageing and cellular damage proposes a commonality to these diseases.[2,3] Nutritional modulation seems to be one of the main approaches to successful ageing through prevention, slowing progression or minimizing disability.

The Recommended Dietary Allowance (RDA) of no more than 20% protein, no more than 30% fat and the remainder as carbohydrate is a reasonable beginning, but this must be modified according to the needs of the individual based on genetics, risk factors, activity level, laboratory values, anthropometric measurements, organ function, overall health or disease, recent surgery or injury, and the quality and source of the macronutrients.[4] The RDAs are inadequate guidelines for determining standards for nutrient intake for individuals. There are no specific separate recommendations for the elderly. Most well-developed industrial societies provide adequate macronutrients (fat, carbohydrates and protein) and obesity tends to a major problem with macronutrient (caloric) excess. Based on animal studies, it appears that caloric restriction in industrial societies would prolong life.[5,6]

However, isolated groups of people do not receive adequate amounts. There is a high prevalence of undernutrition in urban, homebound older adults. Forty-five per cent of those over 85 are frail or vulnerable and at increased risk of adverse health out-comes. The frailty of old age is worsened by a poor diet: Ritchie et al.[7] found that frail adults older than 65 had more than one index of poor nutritional status based on body mass index, dietary intake analysis and serum albumin status. Up to 50% of the elderly in the USA have some degree of malnutrition. In the world, protein-calorie malnutrition is the most common nutritional 'dis-ease'.[8,9] Nitrogen balance studies are the best way to assess protein status. Based on studies of young, healthy individuals, the US RDA is 0.8 g/kg body weight per day. A large proportion of homebound or hospitalized elderly people do not meet this amount and are in negative nitrogen balance. Nitrogen balance studies on those over the age of 60 recommend 1.0–1.25 g of high-quality protein per kilogram of body weight per day.[10]

The ideal proportion of macronutrients has yet to be determined and degenerative diseases of the elderly can significantly modify the RDA. For example, a low albumin level (the major serum protein) is a good predictor of poor outcome (shortened lifespan). This person would require high-quality protein intake along with cofactors necessary for protein digestion and absorption, and additional carbohydrate to spare lean muscle losses.[8] This is typically done for those with wasting diseases such as cancer. Those with renal diseases will be put on lower protein diets. Those with osteoporosis or gouty arthritis are restricted in animal proteins, but encouraged to switch to plant protein sources. Those with gastrointestinal disorders may have to switch temporarily to a liquid protein beverage supplying branched-chain amino acids to enhance bioavailability to and through the damaged gut mucosa.[11] Similar modifications are made for fat and carbohydrate depending on the needs of the individual.[12] The reader is encouraged to research the current information available to determine the specific macronutrient needs based on the status of their patient, since this discussion is beyond the scope of this chapter.

Micronutrient deficiencies are very common among the elderly. Nutrient intake among unhealthy elderly showed significant vitamin deficiencies well below the RDA compared with healthy elderly.[13] An increase in some micronutrients (vitamins, minerals, trace elements, phytonutrients) might enhance tissue function and longevity. Micronutrients supply the coenzymes and cofactors for every system of the body. One isolated micronutrient deficiency (or toxicity) can lead to biochemical dysfunction, functional impairment and death. The reasons for nutrient deficiencies included inappropriate food intake, chronic illness, taking multiple medications, poverty, social isolation and oral health problems. Many diseases and medications alter the absorption and metabolism of both macronutrients and micronutrients.

Chronic illness, disuse of the brain and muscle, and abuse of organs through inappropriate diets and exposure to environmental toxins (xenobiotics) accelerate biological ageing. Some have suggested that ageing occurs as mitochondrial dysfunction and DNA mutations accumulate.[3,14,15] Mutations of mitochondrial DNA have been associated with many human diseases.[16] When mitochondrial dysfunction is present or the ratio of toxic factors to normal mitochondrial function is imbalanced, there is incapacity in mental, physical and social ability.[17] Twenty-seven per cent of elderly patients with myopathies were found to have mitochondrial disease.[18]

There are over 1×10^{17} mitochondria in the adult human, with each one containing 17 000 electron transport chains. Up to 75% of the volume of some cells is comprised of mitochondria.[15] Neurons, skeletal and cardiac muscle have high mitochondrial mass because of their high energy needs.[16] Mitochondria are involved in cell metabolism, produce energy in the form of adenosine triphosphate (ATP), influence cell death and contribute to human genetics. Oxygen and oxidation are essential for life and energy production. The mitochondrial electron transport chain burns 85–95% of the inhaled oxygen to make ATP by oxidative phosphorylation in the Krebs cycle.[16]

Most of the oxygen consumed during energy metabolism in the mitochondria combines with

hydrogen to produce water. During ATP production, 1–5% of the inhaled oxygen passing through the mitochondria will form oxygen-containing free radicals called reactive oxygen species (ROS) due to electron 'leakage' at various steps in the electron transport chain.[14,19] The faster the mitochondria are working to produce energy, the more free radicals they produce.[20] ROS is a major metabolite in the human body.

The body also make's ROS to kill bacteria, fungi and viruses through the macrophages[21] and eosinophils. Free radicals are produced by external factors such as heat, ionizing radiation, cigarette smoke, environmental pollutants, alcohol and some medications. As the liver detoxifies toxins and inflammatory products, it produces ROS. Many viral infections generate ROS.[22] This system is harmful if activated excessively. Rheumatoid arthritis, for example, is a chronic inflammatory condition that generates ROS which contributes to joint damage and pain.[2]

A free radical is a highly chemically reactive molecular structure that contains at least one unpaired electron in its outer shell. The ROS include superoxide radicals and hydrogen peroxide. When these free radicals interact with a transition metal, especially iron and copper, they form the very reactive hydroxyl radical. Iron stores increase as we age. Iron accumulation and excess dietary iron have been associated with oxidative DNA damage, increased hydroxyl radicals, decreased antioxidants, activation of gene transcription and cancer tumour formation.[23] The superoxide radicals can combine with nitric oxide (NO) to form the very reactive peroxynitrite.[2] Its metabolites have been measured in chronic inflammatory disease, arthritis, heart disease, inflammatory bowel disease and adult respiratory distress syndrome. These free radicals then produce substances that can act as mutagens, inactivate enzymes, decrease membrane fluidity, and form cross-linkages called advanced glycosylation end-products.[2]

ROS and NO want electrons. If there are no electrons to donate from redox agents (antioxidants), they will attack and damage almost anything to get them. Mitochondrial DNA is at greatest danger of damage because the DNA is not covered in protective histones and they are on the inner membrane close to the sites of free-radical production. ROS can activate a transcription factor that results in genetic changes.[22] Mitochondrial DNA repair is not efficient. Human mitochondrial DNA has a mutation rate of 10–20 times that of nuclear DNA;

40–60% of the mitochondrial DNA must mutate before a disease is expressed.[14,16,19,24,25]

A lipid-rich membrane protects cells against toxins and carcinogens. The ROS attack and break the double bonds of the polyunsaturated fatty acids through a series of events called lipid peroxidation. Mitochondrial membranes are high in polyunsaturated fats. Both membrane damage and mutated mitochondrial DNA increase the leakage of electrons.[2] The release of small proteins from the damaged mitochondrial membrane signals cell suicide, called apoptosis. This becomes a self-perpetuating situation. Mitochondrial damage, free radicals, increased cytosolic calcium and toxins all contribute to cell death and increase the activity of one another.[26] As more cells are triggered to commit suicide, then illness, disease or death occurs.

The degree of organ dysfunction depends on the tissue's energy requirements. Initially, the individual may have no symptoms. Mutated mitochondrial DNA was found in clinically unaffected muscle, indicating that there is some tissue-specific threshold before disease is expressed.[16,27] As ATP synthesis is decreased, it can lead to complaints of chronic fatigue, muscle weakness, behavioural disorders, personality changes, mental retardation, ataxia, seizures, myoclonus and dementia.[14,22,24] Elderly patients with prominent mitochondrial abnormalities shared a common feature of insidious proximal muscle weakness.[18] As the antioxidant system is damaged, the protective antioxidants are depleted or the number of oxidants increases, the person can develop a significant disease or have a catastrophic life-threatening event. The individual declines quickly because they have no more antioxidant reserves. Cataracts, liver disease, heart disease, diabetes mellitus, neuropathies, myopathies, arthritis and all of the cancers have been associated with mitochondrial dysfunction. Neurological illness and myopathy are common features of mitochondrial DNA mutation. Deafness, cardiomyopathy and diabetes in someone with brain or muscle signs and symptoms should alert the physician to a potential mitochondrial disease.[24]

There is no way to stop the oxygen reduction and the production of free radicals, but there is a defence against the damage. The body has many antioxidant systems, but if any system becomes dysfunctional, there is less flexibility to deal with additional toxic exposure.[2] To age successfully a person must lower oxidative stress, modify and improve mitochondrial functions, and normalize inter-cellular communications through dietary antioxidants, environment and lifestyle choices.[2,28]

Normally, superoxide dismutase (SOD), unbound or bound to copper, zinc or manganese, transforms superoxide to hydrogen peroxide. Glutathione peroxidase with selenium and glutathione (GSH) change the hydrogen peroxide into water. Glutathione transhydrogenases reconvert vitamin E, ascorbate and the carotenoids after oxidation. Glutathione reductase ensures that adequate supplies of reduced glutathione (GSH) are present in the cell. Glutathione transferase normally rapidly removes oxidized glutathione (GSSG) from the cells to prevent its toxic effects on cellular function.[29]

Alzheimer's disease, Parkinson's disease (PD) and other common neurodegenerative diseases are not inevitable consequences of ageing. The mitochondrial DNA can be damaged at any time and lead to disease expression. Mutations in the superoxide dismutase gene account for 20% of all familial cases of amyotrophic lateral sclerosis.[30] The mutated SOD has a shorter half-life and a reduced capacity for clearing ROS. Mice that produce excess SOD are resistant to neurodegeneration.[26]

Neurodegenerative initiating events include chronic inflammation, ischaemia,[31] oxidative damage and apoptotic cell death.[32] A patient who had no family history of neurological diseases began exhibiting personality and aggressive changes at the age of 40. Autopsy revealed a decrease in brain volume with loss of neurons. About 87% of the cerebral cortex and cerebellum had pathogenic mitochondrial DNA mutations. On autopsy of non-clinical cases of PD, mitochondrial DNA-induced defects were found to be most severe in the substantia nigra. Elevated iron levels, inhibition of mitochondrial function, oxidative damage, apoptotic cells, advanced glycoslyation end-products, lipid peroxidation and decreases in GSH antioxidant defences have all been found in PD.[16,26,31,33,34] Advanced glycosylation end-product formation is irreversible and leads to oxidant-damaged protein. Damaged or mutant proteins, transition metals and amyloid are deposited when the substantia nigra fails to process them.[34] Clinical PD is expressed at this point.

The mitochondria appear to be the most susceptible to GSH depletion. The GSH/GSSG ratio is normally very high in the mitochondria to help to control the high flux of oxygen radicals from oxidative phosphorylation activities. The ratio of the GSH to GSSH may be a sensitive and early indicator of oxidative stress.[35] In patients dying of PD and other neurodegenerative disorders, substantia nigra GSH levels were decreased by 40% compared with controls and GSSH were marginally elevated in 29%.[36] The patients made adequate GSH, but there was an increased formation of GSSG and decreased recyling of GSH.[37]

It is estimated that the average person ingests about 150 mg glutathione per day, but the majority is made in the liver. Increasing dietary sources of glutathione would augment antioxidant defences and improve the cells' response to toxins. Advanced glycosylation end-product formation can be inhibited by GSH and *N*-aceytlcysteine.[38] Supplementation is recommended daily as reduced GSH at 15 mg/kg body weight, as *S*-adenosylmethionine (SAMe) at 1600 mg or as its precursor *N*-acetylcysteine[22] at 20–200 mg[39] up to 600 mg.[35] Oral ascorbate both protects GSH and is protected by GSH. Supplementation of ascorbate at 200 mg and selenium at 100–500 μg daily will improve GSH status.[35,39]

Several antioxidants have been measured as being low in those who have PD.[40] An intake of 200–400 IU/day of vitamin E lowered the risk of PD.[41] The cerebellum has the highest concentrations of vitamin E and is depleted the most rapidly when a deficiency is induced. Excess iron significantly decreases vitamin E levels.[23] Perkins *et al.* found that poor memory is associated with low levels of vitamin E.[42] A mixture of supplemented antioxidants including vitamin E significantly reduced indices of oxidative stress *in vivo* compared with a placebo group[20] and prevented cell death and neuronal damage *in vitro*.[33]

The effectiveness of antioxidants is related to the stage of the disease. Treatments with vitamin E in the early stages seem to improve the symptoms of PD and Alzheimer's disease.[29] Vitamin E therapy slows the progression of both diseases and the need for medication is delayed. Vitamin E should be tried immediately there is any evidence of neurodegenerative decline, at 1200–2000 IU/day as a safe and cost-effective dose.[43,44] High doses up to 2000 IU/day significantly increased the brain and liver content in diseased individuals. Long-term therapy is needed to reach maximal concentrations within the brain, but this dose is relatively safe for up to 2 years. Vitamin E up to 3200 IU/day has been used therapeutically in neurodegen-

erative disorders, but there can be a risk of bleeding tendencies and increased myocardial infarction in cigarette smokers at these levels.[43]

Vitamin E and selenium slowed the rate of death in mice exposed to herbicides known to induce oxidative stress compared with non-supplemented controls.[45] Wild mice survived significantly longer after herbicidal exposure compared with genetically GSH-deficient mice.[45] SOD administered to rats decreased brain oedema and intracranial pressure, and increased the cerebrospinal fluid white blood cell count. Administration of intravenous arginine worked similarly to SOD, and also increased the antioxidant nitric oxide synthase inhibitor and reversed the increase in regional cerebral blood flow. The untreated control group had no beneficial changes.[46] Late-stage disease showed no improvement on antioxidant administration. At the time of diagnosis more than 80% of the neurons in the substantia nigra have degenerated and antioxidants will not salvage damaged neurons.

Acetyl-L-carnitine is a metabolic cofactor necessary to move fatty acids into the mitochondria for use as a source of energy for the nerve cells. It also supplies acetyl equivalents for the production of acetylcholine, a neurotransmitter necessary for nerve function. Acetyl-L-carnitine improves aerobic processes and increases electron transport chain activity at doses of 150–200 mg/day.[39] Alzheimer's patients showed a slower rate of deterioration and slight improvement with supplements of 1.5–3 g/day of acetyl-L-carnitine.[47]

Those with high dietary intakes or high serum concentrations of antioxidant vitamins have a 20–40% lower risk of coronary heart disease.[48] Vitamin deficiencies, low vitamin intake and elevated blood homocysteine are associated with coronary artery disease. When vitamins B_6, B_{12} and folic acid are present, homocysteine can be metabolized from methionine and made into cystathione or further metabolized and excreted in the urine. Cystathione can be used to supply cysteine for glutathione production. Blood homocysteine is rapidly oxidized, releasing NO. The longer the duration of exposure and the higher the concentrations of homocysteine, the greater the biochemical damage inflicted. The harmful effects can be cumulative and the clinical consequences progressive.[49,50]

Vitamin deficiencies account for two-thirds of all the cases of hyperhomocysteinaemia and supplementation can normalize elevated levels. The vascular toxicity of homocysteine is related to the production of NO, the presence of toxins from certain drugs and cigarette smoke which depletes the vitamin cofactors, activation of the inflammatory cascade, initiation of lipid peroxidation at the endothelial plasma membrane, and oxidation of low-density lipoprotein (LDL). Byproducts of homocysteine oxidation may become incorporated into the mitochondria and impair oxidative phosphorylation, leading to fatigue, weakness and clinical cardiovascular disease.[50]

Vitamin E inhibits oxidation of LDL-cholesterol in plasma. It is recommended to reduce the vascular lipid peroxidation and protect the plasma membrane.[51] The stable tocopheroxyl radical which forms is converted back to tocopherol in the presence of GSH or ascorbic acid. Vitamin C deficiency promotes atherosclerotic lesions and supplementation leads to regression. Betacarotene protects against endothelial damage.[41]

Significant age-related changes occur in vision. Cataracts form when denatured proteins are deposited in the lens of the eye. Much of that protein denaturation is related to oxidative damage associated with exposure to ultraviolet rays in sunlight.[52] Antioxidants such as vitamins C and E, and the carotenoids can delay the onset of age-related lens changes. The human lens normally contains a large amount of ascorbic acid and ascorbic acid protects against experimentally induced oxidative damage. In a group of women aged 56–71 who regularly took vitamin C for 10 years, there was a 77% lower prevalence of early opacities and an 83% lower prevalence of moderate opacities compared with women who did not use vitamin C supplements. Those who supplemented for less than 10 years did not achieve these benefits.[53]

Free radicals produced by tobacco smoking are involved in bone resorption.[54] In a prospective study of over 66 000 women aged 40–76, current smokers with the lowest intake of antioxidants had the greatest risk for hip fractures. Those with the highest intakes had the lowest incidence.

Food may exert positive or negative effects on the balance of oxidant damage and defence. Overeating results in increased free-radical generation. Yu and McCarter found that caloric restriction extended lifespan by decreasing oxidative stress and and increasing antioxidant defences and repair.[5,6] Antioxidant capacity was increased in a diet high in fruit and vegetables compared with one low in fruit and vegetables.[55] Elderly people between the ages of 65 and 90 who were free of significant cognitive impairment were

examined for dietary content and cognitive performance. Those who performed with no errors on the tests were found to eat a diet with less fat, saturated fat and cholesterol, and more fruits and vegetables, fibre, vitamins (especially folate, vitamins C and E, and betacarotenes) and minerals (iron and zinc).[56]

Several types of diet have been examined as to their life-enhancing qualities. There is a significant inverse relationship to per capita consumption of fresh fruits and vegetables with coronary heart disease. Those who eat diets rich in fruits and vegetables have lower incidences of cancer and heart disease.[41,57] Vegetarians eat more fruits, vegetables and fibre, and less saturated fat and cholesterol. They receive adequate protein, but may be deficient in iron and vitamin B_{12}. Since iron has been associated with accelerated oxidation, this may or may not be beneficial. Vegetarians tend to live healthier lifestyles in general, with more exercise, less alcohol and little smoking. Vegetarians generally have a longer lifespan, with less risk of atherosclerosis and heart disease, bowel and lung cancers, obesity, constipation, hypertension and type II diabetes.[58]

Lasheras et al. studied the diets of non-smoking elderly people aged 65–95 years in northern Spain. Those who followed a Mediterranean-type diet tended to have a longer and healthier life with less cardiovascular diseases and cancer.[59] Those who lived the longest ate more olive oil, cereals, legumes, fruit and vegetables, and less meat and milk than northern Europeans. The type of diet had a significant effect on survival rates for the elderly under the age of 80. Consumption of dairy products was the only dietary factor related to a significant increase in mortality in the over-80 age group. This was thought to be related to the high saturated fat and higher lipid content of the diet. The Lyon Diet Heart Study studied the recurrence rate after a first myocardial infarction in those following the Mediterranean diet compared with the prudent diet similar to that recommended by the American Heart Association.[60] At the end of 27 and 46 months, there was a clear protective effect and decreased incidence of recurrent infarcts in the Mediterranean diet group. Many reasons have been proposed for the benefit of the Mediterranean diet. This diet is very high in plant foods containing flavonoids compared with traditional Western diets.

The US government actively endorses increased consumption of fruits and vegetables to improve public health as they are well-recognized as major dietary factors to prevent chronic disease. Cancer risk is reduced with vitamin C intake and when more fruits and vegetables are eaten.[61] Plants contain vitamins which are known antioxidants. Several plant nutrients, such as the carotenoids, the phenolics such as the flavonoids and the saponins have antioxidant potential. These occur naturally in legumes, grains, vegetables, fruits, nuts and seeds. Some plant foods contain more than one of these compounds and some contain only one.[62] The exact components that protect against disease have not been identified, so eating a wide variety of plant foods is recommended for the best health effects, by obtaining all of the possible plant nutrients.

Consumption of flavonoids found in fruits and vegetables appears to protect against heart disease and cancers, and dietary content predicts the risk of ischaemic heart disease and stroke.[60,63] The flavonoids include quercetin, myricetin, kaempferol and rutin. Tea, onions, apples, red wine, grapes and berries all contain high amounts of flavonoids. The flavonoids are considered one of the most important antioxidant categories in the human diet[14] because they are excellent hydrogen donors. Along with vitamin C, they protect LDL-cholesterol from oxidative damage. Human lymphoctyes were pretreated with various flavonoids and vitamin C and then exposed to hydrogen peroxide. The vitamin C provided definite protection against oxidative DNA damage and the flavonoids clearly acted as antioxidants.[63] Quercetin inhibits free-radical activity and protects and regenerates oxidized vitamin E.[60] The effects of vitamin C and quercetin tend to be synergistic.

Black, green and oolong tea are rich in flavonoids. Tea components appear to have greater antioxidant potency than vitamins C, E and betacarotene.[64] Tart cherries contain flavonoids such as anthocyanins which reduce the incidence of inflammation and chronic diseases including cancer and cardiovascular disease. Maritime pine bark, grape seed extract and red wine contain proanthocyanidin complexes subgrouped as polyphenolic tannins.[65] Antioxidant assays indicated that the activities of anthocyanins are comparable to those of commercial antioxidants such as BHA and BHT and superior to vitamin E at certain concentrations.[64]

The lesser periwinkle plant (*Vinca minor*) contains flavonoids and alkaloids. Vinpocetine, one of the alkaloids, has been used beneficially to treat stroke patients with vascular dementia.[47,66] Vinpocetine increases cerebral blood flow, scavenges hydroxyl radicals and raises ATP levels in nerve cells. For clinical effects to be noted, it was used at 15–45 mg/day. Silymarin or milk thistle is high in flavonoids that enhance SOD activity in the liver cell mitochondria[67] and alter the structural membrane of liver cells to prevent toxins from penetrating.[66] It has been used to decrease oxidative stress related to toxic liver diseases and biliary problems.

Gingko biloba extracts appears to improve concentration and memory deficits due to atherosclerosis.[66] The flavonoid constituents contribute mainly free-radical scavenging and other antioxidant effects. The terpenes in gingko biloba protect against cerebral lipid peroxidation, oedema and oxidative stress.[47] Clinical benefit was achieved at doses of 160–300 mg/day of a 24:6 (gingko heterosides to terpenes) standardized extract. The typical daily dose is 120 mg twice daily. An increased bleeding tendency may occur.

Supplementation may be warranted when the diet is known to be poor in antioxidant nutrients or when the level of oxidative stress surpasses the body's antioxidant defence capacity.[39,68,69] Lipoic acid is a highly absorbable, safe and effective antioxidant which readily crosses the mitochondrial membranes. Lipoic acid has beneficial effects on gene expression, scavenges free radicals, regenerates ascorbic acid and vitamin E after oxidation, helps to elevate intracellular glutathione and can regenerate coenzyme Q, NADPH and NADH indirectly through glutathione. At a daily dose of 50–200 mg, lipoic acid appears to be beneficial in treating polyneuropathy, cataracts and diabetes, and improving blood flow and reducing ischaemia after heart attacks.[39,70] Coenzyme Q10 is located largely in the mitochondria as a key electron transport carrier. Without this coenzyme, lactic acid is produced, which reduces the pH and causes muscle pain. It has been shown to improve aerobic cardiac and muscle capability at daily doses of 20–300 mg.[39]

Patients with late-stage degenerative diseases suffer significant wasting and weight loss. Preserving muscle mass is as important as improving antioxidant status. Protein needs can be met by using high-quality, digestible sources. Emphasis is often placed on animal products such as milk and meat,[71] but legumes, grains, nuts and seeds should also be recommended since they provide protein, essential fatty acids and high concentrations of antioxidants. By recommending a more plant-based Mediterranean-type diet, many of the disease-promoting foods will be eliminated, while providing the nutrients that promote 'successful ageing'.[60] In the long run, the key may not be the amount or proportion of macronutrients ingested, but the type and quality of the macronutrients: starches not sugar, cold-pressed essential oils not rancid saturated fats, more plant proteins and less animal protein.[12] A wide variety of micronutrient-dense, fresh, unadulterated, unprocessed, whole foods will allow people to age as healthy, physically and mentally functional individuals until they ease gently into biological cessation.

References

1   Rowe JW, Kahn RL. Human aging: usual and successful. Science 1987; 237: 143–149.
2   Beckman KB, Ames BN. The free radical theory of aging matures. Physiol Rev 1998; 78: 547–581.
3   Harman D. Aging: a theory based on free radical and radiation chemistry. J Gerontol 1956; 2: 298–300.
4   Barrocas A, Belcher D, Champagne C, Jastram C. Nutritional assessment practical approaches. Clin Geriatr Med 1995; 11: 675–708.
5   McCarter RJM. Role of calorie restriction in prolongation of life. Clin Geriatr Med 1995; 11: 553–565.
6   Yu BP. Aging and oxidative stress: modulation by dietary restriction. Free Rad Biol Med 1996; 5: 651–668.
7   Ritchie CS, Burgio KL, Locher JL et al. Nutritional status of urban homebound older adults. Am J Clin Nutr 1997; 66: 815–818.
8   Lipschitz DA. Approaches to the nutritional support of the older patient. Clinics in Geriatr Med 1995; 11: 715–724.
9   Sullivan DH. The role of nutrition in increased morbidity and mortality. Clin Geriatr Med 1995; 11: 661–674.
10 Evans WJ. Exercise, nutrition, and aging. Clin Geriatr Med 1995; 11: 725–734.
11 Mahan LK, Arlin M. Krause's Food Nutrition and Diet Therapy. 8th edn. Philadelphia, PA: WB Saunders, 1992.
12 Chernoff R. Effects of age on nutrient requirements. Clin Geriatr Med 1995; 11: 641–651.
13 de Jong N, Chin A Paw MJM, de Groot LCPGM et al. Functional biochemical and nutrient indices in frail elderly people are partly affected by dietary supplements but not by exercise. J Nutr 1999; 129: 2028–2036.
14 Halliwell B. Antioxidants and human disease: a general introduction. Nutr Rev 1997; 55(1): S44-S52.
15 Mendell JR. Mitochondrial myopathy in the elderly: exaggerated aging in the pathogenesis of disease. Ann Neurol 1995; 37: 3–4.
16 Schapira AHV, Gu M, Taanman J-W et al. Mitochondria in the etiology and pathogenesis of Parkinson's disease. Ann Neurol 1998; 44 (Suppl 1): S89–S98.
17 Gutierrez-Robledo LM. Invited comment. Nutr Rev 1997; 55(1): S74–S76.
18 Johnston W, Karpati G, Carpenter S et al. Late-onset mitochondrial myopathy. Ann Neurol 1995; 37: 16–23.
19 McCardle WD, Katch FI, Katch VL. Exercise Physiology: Energy, Nutrition, and Human Performance. 4th edn. Baltimore, MD: Williams & Wilkins, 1996.
20 Chao W-H, Askew EW, Roberts DE et al. Oxidative stress in humans during work at moderate altitude. J Nutr 1999; 129: 2009–2012.
21 Christen S, Woodall AA, Shigensaga MK et al. Alpha-tocopherol traps mutagenic electrophiles such as NO_x and complements alpha-tocopheral: physiological implications. Proc Natl Acad Sci USA 1997; 94: 3217–3222.
22 Palmer H, Paulson E. Reactive oxygen species and antioxidants in signal transduction and gene expression. Nutr Rev 1997; 55: 353–361.
23 Yano T. Stimulating effect of excess iron feeding on spontaneous lung tumor promotion in mice. Int J Vit Nutr Res 1995; 65: 127–130.
24 Leonard JV, Schapira AVH. Mitochondrial respiratory chain disorders. I: Mitochondrial DNA defects. Lancet 2000; 355: 299–304.
25 Linnane AW, Marzuki S, Ozawa T, Tanaka M. Mitochondrial DNA mutations as an important contributor to ageing and degenerative diseases. Lancet 1989; i: 642–645.
26 Jenner P, Olanow CW. Understanding cell death in Parkinsons' disease. Ann Neurol 1998; 44(Suppl 1): S72–S84.
27 Nelson I, Hanna MG, Alsanjari N et al. A new mitochondrial DNA mutation associated with progressive dementia and chorea: a clinical, pathological, and molecular genetic study. Ann Neurol 1995; 37: 400–403.
28 Bland J. The use of complementary medicine for healthy aging. Altern Ther 1998; 4(4): 42–48.
29 Vatassery GT. Vitamin E and other endogenous antioxidants in the central nervous system. Geriatrics 1998; 53(Suppl 1): S25–S27.
30 Morrison BM, Hof PR, Morrison JH. Determinants of neuronal vulnerability in neurodegenerative diseases. Ann Neurol 1998; 44(Suppl 1): S32–S44.
31 Ste-Marie L. Hydroxyl radical production in the cortex and striatum in a rat model of focal cerebral ischemia. Can J Neurol Sci 2000; 27: 152–159.
32 Folstein M. Nutrition and Alzheimer's disease. Nutr Rev 1997; 55: 23–24.
33 Dexter DT, Holley AE, Flitter WD et al. Increased levels of lipid hydroperoxides in the parkinsonian substantia nigra: an HPLC and ESR study. Mov Disord 1994; 9: 92–97.
34 Miller JW. Vitamin E and memory: is it vascular protection? Nutr Rev 2000; 58: 109–111.
35 Kidd P. Glutathione: systemic protectant against oxidative and free radical damage. Altern Med Rev 1997; 2: 155–176.
36 Sian J, Dexter DT, Lees AJ et al. Alternations in glutathione levels in Parkinson's disease and other neurodegenerative disorders affecting basal ganglia. Ann Neurol 1994; 36: 348–355.
37 Sian J, Dexter DT, Lees AJ et al. Glutathione-related enzymes in brain in Parkinson's disease. Ann Neurol 1994; 36: 356–361.
38 Munch G, Gerlach M, Sian J et al. Advance glycation end products in neurodeneration: more than early markers of oxidative stress? Ann Neurol 1998; 44(Suppl 1): S85–S88.
39 Ames B. Micronutrient deficiencies: a major cause of DNA damage. Ann NY Acad Sci 1999; 889: 87–106.
40 Jenner P. Oxidative damage in neurodegenerative disease. Lancet 1994; 796–798.
41 Wolf G. Gamma tocopherol: an efficient protector of lipids against nitric oxide-initiated peroxidative damage. Nutr Rev 1997; 55: 376–378.
42 Perkins AJ, Hendrie HC, Callahan CM et al. Association of antioxidants with memory in a multiethnic elderly sample using the Third Health and Nutrition Examination Survey. Am J Epidemiol 1999; 150: 37–44.
43 Handelman GJ. High-dose vitamin supplements for cigarette smokers: caution is indicated. Nutr Rev 1997; 55: 369–378.
44 Vatassery GT, Bauer T, Dysken M. High doses of vitamin E in the treatment of disorders of the central nervous system in the aged. Am J Clin Nutr 1999; 70: 793–801.

45 Cheng WH, Valentine BA, Xin GL. High levels of dietary vitamin E do not replace cellular glutathione peroxidase in protecting mice from acute oxidative stress. J Nutr 1999; 129: 1951–1957.

46 Koedel U, Bernatowicz A, Paul R et al. Experimental pneumococcal meningitis: cerebrovasular alteration, brain edema, and meningeal inflammation are linked to the production of nitric oxide. Ann Neurol 1995; 37: 313–323.

47 Kidd PM. A review of nutrients and botanicals in the integrative management of cognitive dysfunction. Altern Med Rev 1999; 4: 144–161.

48 Buring JE, Hennekens CH. Antioxidant vitamins and cardiovascular disease. Nutr Rev 1997; 55(1): S53–S60.

49 Krumdieck CL, Prince CW. Mechanisms of homocysteine toxicity on connective tissues: implications for the morbidity of aging. J Nutr 2000; 130: 365S–368S.

50 Welch GN, Loscalzo J. Homocysteine and atherothrombosis. N Engl J Med 1998; 338: 1042–1050.

51 Halliwell B. Establishing the significance and optimal intake of dietary antioxidants: the biomarker concept. Nutr Rev 1999; 57: 104–113.

52 Rosenberg IH. Nutrition and senescence. Nutr Rev 1997; 55(1): S69-S77.

53 Jacques PF, Taylor A, Hankinson S et al. Long-term vitamin C supplement use and prevalence of early age-related lens opacities. Am J Clin Nutr 1997; 66: 911–916.

54 Melhus H, Michalsson K, Homberg L et al. Smoking, antioxidant vitamins, and the risk of hip fracture. J Bone Miner Res 1999; 14: 129–135.

55 Jacob RA. Evidence that diet modification reduces in vivo oxidant damage. Nutr Rev 1999; 57: 255–258.

56 Ortega RM, Requejo AM, Andres P et al. Dietary intake and cognitive function in a group of elderly people. Am J Nutr 1997; 66: 803–809.

57 Goodwin JS, Brodwick M. Diet, aging, and cancer. Clin Geriatr Med 1995; 11: 577–589.

58 Walter P. Effects of vegetarian diets on aging and longevity. Nutr Rev 1997; 55(1): S61–S68.

59 Lasheras C, Fernandez S, Patterson AM. Mediterranean diet and age with respect to overall survival in institutionalized, non-smoking elderly people. Am J Clin Nutr 2000; 71: 987–992.

60 Trichopoulou A, Vasilopoulou E, Lagiou A. Mediterranean diet and coronary heart disease: are antioxidants critical? Nutr Rev 1999; 57: 253–255.

61 Lamson DW, Brignall MS. Antioxidants and cancer therapy II: quick reference guide. Altern Med Rev 2000; 5: 152–163.

62 Beecher GR. Phytonutrients' role in metabolism: effects on resistance to degenerative processes. Nutr Rev 1999; 57(9): S3–S6.

63 Noroozi M, Angerson WJ, Lean MEJ. Effects of flavonoids and vitamin C on oxidative DNA damage to human lymphoctyes. Am J Clin Nutr 1998; 67: 1210–1218.

64 Balentine DA. Role of medicinal plants, herbs, and spices in protecting human health. Nutr Rev 1999; 57(9): S41–S45.

65 Fine AM. Oligomeric proanthocyanidin complexes: history, structure, and phytopharmaceutical applications. Altern Med Rev 2000; 5: 144–151.

66 Gruenwald J, Brendler T, Jaenicke C. PDR for Herbal Medicines. 1st edn. Montvale, NJ: Medical Economics Co., 1998.

67 Feher J, Lengyel G, Blazovics A. Oxidative stress in the liver and biliary tract diseases. Scand J Gastroenterol 1998; 228: S38–S46.

68 Jacob RA, Burri BJ. Oxidative damage and defense. Am J Clin Nutr 1996; 63: 985S–990S.

69 Oakley GP. Eat right and take a multivitamin. N Engl J Med 1998; 338: 1060–1061.

70 Nichols TW. Alpha-lipoic acid: biological effects and clinical implications. Altern Med Rev 1997; 2: 177–183.

71 Riviere S, Gillette-Guyonnet S, Nourhashemi F, Vellas B. Nutrition and Alzheimer's disease. Nutr Rev 1999; 57: 363–367.

27

Complementary and alternative medicine and the older patient

Luba Plotkina, Sheldon Freelan and Michael Smith

Many clinical conditions that affect older persons are best managed by a health-care team. In this manner, the unique skills of each health-care provider may be employed. For example, although other health-care professionals may receive some training in spinal manipulative therapy, chiropractors are best trained in this skill and therefore are the best qualified to deliver this type of manual therapy. Similarly, students of other health disciplines receive extensive training in particular therapeutic approaches, while other students may receive only a preliminary introduction to such skills. Such skills include the use of botanical and homoeopathic medicines, acupuncture and the prescription of orthotic foot braces. This chapter will provide the reader with a description of the more commonly encountered complementary and alternative medical (CAM) disciplines, namely naturopathy, homoeopathy and podiatry.

Homoeopathy

The World Health Organization (WHO) cited homoeopathy as one of the systems of traditional medicine that should have been integrated world-wide with conventional medicine in order to provide adequate global health care by the year 2000.[1] Although the essential concept of homoeopathy has been in existence for thousands of years, homoeopathy was first tested and established as a medical science by the German physician Samuel Hahnemann in 1796.[2,3] Today, homoeopathy is used by more than 500 million people around the world, particularly for those chronic conditions that fail to respond to conventional treatments.[2-7] Although practised world-wide, homoeopathy is most popular in Europe, Latin America and Asia.[2-4]

The word homoeopathy is derived from the Greek words *homoios*, meaning similar, and *pathos*, meaning suffering.[2] The core of homoeopathy is the Law of Similars, meaning that which causes an illness can also be used to heal that illness.[2-7] Hence, the homoeopathic approach to the treatment of illnesses is the utilization of highly diluted, specially energized plant, mineral or other natural substances, similar to the ones that cause the disease, to stimulate the body's self-healing abilities.[2-7] Medicines are chosen for their ability to cause, in crude doses, the symptoms similar to those that the person is experiencing.[2-4] Since symptoms are the effort by the individual to re-establish homoeostasis or balance, it is logical to seek a substance that would, in crude doses, cause similar symptoms. Thus, homoeopathic medicines work with, rather than against, the individual's natural defence mechanisms.[2-4] It should be noted that homoeopathic medicines are manufactured by pharmaceutical companies, which must follow specific guidelines, and are further regulated by the American Food and Drug Administration (FDA).[2-4]

Principles of homoeopathy

The principles of homoeopathy are based on four criteria:[2-4]

- the law of similars
- testing in healthy persons
- single remedy
- optimum dose.

The law of similars is also used in some conventional medical therapies, such as immunizations and allergy treatment. These treatments, however, are not purely homoeopathic because a true homoeopathic medicine would be individually prescribed, given in smaller doses and used to treat specific clinical conditions to prevent disease.

In many ways, homoeopathy is similar to traditional Chinese medicine, ancient Ayurvedic medicine and, to a lesser extent, modern allopathy. Homoeopathy is what Hippocrates advocated when he said that it is not as important what sickness a person has, as it is important to know how to treat the person who is sick. Homoeopathy promotes the idea of a vital force which governs the activities of the organs and systems, genetic make-up, immunity and predisposition to diseases.[2–7] Homoeopathy, therefore, encompasses the teachings of both ancient and modern medical thoughts.

The homoeopathic approach considers the entire person and not only the disease. For this reason, the initial contact, history taking and interview with a homoeopathic physician can be a unique experience, requiring as much as an hour or more. The homoeopathic physician asks questions not only about the chief complaint but also about the patient's emotional state, mood, affect, likes, dislikes, sexual activities, diet, level of energy and personality, and explores any traumas in the person's life. This detailed and comprehensive interview provides the homoeopathic doctor with an excellent platform or profiling form from which to build a complete record of the patient's physical, mental and emotional state.[2–4]

In essence, homoeopathy is comprised of two disciplines: toxicology and history taking.[2–4] First, homoeopaths identify the specific physical, mental and emotional symptoms that various substances cause in overdose. Secondly, the homoeopath interviews a patient in great detail to discover the totality of the physical, emotional and mental symptoms that the person is experiencing. The homoeopathic physician then combines this information to determine the substance(s) that would cause the similar symptoms to those of the patient and then provide that substance in small, specially prepared doses.[2–4]

There has been some scientific research supporting the efficacy of a homoeopathic approach. The Lancet[8] published a review of 89 double-blind, randomized, placebo-controlled clinical trials. The authors of that study concluded that the clinical effects of homoeopathic medicines were greater than those of the placebos.[8]

The relevance of homoeopathy to health promotion

Modern medicine is costly and often ineffective in

treating many common acute and chronic diseases. Traditionally, allopathic medicine has emphasized disease treatment, symptom suppression, and the control and management of illness. Current thinking in health care, however, also emphasizes the importance of health promotion. It is the goal of the homoeopathic physician, therefore, to assist the patient to improve his or her physical, mental, emotional and spiritual dimensions of health.[2–4] Indeed, this should be the goal of all health-care providers.

Summary

Homoeopathy assesses the whole person, rather than simply his or her parts. The homoeopathic approach attempts to stimulate a person's own immune system for the resolution of the chief complaint, rather than by simply controlling or suppressing symptoms. For this reason, homoeopathy is very effective in addressing many modern illnesses, which are usually complex in nature.[2–4]

Today, numerous conditions of deficient or overreactive immune systems have reached epidemic proportions. More and more viral and bacterial infections cannot be cured by conventional medications. Allergies, starting at an early age, are much more common and are often incurable with conventional therapies. Since there are no age restrictions or other limitations to who may benefit from homoeopathy, any acute or chronic condition, emotional disorder and injury can be addressed by homoeopathic remedies, which are gentle, safe and effective.[2–4]

Podiatry

Foot care of the geriatric patient, for the most part, is nothing more than the worsening of an accumulation of a lifetime of pedal problems.

The podiatrist, or Doctor of Podiatric Medicine, is the specialist most qualified, and therefore responsible, for the care of the foot and its myriad of problems. He or she is concerned with the examination, diagnosis, treatment and prevention of foot disorders by palliative, medical, mechanical, surgical and other means. In terms of educational background, a podiatrist usually has at least a bachelors degree, followed by a 4 year programme in podiatric medicine from an accredited college and, in most cases, a 1, 2 or 3 year postgraduate residency.

Other health-care professionals, including chiropractors or family physicians, often consult with a podiatrist for the treatment for a variety of foot problems arising from infancy to old age. At the latter part of the age spectrum, a podiatrist encounters patients with the usual array of podiatric problems complicated by circulatory impairments, degenerative joint diseases and the ravages of the ageing process.

As one grows older, it is not uncommon to see nails thicken, corns and calluses worsen, digits stiffen, and joints become less and less functional. These, and other foot symptoms, can have their own inherent problems for patients.

The thickening or hardening of nails may be related to a person's visual impairment, and thus he or she may not be able to cut the nail properly, or it may be related to the person being unable to reach their nails because of dizziness or arthritic limitations. The thickened nails may also cause considerable discomfort either from shoe pressure or from having become ingrown over time. In some cases, simple periodic palliative care is indicated, whereas other cases require permanent partial or total nail removal in order to achieve a solution for an individual patient.

Most of the lump and bump foot problems (corns, calluses, hammertoes and bunions) are caused indirectly by inherited bone structure. These conditions worsen over time, and are further adversely affected by shoes, occupation and attention (or lack thereof) to these problems earlier in life. Added to this is the gradual lose of the fat pads of the feet with age, resulting in even more pressure and discomfort to an already uncomfortable situation.

Arthritis, together with biomechanical changes in bone structures, may also create a situation where simple shoe advice, or even orthotic therapy, may not suffice, and surgical intervention may be required, provided the patient's general health allows for it. The purpose of the surgery, in general terms, would be to remove pressure on areas of the foot created by such deformities as hammertoes or bunions, and to remove the source of the adjacent dorsal, plantar or interdigital hyperkeratotic excrescences.

Feet should not hurt

Almost everyone can walk for exercise for their general good health. Walking is an aerobic exercise, and thus is very beneficial in terms of physical and mental health. However, many people often do not walk because their feet hurt.

The aetiology of foot pain can be from multiple sources:

- Persons who work all of their lives in good, supportive shoes may retire to their homes and spend much of the time in (unsupportive) sock feet or slippers. Wearing a good supportive shoe again, even at home, may solve some of the problems of sore feet.
- Feet do not grow longer with age, but they do become wider. Properly fitting shoes, with special attention to width as well as length, may solve much of a person's foot pain.
- Many shoes manufactured today are not properly supportive. Ensuring that a shoe has a solid counter (heel) and shank (bottom of shoe), together with flexibility at the metatarsal–phalangeal joints, may also solve some the problems of sore feet.
- Where a biomechanical problem is evident, a referral to a podiatrist is in order. This is because the majority of corrective devices often suggested for older persons to use for their foot ailments have a very limited ability to solve the underlying problem.

A proper orthotic foot brace fitting is conducted as follows:

- standing angle and base of gait radiographs with specific measurements for rearfoot and forefoot deviations
- a biomechanical examination and evaluation, including all lower extremity ranges of motion and limitations, as well as varus and valgus deformities of the rearfoot, forefoot and the first ray position and range of motion
- non-weight-bearing plaster of Paris, subtalar neutral position casts
- use of an accredited laboratory which is able to assimilate the information and casts provided into a prescription device which will correct the underlying biomechanical function and provide preventive support.

Summary

A podiatrist and other CAM practitioners can set a high standard for interdisciplinary co-operation and referral. With clinical experience, it becomes apparent that patients respond best when treated by the practitioner most likely to achieve the most effacious clinical results in a specific clinical situation. A patients whose general alignment is maintained by the chiropractor will have better clinical results from podiatric orthotics and, conversely, a patient using an orthotic device will better maintain their chiropractic adjustments, which will also be more therapeutic. It is gratifying to be a hero to a patient, either for something you have done for them while directly under your care, or because you have referred them to the most appropriate health-care provider.

Naturopathic medicine

Naturopathic medicine is an eclectic form of health-care that uses a number of complementary and alternative therapies rather than just one specific modality. As with many other holistic practices, the therapies used are determined both by the patient and by the presenting disease, with treatment plans being tailored to the individual's need. For general information on naturopathy, the reader is referred to refs 9–20.

The terms used to describe both the practice and practitioners vary between geographical locations and are largely determined by the legislation of each jurisdiction. Within the licensed jurisdictions in North America, the term naturopathy has largely been replaced by naturopathic medicine, with the practitioners being referred to as naturopathic doctors or naturopathic physicians. The term naturopathy is still largely used in the remaining areas, and is still the term of choice in Europe and Australasia. This discussion will focus primarily on the practice of naturopathic medicine in the regulated jurisdictions of North America.

Philosophy

Naturopathic medicine is practised in North America according to six principles:

- *Vis Medicatrix Naturae* (the healing power of nature): This principle is based on the belief that, within certain limits, the body has an innate ability to heal itself. The role of the naturopathic doctor is to support and offer therapies that do not block this process.
- *Docere* (doctor as teacher): Naturopathic doctors take this translation literally, with the practitioner taking on the role of educator in encouraging patients to take responsibility for their health. Great importance is placed on the healing benefit of the therapeutic encounter.
- *Primum non nocere* (first do no harm): As with other health-care practices, this principle is fundamental to naturopathic practice.

- *Tolle causum* (treat the cause): This principle recognizes that illness and disease are not without an aetiology. Causes may be multifactorial, affecting the body, mind and spirit. Until the cause is addressed, the condition cannot effectively be treated.
- Holistic approach: This approach is based on the assumption that health, or the lack of it, is not an isolated incident in a person's life. The approach for each person must be individualized and must consider all of the presenting systems and causative factors.
- Prevention: Naturopathic doctors consider prevention of disease and promotion of health maintenance to be primary objectives. Prevention is truly best medicine for good health.

Practice

Today, naturopathic medicine (or naturopathy) is practised throughout the English-speaking world, most notably the USA, Canada, the UK, Australia and New Zealand. While both the legislation and beliefs of each jurisdiction affect the practice, a theme common to all is the eclectic nature of treatment protocols. Especially in North America, naturopathic doctors are commonly referred to as the general practitioners of the complementary and alternative health-care world. While therapies used by naturopathic doctors differ between jurisdictions, the core modalities in North America are diet modification and the use of nutritional supplements, herbal (botanical) medicine, homoeopathy, hydrotherapy, bodywork including spinal manipulation, and lifestyle counselling. In some Canadian provinces and American states, traditional Chinese medicine and acupuncture are also practised by naturopathic doctors and core treatment modalities. These individual therapies are discussed in detail in other chapters of this book. The combination of these therapies is considered by naturopathic doctors to be more effective than individual options.

It is important to note that the practice of naturopathy outside North America is not as diverse. In the UK, the practice focuses on the use of nutritional and dietary modifications, hydrotherapy and bodywork (including osteopathic manipulation). The role of the Heilpraktiker, a natural health-care practitioner in Germany, and other practices of mainland Europe, are also often included within the term naturopathy. At present, there are very little formal associations between practitioners trained in North America and those practising in other parts of the world.

Even given this central eclectic theme, it is becoming increasingly popular within the profession to specialize in one or a few therapies. This can often lead to difficulty in distinguishing between naturopathic doctors and other complementary health-care providers such as homoeopaths and herbalists. In addition to the formalized eclectic approach and the core naturopathic principles, another definitive distinction can be arrived at by considering and licensing requirements that exist in the specific jurisdiction.

While naturopathic medical care is partly reimbursed through the provincial health-care plan in British Columbia, this is currently the exception to the rule. As with other forms of complementary and alternative care, third-party organizations such as insurance companies are increasingly including naturopathic medicine within their benefit plans.

Professional/educational requirements

With the possible exceptions of chiropractic, acupuncture and therapeutic massage, naturopathic medicine is the most regulated complementary profession in North America. While not universally legislated for, it is a licensed or regulated primary health-care profession in four Canadian provinces, 11 US states and Puerto Rico (Table 27.1). In general, licensing in one of the regulated jurisdictions requires completion of a common licensing examination, the Naturopathic Physicians' Licensing Examination (NPLEX), accepted by all jurisdictions, often together with a second set of local licensing examinations. The scope of practice permitted varies according to the jurisdiction, with some regions simply recognizing the existence of the profession while others offer a broad scope of practice including such practices as minor surgery, aiding in childbirth and limited prescribing of prescription medication.

While many North American institutions teach naturopathy, candidates from only five naturopathic medical schools are permitted to sit the NPLEX to become licensed in the regulated jurisdictions (see Appendix 27.1). Two of these colleges (Bastyr University and Bridgeport University) are accredited as universities or university-based programmes, with the other three institutions being recognized as either full members or candidates for accreditation by the Council on Naturopathic Medical Education (CNME). The naturopathic doctor programme within these five schools is a 4 year full-time graduate programme. In addition to training in the therapeutic modalities, courses familiar to conventional medical practice (e.g. physical and clinical diagnosis, pathology and anatomy) are taught.

In most jurisdictions where naturopathic medicine is regulated, practitioners can use the title 'Dr'. The Canadian and US national professional bodies are noted in Appendix 27.2.

Evidence

Naturopathic medicine shares a number of issues with other complementary therapies when it comes to evaluating efficacy and safety. As with other complementary therapies, the majority of evidence supporting naturopathic medicine is primarily empirical and/or folkloric in nature. Objectively and effectively evaluating this form of evidence can be particularly challenging. While there are appreciable amounts of scientific evidence from animal and *in vitro* studies, there is still a paucity of information from clinical trials conducted on humans. What 'quality' information does exist primarily comes from a few specific therapies such as acupuncture, the use of clinical nutrients and herbal medicine.

A challenge unique to naturopathic medicine is in evaluating the eclectic approach of the discipline. Most information comes from individual therapy techniques and not the integrated approach used by naturopathic doctors. The evidence supporting the use of more than one complementary therapies is often empirical in nature. This situation is dynamic, with naturopathic colleges conducting clinical research, either on site or as a partner, on this integrated treatment model. Cur-

Table 27.1 Jurisdictions in which naturopathy and naturopathic medicine is regulated

Canada	USA
British Columbia	Alaska
Manitoba	Arizona
Ontario	Connecticut
Saskatchewan	Hawaii
	Maine
	Montana
	New Hampshire
	Oregon
	Puerto Rico
	Utah
	Vermont
	Washington State

rently, naturopathic medical colleges are involved in research projects in many areas such as women's health and pregnancy, human immunodeficiency virus (HIV) and immune-based conditions. Given the fact that unconventional medicine is complementary rather than alternative in nature, this integrated research being conducted by naturopathic medical colleges is particularly topical.

This participation in research, and the increasing importance placed on it by members of the profession, plays a strong role in developing standards of practice and in shaping the future face of the profession. A detailed research project investigating attitudes among licensed Canadian naturopathic doctors identified a growing dichotomy in the profession, with one group holding and basing their practice on the traditional 'holistic' principles and the other following more scientific beliefs. It is highly likely that this professional evolution will impact on both clinical practice and the recruitment of students to the naturopathic colleges.

Summary

Naturopathic medicine is an eclectic practice that, unlike most other forms of complementary therapies, is partially regulated by law. Central to treatment protocols is a belief that the body has an innate healing ability, which can be reinforced by using multiple complementary therapies. Naturopathic doctors in the licensed jurisdictions are sufficiently trained to participate in and augment the primary health-care team. The fact that naturopathic medicine is legislated in a number of jurisdictions has resulted in the existence of relatively uniform standards of practice and education. Naturopathic medicine is a dynamic health-care discipline that is adapting to different evidence sources.

The increasing popularity in of CAM poses new challenges for the provision of conventional health care. In response, members of the conventional health-care team will have to evolve to accommodate these changes in order to provide safe and effective treatment for their patients. Given that naturopathic medicine is one of the few holistic professions to have both established professional and educational criteria, its interaction with members of the conventional health-care team could prove beneficial in the development of primary health-care in North America and elsewhere in the world.

References

1 World Health Organization. Discussion Document on the Concept and Principles of Health Promotion. Geneva: WHO, 1984.
2 Roberts AR. The Principles and Art of Cure by Homeopathy. New Delhi: B Jain Publishers, 1994.
3 Hahnemann S. Organon of Medicine. New Delhi: B Jain Publishers, 1996.
4 Sankaran R. Homeopathy: The Science of Healing. New Delhi: B Jain Publishers, 1995.
5 Ullman D. Conventional Medicine. Alive: Can J Health Nutr 1995: 40–41.
6 Vithoulkas G. The Science of Homeopathy. New York: Grove Press, 1981.
7 Dookhan-Khan B. The Effectiveness of Health Promotion: Canada and International Perspectives. Toronto: Centre for Health Promotion, University of Toronto.
8 Homeopathy Today. Alexandra, Va: National Centre of Homeopathy, 1997–1998.
9 Boon H. Canadian naturopathic practitioners: holistic and scientific world views. Soc Sci Med 1998; 46: 1213–1225.
10 Cody G. History of naturopathic medicine. In: Pizzorno J, Murray M, eds. Textbook of Natural Medicine. 2nd edn. New York: Churchill Livingstone, 1999: 17–41.
11 Bradley R. Philosphy of naturopathic medicine. In: Pizzorno J, Murray M, eds. Textbook of Natural Medicine. 2nd edn. New York: Churchill Livingstone, 1999: 41–50.
12 Ernst E. Towards quality in complementary health-care: is the German 'Heilpraktiker' a model for complementary practitioners. Int J Qual Health Care 1996; 8: 187–190.
13 www.naturopathic.org
14 info@naturopathicassoc.ca
15 Bergner P, Calabrese C, Rogers C, Weeks J. Safety, effectiveness and cost effectiveness in naturopathic medicine. Seattle, WA: American Association of Naturopathic Physicians, 1991.
16 Board of Directors of Drugless Therapy Naturopathy. Naturopathic Application to the Health Professions Regulatory Advisory Council. Toronto: HPRAC, 1994.
17 Einarson A, Lawrimore T, Brand P et al. Attitudes and practices of physicians and naturopaths toward herbal products, including use during pregnancy and lactation. Can J Clin Pharmacol 2000; 7: 45–49.
18 Gallo M, Sarkar M, Au Waiszu et al. Pregnancy outcome following gestational exposure to echinacea. Arch Intern Med 2000; 160: 3141–3143.
19 Astin J. Why patients use alternative medicine: results of a national study. JAMA 1998; 279: 1538–1553.
20 Calabrese C, Berman S, Babish J et al. A phase 1 trial of andrographolide in HIV positive patients and normal volunteers. Phytother Res 2000; 14: 333–338.

Appendix 1: naturopathic colleges

Bastyr University
14500 Juanita Dr. NE, Bothell, WA 98011, USA
Tel: +1-425-823-1300
Website: www.bastyr.edu

Canadian College of Naturopathic Medicine
1255 Sheppard Ave East, North York, Ontario, Canada M2K 1E2
Tel: +1-416-498-1255
Website: www.ccnm.edu

National College of Naturopathic Medicine
049 SW Porter Street, Portland, OR 97201, USA
Tel: +1-503-499-4343
Website: www.ncnm.edu

South West College of Naturopathic Medicine & Health Sciences
2140 E Broadway Street, Tempe, AZ 85282, USA
Tel: +1-602-858-9100
Website: www.scnm.edu

University of Bridgeport, College of Naturopathic Medicine
60 Lafayette Street, Bridgeport, CT 06601, USA
Tel: +1-203-576-4109
Website: www.bridgeport.edu/naturopathy

Appendix 2: national professional organizations

American Association of Naturopathic Physicians
601 Valley Street, Ste 105, Seattle, WA 98109, USA
Tel: +1-206-298-0126
Fax: +1-206-298-0129
Website: www.naturopathic.org

Canadian Naturopathic Association
1255 Sheppard Ave East, North York, Ontario, Canada M2K 1E2
Tel: +1-416-496-8633
Website: info@naturopathicassoc.ca

28

Strength training for seniors

Joseph J Piccininni

Of the four principal components of physical fitness–cardiovascular endurance, flexibility, muscular endurance and muscular strength – it is the last of these that may be the most neglected by seniors and those health-care professionals who provide services for them. There is also no doubt that seniors, either healthy or recovering from illness or injury, can derive important benefits from an exercise programme designed to increase muscular strength. Indeed, much of the recent literature in the field supports the importance of strength-building exercise for the elderly.

Current research in the field has offered support for several different central themes regarding the importance of muscle-strengthening exercise for older people. As people age, they have a tendency to lose both muscle mass and muscle strength. These losses can have negative effects on both functional abilities and quality of life.[1–3] Increases in muscular strength can result in improvements in activities of daily life (ADLs), quality of life and balance, which may decrease the likelihood of injurious falls. Regular performance of resisted or muscle-strengthening exercises is therefore important to counter these effects.

The skeletal muscles of seniors can and do hypertrophy and become stronger in response to regularly performed strengthening exercise. Psychological and social benefits can also result from a well-planned exercise programme. Increasing strength may also reduce the risk of injurious falls, improve posture, enhance quality of life through decreased levels of fatigue and increased functional ability, lessen the chance of injury, increase overall health, self-confidence, and strengthen bones.[4] These and other results are well documented by researchers.

Rantanen et al. studied elderly persons and found that those with the greatest losses in muscle strength reported more increase in motor problems.[5] Krebs et al. found that decreased muscle strength impedes the performance of ADLs such as gait and those with the greatest strength losses reported more difficulties with motor activities. They investigated the use of moderate-intensity resisted exercise on a group of elders with functional limitations. Resistance was provided by using elastic tubing and the subjects exercised their lower bodies three times weekly. Their research indicated that, after 6 weeks of exercise, the subjects in the experimental group increased their strength significantly and this increase had a positive effect on gait stability.[6] Other researchers also found that exercise can be used effectively to increase the strength of seniors' leg muscle strength and that this gain is associated with improvements in daily activities such as gait speed, rising from a chair and stair climbing.[7–9] Psychological changes such as improved confidence were also made following the period of strength training.[7,10,11] In addition to this, some researchers found that improved balance was also one of the outcomes of a resisted training programme.[12] The effect of progressive resisted training on depression in elders was also studied. Singh et al. reported that resisted training can serve as an effective antidepressant while also being responsible for positive changes in strength, morale and quality of life.[13]

There is little doubt that resisted training exercises can be effective in increasing the muscular strength of seniors. Fiatarone et al. studied a group of frail older patients with a mean age of 87 and a maximum age of 98 years. After only 10 weeks of a resisted training programmme, they found increases in muscle strength of up to 113% with concomitant improvements in gait velocity, stair climbing and spontaneous physical activity. In addition, they found increases in the measurement of the cross-sectional area of the thigh muscles which were likely to be due to muscle hypertrophy in response to the training stimulus. From the results of this and similar studies, it would appear that the skeletal muscles of older people respond to resisted exercise in much the same way as those of younger adults.[14]

Resisted exercise programmes designed to increase muscular strength need not be complicated or dependent on access to a fitness facility. McCool and Schneider have shown that home-based low-technology strengthening programmes designed and prescribed by general practitioners can be effective at increasing muscle strength and improving functional task performance.[15]

In order to design a safe and effective strength exercise programme for seniors, the clinician must understand and be able to apply several key exercise physiology principles.

Basic principles: a brief review

The term 'exercise' is broad in meaning and has many modes. In general, exercise can be divided into five types. Each type of exercise has the capacity to cause improvements in the following areas:

- cardiovascular endurance
- muscular strength
- flexibility or range of motion
- muscular endurance
- proprioception, recruitment, balance and co-ordination.

Exercise principles

This section is adapted from JJ Piccininni, A Clinical Guide to Planning and Prescribing Exercise, 2nd edn, 1998, with permission of the author.[16]

Overload

The main goal of exercise is to cause biological adaptations for the purpose of improving the performance of a specific task. In order to cause beneficial biological adaptations, it is necessary to tax the body's systems to a point near their present maximal levels.

Cells, tissues, organs and systems adapt to loads that exceed what they are normally required to do. Once an adaptation has taken place in response to a specific load or stimulus, then to induce further changes, the load must be progressively increased.

Exercise, if it is done to achieve physiological gains, never becomes easy. As one adapts, the workload must continually be increased if further gains are required.

Adaptation response

The term adaptation response refers to the body's ability to respond physiologically to and compensate for the physical demands imposed during exercise activity. Appropriate balance between stressing a particular system or tissue and avoiding overworking it must be maintained. Adaptation occurs only in the cells of those systems that are stressed. There appears to be no (or at best, very little) carryover between stressed and non-stressed tissues.

The body, in response to exercise, and in anticipation of the next bout of exercise or heavy work, makes compensatory changes in the form of biological adaptations. If the next session does not occur soon enough, the adaptations are lost. The body will try to adapt by the easiest methods first; it will use the resources that already exist. With strengthening exercises, this means that neuromuscular improvements will precede hypertrophic changes.

Exercise specificity: SAID

This principle is of cardinal importance for exercise programmes, work-related injury rehabilitation and sports injury rehabilitation. The acronym SAID stands for specific adaptation to imposed demands. It reminds exercise prescribers that, in response to the exercise or physical activity demands imposed on the body, the body will make specific and predictable adaptive responses.

Exercise overload must be specific to the desired effect. Adaptation can be directed towards certain results on combinations thereof. Overload results in adaptations to those cells, tissues, organs or systems that have been overloaded. The resulting adaptation is dependent upon the type and amount of overload.

The adaptations made by the body in response to exercise loads are specific to the structures and functions that are loaded. Training and conditioning effects are specific to the energy supply systems that have been utilized. Adaptations are also specific to:

- muscle groups used
- joint action(s)
- type of contraction (concentric, eccentric, isometric)
- the speed of contraction
- patterns of movement.

This information is crucial to the design of a programme intended to allow a patient to return to work, sport, etc. The exercises must eventually simulate the actions necessary for the activities, but must also approach the loads that will be experienced.

When prescribed exercise loads are applied, they should be:

- specific to the desired effect
- appropriate to the individual in terms of type of stimulus (frequency, intensity, duration, type).

When clinicians develop a programme, they should know in advance what changes will result. Application of this SAID principle allows this prediction to be quite accurate. Conversely, if the practitioner knows what physical capacities a patient needs, he or she should be able to develop a programme of exercise to prepare the body to meet those capacities.

Rest and recovery

In response to a training stimulus at the threshold level, or greater, the overloaded systems of the body will undergo some degree of breakdown. These can occur at various levels, including the subcellular, cellular and tissue. The result of this breakdown is a temporary reduction in the functional ability of the cell, tissue, organ or system.

Following exercise, a period of rest is necessary. During this rest period, the body makes adaptations to the exercise load by resynthesizing the necessary proteins to a higher level than prior to the overload. In addition, wastes are removed and nutrients and energy stores are re-established.

This recovery can take normally 12–48 h. The time required for recovery is dependent upon both the intensity and volume of the exercise session. As the intensity and/or volume of exercise increases, so must the allowed rest time. Levels of fatigue and energy store depletion vary with intensity and volume. Chronic

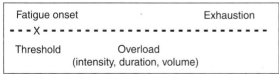

Figure 28.1 Initial fatigue may correspond with the threshold at which an adaption response is stimulated. As exercise overload progresses toward exhaustion, greater recovery time is required

overloading without sufficient rest can result in overtraining, which may can be counterproductive or may even lead to injury. Exercise designed to increase muscle strength should produce some level of fatigue. Complete exhaustion of the muscle is not, however, necessary or even beneficial (see Figure 28.1).

Exercise stimulus

The performed exercise will stimulate various physical responses. Some of these responses are short term or of brief duration, while others are long term. Characteristics of the exercise load that act as stimuli for both the type and magnitude of training effects are:

- intensity (speed, resistance, caloric cost)
- duration of the exercise session (minutes)
- exercise frequency (number of sessions per week)
- length of the programme (number of weeks, months)
- pattern of the exercise (continuous, interval, etc.)
- exercise mode (running, cycling, swimming, walking, etc.)

Any change in an individual's activity level will stimulate an adaptive response. An increase in activity level will improve conditioning, while a decrease in activity level will result in deconditioning. To stimulate conditioning adaptation, overload is required.

The three key stimulus components or variables of exercise programmes are frequency, intensity and duration. Unless all three reach threshold levels, it is unlikely that positive functional gains will be made. Exercise stress which is below the threshold level causes little or no change.

The overload exercise programme designed to produce adaptation is a combination of these stimulus components. Progressions in the programme can be made by increasing one or a combination of the exercise frequency, intensity and duration. However, the nature of the adaptive response will differ and is dependent on whether the increase in exercise volume is due to an increase in intensity as opposed to frequency or duration. Unless all three variables reach the threshold levels, beneficial adaptation in response to the exercise is unlikely.

Maintaining conditioning

If the exercise training stimulus is stopped, reduced or altered, the training or conditioning effects which have been gained will eventually decline. For example, the required rest, following an injury, will allow for tissue healing to begin, but will also result in a diminishing of physical capabilities.

The training or conditioning effects can, however, be maintained for up to a few months if the exercise frequency is reduced to one-third and exercise intensity and duration are maintained. This would be difficult to accomplish following a moderate or severe soft-tissue injury since, even if the patient could maintain the required frequency, he or she would probably have to reduce greatly both the intensity and duration of daily activities.

For periods of up to 2 or 3 weeks, conditioning effects can be maintained if exercise duration is reduced to two-thirds, but the activity intensity and frequency are maintained at the levels that produced the training effects. Once again, this might be a difficult requirement to meet in the first few days or weeks following a soft-tissue injury. It would mean that the injured worker, for example, would continue to work every day, doing full duties, but for only two-thirds of his or her regular hours.

Individualizing the exercise programme

Each person presents with a unique set of circumstances and conditions to the clinician. A 'cook book' approach to exercise planning and prescription, whereby a standard set of exercises and progressions is applied to every patient presenting with like diagnoses, may work with some patients. For others, it will be ineffective and for another group, this approach may even be unsafe. A properly planned, prescribed and performed exercise programme will facilitate the safe return of patients to their physically demanding ADLs.

Patients, even if they do not participate in sports, can be considered as 'industrial athletes'. Just like competitive professional athletes, these patients rely on their bodies being able to perform at a given functional level in order to earn a pay cheque. Just as athletes need to have individualized exercise programmes, so too does the industrial athlete patient require a specific and unique programme both to address the diagnosed condition and to prepare him or her to meet the demands of work. Elderly people also have unique sets of activities that they must or would like to be able to perform. A well-designed, individualized exercise programme can enhance the abilities of older patients in the performance of these tasks.

Clinicians should work hard to create an individual programme for each patient. There are many factors to be understood and considered when taking this approach. Some of these are concerned with exercise programme planning and development, while others relate to programme modification and progression. Some factors to be considered are:

- diagnosis
- patient's age
- psychosocial factors
- physical demands or ADLs
- assessed physical deficits
- patient's daily schedule
- health history and current health status
- exercise history and current exercise status
- time since injury onset
- return to work (or sport) schedule/plans/goals
- patient's response to the exercise programme
- patient's rate of progress
- patient compliance/voluntary effort
- programme intensity
- patient's knowledge level/educational needs
- patient's educational interests/goals
- patient's exercise skill level and co-ordination
- patient likes and dislikes
- patient's access to equipment and facilities.

Individual decisions must be made for each patient which are specific to the programme designed for that individual. These include:

- selection of exercise types (endurance, strength, range of motion)
- selection of each specific exercise (curls, sit-ups, etc.)
- order of exercise performance
- prescribed frequency (days/sessions per week)
- prescribed intensity (caloric cost/minute or percentage effort)
- prescribed session duration
- programme length (number of days/weeks)
- prescribed technique (slow/controlled, dynamic/ballistic)
- selected modes of exercise (running, walking, cycling, swimming)
- prescribed pattern (continuous or intervals)
- time of day for exercise performance
- selected equipment (free weights, Theraband, machines).

Exercise equipment selection

Several various types of equipment can be used for strength-building exercises. Each has advantages and disadvantages. Free weights are the most common equipment used and include dumbbells, barbells, sand bags and medicine balls. These are available in very light weights beginning at less than 2 kg. Dumbbells, or single hand weights, are very useful for home programmes since they are extremely versatile and can be acquired at minimal cost.

Elastic bands and tubing are also very versatile materials for muscle-strengthening exercise programmes. They are inexpensive and portable, and can be purchased in various lengths. Exercises can be devised for every part of the body using tubes and bands. A variety of handles, loops, bars, etc., can be attached to customize the set-up for the patient. Tubes and bands are available in various resistance levels which are usually colour coded. As strength increases or when more resistance is required the material can also be doubled or combined with other pieces to increase the resistance.

As with any type of exercise equipment, caution should be applied when using resistive tubes and bands. Wherever the material is fixed to another object, the point of attachment must be checked for its security. The material requires some care and should not be exposed to harsh chemicals or excessive sunlight. Resistive tubes and bands should be inspected regularly for signs of wear.

Large pieces of equipment that provide isotonic or isokinetic resistance are available at most fitness facilities and many community centres. These may prove to be safer than free weights although the cost of accessing them is a disadvantage for some. In addition, they are usually much less versatile than free weights or resistive tubes and bands.

Ten factors to consider when selecting resisted exercise equipment are:[17]

- expense
- safety
- ease of use
- ease of instruction
- effectiveness for home programme
- versatility
- simulation of ADLs
- quantification of work or improvement
- usefulness for proprioception, balance and recruitment exercise
- accuracy of resistance adjustment.

Preparticipation screening for health risks

Resisted exercises used to build muscular strength are relatively safe. As with any activity that will overload a physiological or anatomical system, there is some risk of injury. The incidence of injury resulting from strengthening exercises can be minimized by appropriate patient education and by the use of an effective preparticipation screening procedure.

The American College of Sports Medicine (ACSM) recommends that screening procedures for exercise programme include four components: (i) those with medical contraindications to exercise, or a specific type of exercise, should be identified; (ii) those who are at increased risk for disease because of age, symptoms and other risk factors should undergo a medical evaluation and may need testing before beginning their programme; (iii) persons with significant disease may be required to participate in an exercise programme under medical supervision; and (iv) those people with other special needs should be identified.[18]

Sample exercise programme

The following exercises represent a selection of exercises that can be done with resistance of several forms including free weights, elastic tubes and bands, body weight and exercise machines. Note that not every exercise in this sample selection is suitable for use with every resistance option listed above. This battery of exercises will address all of the major muscle groups of the body. Many of these exercises can be done in a seated position, so even those with some balance problems may still be able to do some of them. These selected muscle-strengthening exercises are:

- one-quarter to one-half squats (quadriceps and hip extensors)
- hamstring curls or resisted knee flexion (hamstrings)
- military or overhead press (deltoids, trapezius, triceps)
- seated rowing or seated horizontal pulls (forearm, elbow flexors, rhomboids)
- pull-downs (latissimus dorsi, elbow flexors)
- biceps curls (elbow flexors)
- triceps press (elbow extensors)
- sit-ups: one knee bent, one knee flexed, hands at the sides and raise the scapula (trunk flexors); this position, or alternatively with the hands under the lumbar spine, is optimal for maintaining the neutral lumbar lordotic curve[19]

- four-point kneeling hip/knee extension (lumbar and hip extensors).

Exercises to address a specific concern may also be added. For example, if one or more of the rotator cuff muscles is weak, resisted glenohumeral rotation exercises may be included in the programme.

Suggestions for a successful strengthening programme

- Appropriate patient education is critical. Cognitive, affective and psychomotor learning is recommended. Patients should be taught why the exercise programme is important, how often to do the exercises and what the signs of injury or overuse are.
- Patients must use the correct technique to perform the exercises. Posture and movement are both important.
- A Patient log book may be used to record the exercises and other notes and comments. The log book can serve as a reminder of key information and technique points. It can also be a patient-completed record of the exercises done and the resistance used for each exercise.
- Small and frequent changes should be made to the programme. Increases may involve adding one or two repetitions to each set of exercises, adding sets or adding resistance. This will minimize the chance of injury and will also encourage the patient as progress is made.
- The patient should be informed about delayed onset muscle soreness (DOMS) which frequently accompanies a resisted exercise programme. Continued low-level exercise, as opposed to rest, seems to be the best way to deal with DOMS.
- The development and schedule of the programme should be negotiated with the patient, not imposed. This will make the patient a partner with the clinician in formulating the exercise plan.

References

1 Astrand PO. J.B. Wolffe Memorial Lecture. Why exercise? Med Sci Sports Exerc 1992; 24: 153–162.
2 Graves JE, Pollock ML, Carroll JF. Exercise, age, and skeletal muscle function. South Med J 1994; 87(5): S17–S22.
3 Gleberzon B, Annis R. The necessity of strength training for the older patient. J Can Chiropractic Assoc 2000; 44: 98–102.
4 American College of Sports Medicine. American College of Sports Medicine Position Stand. Exercise and physical activity for older adults. Med Sci Sports Exerc 1998; 30: 992–1008.
5 Rantanen T, Guralnik JM, Sakari-Rantala R et al. Disability, physical activity and muscle strength in older women: the women's health and aging study. Arch Phys Med Rehabil 1999; 80: 130–135.
6 Krebs DE, Jette AM, Assmann SF. Moderate exercise improves gait stability in disabled seniors. Arch Phys Med Rehabil 1998; 79: 1489–1495.
7 Chandler JM, Duncan PW, Kochersberger G, Studenski S. Is lower extremity strength gain associated with improvement in physical performance and disability in frail, community-dwelling elders. Arch Phys Med Rehabil 1998; 79: 24–30.
8 Sauvage LR, Myklebust BM, Crow Pan J et al. A clinical trial of strengthening and aerobic exercise to improve gait and balance in elderly male nursing home residents. Am J Phys Med Rehabil 1992; 71: 333–342.
9 Evans WJ. Exercise training guidelines for the elderly. Med Sci Sports Exerc 1999; 31: 12–17.
10 Lord SR, Lloyd DG, Nirui M et al. The effect of exercise on gait patterns in older women: a randomized controlled trial. J Gerontol A Biol Sci Med 1996; 51(2): M64–M70.
11 Tsutsumi T, Don BM, Zaichkowsky LD, Delizonna LL. Physical fitness and psychological benefits of strength training in community dwelling older adults. Appl Hum Sci 1997; 16: 257–266.
12 Judge JO, Underwood M, Gennosa T. Exercise to improve gait velocity in older persons. Arch Phys Med Rehabil 1993; 74: 400–406.
13 Singh NA, Clements KM, Fiatarone MA. A randomized controlled trial of progressive resistance training in depressed elders. J Gerontol A Biol Sci Med 1997; 52(1): M27–M35.
14 Fiatrone MA, O'Neill EF, Ryan ND et al. Exercise training and nutritional supplementation for physical frailty in very elderly people. N Engl J Med 1994; 330: 1769–1775.
15 McCool JF, Schneider JK. Home-based leg strengthening for older adults initiated through private practice. Prev Med 1999; 28: 105–110.
16 Piccininni JJ. A Clinical Guide to Planning and Prescribing Exercise. 2nd edn. Toronto: Rehabilitation Clinic CMCC, 1998.
17 Piccininni JJ. Prescribing strengthening exercises for my patients: which equipment should I select? J Can Chiropractic Assoc 1994; 38: 223–226.
18 American College of Sports Medicine. ACSM's Guidelines for Exercise Testing and Prescription. 6th edn. Philadelphia, PA: Lippincott, Williams & Wilkins, 2000.
19 McGill SM. Low back exercises: prescription for the healthy back when recovering from injury. In: American College of Sports Medicine. ACSM's Resource Manual for Guidelines for Exercise Testing and Prescription. 3rd edn. Baltimore, MD: Williams & Wilkins, 1998: 116–126.

29

Spinal rehabilitation and stabilization for the geriatric patient with back pain

David Byfield

Western societies are experiencing a rapid ageing of their populations. Current reports indicate that by the year 2050 approximately 25% of the population will be over the age of 65 years.[1] Furthermore, baby boomers are now turning 50 years old, making this a dominant social group who may very well dictate and initiate much-needed changes in health-care delivery. This has already been observed as an increase in the use of complementary and alternative medicine in both the USA and the UK.[2] It also appears that, as a result of this shift in demographics, the health-care needs for this group, and society as a whole, may very well be dramatically redefined. This dramatic demographic swing may influence epidemiological perspectives, particularly with respect to common musculoskeletal conditions such as chronic low back and neck pain, which are recognized as leading causes of chronic disability.

Research has shown that 60–80% of the population suffers from back pain at some time during their lives.[3,4] At any given time, approximately 10–30% of the population is experiencing chronic neck pain, with its incidence increasing equally in both men and women as they age.[5,6] It therefore stands to reason that health-care providers, and the health-care industry in general, must be concerned about the future cost of back pain disability and its potential socioeconomic burden. Strategies to reduce this burden have been suggested and progress has been made with the publication of various international guidelines for the management of both acute and chronic back pain.[7,8] Furthermore, the recent publication of occupational health guidelines for back pain in the UK demonstrates

a clearer view of the underlying mechanisms responsible for back pain and signifies a serious shift in management and prevention protocols.[9] The implementation of these protocols becomes the next challenge to the health-care community as a whole.

Back pain in the elderly

Back pain is extremely common in the elderly, even though there is a widespread impression that back pain is considered chiefly a problem of working people. Edmond and Felson,[10] for example, reported that back pain is extremely common among the elderly. Their findings support previously documented evidence by Bresslar et al.,[11] who conducted a systematic review of the literature regarding the prevalence of low back pain among older persons. They concluded that there is a widespread underestimation of the older population in the back pain literature and that the prevalence of low back pain in this population (> 65 years) is not known.[11] More specifically, Edmonds and Felson,[10] in a study of subjects aged 68–100 years, demonstrated that women (53%) reported more back pain than men (42%), although age itself did not seem to influence the prevalence of reported back pain. These findings may influence low back management strategies and future guideline reviews and implementation, particularly as the population continues to age at its current rate.

Even though the jury may still be out regarding the nature of back pain and the elderly, there is certainly a need to develop more appropriate functional management protocols for this group of persons. Mayer *et al.*[12] echo this view in a recent presentation to the American Spine Society wherein the researchers called for enhanced opportunities for older workers following spinal disorders, especially in light of the ageing of working populations across the industrialized world. They found that age appears to be a potent influence on outcomes as older individuals had higher disability levels and lower scores on functional testing, even after a comprehensive rehabilitation programme for chronic low back pain.[12] These cases may require behavioural strategy interventions to monitor progress for a more positive outcome.

Osteoporosis and the geriatric patient

The relationship between osteoporosis and the rehabilitation of older persons must be explored. Osteoporosis is an increasing public-health problem that may cause loss of life or contribute to a reduction in quality of life of surviving sufferers.[13–15] It is considered a common metabolic disease, affecting approximately 25 million Americans annually.[16] Osteoporosis is characterized by low bone mass and deterioration of the foundational architecture, leading to skeletal fragility and increased risk of fracture.[15] Furthermore, osteoporosis affects one-third of all postmenopausal women, resulting in 1.5 million fractures annually.[16] The annual cost in the USA has been estimated to be approximately $20 billion.[1,17] This has significant social implications, especially as the population is generally living much longer. The mortality rate related to osteoporosis is a staggering 20% at 6 months postfracture, with 50% of these individuals suffering a significant decline in physical activity and permanent disability.[13] It has also been reported that 20–30% of these individuals are institutionalized, which creates additional stresses for this group of people and their families.[13] This would suggest significant implications with respect to exercise choices, duration and frequency. It has also been recently reported that vertebral fractures are a common accompaniment to ageing, which can, in turn, have significant impact on both the functioning abilities and well-being of older patients.[18] In one study,[18] researchers found that 39% of both men and women had evidence of prior vertebral fracture which, as the authors discussed, has substantial implications for the comfort and health of ageing individuals. This may influence any proposed interventions and clinical management of this particular age group.

Rehabilitation and the older patient

Regardless of the above scenario, the benefits of exercise appear to be greater than any deleterious effects. The overriding consideration for treating spinal problems among the elderly is preventing functional decline. It has been shown that those who remain functional and active have the best opportunity for more productive living.[19] The key is to prescribe the most appropriate programme to suit the patient's needs and abilities, taking into consideration any underlying contraindications and pathology. This requires a comprehensive assessment of the patient's health status before embarking on any specific programme. Positive outcomes have been reported on the effects of a training programme including muscle strength, stabilization and balance for osteoporotic patients.[20,21] Depending upon the age of the patient, the objective, through structured exercise, is to stimulate maximum bone mass during adolescence, achieve small increases in the middle adult years and, most importantly, conserve bone mass in older adults. This may be accomplished by reducing the risk of falls, improving balance, promoting postural awareness and improving overall mobility by way of specific individualized exercise regimens.[15] There is scientific support that continued exercise into old age may help to preserve bone density gained during activities in youth.[22] Although there is still no evidence that exercise prevents falls and fractures in the elderly, epidemiological studies consistently demonstrate that both past and current physical activity protects against hip fracture, reducing the risk by up to 50%.[23]

All relative contraindications must be taken into consideration, with particular reference to medication usage as well as other nutritional concerns, as part of health-status assessment, including alcohol and smoking habits. Particular care must be taken with those patients receiving long-term oral steroid therapy who may be enrolled in a rehabilitation programme.[24] Moreover, patients who are long-term corticosteriod users should be receiving vitamin D and calcium treatments in an attempt to prevent steroid-induced osteoporosis.[25] Therefore, it would be advisable to ensure that appropriate documentation is established and maintained, and that other health-care professionals are alerted to the planned rehabilitation programme. This may encourage feedback and alert other clinicians to any other underlying conditions that may influence programme compliance and patient motivation. It should also be noted that osteoporosis, although predominantly affecting older females, can also be found in males and patients of all age groups. The safety of patients is vitally important when dealing with these conditions and their needs must come first.

Functional rehabilitation and back pain

Active functional rehabilitation has emerged as an effective management intervention for subacute and chronic mechanical neck and back pain.[7,26–46]. Exercise programmes that emphasize a graded return to normal activity have a significant effect on disability, coping-with-life abilities and lost work time.[47] A study by Klaber Moffett et al.[47] involving patients up to 60 years of age demonstrated results that were consistent with an earlier study involving patients with chronic back pain participating in a similar exercise programme.[28,48] The Klaber Moffett study programme consisted of eight 1-h-long evening classes over 4 weeks and included stretching, low-impact aerobics and strengthening exercises aimed at the main muscle groups. Many of these low-intensity exercise programmes have been shown to be cost-effective and have gained significant support in the literature, particularly when comparing long-term gains in self-perceived disability.[49] Protocols specifically designed to address endurance, strength, flexibility, co-ordination and balance, which would accommodate the older age groups, have been supported by well-conducted clinical research trials.[38] Furthermore, there is promising evidence regarding the importance of both the strength and endurance characteristics of soft tissues required for spinal stability and optimal function. Panjabi[50] eloquently described a model for spinal stability that incorporated three important components, which includes: (i) neural (nervous system), (ii) passive (ligaments), and (iii) active (muscles) subsystems, all functioning in harmony. Moreover, it is now well known that most back injuries are not due to frank trauma but more likely to be the result of trivial events and associated motor control errors causing inappropriate muscle activation and aberrant joint motion.[51,52]

Considerable functional demands are placed upon stabilizing muscle groups during the performance of common activities of daily living (ADLs), regardless of the age of the individual. This warrants serious objective consideration during assessment and any recommendations for functional restoration programmes. For example, recent research has determined that the normal strength ratio relationship between the extensors and flexors is 1.7:1 in the cervical spine and 1.4:1 in the lumbar spine.[6,29,53,54] From a clinical perspective, this ratio appears to be only 1:1 in most chronic neck and back pain patients, which undoubtedly contributes to a patient's overall fatigue and chronic dysfunction.[35,55] This functional instability may contribute significantly to the high prevalence of both conditions sampled in the population.

There is a hierarchy describing descending muscular strength values for both the cervical and lumbar spines, with the extensors dominating the picture due, in part, to heavy postural demands and their natural role in bipedal stance and the performance of normal daily activities. Moreover, it is also becoming more apparent that muscle group recruitment patterns, reaction times and other aspects of the somatosensory system are impaired in patients with back pain compared with a healthy population. This finding warrants further clinical assessment.

Recent evidence has demonstrated that active rehabilitation protocols are an effective method for the restoration of lost functional capacities of both the cervical spine and shoulder region for patients with chronic neck pain and mechanical low back pain.[40] These functional capacities include range of motion, flexibility, strength, endurance and proprioception for the purpose of managing daily tasks and activities at the workplace and at home. Rehabilitation of the cervical spine should address specific functional demands required by each individual patient, and incorporate principles of muscle and exercise physiology and neural adaptation. Therefore, a successful rehabilitation programme should include progressive submaximal resistance training with predetermined dosage (number of repetitions and resistance) and goals, as well as adequate resistance for either strength or endurance, and be of sufficient duration (number of sessions or weeks) required for physiological remodelling. In addition, sensorimotor training (balance, reaction timing and position sense) should be integrated into this management scheme to address eye–head–neck co-ordination, which is often impaired in patients with chronic neck pain. A relative disregard for pain, while establishing reasonable programme goals, is also considered on essential feature of a successful programme. This chapter will focus on the essential features of a low-technology, evidence-based rehabilitation programme for patients with chronic neck and back pain.

It should also be noted that the benefits of exercise are numerous and should always be considered when managing patients of any age with musculoskeletal dysfunction, including:

• improved strength and flexibility
• improved respiratory and circulatory function
• increased preservation of bone mass
• general well-being
• confidence and motivation
• independent activity.

Rehabilitation and the elderly

It is well known that physical ability decreases with age; however, the impact of age-induced changes on rehabilitation is often overestimated.[56] The elderly may enrol in endurance training with little adverse effects on their joints and tendons. It has also been demonstrated that weight training increases muscle force even among people well into their eighties. Any rehabilitation programme should take into consideration the patient's physical, psychological and social background. This incorporates the principles of the biopsychosocial model of pain and contemporary management protocols. In order to obtain optimal results, specific goals for the rehabilitation programme must be adapted accordingly. The goals and needs of a geriatric rehabilitation programme are likely to be different from those of a younger group, although there is considerable overlap dealing with functional restoration in both groups. The issue of adequate bone mass is paramount in this discussion, as well as the age at which this should be maximized and maintained. Issues of endurance, strength, flexibility and co-ordination are similar but tailored to ADLs. Moreover, it is very important that older patients are not denied rehabilitation based upon age alone.

Research has shown that healthy men and women maintain comparable levels in isometric strength, isometric endurance and range of motion in the cervical spine up to and including the sixth decade.[6] McGill[51] has also reported that endurance of the back muscles is of primary concern in any exercise programme, rather than absolute strength. Functional spinal sta-

bility is required during the performance of most normal daily activities. Moreover, the emphasis in rehabilitating the older patient is on early and sustained activity.

Low back rehabilitation programme

The cornerstone of low back rehabilitation is extensor musculature endurance and motor control.[51,52] Strength should not be ignored; however, is it more important to enhance the stabilization of the lower back. This will better enable an individual to sustain a variety of trunk postures over long periods without fatigue.[52] The deep extensor muscles play an important role in enhancing spinal segmental support and movement control, which may be impaired in those individuals experiencing chronic recurrent mechanical low back pain.[52] This may also explain the high prevalence of neck pain, as the lumbar spine and cervical spine exhibit similar neuroanatomy and functional physiology. It is a well-established fact that poor endurance is a good predictor of future low back pain episodes.[55] It is also well established that muscle reaction times, muscle co-ordination and position sense are all impaired in patients experiencing recurrent episodic low back pain, which may imply some motor control irregularity.[52] Jull and Richardson[52] propose specific exercises designed to retrain the co-contraction of the deep muscles (transversus abdominus and the multifidus) to re-establish spinal stability and reduce neuromuscular impairment and to provide pain control.

It is important to include a number of functional components in any rehabilitation programme, regardless of the age of the patient. The programme needs to be designed based upon the patient's individual requirements in order to maintain his or her ADLs. Stretching exercises, once the mainstay of most low back programmes, are highly inadequate to generate a training stimulus and response within the neuromusculoskeletal system during functional recovery. The role of static stretching protocols has recently been questioned and proposals to abandon its current use in light of recent evidence have been highlighted and replaced by more dynamic stretching skills.[57] Nevertheless, programmes must adhere to the principles of muscle physiology and training, and (i) address functional loss, (ii) establish training objectives, and (iii) reach sufficient intensity, dosage and duration. To avoid tissue stress and control potential tissue reactions the programme also needs to be submaximal but progressive over at least an 8–12 week period.

With that in mind, the proposed rehabilitation programme will consist of five main areas:

- extensor muscle endurance and co-contraction
- trunk muscle balance
- spinal stabilization
- balance and coordination
- lower limb strength.

This programme is very comprehensive, and includes many aspects of musculoskeletal function and stability that are required during the safe performance of everyday activities. The foundation of this programme is the re-establishment of extensor/flexor balance (1.5:1) and the improvement of overall endurance performance of these muscles. Some studies have demonstrated significant endurance gains (100–150%) over an 8–12 week period.[27] The overall rehabilitation time-frame is an important concern and must be understood by both practitioner and patient. Activity must be consistently sustained over a 2–3 month period in order to demonstrate any functional recovery and ensure effective neural adaptation and response.

The key elements of this programme are:

- dosage (number of repetitions, sets and resistance)
- duration (two or three times per week over 8–12 weeks)
- relative disregard for pain (encourage patients)
- training objectives (effective goal setting)
- programme supervision.

Supervised training has been shown to be far superior to non-supervised efforts: patients tend to achieve much better results when they are under the guidance of a trainer.[58,59] (Many practitioners have found exercise sheets either abandoned in the changing rooms or left homeless in reception.)

Programmes should be flexible enough to allow patients some variety in terms of time and duration, but the programme must cover a specific period in order to achieve a training response and overall improvement in spinal function and stability. This needs to be reinforced with the patient and a commitment to the programme needs to be obtained. This requires the practitioner or trainer to set out a plan for the patient that includes not only the nature of the intended training scheme but also the time-frame during which this will be carried out, including any supplemental home exercises.

Therefore, training strategies for the cervical and lumbar spines would be based upon:

(i) the cervical spine:
  - resistance (full-range strength)
  - progressive, sub maximal
  - speed and co-ordination
  - functional stabilization;

(ii) the lumbar spine:
  - endurance (lifting trunk weight)
  - progressive (30–40% MCV)
  - stability: co-contraction
  - motor control.

This represents the foundation of rehabilitation of both the cervical and lumbar spines. The cervical spine requires full-range submaximal resistance exercises, whereas the lumbar spine requires body endurance to comply with postural demands and negotiating various trunk activities.

The programme has several components to maintain patient interest and to establish a variety of different activities while, simultaneously, achieving a number of training objectives for both the cervical and lumbar spines:

- warm-up period (5–10 min): stationary exercise bike or treadmill
- stretching period for specific muscle groups in each region
- intensive training
- sensorimotor training
- postexercise stretching
- warm-down (5–10 min)
- home exercises (balance and stabilization)
- outcomes management (use of valid and reliable questionnaires to monitor progress and ongoing treatment needs).

The lumbar or cervical programme should be kept within a 60–90 min time frame. It would also be advisable for each patient to complete a Physical Activity Readiness Questionnaire (PAR-Q) before starting a rehabilitation programme in order to manage any potential risks that may occur.[60]

It should be noted that the following programmes are designed for patients to participate in safely up to and including 70 years of age. Beyond this age, modifications must be made to accommodate patients needs and their general health status.

Before starting such a programme the practitioner should:

- decide whether the patient will benefit from participating in the program (benefit versus risk)
- obtain written informed consent
- thoroughly explain and describe the content of the programme
- discuss commitment to complete the desired period of training
- demonstrate some of the equipment and how it is used (Figure A)
- ensure that the patient understands the very low entry level and starting point but also the progressive nature of the training programme (Figure B)
- introduce them to the instructor (if this is someone other than the practitioner)
- contact the patient's general practitioner to inform them of the intended programme and any feedback or advice

- complete the PAR-Q
- establish the patient's entry level
- address any concerns or questions raised by the patient
- encourage the patient at all times to remain active.

Lumbar spine

Part 1

The programme includes a warm-up period, including 5–10 minutes on an exercise bike or treadmill, depending on the patient's level of fitness (Figure 29.1). This is designed to prepare the individual for the intended exercise load and to also relax the patient. This is followed by a 10 min stretching routine of the major muscle groups of the lower back, trunk and lower extremity (Figures 29.2–29.12). These activities should be carried out individually for a 15–20 s period. There are many different stretching exercises that can be included in this section, which are at the discretion of the practitioner. The stretches should

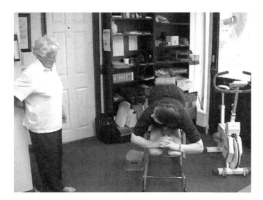

Figure A

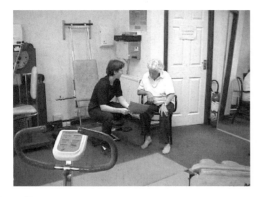

Figure B

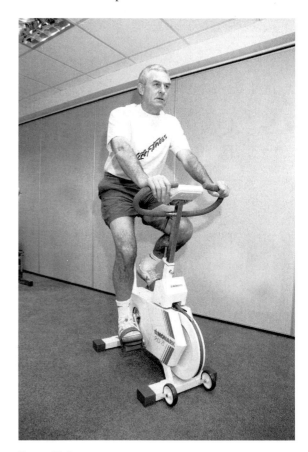

Figure 29.1

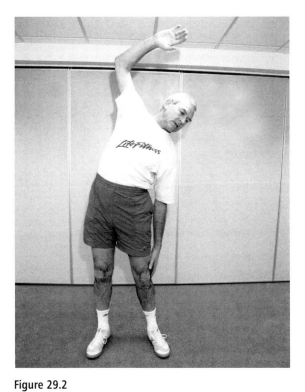

Figure 29.2

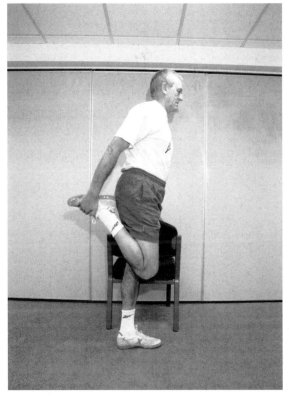

Figure 29.4

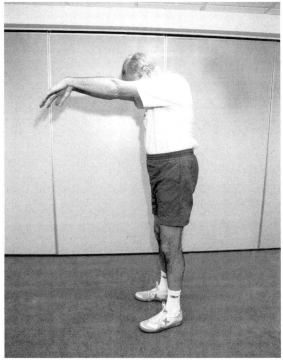

Figure 29.3

Figure 29.5

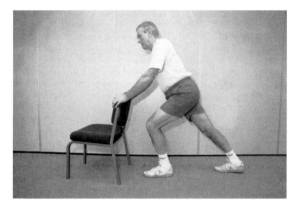

Figure 29.6

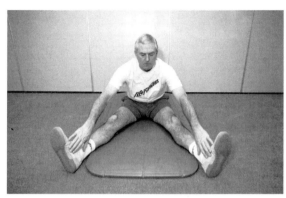

Figure 29.9

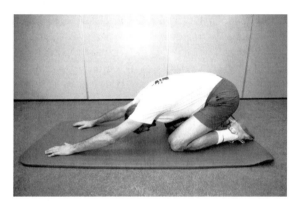

Figure 29.7

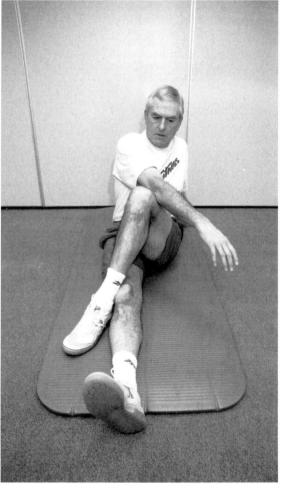

Figure 29.8

Figure 29.10

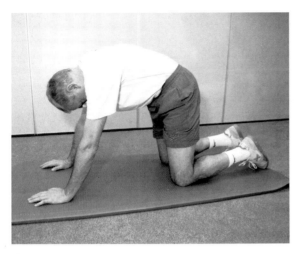

Figure 29.11

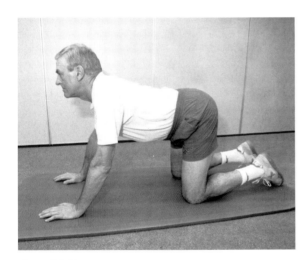

Figure 29.12

be conducted with a goal to increase joint and soft-tissue ranges of motion in preparation for the more demanding aspects of the programme. Although stretching is a common procedure there are some myths to dispel during instruction and subsequent training. There should be no bouncing or excessive end-range pressure during the procedures, as these actions could potentially lead to minor injury.

As mentioned previously, there is still some controversy regarding the therapeutic benefits gained from stretching.[46] Murphy[46] advocates the use of a more dynamic form of stretching which simulates the intended activity. This will be recommended during some of the proposed training programmes for the low back and neck regions. Even though the stretching debate rages on, clinicians should not disregard their patient's desire to stretch, and it is the author's experience that patients 'love to stretch'. The task, however, is to provide a more comprehensive programme to address the rehabilitative process and encourage functional integrity and independence. (The stretches depicted can also be included as part of a home exercise programme.)

Part 2

This component of the rehabilitation programme is the cornerstone of the low back programme. It is designed to focus on improving the overall endurance and stability of the spinal extensor mechanism and to condition the supportive musculature of the trunk and lower extremity. These areas of the body are primarily used in lifting activities. The first step is to establish spinal co-contraction stability and a neutral spine stance.[51] This is accomplished in the quadruped position with the assistance of the instructor (Figure 29.13). The patient is instructed to tilt the pelvis fully forwards (Figure 29.14) and then fully back (Figure 29.15) in order to appreciate the range of pelvic movements. Following this, the patient is instructed to find the mid-way point between these two extremes, which McGill[51] calls the neutral lordosis. The patient is then instructed to move the umbilicus actively upwards and inwards towards the back in order to contract the transversus abdominus, which will cause a co-contraction of the multifidus. This action will stabilize the lumbosacral spine (Figure 29.17). The patient can also be taught this co-contraction posture in the standing, sitting and supine positions as part of their overall rehabilitation and functional recovery. From this position, the patient can be instructed to extend individually the upper extremity (Figure 29.18) and the lower extremity (Figure 29.19) (approximately 18% MVC in the lumbar extensors on one side) and then to do both actions simultaneously (Figure 29.20). According to McGill[51] the combined arm and leg extension produces 27% MVC in the lumbar extensors and 45% MVC in the thoracic extensors of the other side. This is a significant training input. It has to be instructed and rein-

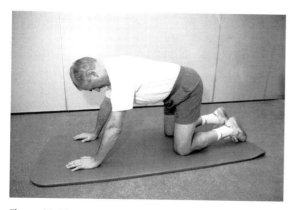

Figure 29.13

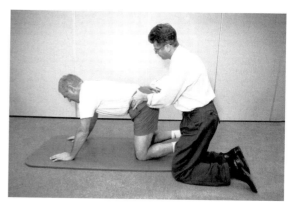

Figure 29.16

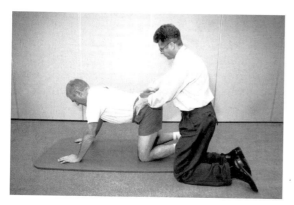

Figure 29.14

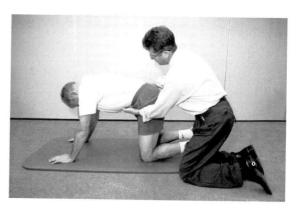

Figure 29.17

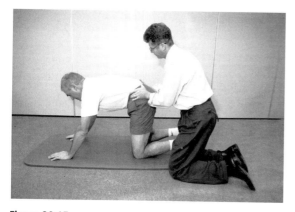

Figure 29.15

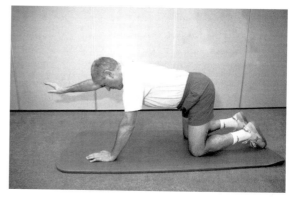

Figure 29.18

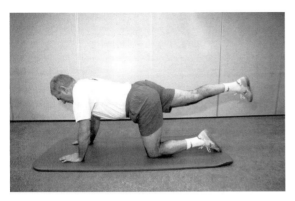

Figure 29.19

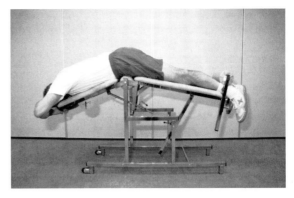

Figure 29.21

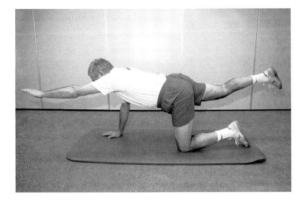

Figure 29.20

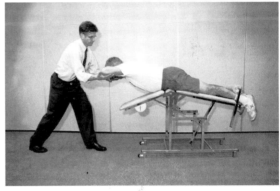

Figure 29.22

forced under direct supervision and practised at home or work on a regular basis to ensure that these skills are learned and reproduced automatically. Constant reinforcement is required to engrain these skills subcortically.

The next stage is to introduce trunk weight endurance conditioning of the spinal extensors. This is achieved by actively extending the trunk against gravity, beginning with sets of 10 repetitions. The patient lies prone on an angle bench with the feet secured under the rear cushion piece for leverage and stability and align the anterior superior iliac spine (ASIS) over the central cushion (Steen Physical, Norway) (Figure 29.21). The patient is instructed to interlace the fingers, place the dorsum of the hands against the forehead and lift the trunk up to a horizontal position and then immediately down to resting posture with the assistance of the trainer during the initial training period (Figure 29.22). Once the patient is

comfortable and confident with these protocols, he or she is instructed to repeat the procedure without supervision (Figure 29.23a). The rear portion of the bench is angled slightly down at the back to help protect the sensitive facet joints during repetitive extensions. The angle of the bench is optimally set at between 30 and 40 degrees, which is the length–strength relationship for the extensors. This is the angle at which both the flexors and extensors of the trunk are at their strongest. The angle is set depending on the entry level, age and ability of the patient. It is advisable to begin the programme at about 15–20 degrees and increase as the patient progresses (Figure 29.23b). The angle may stay the same throughout the programme, depending on the above factors. The important aspect is that the extensor musculature is challenged enough over a sufficient period within the patient's tolerance and abilities. As the patient progresses the flexion angle is lowered until the optimum range is achieved at 30–40 degrees. The patient will continue to complete extension movements at a rate of 15–16/min, which is similar to the average breathing cycle of 15–16 breaths/min. The first training session should complete one or two sets of 10 extensions and subsequent training periods should progress from there. It must be emphasized that progression should not exceed more than 10–15% to avoid overuse and tissue failure. The clinician must keep in mind a number of parameters, such as the patient's age, general health, general fitness, condition and current symptoms, when beginning the programme. It is prudent to begin slowly and work at a steady pace. This may add to compliance and enhance programme effectiveness. Over 8–12 weeks the patient should be able to work up to between eight and 10 sets of 10 back extensions given normal physiological response and adaptation time. This programme should be implemented for those patients up to 70 years of age only.

Next, the patient is instructed to reverse his or her position on the angle bench and initially simultaneously lift the legs to challenge the extensor mechanism further and add to the training effort with the assistance of the trainer (Figure 29.24). The ASIS is once again aligned over the central cushion of the bench. The patient is also instructed to hold on to the side of the bench to assist the lifting mechanism. Initially the patient is assisted in their efforts or, alternatively, he or she may lift one leg at a time depending on the entry-level ability. The patient is instructed to keep both feet together and control movement. A strap can be wrapped around the lower back region to stabilize the spine and avoid any excessive substitution during this exercise. The bench is angled to accommodate the length–strength ratio. This may initially be much less, depending on the ability of the patient. Once the patient has been sufficiently instructed they can perform lower leg lifts unassisted (Figure 29.25a). If the patient is unable to lift both legs at once they should instructed to lift one leg at a time during the programme (Figure 29.25b). As the patient gains strength they may attempt a double leg lift. This should not progress until the patient is capable. The goal is to work up to five sets of 10 repetitions over the length of the programme. The patient maintains a cycle of 15–16 lifts/min during this aspect of the programme. The bench is once again angled to avoid overextension and facet joint irritation. This is particularly important in the older groups owing to normal degenerative

changes associated with the ageing spine. The patient should work up to five sets of 10 repetitions over the course of the programme.

The abdominal musculature plays an important role in low back stability and is included in this programme. The abdominals rank second in strength and endurance requirements, with a ratio of 1.5:1. McGill[51] investigated abdominal exercises for spinal stability and overall muscular challenge. Figure 29.26 illustrates the most advantageous method for challenging the trunk flexors. Note the forearm and hand placed under the back to maintain the neutral spine and spinal stability. The head and shoulders are lifted as the patient breathes out, tucking the chin towards the chest, completing 15–16 repetitions/min, as above. One knee is flexed during the exercise, and this can be alternated between sets. The patient can do these exercises at home on a regular basis to supplement the in-house programme. The patient should work up to five sets of 10 repetitions over the course of the programme. This amount of activity will maintain the appropriate extensor to flexor ratio during training.

The lateral flexors, including the quadratus lumborum (QL), are considered to be one of the most important stabilizers of the lumbar spine.[51] The QL is regarded as the most important stabilizing muscle structure of the lumbar spine because of its anatomical position and infrastructure.[51] It would therefore be prudent to exercise this muscle group appropriately in order to assist lumbar spine stability and eventually to diminish back pain. McGill[51] documented a specific exercise that provides sufficient muscular challenge to limit the biomechanical load on the sensitive spinal structures, which is described as follows.

This part of the programme is very demanding and should only be initiated after the patient is comfortable with the other aspects of the programme and has developed some degree of confidence. The patient lies on his or her side with the feet secured under the rear stabilizing cushion as a lever. The lower leg supports the top leg in order to achieve an effective fulcrum with the patient's arms folded and torso slightly rolled forwards towards the table (Figure 29.27). This avoids substitution by the abdominals during side-body raises which would otherwise confound the exercise. The patient is instructed and assisted to produce a side-body lift (Figure 29.28). This activity is to be performed bilaterally. This is a very demanding activity so it may be advisable to delay introducing this exercise until

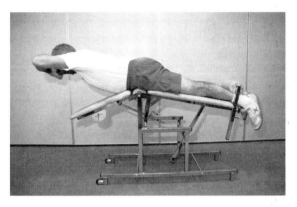

Figure 29.23a

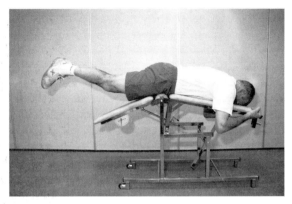

Figure 29.25a

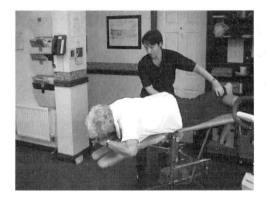

Figure 29.23b

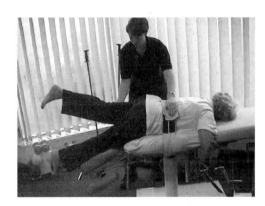

Figure 29.25b

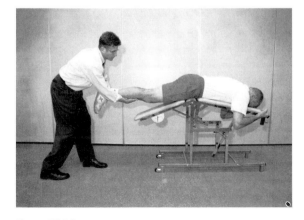

Figure 29.24

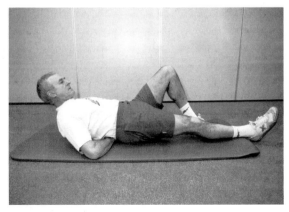

Figure 29.26

later in the programme, at the third or fourth session. The patient should work up to three sets of 10 repetitions for each side during the course of the programme. This should develop and maintain the appropriate strength ratio during training.

Because of the demanding nature of this part of the programme, as well as the need to improve the overall contribution of the QL, the patient is instructed to perform a floor exercise to challenge this muscle group. The patient is requested to lie on the floor in the side posture position supported by the arm with the knees bent to 90 degrees and the hips slightly flexed. The patient is then instructed to lift the pelvis off the floor by contracting the QL closest to the floor (Figure 29.29). This exercise should be performed bilaterally and as a precursor to the more demanding exercise depicted in Figure 29.28. The patient may continue to perform these exercises while at home, starting at three to five repetitions and increasing to 15–20.

This part of the programme will address the strength and endurance of some of the upper and lower limb support musculature to enhance and stabilize the kinetic chains during various activities. These include: the latissimus dorsi, hip abductor and adductors, and the quadriceps. The latissimus dorsi is particularly important in that owing to its anatomical connection with the thoracolumbar fascia it functions to assist during lifting activities by transferring loads between the upper and lower extremity. This may have significant functional implications for geriatric patients with respect to carrying out ADLs and independence. These exercises are also meant to stabilize overall lumbopelvic function. The purpose of these exercises is to develop some strength and endurance of the surrounding soft-tissue structures.

- Lateral pull-downs: These start at the patient's tolerance with regard to weight, depending on equipment, and proceed with sets of 12 repetitions. The patient works up to three sets of 12 repetitions over the training period (Figure 29.30) (Steens Physical, Norway).
- Quadriceps squats: These start at the patient's tolerance with regard to weight, depending on equipment, and proceed with sets of 12 repetitions. The patients works up to three sets of 12 repetitions over the training period. The equipment is set so that the knee angle is < 90 degrees (Figure 29.31) (Steens Physical) in order for full extension to occur with-

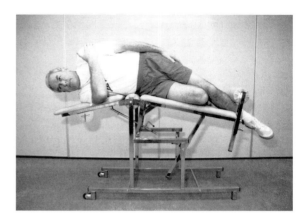

Figure 29.27

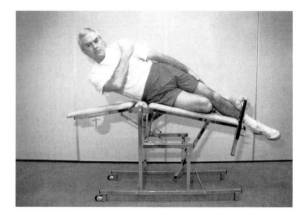

Figure 29.28

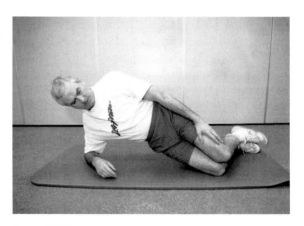

Figure 29.29

out locking the knees (Figure 29.32). If equipment is not available free weights may be used to perform static squats or dynamic lunges to challenge these muscle groups.

- Hip abductor/adductor: These start at the patient's tolerance with regard to weight, depending on equipment, and proceed with sets of 12 repetitions. The patients works up to three sets of 12 repetitions over the training period (Figures 29.33, 29.34) (Steens Physical).

The patient should warm down with stretching and cycling or treadmill walking as per the beginning of the programme to relax the muscle groups that have been under load. The stretching exercises can be advised as home exercises. It is important to inform the patient that they may experience some soreness as a result of these activities. Appropriate protocols should be explained to minimize these potential detrimental side-effects. Patients should also be encouraged to continue and complete the programme with a view of proceeding to lifelong activity and exercise once rehabilitation has been adequately achieved.

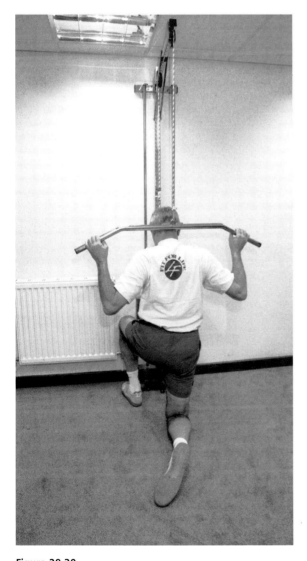

Figure 29.30

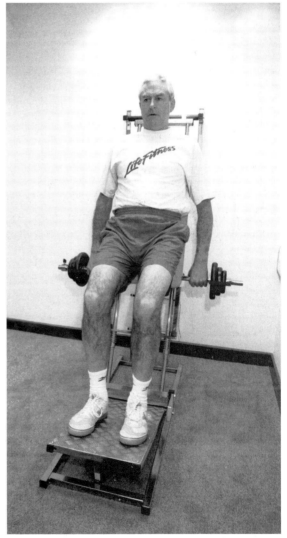

Figure 29.31

Balance and co-ordination exercises will be discussed later in the chapter.

Cervical spine

The cornerstone of the cervical spine programme is strength training.[40] Even though the cervical spine muscles only represent 7–8 % of total body weight, compared with 65–70% for the lumbar musculature, they are twice as strong overall. The postural demands placed on the cervical muscles are significantly different to those placed on the lumbar muscles, as the former muscle group must balance the weight of the head against gravity during all ADLs. Both men and women retain strength and endurance values until the sixth decade of life and, as is the case with the lumbar spine, there is a strength hierarchy that must be balanced to achieve optimal function. In terms of strength, the extensor group dominates, primarily because of its role in posture, followed by the lateral flexors, and the flexors, respectively.[36]

The muscles of the cervical spine must not only meet significant strength requirements during normal daily activities, but they are also crucial for balance and position sensing. These abilities must be retrained, particularly among patients experiencing chronic neck pain or post-whiplash injury.[46]

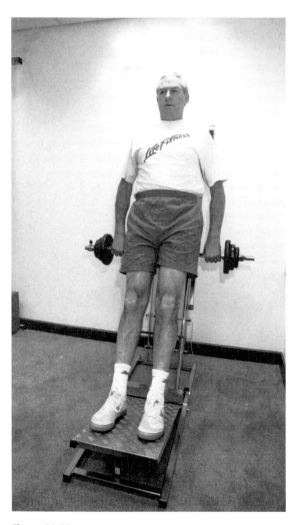

Figure 29.32

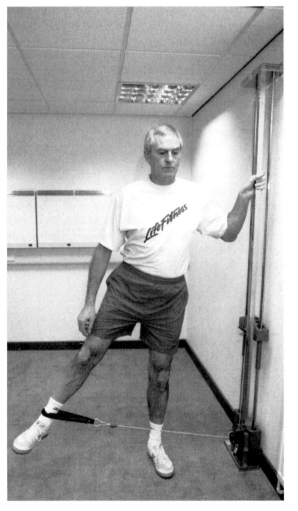

Figure 29.33

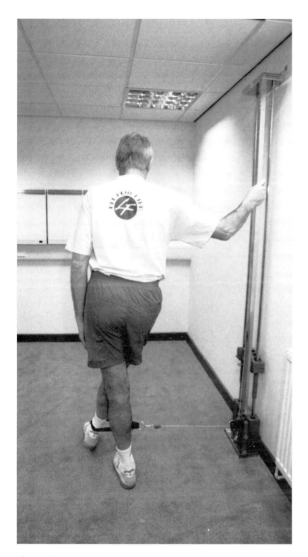

Figure 29.34

There are no specific age barriers associated with this strength training for the cervical spine. Jordan et al.[6] investigated the physical characteristics of both healthy and non-healthy subjects and found that isometric strength and endurance values were well maintained up to and including the sixth decade of life in both men and women. According to these results, individuals in their fifties could train at essentially the same level as people in their twenties. This creates a more flexible and safer approach to rehabilitation for a wide range of patients, including those in the geriatric age groups. Certain aspects, such as facet degen-

eration, must be taken into consideration as this process increases in both gender as part of the natural ageing of the cervical posterior zygapophyseal joints. Simply restricting the overall range of extension should accommodate these specific joint changes.

The cervical programme is very similar in structure and time to the lumbar spine protocols. The programme consists of the following:

- warm-up period: stationary exercise bike or treadmill
- stretching: general upper back and neck procedures
- intense cervical strength conditioning
- upper back and shoulder strength and conditioning exercises
- balance and position sense procedures
- postexercise stretching
- warm-down: exercise bike or treadmill
- outcomes management.

Part 1 (warm-up)

The warm-up is designed to prepare the upper back and neck regions for a training encounter. The bike or treadmill is not used for cardiovascular training, but a PAR-Q should be obtained before starting the exercise. The warm-up on the bike should be for approximately 10 min (Figure 29.1). The patient may need to build up to this amount over a period of time.

The stretching procedures are designed to isolate the soft tissues and joints of the upper back and neck bilaterally. Patients should be sitting during the performance of most of these exercises and they should be instructed to hold the stretch for about 15–20 s without any bouncing or excessive pulling. The patient should proceed through the stretches methodically and systematically, learning the techniques properly so that they can be used as a home programme.

A sample of the specific stretches is shown in Figures 29.35–29.41. Stretches can be added or deleted depending on the patient's tolerance. It is essential not to overstress the passive structures and to stay within tissue tolerance. Proper technique is also very important in learning the correct approach to these warm-up exercises.

At this stage, the patient should also be shown the cervical stability and quadruped posture in order to begin re-educating cervical musculature. The patient is instructed to adopt the quadruped position (Figure 29.42). The patient is then instructed to tuck the chin

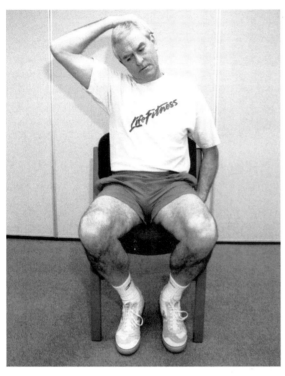

Figure 29.35

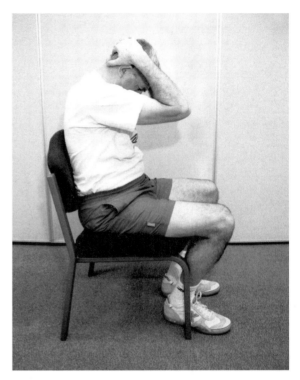

Figure 29.37

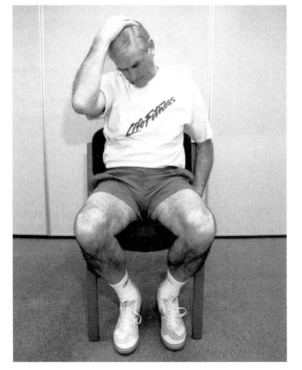

Figure 29.36

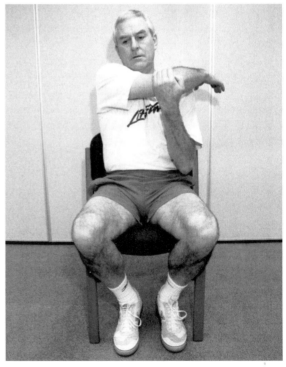

Figure 29.38

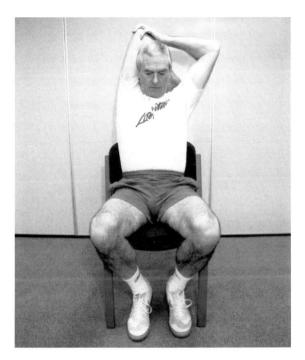

Figure 29.39

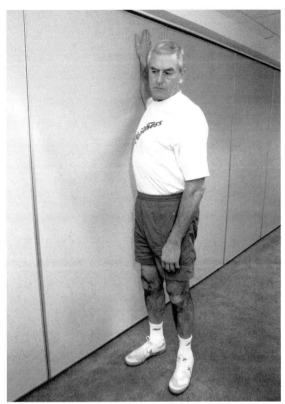

Figure 29.41

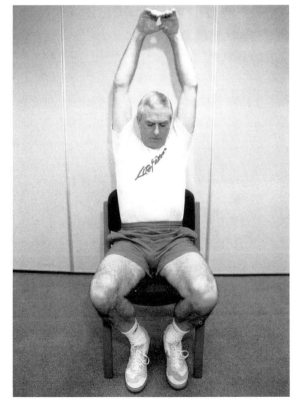

Figure 29.40

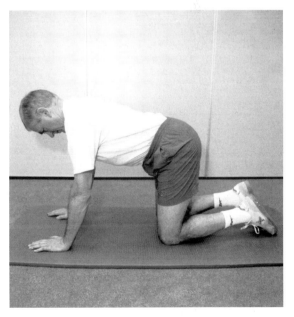

Figure 29.42

in (double chin) but not to flex the head to the chest (Figure 29.43). Tucking the chin in activates the deep neck flexors, which assists in stabilizing the cervical spine. (Note the position of the arms and the alignment of the head and upper back). The patient should be instructed to perform this activity during each training session and at home. They may also perform simple tasks from this position, as described in Figure 29.18. The patient may also adopt the neutral spine posture for the lumbar spine by co-contracting the deep stabilizing muscles at the same time. This may potentially increase central nervous stimulation and enhance the training response.

Part 2 (full-range strength training)

The key to the cervical spine is progressive submaximal full-range strength training of all the cervical spine musculature according to the strongest to weakest hierarchy. This is best accomplished using equipment specifically designed and appropriately tested for this task, and the equipment should provide sufficient resistance in all planes of motion. The equipment selected should also be flexible enough to adapt to a variety of patient types of all age groups (Figure 29.44; Steen Physical, Norway). The equipment shown in Figure 29.40 is widely used and has been employed in a number of research projects comparing various treatment protocols for patients with chronic neck pain or post- whiplash injuries.[40] This equipment is adaptable to persons of all shapes and sizes because it has a well-engineered seat and resistance arm. (Figure 29.44). Other equipment may be used, such as Therabands or simple isometric exercises, but it is the authors' opinion that these procedures do not provide a large enough training stimulus for the cervical musculature.

The length–tension relationship (point of maximum isometric contraction strength) for the cervical spine is considered to be 30 degrees of extension from the neutral for the extensors and 45 degrees for flexion from the neutral for the flexors.[40] The relative strength ratio between extensors and flexors is considered to be 1.7:1 under normal conditions. This ratio must always be kept in mind when structuring an individual programme. Most patients who are symptomatic have a 1:1 extensor to flexor ratio, which is inadequate in terms of overall support and stability. Relative weight values have been modified to accommodate the older age group.

Sidebending to the right and left (lateral flexors)

The patient is instructed to sit facing forwards with the feet flat on the floor, grasping the handles near the seat to encourage good posture and muscle group isolation and reduce other muscle recruitment. The resistance arm pad is placed so that the bottom of the pad is just touching the side of the head above the ear. This can be accomplished by adjusting the resistance arm height and length. Next, the patient is instructed to side-bend the head towards the left shoulder (Figure 29.45). Initially, this should be performed with no resistance except for the weight of the arm (0.5 kg). This prepares the muscle groups for activity and also provides the patient with appropriate instruction as they learn the protocols. The patient should then allow the apparatus to return to the neutral position. One set of 12 repetitions is performed with no weight. Following this, the patient is instructed to repeat the same procedure, but this time with an appropriate starting weight. This will depend on a number of factors, including the patient's presenting condition, pain level and confidence. This will take a certain amount of clinical judgement, but the exercise should start at a lower weight and progress slowly. One should aim at starting at 1–2 kg for women and 2–3 kg for men, or at patient tolerance. It should be kept in mind that this is highly variable. Weight should be added progressively over the programme period at a rate no greater than 10–15%/week, starting at one set of 12 repetitions with increasing weight to a frequency to three sets of 12 repetitions. Programme length and progression will be individually based upon a number of factors, including pain levels, perceived disability and motivation. There may be some drop off in terms of patient compliance over the course of the programme, but the practitioner should emphasize the importance of patient commitment to the programme. Both left and right lateral flexion should be performed, incorporating the same procedure. It may be wise to assist the patient in the initial few sets by helping the him or her to push the resistance arm. This may be especially important in the initial phase of the programme in order to build the patient's confidence and trust.

Forward flexion (neck flexors)

To train the neck flexors the patient must be seated facing the resistance pad which is placed directly against the forehead. Releasing the pin under the seat and swivelling the apparatus into its new position changes the

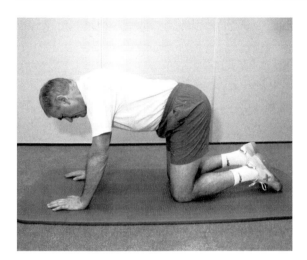

Figure 29.43

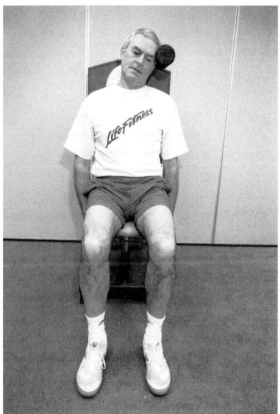

Figure 29.45

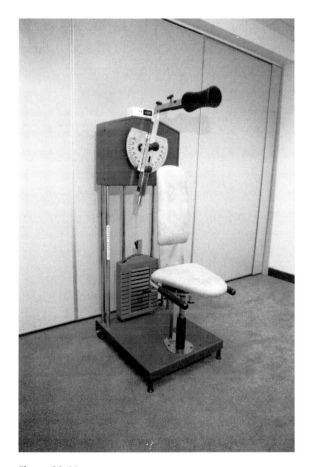

Figure 29.44

seat orientation. The patient is instructed to retract his or her chin in and then flex the head forwards, moving the pad towards the chest (Figure 29.46). This procedure activates the deep neck flexors that assist in stabilizing the cervical spine. The first set of 12 repetitions is without weight, as above. The next set is with weight, starting at 0.5–1.0 kg for women and 1.0–2.0 kg for men, or at patient tolerance. The patient is instructed to perform one set of 12 repetition throughout the entire programme since they are well down on the strength hierarchy. Weight should be added progressively and submaximally for all ranges of motion, keeping the strength ratio in mind at all times. From a clinical perspective, this may have to be reversed, particularly when dealing with chronic post-whiplash patients. The deep neck flexors have been shown to be much weaker than the extensors.[5] For these cases, flexors would be trained up to three sets of 12, while only one set of 12 repetitions is required for the extensors. Once the appropriate ratio

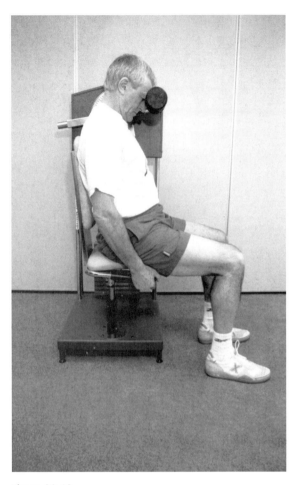

Figure 29.46

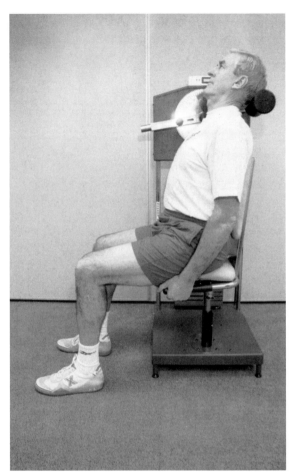

Figure 29.47

has been established, the programme can be further modified to accommodate the patient's other needs. It may be wise to help the patient in the initial few sets by assisting the movement of the resistance arm.

Extensions (extensor muscles)

The extensors generally are the most important muscle group in the upper back and neck region. Their function is to stabilize and maintain postures for a considerable time during the performance of various daily activities. The extensors have been reported to be weaker in patients presenting with chronic neck pain and headaches.[5] The seat is swivelled around to place the resistance pad against the back of the head. The cushion is placed above the external occipital protuberance (EOP) while the head is held in the neutral posture. The patient is instructed to extend the head and look up at the ceiling in order to engage the upper back extensor mechanism (Figure 29.47). The initial set is performed with no weight, as described above, followed by resistance for the next set. The next set is with weight starting at 1.5–2.0 kg for women and 2.0–3.0 kg for men, or at patient tolerance. It may be wise to limit the amount of extension to avoid stressing the posterior facets, which are prone to degenerative changes in both gender with advancing age. It my also be wise to guide the resistance arm as the patient extends his or her head in order to provide a training distance in the initial phase of the programme. This may be particularly important if the patient is struggling to push the preselected weight.

Part 3

This part of the programme will address the strength and endurance of some of the upper back and neck support musculature to enhance and stabilize the kinetic chains during various activities. The muscle include the upper trapezius, latissimus dorsi, deltoid, anterior chest wall (pectoralis major) and the interscapular musculature (rhomboids). The latissimus dorsi, owing to its anatomical connection with the thoracolumbar fascia, assists during lifting activities by transferring loads between the upper and lower extremity. This may have significant functional implications for geriatric patients with respect to carrying out ADLs and independence. These exercises are also meant to help to stabilize the upper back and neck region and to assist in lumbopelvic function. The key in this section of the programme is to develop some strength and endurance in the surrounding soft-tissue structures. In general, weight magnitudes should be kept in the 1–6 kg region, working within the patient's initial tolerance and then increasing submaximally and progressively through the programme. Small, hand-held free weights are optimal for this section of the programme.

- Lateral pull-downs: These start up at the patient's tolerance with regard to weight, depending on the equipment selected, and proceed with sets of 12 repetitions. The patient works up to three sets of 12 repetitions over the training period (Figure 29.30). The bar should be brought down behind the head at a rate of 15–16 repetitions/min. Both positive and negative contractions are emphasized.
- Shoulder rolls: These start the patient's tolerance with regard to weight, depending on equipment, and proceed with sets of 12 repetitions. The patients works up to three sets of 12 repetitions over the training period (Figure 29.48).
- Shoulder abductions: These start at the patient's tolerance with regard to weight and proceed with sets of 12 repetitions. The patient works up to three sets of 12 repetition over the training period (Figure 29.49).
- Anterior chest wall (supine flies): These start at the patient's tolerance with regard to weight depending on equipment and proceed with sets of 12 repetitions. The patient works up to three sets of 12 repetitions over the training period (Figure 29.50).
- Interscapular (reverse prone Flies): These start at the patient's tolerance with regard to weight depending on equipment and proceed with sets of 12 repetitions. The patient works up to three sets of 12 repetitions over the training period (Figure 29.51).

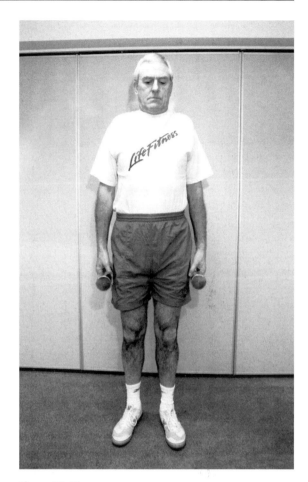

Figure 29.48

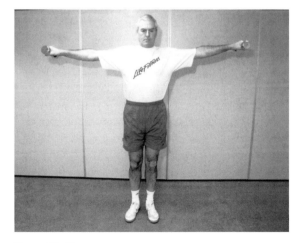

Figure 29.49

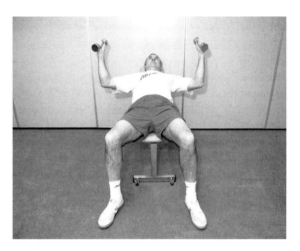

Figure 29.50

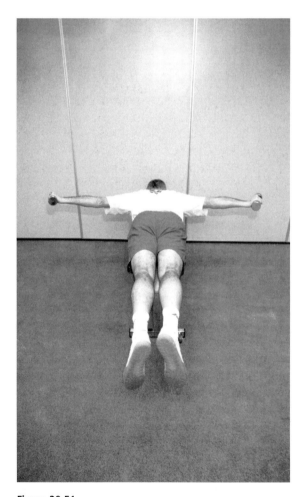

Figure 29.51

Part 4 (warm-down)

The patient should warm down with stretching and cycling or treadmill walking as performed at the beginning of the programme to relax the muscle groups that have been under load. The stretching exercises can be advised as home exercises. The patient should be warned that they may experience some soreness. Strategies to minimize this side-effect should be explained to the patient. Patients should also be encouraged to continue and complete the programme with the ultimate goal of lifelong activity and exercise even after successful rehabilitation has been adequately achieved.

Balance and co-ordination exercises will be discussed in more detail in the next section of the chapter.

Functional spinal stabilization and sensorimotor training: protocols and rationale for the older population

Spinal stabilization exercises and sensorimotor training are important components of any rehabilitation program, regardless of age. These activities are very practical and cost-effective methods to assist functional recovery in patients with subacute, chronic and/or recurrent back and neck pain.[61] They are based on the Panjabi's concept of spinal stabilization with its three components:[50] (i) the active component, consisting of the deep small muscles surrounding the spine; (ii) the passive component, which is made up of the ligament structures that act as transducers; and (iii) the central nervous system (CNS) which acts as the controlling component. Dysfunction, injury or disease to any of these three components may lead to spinal instability.[51] As mentioned previously, most back pain is not the result of frank trauma but more likely to be due to trivial movement caused by a breakdown in the stability system secondary to motor control error.[51,52] For example, the spinal column devoid of muscles buckles at a very low force of 90 N. Normally, with muscles intact, the spinal column can handle up to 20 times that level of compression. According to Panjabi, 'this large load carrying capacity is achieved by the participation of well-co-ordinated muscles surrounding the spinal column'.[50]

The goal of spinal stabilization is to train and improve motor control and stability, and to activate the maximum number of motor units possible in the target muscle, while minimizing the joint load in order to meet the variety of demands of daily activities.[51] In the older populations these exercises are specifically designed to improve balance and to reduce the number of potentially dangerous falls. They also provide another way of managing patient care and promoting independent activity.

Sensorimotor training is a method of stimulating the CNS through a bombardment of afferent impulses. The CNS depends on afferent input from the periphery to order appropriately movement patterns that are harmonious and co-ordinated and that provide stability to the musculoskeletal system. With sensorimotor training, an attempt is made to facilitate the automatic or reflexogenic reactions that the locomotion system creates in response to unexpected stimuli from the periphery. In neck training an attempt is also made to improve the efficiency of the reflexes that govern eye–head–neck–upper extremity co-ordination, which is an important aspect of normal neck function.

As a rule, training should progress from stable to labile surfaces and from simple to complex activity, to provide maximal train stimulus. During training attention should be paid to correct posture, which should be maintained throughout.

Correction should begin at the feet and gradually extend proximally:

- feet
- knees
- hips
- pelvis
- spine
- shoulders
- head.

These training systems are meant to be extremely flexible and entirely based upon patient indications and needs.

See Liebenson[37] and Murphy[62] for further reading and references regarding spinal stabilization and sensorimotor training for both cervical spine and lower back rehabilitation.

Stabilization protocols

The main aims of low back stabilization are to increase the co-contraction ability and endurance of the multifidus and transverse abdominus muscles, together with their speed of contraction.[52] The strength and endurance of the surrounding phasic and postural muscles are also addressed, as described in detail earlier in the chapter.

Duration of exercises

It is important that the duration of stimulation during training be of sufficient length to challenge the capacity of the CNS to maintain and improve overall stabilization. In general, the patient should perform the maximum number of repetitions that he or she is capable of performing while maintaining stability. The number of repetitions is gradually increased until 10 repetitions can be performed with good stability, after which time the patient is ready to progress to the next level of difficulty. This is usually set at about 1–2 min of uninterrupted activity. Once the exercises can be performed under supervision in the office, the patient may perform them as a home routine, having mastered the psychomotor skills and become able to execute the protocols safely and confidently.

General points

Initially, the patient should only feel a mild 'burn' in the large muscles, while feeling no strain in the spinal regions. A key point is the emphasis on maintaining the spine in the functional range during training. Patients will progress at different rates depending on their entry level and any other confounding factors with respect to their age, level of fitness and overall health. Sessions may vary from 5 to 10 min as part of the overall rehabilitation programme, as outlined throughout this chapter.

Time factor and goals of sensorimotor training

The exercises can be performed on a daily basis for endurance and stability, or three times per week for strengthening. A total of 2–3 months may be required to achieve a physiological response and training adaptation, whether the objective is strength, endurance, balance or stability. At all times the patient must feel comfortable and confident to continue the protocols unsupervised. In order to ensure this that is the case, instruction given to the patient should begin from very simple exercises (illustrated below) to those that are more complex. One of the most important factors is to establish functional objectives and to work systematically towards them with the patient. These objectives or goals are based solely upon the demands placed on the individual in order for them to carry out their ADLs in as efficient and confident a manner as possible.

The goals of training are:

- to achieve automatic control of muscle function, specifically those muscles responsible for posture and gait
- to increase the stimuli from the peripheral structures (skin, joints and muscles) in order to increase activity of subcortical regulatory centres, thereby increasing the likelihood of automated muscle action
- to improve the efficiency and effectiveness of common movement patterns in which the cervical spine and upper extremities engage on a regular basis
- to improve the efficiency of the reflexes those govern eye–head–neck–upper extremity co-ordination.

Exercise tracks

Lumbopelvic range of motion

Patients experiencing low back pain often find it hard to control simple movements in this region. This exercise promotes and explores the functional range of lumbopelvic motion and decreases patient anxiety regarding movement. The patient is instructed how to perform anterior and posterior pelvic tilts, after which they are taught to perform these tilting movements in a variety of different positions. These positions include: supine, prone, quadruped, kneeling seated and standing, as illustrated in Figures 29.14–29.17. These protocols are the foundation for this part of rehabilitation and require time to learn and perform efficiently.

Abdominal hollowing (tummy tuck)

The patient is taught to how to co-contract the transverse abdominus and lumbar multifidus muscles by actively pulling the navel inwards and slightly upwards towards the spine. The patient should learn this skill in all static and dynamic postures, including sitting, standing, lifting, walking and when rising from a seated to a standing position. This exercise establishes and promotes spinal stability and it has been suggested that it should form the basis of all spinal stabilization exercises, both for endurance and for strength.[51,52] The most common position in which to learn this skill is to place the patient in either the supine or the prone posture. The patient is taught to perform abdominal hollowing by actively drawing the navel in towards the spine and upwards towards the lower ribs (Figure 29.17). This is described in detail earlier in the chapter.

Patient assessment

Sensorimotor assessment methods

Functional assessment is subjective and a number of functional tests may help in selecting patients who may benefit from sensorimotor training. A general impression can also be gained of a patient's kinaesthetic awareness by simple observation. For example, many patients may not be able to perform a pelvic tilt exercise or may seem generally uncoordinated. This may be particularly evident among older persons. This is a clinical assumption and it is the author's opinion that some sort of sensorimotor training should be included in all rehabilitation programmes, regardless of age. The level of intensity and difficulty must be developed according to the patient's current capabilities. It is important to start at a very low level of activity and progress over time, once the initial skills have been thoroughly mastered. Patient confidence is paramount in any exercise programme.

Simple assessment protocols may be used during patient investigation to determine the need for spinal stabilization and sensorimotor training. Simply asking

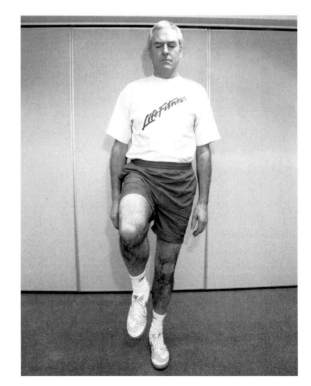

Figure 29.52

the patient to stand alternately on one leg and then the other with the eyes open and then closed and observing their response may be adequate to evaluate the balancing system (Figure 29.52). More elaborate investigational tests, used to isolate those persons requiring additional rehabilitation, are performed by eliminating auditory and visual input (Figure 29.53). Patient selection for these assessment procedures needs to be based upon a number of clinical factors, including general fitness and age. Assessing the patient while he or she is sitting may sufficiently challenge important functional systems (Figure 29.54). The patient is requested to maintain bilateral arm position while rotating the head and neck fully in directions with the eyes both open and closed. Any deviation in the arm position is considered to indicate some functional loss.

Indications for use

Sensorimotor stimulation is beneficial when used as part of any exercise programme, in that it helps to improve muscle co-ordination and motor programming or regulation and increase the speed of muscle activation.

The sensorimotor approach is not a rigid programme or system. It can be used in all types of cases and can be tailored to each individual patient's needs and age group. The exercise protocols should be flexible to meet the patient's abilities and level of motor performance. Safety should always be considered when developing an individualized programme.

Clinical Indications for sensorimotor training

- unstable knee
- sprained or unstable ankle
- chronic back and neck pain
- faulty posture
- faulty movement patterns
- prevention and treatment of ataxia.

These signs should not be seen as outright indications, as they may normalize with the correction of joint and muscle dysfunction.

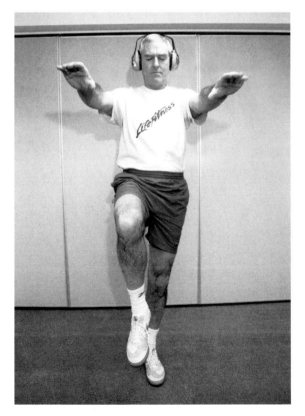

Figure 29.53

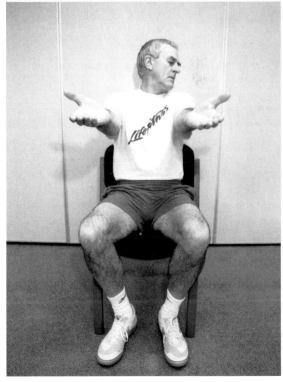

Figure 29.54

Exercise gym balls and rocker board

Some exercises can be combined with gym balls and rocker boards to introduce a labile surface for important sensorimotor training. This will place more demand on the spinal stabilization system and challenge the nervous system that controls motor behaviour and movement co-ordination. These elements of control and reaction times seem to be impaired in patients suffering from recurrent back pain. This would necessitate appropriate strategies to address these important deficiencies.

These exercises and associated equipment can add some fun to the programme and stretching exercises can be done using the gym ball to help the stretch. Back extension endurance exercises similar to those on the angle bench can also be performed on a gym ball, together with other extensor exercises, to add some variety to the overall programme.

Sensorimotor training: low back (rocker board)

Rocker boards are used as a liable surface. The rocker board is unstable in only one plane. The patient stands on the board in various directions to control the plane of stability. The exercises proceed from eyes open to eyes closed and from two-legged standing to single-leg stance. To elicit a faster reflexive response, the patient can also be pushed gently about the torso and shoulders by the trainer. Overhead arm movements, as well as catching a ball and turning the head, are other methods to vary the centre of gravity and make the programme more interesting. Mixing labile and stable surfaces are ways of making the ability to control stability more difficult.

The following rocker-board exercises are recommended as entry-level training for older age groups. These exercises include all axes of motion both assisted and unassisted:

- The patient is requested to balance their weight centrally on the rocker board using ski poles or balance sticks (Figure 29.55). From this position the patient is requested to move the front edge of the rocker board to just meet the floor and then back to neutral. He or she is requested to repeat this up to 10 times forwards and then backwards, using the poles to assist balance. The patient should progress to 20 repetitions.
- As the patient progresses through the exercises in Figure 29.55 and develops more skill he or she can move to unassisted protocols depicted in Figure 29.56. Here

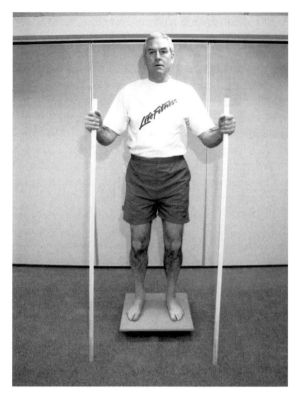

Figure 29.55

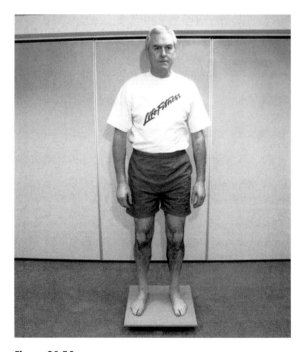

Figure 29.56

the patient is requested to move the front edge of the board towards but not touching the floor from neutral and back to neutral up to 10 times (Figure 29.56). The patient is then instructed to move the board backwards and repeat up to 10 times, progressing over time to a maximum of 20 repetitions.

- The patient is instructed to turn the board 90 degrees and balance in a lateral direction both assisted and unassisted for approximately 2 min (Figure 29.57). The goal during this exercise is to maintain central balance with good posture and central gaze for 1 min, progressing to a maximum of 2 min.
- The patient is then instructed to position the board diagonally in both directions and attempt to maintain balance for 1 min, progressing to a maximum of 2 min of effort in total (Figure 29.58).

Cervical spine stabilization

The mechanisms by which the cervical spine maintains its stability does not operate in isolation from the rest of the body but, rather, are simple localized manifestations of the whole-body stabilization system that is co-ordinated by the CNS. When training the system, it is best to locate certain parts of the system where function may be impaired, followed by integrating these parts with the whole. The cervical spine is a both reflex-orientated and a strength-orientated system, and this should be considered during rehabilitation.

Head and neck stability

Several muscles are important for maintaining head and neck stability, including:

- posterior intersegmental muscles (multifidi and suboccipitals)
- deep neck flexors (longus capitis and colli)
- lower cervical/upper thoracic extensors (semispinalis cervicis and longissimus cervicis)
- scapula stabilizers (middle and lower trapezius and serratus anterior).

Eye–head–neck co-ordination

Several important functional reflexes co-ordinate head, eye and neck movement, including:

- cervico-ocular reflex
- vestibulo-ocular reflex
- cervicocollic reflex
- vestibulocollic reflex
- optokinetic reflex to monitor smooth pursuit and saccades.

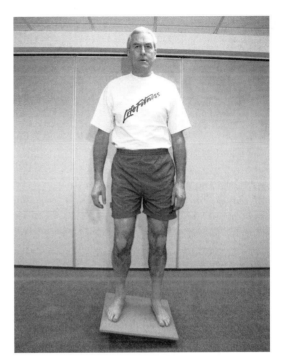

Figure 29.57

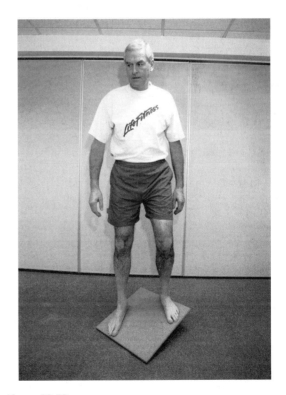

Figure 29.58

Cervical stabilization tracts

- Cervical brace position: The chin is slightly tucked in and the cervical spine elongated. This action is very subtle and places the head in a neutral posture. This activity forms the basis for all the other exercises illustrated earlier in the chapter (Figures 29.42, 29.43). The exercise progresses up to 15–20 s.
- Quadruped book balance: This is the same as above, but a small, very light, hard backed book is placed on the back of the patient's head (Figure 29.59). The patient holds the position until loss of stability or shaking occurs. The exercise progresses up to 15–20 s. The patient may progress to a slightly heavier book to assist and maintain overall strength gains derived from other sections of the programme.
- Single arm raises: The quadruped position is adopted and the patient is instructed to raise one arm overhead as high as possible without losing stability. Alternate arm raises further the facilitation of the middle and lower trapezius. The patient is instructed to open fingers as wide as possible (Figure 29.60).

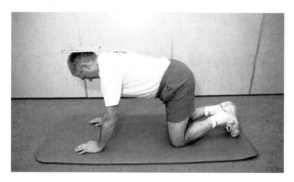

Figure 29.59

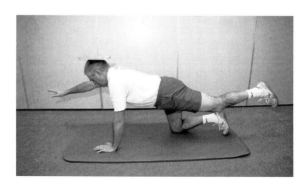

Figure 29.60

- Single leg raise: The quadruped position is adopted and the patient is instructed to raise one leg behind as high as possible without losing stability. The legs raises are alternated. This is illustrated in Figure 29.19 and can be performed with or without a book for balance. The patient progresses up to 15–20 s of balanced effort.
- Cross crawl: The quadruped position is adopted and the patient instructed to raise one arm and the opposite leg within his or her functional range of movement without losing stability, and alternate (Figure 29.61). Once the patient can maintain stability with the single arm raise, single leg raise and cross-crawl, these can be performed with the use of a book.

Gym balls: cervical and lumbar rehabilitation

The introduction of gym balls to vary the exercise surface and challenge the nervous system is another method of stimulating the nervous system while providing an environment for all ages to engage in various aspects of functional rehabilitation and additional sensorimotor training. The following exercises are only an example of a vast number of possible protocols using a gym ball during rehabilitation management. The key is to be creative and work within the patient's capabilities and needs.

- The patient is instructed to sit and balance on the gym ball, focus on a point on the wall and move laterally while maintaining central gaze in both left and right directions (starting at five repetitions and progressing up to 20 repetitions) (Figure 29.62). The patient is asked to move laterally in both directions and, once this skill has been mastered, to attempt

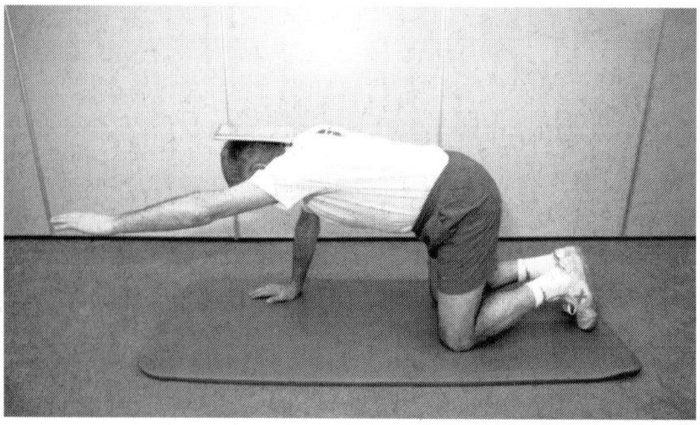

Figure 29.61

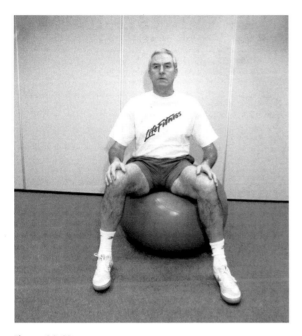

Figure 29.62

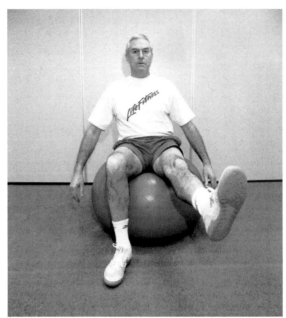

Figure 29.63

clockwise and counterclockwise movements while maintaining central gaze. Supervision is necessary until performance is safe and effective.

- The patient, following progression from the exercise described in Figure 29.62, is requested to lift one leg off the floor and eventually the opposite arm while maintaining a central gaze in order to challenge the CNS and promote sensorimotor training (Figure 29.63). The patient learns to hold these postures for 5–10 s, progressing to 15–20 s.

The following exercises are examples of entry-level ball exercises that may be incorporated as an adjunct to the more demanding elements of the overall rehabilitation programme or added to a home programme.

- The patient is instructed to balance over the ball and perform a trunk lift (Figure 29.64). This exercise may be used as an entry-level method to train both the extensors and balance systems. The patient should start at 5–10 repetitions, progressing to 25–30 to place more demand on the spinal extensor mechanism.
- The patient is instructed to balance supine on the ball, establish balance and perform trunk flexion exercises both to train the abdominal musculature and to stimulate balance systems (Figure 29.65). The patient should progress from 5–10 repetitions to 15–20 repetitions.

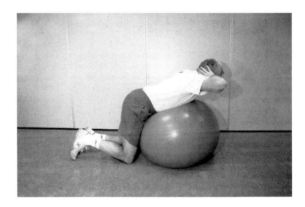

Figure 29.64

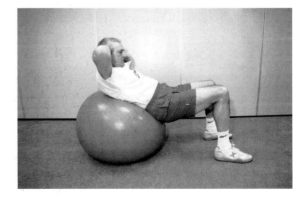

Figure 29.65

- The patient is instructed to balance supine on the floor with the feet securely positioned and lift the pelvis initially with the knees bent (Figure 29.66) and then with the knees extended (Figure 29.67), placing additional demand on the stabilizing structures.
- Pelvic stabilization without a gym ball: The patient initiates the exercise depicted in Figure 29.68 and progresses to the more demanding protocol shown in Figure 29.69. Once again, the patient is instructed to start at a low level of activity and progress in both numbers of repetitions and time. The patient is also instructed to chin tuck and tummy tuck during the performance of these exercises to maximize their effectiveness during training.

These are just a few of the many possible exercises that can be added to a programme to provide variety and motivation. The exercises illustrated above are foundational and should be mastered before progressing to more demanding activities.

Summary

This chapter has presented a specific approach to geriatric rehabilitation for both neck and low back pain. Several issues have been raised with respect to patient safety during any rehabilitation programme. The programmes are supported by a substantial evidence-base with respect to the selection of activities for patients presenting with chronic forms of back pain. Special considerations were noted with respect to the age of the patient and the possibility of underlying osteoporosis that may warrant clinical vigilance. Nevertheless, this chapter has emphasized the importance of maintaining and sustaining levels of activity in order to prevent functional decline for those practitioners dealing with elderly patients now and in the near future.

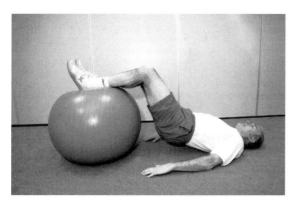

Figure 29.66

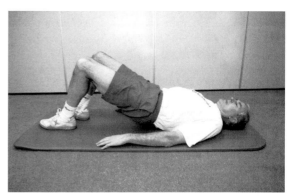

Figure 29.68

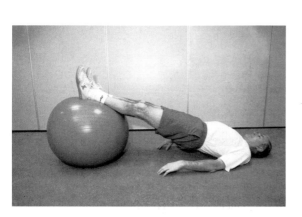

Figure 29.67

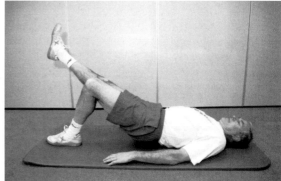

Figure 29.68

Acknowledgements

We would like to acknowledge Annabel Kier-Byfield DC for her assistance during the preparation of this chapter and Mike Davies of Media Services at the University of Glamorgan for the photographic work and figure preparation. We would also like to thank Gordon King DC as the model used in most of the photographs and Jeffrey Shurr DC for providing additional photographs of his rehabilitation clinic. We acknowledge Active Care Solutions, UK, for supplying the rehabilitation equipment described in the programme.

References

1 Jenkins EA, Cooper C. The epidemiology of osteoporosis: who is at risk? J Musculoskeletal Med 1993; 10(3): 18–33.

2 Eisenberg DM, Davis RB, Ettner SL *et al.* Trends in alternative medicine use in the United States, 1990–1997. JAMA 1998; 11: 1569–1575.

3 Burton CV, Cassidy JD. Economics, epidemiology, and risk factors. In: Kirkaldy-Willis WH, Burton CV, eds. Managing Low Back Pain. 3rd edn. London: Churchill Livingstone, 1992: 1–6.

4 Cassidy JD, Thiel HW, Kirkaldy-Willis WH. Side posture manipulation for lumbar intervertebral disk herniation. J Manipulative Physiol Ther 1993; 16: 96–103.

5 Jordan A, Oestergaard K. Rehabilitation of neck/shoulder patients in primary health care clinics. J Manipulative Physiol Ther 1996; 19: 32–35.

6 Jordan A, Mehlsen J, Oestergaard K. A comparison of physical characteristics between patients seeking treatment for neck pain and age-matched healthy people. J Manipulative Physiol Ther 1997; 20: 468–475.

7 Waddell G. Modern management of spinal disorders. J Manipulative Physiol Ther 1995; 18: 590–596.

8 Manniche C *et al.* Low-back pain: frequency, management and prevention from an HAD perspective. Dan Health Technol Assess 1999; 1(1).

9 Waddell G, Burton AK. Occupational Health guidelines for the Management of Low Back Pain at Work – Evidence Review. London: Faculty of Occupational Medicine, 2000.

10 Edmond SL, Felson DT. Prevalence of back symptoms in elders. J Rheumatol 2000; 27: 220–225.

11 Bressler HB, Keyes WJ, Rochon PA, Badley E. The prevalence of low back pain in the elderly. Spine 1999; 24: 1813–1819.

12 Mayer T *et al.* The effect of age on outcomes of tertiary rehabilitation for chronic disabling spinal disorders. Proceedings of the North American Spine Society, New Orleans, 2000.

13 Anderson GBJ, Weinstein JN. Focus issue on osteoporosis. Spine 1997; 22(24s): 1s.

14 Glaser DL, Kaplan FS. Osteoporosis. Definition and clinical presentation. Spine 1997; 22(24s): 125–165.

15 Bennell K, Khan K, McKay H. The role of physiotherapy in the prevention and treatment of osteoporosis. Manual Ther 2000; 5: 198–213.

16 Mannello DM. Osteoporosis: assessment and treatment options. Top Clin Chiropractic 1997; 4(3): 30–33.

17 Cooper C, Melton LJ. Magnitude and impact of osteoporosis and fractures. In: Marcus R, Feldman D, Kelsey J, eds. Osteoporosis. San Diego, CA: Academic Press, 1996.

18 Pluijm SMF *et al.* Consequences of vertebral deformities in older men and women. J Bone Miner Res 2000; 15: 1564–1572.

19 Sarkisian CA, Liu H, Guterrez PR *et al.* Modifiable risk factors predict functional decline among older women: a prospectively validated clinical prediction tool. The Study of Osteoporotic Fractures Research Group. J Am Geriatr Soc 2000; 48: 170–178.

20 Kronhed AC, Moller M. Effects of physical exercise on bone mass, balance skill and aerobic capacity in woman and men with low bone mineral density, after one year of training – a prospective study. Scand J Med Sci Sports 1998; 8: 290–298.

21 Malmros B, Mortensen L, Jensen MB, Charles P. Positive effects of physiotherapy on chronic pain and performance in osteoporosis. Osteoporosis Int 1998; 8: 215–221.

22 Karlsson MK, Linden C, Karlsson C *et al.* Exercise during growth and bone mineral density and fractures in old age. Lancet 2000; 355: 469–470.

23 Kannus R. Preventing osteoporosis, falls, and fractures among elderly people. Promotion of lifelong physical activity is essential. BMJ 1999; 318: 205–206.

24 Buckley LM, Marquez M, Feezor R *et al.* Prevention of corticosteroid-induced osteoporosis: results of patient survey. Arthritis Rheum 1999; 42: 1736–1739.

25 Amin S, LaValley MP, Simms RW, Felson DT. The role of vitamin D in corticosteroid-induced osteoporosis: a meta-analytic approach. Arthritis Rheum 1999; 42: 1740–1751.

26 Fitz-Ritson D. The chiropractic management and rehabilitation of cervical trauma. J Manipulative Physiol Ther 1990; 13: 17–21.

27 Manniche C, Lundberg E, Christensen I *et al.* Intensive dynamic back exercises for chronic low back pain: a clinical trial. Pain 1991; 47: 53–63.

28 Frost H, Lamb SE, Klaber Moffett JA *et al.* A fitness programme for patients with chronic low back pain: 2-year follow-up of a randomised controlled trial. Pain 1998; 75: 273–279.

29 Manniche C, Jordan A. Editorial. Spine 1995; 20: 1221–1222.

30 Vernon HT, Piccininni J, Kopansky-Giles D, Fuligni S. Chiropractic rehabilitation of spinal pain patients: principles, practices and outcome data. J Can Chiropractic Assoc 1995; 39: 147–153.

31 Bendix T, Bendix AF, Busch E, Jordan A. Functional restoration in chronic low back pain. Scand J Med Sci Sports 1996; 692: 88–97.

32 Bronfort G, Goldsmith CH, Nelson CF *et al.* Trunk exercise combined with spinal manipulative or NSAID therapy for chronic low back pain: a randomized, observer-blinded clinical trail. J Manipulative Physiol Ther 1996; 19: 570–582.

33 Deutsch FE. Isolated lumbar strengthening in the rehabilitation of chronic low back pain. J Manipulative Physiol Ther 1996; 19: 124–133.

34 Gluck NI. Passive care and active rehabilitation in a patient with failed back surgery syndrome. J Manipulative Physiol Ther 1996; 19: 41–47.

35 Jordan A, Manniche C. Rehabilitation and spinal pain. J Neuromuscuskeletal Syst 1996; 4: 89–93.

36 Jordan A, Oestergaard K. Implementation of neck/shoulder rehabilitation in primary health care clinics. J Manipulative Physiol Ther 1996; 19: 36–40.

37 Liebenson C. Rehabilitation and chiropractic practice. J Manipulative Physiol Ther 1996; Feb; 19: 134–140.

38 Bentsen H, Lingarde F, Manthorpe R. The effect of dynamic strength back exercise and/or a home training program in 57-year-old women with chronic low back pain. Results of a prospective randomised study with a 3-year follow-up period. Spine 1997; 22: 1494–5000.

39 Ammendolia C. Rehabilitation of the older patient: a case report. J Can Chiropractic Assoc 1998; 42(1): 42–45.

40 Jordan A, Bendix T, Nielsen H *et al*. Intensive training, physio-therapy, or manipulation for patients with chronic neck pain. A prospective, single-blinded, randomized clinical trial. Spine 1998; 23: 311–319.

41 Randlow A, Ostergaard M, Manniche C *et al*. Intensive dynamic training for females with chronic neck/shoulder pain. A randomized controlled trail. Clin Rehabil 1998; 12: 200–210.

42 Skargen EI, Carlsson PG, Oeberg BE. One-year follow-up comparison of the cost and effectiveness of chiropractic and physiotherapy as primary management for back pain. Subgroup analysis, recurrence, and additional health care utilization. Spine 1998; 23: 1875–1883.

43 Carpenter DM, Nelson BW. Low back strengthening for the prevention and treatment of low back pain. Med Sci Sports Exerc 1999; 31(1): 18–24.

44 Kankaanpaa M, Taimela S, Airaksinen O, Hanninen O. The efficacy of active rehabilitation in chronic low back pain. Effect on pain intensity, self-experienced disability, and lumbar fatigability. Spine 1999; 24.

45 Manniche C, Bendix T. Non-surgical treatment strategies. Rheumatol Eur 1999; 28(1): 19–21.

46 Murphy DR. Chiropractic rehabilitation of the cervical spine. Invited Paper. Sky City Conference Centre, Sky City Theatre, May, 1999.

47 Klaber Moffett J *et al*. Randomised controlled trial of exercise for low back pain: clinical outcomes, costs, and preferences. BMJ 1999; 319: 270–283.

48 Frost H, Klaber Moffett JA, Moser JS, Fairbank JC. Randomised controlled trial for evaluation of fitness programme for patients with chronic low back pain. BMJ 1995; 310: 151–154.

49 Mannion AF, Muntener M, Taimela S, Dvorak J. A randomised clinical trial of three therapies for chronic low back pain. Spine 1999, 24: 2435–2448.

50 Panjabi MM. The stabilising system of the spine. Part 1. Function, dysfunction, adaptation and enhancement. Part 2. Neutral zone and instability hypothesis. J Spinal Disord 1992; 5: 383–397.

51 McGill S. Low back exercises: evidence for improving exercise regimens. Phys Ther 1998; 78: 754–765.

52 Jull GA, Richardson CA. Motor control problems in patients with spinal pain: a new direction for therapeutic exercise. J Manipulative Physiol Ther 2000; 23: 115.

53 Highland TR, Dreisinger TE, Vie LL, Russel GS. Change in isometric strength and range of motion of the isolated cervical spine after eight weeks of clinical rehabilitation. Spine 1992; 17: 77–82.

54 Berg H, Tesch P, Berggren PT, Tesch PA. Dynamic neck strength training effect on pain and function. Arch Phys Med Rehabil 1994; 75: 661–665.

55 Biering-Soerensen F. Physical measurements as risk indicators for low back trouble over a one year period. Spine 1984; 9: 106–119.

56 Frischknecht R. Rehabilitation of the elderly – are there limits? Proceedings of the Association of Swiss Chiropractors Continuing Education Program, Montreux, Switzerland, 1999.

57 Murphy DR. Dynamic range of motion training: an alternative to static stretching. Chiropractic Sports Med 1994; 8(2): 59–66.

58 Harkapaa K, Jarvikoski A, Mellin G, Hurri H. A controlled study on the outcome of inpatient and outpatient treatment of low back pain. Part 1. Scand J Rehabil Med 1989; 21: 81–89.

59 Reilly K, Lovejoy B, Williams R, Roth H. Differences between a supervised and independent strength and conditioning program with chronic low back symptoms. J Occup Med 1989; 31: 540–550.

60 Physical Activity Readiness Questionnaire. Canadian Society for Exercise Physiology Review, 1994.

61 Liebenson C. Rehabilitation of the Spine: A Practioner's Guide. London: Williams & Wilkins, 1996.

62 Murphy D. Conservative Management of Cervical Spine Syndromes. London: McGraw-Hill, 2000.

Further reading

Melton JL. Epidemiology of Spinal osteoporosis. Spine 1997; 22(24s): 2s–11s.

Morris CE. Chiropractic rehabilitation of a patient with S1 radiculopathy associated with a large lumbar disk herniation. J Manipulative Physiol Ther 1999; 22: 38–44.

Occupational Health Guidelines for the Management of Low Back Pain at Work – Principal Recommendations. London: Faculty of Occupational Medicine, 2000.

30

Prevention and health promotion in the older patient

Lisa Killinger

As discussed in earlier chapters of this textbook, the geriatric population is the fastest growing segment of the world's population. It is simply unprecedented in world history that the oldest segment of the population is truly 'where the action is'. Remarkably, the fastest growing subset of 'geriatric' patients is those over the age of 85. Older persons accounted for 37% of all hospital stays throughout the mid-1990s in the USA,[1] and health-care utilization and needs are expected to rise as the population continues to live longer lives.[2]. Since the geriatric population accounts for over one-third of all health-care expenditure, health-care systems and professionals are scrambling to develop the training and resources to provide more effectively for the health-care needs of older patients.[1,2]

According to recent statistics, elderly patients with chronic problems have a disproportionately higher cost associated with their care[3] and chiropractors are caring for a significant number of these older patients.[4] In chiropractic practice, geriatric patients often present with one or more chronic health problem.[3,5] The most recent report on chiropractic practice indicates that over one-third of the patients in the typical chiropractic practice are over the age of 50, and nearly half of these patients are over the age of 65.[4] Given the complexities of geriatric health-care and the rapid expansion of society's need for such care, chiropractors must obtain the education and practical skills required to deliver competent care to this important patient population.[6–8] Hopefully, this textbook and this chapter can contribute to the educational base of chiropractors who care for older patients.

If there is one aspect of geriatric patient care that a chiropractor should become an advocate of, an expert in and a champion of, it is health promotion and prevention (HPP). The literature on health promotion indicates that greater age is associated with higher levels of compliance with health promotion recommendations.[9,10] Whereas health-care systems often focus on providing crisis intervention for older patients, HPP is an area of increasing interest.[11,12]

Literature on health promotion, prevention and chiropractic

The Healthy People 2010 document states that the goals of geriatric health-care professionals must be to promote wellness and recommend preventive practices for older patients. The overall goal of the Healthy People 2010 effort is to add quality to years of life for all persons.[13] Chiropractic has, since its inception, championed efforts to improve quality of life and help patients to achieve optimal wellness. Recently, a 'wellness' movement has been gaining momentum within the chiropractic profession, a trend that is reflected in the health promotion-related topics surfacing in chiropractic literature.[14] There have been several recent articles on HPP in chiropractic geriatric practice. Chiropractors are, currently engaged in a significant level of HPP activity, in addition to providing other primary-care services.[15–17] Chiropractors recommend exercises to nearly 70% of their patients.[17] One important point made by Rupert *et al.* is that the term 'maintenance care', which may be used interchangeably with 'health promotion' in chiropractic practice, relies on manual procedures at its core, with the addition of exercise, dietary counselling and other related interventions, as appropriate in each patient's case.[17] Interestingly, in this study, patients who had been under chiropractic maintenance care for several years reported a decreased use of cigarettes and non-prescription drugs, and had 50% fewer visits to medical providers than the general population.[17] The latter piece of data may indicate that chiropractic management may be replacing some medical care.

Rupert *et al.* also present the results of their survey on the attitudes of US chiropractors to HPP: the amount of HPP services and income generated from providing HPP in chiropractic offices may be second only to those from the treatment of low back pain. They also suggest that the level of HPP services provided by chiropractors may surpass that of other physicians[16] It is clear from this study that the vast majority of chiropractors surveyed felt that diet, exercise and lifestyle changes were all essential components of chiropractic preventive maintenance care.[16]

In Part II of their article, Rupert *et al.* focus not only on the HPP activities that chiropractors believe are important, but those that are actually incorporated into practice.[17] The study confirms previous articles that indicate that chiropractors do engage in HPP activities, such as screening and patient counselling related to issues such as diet, exercise, smoking and alcohol use.[18,19]

Definition of prevention

Traditionally, preventive practices are divided, for the sake of discussion, into three categories:[20,21] primary, secondary and tertiary prevention.

Primary prevention essentially means those activities or practices that help the patient to avoid developing a disease state altogether.[21] Primary prevention is essential, and includes the best strategies to maintain wellness in patients. Chiropractors, interested and engaged in primary preventive practices in their practice, naturally strive to have a positive impact on the wellness and health of their patients over their lifetimes. Although there have been be scientific studies documenting the effects of long-term regular chiropractic care on overall health status, the lack of proof is not equal to disproof of the theory that regular chiropractic care, in and of itself, may be a type of preventive health practice. On a personal note: this author has four children who have essentially never taken any medication or drugs of any kind. The only 'health care' that they have received in the past 17 years is regular chiropractic adjustments. These four children have been extremely healthy, and if any of them ever have a sniffle they ask to be adjusted, and almost instinctively drink more fluids and take more rest. This speaks to the attitude of persons who have been raised in an environment of health promotion and prevention, rather than symptom management (as is common in mainstream medicine). The author's family may have just been very fortunate, but it seems that chiropractic management has served then well. Although this sample size of four is very small, there are thousands of chiropractic families with similar experiences, wherein chiropractic care has always been used as the primary, in-house prevention strategy.

Secondary prevention includes any activities or practices that help to identify conditions early so that the negative impact on the patient's health status will be minimal.[21] Many conditions, with early detection, are completely reversible. Identifying disease states early could mean the difference between a simple outpatient procedure (such as a biopsy or removal of a precancerous skin lesion) and death (should the cancerous lesion go undetected and metastasize).

In a chiropractic practice, secondary prevention could include early scoliosis screenings to determine imbalances that could result in potentially devastating pain and disfigurement, without proper management. Another example would be regular chiropractic examinations to determine the presence of spinal misalignments. Chiropractors may also choose to recommend a range of evidence-based health screenings such as regular breast self-examination, prostate examinations and blood-pressure screenings.

Tertiary prevention essentially means preventing or lessening the impact of the disease or condition once it becomes clinically apparent.[21] Tertiary prevention focuses more on maintaining functional status and independence in a diseased state, or delaying progression of the condition.

Tertiary prevention services to retard the progression of established disease and disability are a major health promotion challenge, particularly in geriatric practice.[22]

An example of tertiary prevention would be to use diet and exercise to minimize the negative impact of diabetes on a previously diagnosed patient. Another example might be to use chiropractic care to decrease the musculoskeletal pain and increase joint motion in a patient who has an extremely compromised health status due to arthritis, acquired immunodeficiency syndrome (AIDS) or other disease states.

Prevention terminology may be summarized as follows:

- primary prevention: prevention of disease
- secondary prevention: early detection of disease
- tertiary prevention: lessening the impact of disease, once detected.

Geriatric HPP programmes generally include the categories:[20]

- health screening
- physical activity programmes
- programmes for chronic disease prevention
- nutritional screening and education
- health risk assessment and information sharing on chronic and age-related conditions
- mental health screening, education and referral
- home injury prevention
- counselling about health services
- gerontological counselling.

Many of these activities are commonly carried out in some chiropractic practices. According to several recent articles,[15–18] most chiropractors routinely perform physical assessments on their patients, provide nutritional counselling, recommend physical activity programmes, etc. In the discussion that follows, the author will propose several additional types of health promotion and prevention activities easily incorporated into chiropractic practice, and discuss how these might impact the overall health status of the patient. Although musculoskeletal health may be a common thread in chiropractic practices, owing the chief complaints and needs of patients, this chapter will also propose a broader view of health and health promotion in the hope of helping patients to realize a greater wellness potential into their later years.

The role of the chiropractor in prevention

Philosophical perspectives

Chiropractors have a range of views on their role as health-care providers. Some doctors of chiropractic feel that the role of the chiropractor is to find and correct the vertebral subluxation complex (subluxation-based practice). This view was popularized by one of the profession's developers, BJ Palmer.[23] In this view the chiropractor's contribution to the patient's health is the chiropractic adjustment, and only the adjustment. In this philosophical model, the chiropractor's

goals have little or nothing to do with the patient's symptoms or conditions. In adjusting the patient, conditions may improve, yet the subluxation-based chiropractor's only concern is whether the subluxation had been removed, theorizing that the patient's potential for optimal neural flow was hence maximized. Many doctors of chiropractic practice quite successfully with this philosophical foundation to their patient care practices.

Other chiropractors take on a more active role in prevention and health promotion. In such chiropractic practices, the chiropractor may not only adjust their patients, but also counsel patients on diet, exercise or other lifestyle changes that would be appropriate to improve their overall health. This view may be more in line with the writings of the founder of chiropractic, DD Palmer, who emphasized that three main entities influence health: thoughts, traumas and toxins.[24]

Some chiropractors feel that their only appropriate role is to relieve musculoskeletal complaints such as back pain through chiropractic adjustment and perhaps other adjunctive therapies.[25] This type of care might be referred to as condition-based care. Condition-based chiropractors feel that it is important to restrict their role to the care of conditions for which scientific evidence has shown chiropractic to be an effective treatment. For example, chiropractic care has been shown to be an effective treatment choice for the care of low back pain, and some chiropractors focus their practices on the care of that condition. This view may, in essence, restrict the profession's scope of practice to specific systems, placing it within the current health-care system as a limited medical specialty.[26]

Interestingly, whatever the philosophical view of the chiropractor, the vast majority of the patients who seek chiropractic care come in with a chief complaint of back pain.[27–29] During the course of chiropractic care, other health improvements (besides the relief of the initial musculoskeletal complaint) may be observed in spite of the chiropractor's view of his or her role in the patient's health-care. Since the early 1990s, chiropractic (and alternative health care in general) has grown in popularity[28] to the point where chiropractic is increasingly being viewed as a part of the mainstream health-delivery system.[30,31]

According to the Council on Chiropractic Education, chiropractors are trained to be primary contact providers. This includes providing patient education in HPP, health screening assessment, and the diagnosis, treatment, management and reassessment of common problems, both acute and chronic.[32] Although chiropractic patients present with musculoskeletal problems most of the time, the approach to care is patient centred, geared towards treating and caring for the patient rather than the condition.[33] Chiropractic education complements this health-care approach.

The patient's health and well-being are of primary importance to both the chiropractor and the patient. The philosophical language used by a chiropractor to describe his or her role is of less significance (at least to the patient as the consumer of chiropractic services). The chiropractor, whatever his or her philosophical perspective, must engage in activities that they feel will most effectively increase the patient's wellness potential, whether the patient is 20 years old or 80 years old. The fastest growing age group in today's society comprises people aged over 80.[34] Furthermore, the doctor of chiropractic, other health-care providers and the patient should all work together towards establishing a plan for achieving optimal wellness and preventing disease: 'The clinician and patient should share decision-making' – this was a principal finding of the US Department of Health and Human Services Task Force's guide to clinical preventive services.[21]

In the next sections, several major health concerns of elderly persons will be discussed, followed by a description of primary, secondary and tertiary preventive strategies that can be incorporated into chiropractic practice to promote optimal health and prevent disease.

Principal health concerns in the elderly

It is often forgotten that chiropractic patients are people who have the same general health concerns as the population at large. Chiropractic practice and chiropractic patients do not exist in a vacuum, free from the epidemiology of the nations in which they live. Therefore, when discussing general health issues, the statistics apply to all patients and a clinician must be aware of the bigger picture of geriatric health.

The statistics on the major causes of mortality and morbidity in the elderly patient tell a tale about the need for better health promotion and prevention. On reviewing the following list of major causes of death and disability, the reader should consider how these conditions might have been prevented through health promotion or prevention-type health interventions, or changes in health habits and lifestyle.

(i) Top three causes of mortality in the geriatric patient:[22,35]
 • heart disease
 • cancer
 • stroke.
(ii) Common causes of morbidity in the elderly:
 • arthritis
 • diabetes
 • osteoporosis
 • falls.

Upon examination of these lists, it becomes apparent that older patients seen in chiropractic practices are likely to present with serious health concerns, in addition to their chief complaints. Patients who present with a musculoskeletal complaint, or who attend for wellness or maintenance care, may also have heart disease, arthritis or diabetes. A choice must therefore be made about the role that the practitioner will play in the patient's overall health-care, as well as the clinician's level of involvement.

Specific health concerns and strategies for prevention

Heart disease and hypertension

Among persons aged 65 years and older, heart disease is the leading cause of both death and hospitalization in the USA. It is also the second or third leading cause of disability in the geriatric population.[22] Heart disease is a major health problem in many industrialized nations, caused in part by sedentary lifestyle, obesity, smoking and dietary factors. Although smoking is a major contributing factor, and a preventable risk factor for heart disease, the discussion focuses on the importance of smoking cessation as it relates to stroke. In this section, risk factors, dietary factors and other lifestyle factors will be discussed.

Risk factors of heart disease and hypertension include a family history of heart disease, high cholesterol, high blood pressure, smoking, overweight, and excessive consumption of saturated fat and cholesterol[21,22] (see also Chapter 15).

The scientific literature strongly supports several dietary recommendations in persons with heart disease.[36–41] Various diets have been studied in the prevention of heart disease, including the Mediterranean diet (a diet high in fish, fruits, vegetables, omega-3 fatty acids, and fibre, and low in red meats),[36] low-sodium diets,[37] low cholesterol diets,[38] high-antioxidant diets,[40,41] and high-fibre diets.[38] Although these studies all offer pieces of information about appropriate nutrition for geriatric heart patients, a good general discussion of the 'modified food pyramid for people over 70 years of age' is found in Russell's 1999 article in the Journal of Nutrition.[42]

One area in which the scientists seem to agree is on the value of exercise for older patients with heart disease or the risk factors of heart disease.[11,21,43] Previous chiropractic articles have also addressed the importance of exercise in the management of older patients.[44–47] A clear and concise guide to appropriate exercise for older persons has been developed by, and can be obtained at no cost from, the US National Institute on Aging.[48]

In light of the evidence, some primary prevention strategies for the prevention of heart disease are to: limit alcohol use, quit smoking, use less salt, lose weight, if overweight or obese, choose lower fat foods, eat more fruits, vegetables and whole grains, lower the intake of cholesterol and exercise.

Further discussion on this topic is provided in the form of case studies that were actually cared for in chiropractic practice. Minor revisions have been made to the cases in some instances. On reviewing these cases, the reader may observe similarities between the cases presented here and the patients that may be seen in everyday practice.

Case study: Aisha's ear ache

Aisha, a 76-year-old African-American woman, presents with a chief complaint of left ear pain. She first noticed the pain yesterday afternoon, but hoped that it would go away overnight. She states that the pain is in her left ear, but also bothers her left jaw, cheek and the left side of her neck. The pain is reported as a '3' on a 10 point visual analogue scale, but it worsened to a '7' when she was out in the yard shovelling snow today and while walking in the cold from her car to the chiropractor's office.

Aisha recalls eating barbequed pork last night, and thinks that the jaw pain started after that. She reports that she had moderate heartburn after dinner, which is still mild today. She took over-the-counter Tagamet and thinks that may have helped to relieve some of the heartburn.

She also reports that her arms and hands are sore and slightly 'puffy' today. She attributes this to the snow

shovelling, and perhaps the salt and fat content of last night's meal.

What elements of patient's history require further investigation? Before proceeding with the discussion of this case, indicate some areas that should be further investigated.

Discussion

The chiropractic examination on Aisha does not reveal that a jaw or neck problem. Although the patient diagnosed and treated herself for heartburn, it would be wise to investigate this case further. Whether a pain pattern is worse with exertion, there should be some suspicion of possible angina or that a minor heart attack has occurred or is occurring. In women, the pain pattern that the patient experiences during a heart attack may either differ greatly from the typical pain pattern of chest and left arm pain, or the patient may have almost no pain at all. In this case the pain was mostly felt in the jaw area, a presentation which may be confusing to the examining doctor. In Aisha's case, although she was taking Tagamet, and thought it might have been helping, the puffiness experienced the next day is of concern. It is important to note that heart disease is significantly higher in the African American population than in other patient populations.

Management

After a complete examination, the chiropractor strongly suspected that this patient was experiencing a heart attack and/or some level of congestive heart failure. The patient's medical doctor was contacted while the patient was still in the office. When the chiropractor described the patient's symptoms to the nurse, she asked that the patient go straight to the doctor's office. The patient was experiencing a heart attack, and this case was handled as an emergency.

The patient spent the night in hospital and was released after the prescription of several heart medications. Aisha returned to the chiropractic office after 1 month, feeling better, but wanting to continue with chiropractic care. She was counselled on dietary management strategies and an exercise plan was developed with the approval of her medical provider. Exercise is perhaps the single most important lifestyle change for this patient, but should be entered into gradually and cautiously so as not to place undue stress on her heart.

Case study: Charlie's cephalgia

Charles, a 74-year-old African-American male, presents with a chief complaint of headache. He has been waking up with a headache every day for the past 3 weeks. The pain feels like tightness and pressure at the base of his skull and in his eyes, rated as an 8 on a 1–10 scale. The pain is debilitating in the morning, but decreases significantly by lunchtime. He has not taken any medication or sought any other treatment for his headaches.

Five months ago Charlie was started on 25 mg of Capoten (captopril, an angiotensin-converting enzyme inhibitor) twice a day. He has been taking the pills with breakfast and lunch.

His last eye examination was 5 months ago and he reports that he did not need a change in his glasses prescription, nor did he have glaucoma or any other eye-related diseases.

What questions should Charlie be asked?

What examinations or tests should be performed?

Discussion

The chiropractor's first instinct is to adjust the patient. Although an adjustment may be required, there are other health issues that must be investigated. The orthopaedic/neurological examination and a look into the patient's eyes ruled out a space-occupying lesion in the head as a possible aetiology. Since the patient was on blood-pressure medication it would seem appropriate to check his blood pressure. In the course of the examination, this patient was found to have very high blood pressure in the morning. On visits later in the day, the blood-pressure was within the normal range. Recall that the patient reported that he was taking his blood-pressure medication in the morning and at lunchtime. Apparently, this pattern of medication use was allowing the blood pressure to rage out of control during the 16 h between the lunchtime and breakfast doses.

Management

The patient was examined and adjusted for thoracic spine and cervical spine misalignments and subluxations. However, he was not allowed to leave the clinic until his medical doctor was reached by telephone and an appointment made to re-evaluate his medication dosage/use patterns. The patient returned 1 week later, very appreciative that the chiropractor had identified the cause of the severe and debilitating headaches. He valued the fact that the chiropractor identified the problem with his medication and communicated effectively with his medical doctor, and that the proper care was collaboratively implemented.

Cancer

The most common and deadly cancers are:[21,22]

- skin cancer: most common form of cancer; preventable
- lung cancer: leading cause of cancer deaths in geriatrics
- prostrate/breast cancer: second leading cause of death in geriatrics
- colon cancer: third leading cancer incidence in both genders over the age of 55
- ovarian cancer: fourth leading cause of cancer deaths in women
- oesophagus/stomach cancer: seventh and ninth leading causes of cancer deaths

This list illustrates an important point about cancer, which is the second leading cause of death in older persons: most cancers are preventable and are not fatal if treated early. For example, stomach and esophagus cancers, although common in North America, are rare in societies where people do not drink alcohol or use tobacco products.[35] Also, while skin cancer is almost non-existent in women in societies where they avoid exposure to the sun, it is one of most common diseases in the US geriatric population.[35] It is clear that such lifestyle choices as these affect the difference in the health enjoyed (or missed) as a person ages. From the chiropractic perspective, what role should be undertaken in the contribution of cancer prevention? The following sections will review a few types of cancer and propose preventive activities that may be incorporated into chiropractic practice. A summary of cancer symptoms and risk factors is provided in Table 30.1

Table 30.1 Cancer signs, risk factors and recommended screening schedule for geriatric persons

Type of cancer	Risk factors	Symptoms	Recommended screenings
Breast	No children or having first child after one age of 35; family history of breastcancer; high-fat diet, alcohol or caffeine intake; use of oral contraceptives	Lump in breast tissue, change in breast or nipple, i.e. redness, tenderness, etc.	Baseline mammogram at the age of 40; then every other year; monthly breast selr-examination; annual breast examination by doctor.
Testicular	Undescended testicle	Lump in, enlargement of or pain in testicle; ache in groin or lower abdomen, fluid collection in scrotum	Regular (monthly) self-examination; annual testicular examination by doctor
Cervix	Multiple pregnancies, intercourse before the age of 18 or with multiple partners; history of venereal warts or gonorrhoea.	Bleeding between menstrual periods; (post menopausal bleeding); unusual discharge	Annual cervical smear
Prostate	History of venereal disease or prostate cancer; diet high in animal fat or caffeine; vasectomy; age 50+; African-American	Constant pain in low back, pelvis or thighs; difficult, painful or interrupted urine flow; frequent or bloody urination	Annual digital rectal examination; blood tests including prostate-specific antigen or prostate acid phosphatase
Colon	Family history of colon cancer; low-fiber diet, low calcium intake, high-fat diet; chronic constipation	Persistent diarrhoea or constipation, blood in stool; tiredness; loss of weight for no apparent reason; frequent intestinal gas or cramps	Annual faecal occult blood test; sigmoidoscopy every 5 years, colonoscopy every 10 years
Skin	Family history of skin cancer, exposure to the sun or ultraviolet radiation, fair skin, scars from severe sunburn, moles	Change in shape, size, or colour of mole; skin lesion that will not heal, especially on the face, hands, ears or shoulders	Vigilance regarding all moles and skin lesions; annual dermatological examination, especially when suspicious lesions are present
Lung	Smoking, exposure to second-hand smoke, asbestos, pesticides or chemicals; chronic bronchitis, history of tuberculosis	A productive persistent cough; bloody sputum; chest pain	Chest X-ray when clinical signs are present

Skin cancer

Since approximately one in four people over the age of 50 will have at least one incidence of skin cancer in their life, this is a topic worthy of some basic discussion. Over 900 000 new cases of basal and squamous cell carcinoma and 43 000 cases of malignant melanoma were reported in 1997. In the same year, 10 000 deaths occurred in the USA due to skin cancer. Remarkably, skin cancer is 100% curable, if diagnosed early.[21] As the children of the 1960s (the generation of 'sun worshippers') age, the incidence of skin cancers is bound to continue its upward trend.

Simple lifestyle changes can prevent the vast majority of skin cancers. Counselling patients of all ages on minimizing exposure to the sun and other sources of ultraviolet radiation (such as Sunbeds) is an important primary prevention strategy. Patients who work in the sun can be advised to wear light-coloured, long-sleeved shirts, and hats that shade the face, neck and ears, and to apply sunscreen on any exposed skin. Over half of all skin cancers could be prevented by simply practising these preventive measures.[21]

Relative to secondary prevention, it is essential for the chiropractor to note the presence of any suspicious skin lesions (those with irregular borders or colours). Skin lesions located on body parts that have had the highest exposure to the sun, such as the face, hands, ears and shoulders, should be watched for growth or change in character. Early identification of skin cancer is essential, in that often a cancerous lesion can be removed as an outpatient office procedure. If lesions are ignored, serious disfigurement is likely and, in some cases, metastasis is possible, with serious or fatal consequences.

A useful mnemonic for skin cancer examination is:[21]

A: Asymmetry
B: irregular Borders
C: variation in Colour within the same lesion
D: growth in Diameter greater than 6 mm.

Chiropractors are the professionals who may be most likely to see an older patient regularly, and to see the skin of the patient. Any skin lesion should be documented in the patient file (with measurement and description of shape, colour etc.) so that changes in such lesions can be tracked. Chiropractors with some training in the diagnosis of skin disorders can then advise patients with suspicious skin lesions to see a dermatologist whenever cancer is suspected (see also Chapter 17).

Lung cancer

Lung cancer is the most common type of cancer (and cancer-related death) in both male and female older patients, aside from skin cancer.[21,22,35] Smoking is by far the most significant risk factor for lung cancer. It causes more deaths per year than murder, suicide and car accidents combined.[35] Smoking is the habit/ lifestyle choice with the most serious negative health consequences by far, and is the key risk factor for lung cancer, heart disease and stroke, the top three causes of death in older persons.

Smoking cessation is an important topic, one with very real opportunities for chiropractors significantly to influence their patients towards enjoying a healthier existence. But, first, if the reader is a chiropractor and smokes, they should quit. The use of such an extremely harmful drug flies in the face of chiropractic philosophy. Health-care providers (such as chiropractors) cannot, in good conscience, promote a drug-free approach to health care if they routinely choose to use one of the most harmful drug-laden products available. If ever there were a situation where the quotation, 'Physician, heal thyself' applied, it is with doctors who smoke. For those patients who smoke, education is essential in helping to motivate them to quit.

The lifestyle change that potentially has the most positive impact on the patient's health is smoking ces-

sation. However, regular exercise programmes are equally important and pertain to all patients. Patients who have quit smoking report that the most influential factor in their decision to quit was simply that 'their doctor recommended it'.[49] Chiropractors, as members of the largest drug-free health profession, MUST take the time to encourage, request and implore patients to stop smoking. Again, since chiropractors see patients with some regularity, they have the opportunity to remind patients regularly of the importance of quitting, and to support and monitor progress as they do so.

A wealth of material on the risks of smoking and on smoking cessation programmes is available at no cost, through either the American Cancer Society or equivalent agencies in Canada and the UK. For guidelines, suggestions and aids in helping patients to quit smoking, the reader is referred to Solberg's article in the Journal of Family Practice.[49] (Contact information is provided in Appendix 30.1) Chiropractors, who are interested in the overall health of their patients, should make information on smoking cessation and the dangers of smoking available to all patients. It may also be worthwhile to offer incentives to patients who quit smoking. Special recognition of patients who make such important changes in their health habits can help to keep such patients on track, and encourage others to follow in their footsteps.

Regarding secondary prevention of lung cancer, it is important for the chiropractor to recognize the clinical signs that may indicate the presence of cancer. Patients who present with or complain of a persistent cough, especially with blood in their sputum and chest pain, should have a posteroanterior chest X-ray taken to rule out lung cancer. With early detection lung cancer need not be fatal. Early detection of lung cancer is also essential since metastasis from the lung to osseous structures (particularly the thoracic spine) is not uncommon.[21]

Gender-related cancers: prostrate, testicular, breast and cervical cancer

The next most common types of cancer in older persons are the gender-related cancers. Although each of the types listed above is worthy of a full chapter of discussion, they have been grouped together in one paragraph for an important reason. These cancers are generally not fatal if identified early and are relatively simple to screen for. The chiropractors role is simple in the prevention of gender-related cancers. Patients should be asked to report the dates of their most recent screening examination for breast, cervical or prostrate cancer. For women, this means a palpatory breast examination, mammogram and cervical smear. For men this means a digital rectal examination and/or blood test, and self-examination for testicular cancer.[21] Most patients can easily recall such examinations and will be able to report to the chiropractor the month and year of their most recent screening. In addition, the scientific literature suggests that a low- fat diet, high in vitamins and minerals, is an effective prevention strategy for breast cancer.[21,50]

Colon cancer

Colon cancer strikes 1 in every 17 people in the USA, and over 55 000 persons die of colon cancer in the USA each year. The vast majority of colon cancer cases are in people over the age of 50. The scientific evidence is strongly in support of dietary changes for the prevention of colon cancer. This affords chiropractors with the opportunity to participate in the primary prevention of colon cancer, through dietary advice. It has long been understood that a low-fibre, high-fat diet increases the risk of colon cancer, as does alcohol consumption. Conversely, a diet low in fat and high in fibre is preventive for colon cancer. It is simple to advise patients on ways to increase the fibre in their diet. A diet with 30 g or more of fibre per day is optimal.[51] High-Fibre Foods are listed in Table 30.2.

Stroke

Stroke ranks as the third leading cause of death, following heart disease and cancer.[35] Every year over

Table 30.2 High-fibre foods for colon cancer prevention[51]

Fibre rich foods (typical serving)	Fibre content (g)
Wheat-bran breakfast cereals	4–12
Canned beans (chilli or kidney)	9–10
Popcorn	7–9
Seeded berries	5–7
Raisins or mixed dried fruit	3–4
Raw fruits or vegetables	3–5
Wholewheat pasta	4
Buckwheat pancakes	4
Wholewheat bread or bagel	3

150 000 people die and many more are disabled through strokes. Over 130 000 of these deaths are in patients over the age of 65,[35] making this a serious issue in geriatric patient management. Since treatments for stroke are quite limited and costly, prevention is of utmost importance. Prevention of stroke is best accomplished by preventing the two major causes of stroke: atherosclerosis and hypertension. Numerous studies show that physical activity is associated with lower stroke risks.[52–56] Therefore, the most important preventive measure that a chiropractor can suggest for his or her patients is that they begin a regular exercise programme. Walking more than 20 km (12.5 miles) week is suggested as the optimal exercise relative to stroke prevention, although patients may choose other activities and experience equivalent protective effects.[52]

Certain dietary practices have also been shown to have a preventive value against stroke. Diets high in fish and lower in red meats have been associated with a reduced risk of stroke. In general, a diet high in whole grains, fruits and vegetables, higher in vitamins C and B, potassium, calcium and magnesium, and low in fat, calories and meat-based proteins is recommended to reduce the risk of stroke.[57–59] These dietary recommendations may also have value in the prevention of many diseases common in the older patient, so such advice may be useful for the majority of older patients.

Since smoking is a primary risk factor of stroke, it is essential to counsel patients on smoking cessation to decrease their risk of suffering a stroke. Excellent suggestions for incorporating smoking cessation successfully into practice exist in Solberg's 1990 article.[49]

The following case is included to give the reader an example of a patient actually seen in chiropractic practice, and offers an example of chiropractic case-management strategies.

Case study: Mrs Z's bad breakfast

Mrs Z, a 73-year-old housewife who has recently begun chiropractic treatments, is eating breakfast one day and feels dizzy, drops her cup of coffee and loses consciousness. Her visiting grandson revives her and she refuses to go to the hospital. Having rested, she presents to the chiropractor's office later that day. She says she feels fine, although still a little shaky and disorientated after this morning's 'spell'. Mrs Z does not have a history of fainting. She does not smoke, although her husband had smoked two packs a day for the past 50 years. He recently passed away after being diagnosed with lung cancer. Mrs Z is fairly sedentary much of the time, although she does walk once or twice a week (except during the winter months). She has been receiving chiropractic care for a month for the treatment of her headaches. She had not had a history of headaches prior to this year, but now reports occasional severe headaches. She has been undergoing adjustment using the Activator Method Technique, and has had a total of four treatments. She has started to incorporate recommendations for decreasing caffeine consumption and to follow a low-fat diet. She was also advised of the importance of sufficient water and potassium intake, owing to her examination findings as described below. (Her nutritional profile had also revealed that she consumed more than 30% of her calories from fatty foods).

What next?

During a brief physical examination, it is noticed that she is not as 'sharp' as usual, answering hesitantly and having trouble getting her words out. She reports some numbness in her right hand (the same hand that dropped the coffee cup earlier today). Mrs Z says that she wanted to come for a chiropractic treatment because she has had a severe headache since this morning when she woke up. She had trouble filling out her part of the patient information forms today and had to ask the receptionist to help her.

What tests might you perform?

- blood pressure: 160/98 bilaterally
- orthopaedic tests to rule out carpal tunnel
- cognitive: mini-Mental Status examination.

Discussion

The patient was moderately hypertensive, as had been noted on previous visits. There were no clear structural reasons for her hand weakness. Her chief complaint was headache, so it was important to rule out several possible aetiologies, such as tumour, blood sugar problems and blood pressure. However, this patient's pattern of recent, severe, focal, progressively worsening headaches indicated that she may have had a stroke or transient ischaemic attack. This would be consistent with the hand weakness and sudden onset of speech disturbance. Considering the entire clinical picture, a diagnosis of stroke was likely.

Management

This patient was referred for further tests and it was determined that she had suffered a stroke. The medical examination and a battery of tests were performed to assess the severity of the damage and risk for future strokes. The patient was hospitalized overnight and released. After 3 weeks, she returned for her regular chiropractic appointment. Her speech disturbance was no longer evident and she had regained most of the strength in her hand.

Mrs Z will continue to be managed under a low-force chiropractic technique that does not introduce cervical spine rotational vectors (owing to the risks of subsequent strokes). While under chiropractic care, she has been counselled on the dietary management of her blood pressure and an exercise routine was developed. In this case, the patient was advised to work up gradually to walking 3 miles four times per week. In winter months, the patient was advised to walk on a treadmill or ride an exercise bicycle. This patient expressed a strong willingness to take charge of her health to prevent future strokes, and has remained healthy and active for several years following her stroke.

Osteoporosis

A discussion of this condition is essential in relation to chiropractic geriatric practice, for numerous reasons. First, the vast majority of older chiropractic patients enter the chiropractic office with a musculoskeletal complaint.[15] Bone health is essential to musculoskeletal well-being. Secondly, chiropractic care centres around adjustments or manipulative manoeuvres. To provide responsible and safe chiropractic care in geriatric patients, the patient must be empowered to engage in activities and incorporate lifestyle practices that help to maintain optimal bone density.

It is important to understand the impact of osteoporosis on the health status of the elderly patient and the impact of osteoporosis on society. About $10 billion is spent annually in the USA alone for the diagnosis, treatment and rehabilitation related to the 1.3 million-plus fractures sustained in osteoporotic patients.[60] Osteoporosis is one of the most prevalent conditions in elderly patients, particularly females, with over 25 million persons affected in the USA.[60] It is considered a part of 'normal ageing' for a female patient to lose 1% of bone mass per year after the age of 30, about twice the rate of bone loss for men,[61] but pre-

Table 30.3 Osteoporosis risk factors

Preventable risks	Non-preventable risks
Smoking	Familial history of osteoporosis
Excessive alcohol consumption	Fair skinned and/or small framed
Caffeinated beverages	Asian or European descent
Excessive consumption of soft drinks ('pop')	Hysterectomy (female)
Diet high in meat-based protein	Female
Aversion to or avoidance of dairy products	
Sedentary lifestyle	

vention and health promotion can slow or reverse this process in most patients.

Often, patients feel that osteoporosis is hereditary and therefore there is nothing that can be done to prevent the condition from occurring. Although a familial history of osteoporosis is one risk factor for developing the condition, a more complete list of risk factors is given in Table 30.3. It should be noted that the preventable risk factors outnumber those that are out of the patient's control.

Strategies for prevention

The Clinician's Handbook of Preventive Services states simply that:

> The most effective management for osteoporosis is the prevention of osteoporosis through counseling about dietary and behavioral practices to maximize peak bone mass achieved by the third decade of life and to slow the rate of bone loss after that period.[21]

Simple changes in diet and lifestyle, recommended by the chiropractor, can significantly reduce the risk of developing osteoporosis, and in many cases can reverse the bone loss once it is detected.[43,62,63]

Primary prevention

Chiropractors are sometimes perceived (by patients) as 'bone doctors'. Patients should at the very least be able to rely on chiropractors to offer preventive strategies related to musculoskeletal conditions, such as osteoporosis.[46] The scientific literature strongly supports the use of preventive strategies to enhance patients' long-term skeletal health.[11,43,62,63] To prevent osteoporosis

before it develops, the doctor of chiropractic can share information about osteoporosis prevention.

The most important factor relative to osteoporosis prevention is an emphasis on incorporating regular exercise into a patient's life.[43–45,62,63] In chiropractic training, there may be insufficient space to explore sufficiently the specific types of exercise most useful for osteoporosis prevention. A resource with good visual presentation of various exercises appropriate for patients who wish to prevent frailty in their later years is available through the National Institute on Aging.[48] Common sense, combined with basic knowledge of osteoblastic and osteoclastic processes, and the physiology of exercise and bone remodelling, will guide the chiropractor in developing safe and effective exercise-based osteoporosis prevention plans for his or her patients.

Axial loading

The types of exercise that have been shown to have the greatest positive impact on bone density in the axial skeleton (including the spine) are 'axial loading' exercises. In essence, these are exercises that increase the vertical forces on the spine. Examples of such exercises are walking, running, step routines and stair climbing.[11,48]

Nutritional considerations

The scientific evidence is overwhelmingly in support of increasing the dietary intake of both calcium and vitamin D as a preventive measure against osteoporosis and related fractures.[64–67] The US National Institute of Health recommends a daily calcium intake of 1500 mg for persons over the age of 65. This is similar to the recommended daily calcium intake for a pregnant or breastfeeding woman, underlining the importance of educating older patients about a diet high in calcium and vitamin D, along with calcium supplementation.[63,64,67]

Both smoking and excessive alcohol or caffeine consumption increase the risk of osteoporosis, and should be avoided.[63,66] Diets very high in meat-based protein also increase osteoporosis risk, whereas replacing meat with soya-based proteins may help to reduce the risk of osteoporosis.[62,63]

Summary of basics of osteoporosis counselling

- All patients should be counselled about consuming adequate amounts of calcium and vitamin D. All patients should be advised to avoid smoking and excessive alcohol and caffeine intake.

- All patients should be counselled to exercise, unless health complications preclude their safe participation in such activities.
- For all older patients, the risk of falls should be assessed and precautionary measures provided to improve safety.
- Patients should be evaluated for the presence of clinical risk factors to identify those who would benefit from more precise assessment of bone density, closer monitoring and more specific recommendations.

Patients may also ask their chiropractor about hormone-replacement therapy (HRT) or other pharmaceutical interventions for osteoporosis. Although making recommendations about a patient's drug regimen falls outside the chiropractic scope of practice, it is wise for the chiropractor to become familiar with the scientific literature on current drug interventions. The bottom line according to recent literature reviews is that HRT can reduce the risk of osteoporosis and related fractures, and decrease the incidence of heart disease in older females. Further research is needed to explore the possible link between HRT and some specific types of cancer.[68]

Case study: Ruth's tough break

An active, healthy 70-year-old female chiropractic patient sustained a compression fracture of the eighth and ninth thoracic vertebrae while lifting a bulky but lightweight object in her yard so that she could mow the grass beneath it. She felt a sharp pain at that time, which did not remiss for a few days. Worried, she had X-rays taken at her medical doctor's office, and he diagnosed the fractures. However, the medical doctor indicated to the patient that there was nothing he could do about the fractures, but that she should 'be more careful'. He prescribed a pain medication. She presents to a chiropractor's office because she has a great deal of pain around the fracture site, especially when she breathes in deeply.

What should be done? What assessments should be performed? What questions need to be asked?

Discussion

In this case, the patient sustained a fracture in the course of her normal activities. She did not fall from a high place or sustain a trauma that would cause a fracture in healthy bone. Osteoporosis may be a possible of concern. Her X-rays were requested from the medical doctor, and moderate osteoporosis was listed on the radiology report and was clearly visible on the films. To be apparent on plain-film X-rays, a significant amount of demineralization must have already occurred.

An osteoporosis risk-factor form should be completed by the patient, not for diagnosis, but to guide the clinical decision-making process. In this case the following risks were identified. The patient is a fair-skinned, small-framed woman of European descent, with a mother who had severe osteoporosis. She had a complete hysterectomy at the age of 40, she has always disliked milk, even as a child, she drinks five cups of coffee per day and she does not engage in regular exercise.

She had several of the non-controllable risk factors for osteoporosis, such as familial history, fair skin, small frame, hysterectomy and European descent. Thus, she may have had the tendency to develop osteoporosis. However, many habits and practices in this patient could decrease her chances of maintaining healthy bone as she ages (e.g. an aversion to milk and a liking for coffee).

Chiropractic care of this patient

A low-force chiropractic technique can be used to adjust this patient, and because of to the nature of her complaint the ribs should be assessed for malposition. Since ribs are the most common iatrogenic fracture in chiropractic practice, extreme caution should be used, and a light force or instrument-assisted chiropractic method should be employed.

Counselling this patient

This patient can do many things to slow or arrest the further demineralization of her bones. Since she has just sustained a fracture, she may be very motivated to change her lifestyle and habits. In this case, the patient could be encouraged to take calcium and vitamin D supplements, and increase her dietary intake of calcium. She can also be advised on the importance of avoiding a diet high in meat-based protein, and avoiding alcohol and caffeine. She must, above all, begin to participate in regular exercise, such as walking or aerobics classes, and offered a simple free weight-lifting programme, once her pain has subsided from the thoracic spine fractures. Her bone density should be checked regularly to assess the stability or reversal of her osteoporotic state.

Other important prevention topics in chiropractic practice

Automobile safety

Automobile accidents are a frequent cause of injury and disability in older persons. After teenagers, the group most likely to be involved in a car accident comprises persons. As a result of many ageing-related factors, the injuries sustained by older persons in these accidents are much more likely to cause death or serious impairment than the same injuries sustained by younger persons. Of particular concern is head trauma, which is considered to be very life threatening in older patients. However, many vehicle-related injuries can be prevented or their impact minimized through the use of seatbelts. It is that simple. Seatbelts save lives, particularly in children and in older persons. However, older patients did not learn to use seatbelts as children. In fact, they may have spent well over two-thirds of their life before seatbelts were even in common usage. Developing the habit of seatbelt use is a particular challenge to older persons, whereas such habits may be second nature to the generations of the 1970s and beyond. Encouraging seatbelt use is every doctor's responsibility. Counselling on seatbelt use, along with periodic vision and hearing screening, to identify impediments to driving skills, are traditional prevention-related recommendations for geriatric health-care providers.[69] In chiropractic practice, incentives can and should be offered to patients who demonstrate good prevention habits and participation in 'wellness' activities such as seatbelt use. Thus, seatbelt use is a good habit worthy of nurturing and rewarding in older patients.

Many older people continue to drive long after they have lost the ability to do so safely. A patient with poor vision or hearing, slow reaction time or impaired balance and co-ordination (to the extent that his or her driving is affected) should be counselled regarding their decision to continue driving. Voicing an opinion to the patient may prevent severe injury or death due to a driving accident.[44] (see also Chapter 31).

Fall prevention

Falls are a leading cause of disability in the elderly, and the second leading injury-related cause of death in those aged 65 and older. Falls are the leading cause of death in those over 85 years of age.[35] An excellent discussion of the causes, impact and prevention of falls can be found in the earlier chapters of this text (see Chapter 14). Since this is an important area of prevention recommendations, a summary of strategies for fall prevention is given here:.

- exercise: numerous studies have shown that some exercise can help to prevent falls[43,48]
- chiropractic: to restore optimal function of bone and joint structures, and decrease the chance of falls
- safety in the home: the home environment be assessed for safety, and for the presence of objects or conditions that might put a person at risk for a fall. Such hazards should then be removed.

Arthritis

Over 50% of persons over the age of 65 suffer from arthritis.[22,35] The impact of this disease is profound, and the cost in human suffering is immense. Chiropractors, with adjustments as the core of their practices, are well suited to play a role in maintaining or increasing joint mobility. Rao,[5] in 1999, stated that significant numbers of older arthritis patients are seeking out alternative therapies, including chiropractic. Aside from offering chiropractic adjustment, chiropractors may be able to advise the patient in exercise programmes that will contribute to the maintenance of flexibility and function. In this condition, as in others discussed in this chapter, exercise is key to successful patient outcomes.[43,48]

Barriers to incorporating health promotion and prevention into practice

We must seek more effective ways to motivate older persons into sustained participation in meaningful behavioral change. This is no small task!
Robert L Kane MD in 'The public health paradigm'.[20]

There are many reasons for health-care providers failing to incorporate HPP into their practices. The next section will discuss some of these reasons, along with the reasons why patients sometimes do not comply with the HPP recommendations that are provided to them. Following this, strategies to overcome these obstacles will be discussed, in order successfully to promote health and lifestyle changes among older patients.

First, there is the time element. It takes time to assess the patient's health status, to determine appropriate

HPP needs and to engage the patient in effective dialogue about making changes in his or her life to promote wellness. In the current health-care system, the inherent time pressures in the managed care setting are bound to have a negative affect on the amount of HPP activity that providers are willing and able to offer.

Aside from the limitations on time, some chiropractors are overwhelmed by the sheer volume and diversity of literature on various topics. The provider may have difficulty discerning sound prevention recommendations from fads or information from unreliable sources. The flood of information readily available to the patient (and everyone) on the internet and in the popular media, has both empowered and confused the health-care consumer and health-care providers alike. Critically appraising the literature, both popular and professional, is a challenge to all consumers. The author 'weeds out' information that may be unsound or unreliable as follows. If the information is accompanied by a sales pitch or product-ordering information, it is viewed with suspicion. In addition, information found on personal websites of individuals with no credentials should be considered as opinion, unless referenced.

Patients' reasons for not complying with their doctor's sound health-promotion advice are varied and complex (70, 71). In the space below, the reader is asked to consider the different reasons why an older patient may fail to comply with suggestions or recommendations.

Reasons why a patient may fail to comply with suggestions/recommendations:

Patient non-compliance is an important issue and many articles have been written to address this topic.[10,70,72] An excellent discussion of the reasons for patients' non-adherence to health-promotion and disease-prevention regimens can be found in the textbook entitled Behavioral Medicine in Primary Care.[70] Some of the reasons given for non-adherence are:

- poor provider-patient communication about the regimen
- lack of trust and mutual caring in provider–patient relationship
- controlling, paternalistic provider behaviour
- patient's failure to understand costs, benefits and efficacy of regimen
- patient's lack of commitment to regimen
- provider's failure to anticipate and overcome practical barriers to adherence.

Success in incorporating health promotion and prevention into practice

The above list underscores the point that changes in patients' health habits can only result from a combined and well-communicated collaborative effort between doctor and patient. To achieve greater success in patients' incorporation of health and lifestyle changes, the following questions must be considered.

- Was the information given to the patient regarding the desired health/lifestyle changes clear and understandable?
- Does the patient have the support, emotional and otherwise, to succeed in making change?
- Has the patient been offered an acceptable course of action to which commitment to change can (and probably will) be made?
- Does the patient have help in overcoming barriers to incorporating change?
- Is the focus of that change an improvement in the patient's quality of life?
- Are both the doctor and the patient willing to negotiate about the proposed change?
- Have the doctor and the patient collaboratively developed an implementation plan for the health-related change?

If these issues have been addressed, the likelihood of success in incorporating health promotion and prevention into a patient's life is good. It should be emphasized that the doctor's role does not end with simply proposing these lifestyle changes. Rather, the provider's role or responsibility also includes helping the patient to implement these changes in his or her life. Expressing continued encouragement, monitoring patient progress towards change, renegotiating the plan if need be and reconfirming an interest in the patient's quality of life are all essential to incorporating change successfully.[10]

Interventions that address patient's personal health practices are vitally important
A major finding of the *US* Preventive Services Task Force[21]

Patients are most likely to continue with an activity or health habit that they enjoy or have fun doing.[43,72] If a patient hates to swim, yet their doctor has told them that swimming is the key to better health, the patient is not likely to comply. An alternative strategy would be for the same doctor to ask the patient what physical activity they really enjoy (or enjoyed when they were younger or fitter). The doctor may then encourage the patient to set a goal of starting or restarting a programme that includes their favourite activity. For one patient it may be walking by the beach or river, while for another it might be square dancing. If a patient is going to stick with an activity, they are going to have to like it, or else be exceedingly motivated (for health or personal reasons) to adhere to it.

Educating older patients about healthy living and sharing prevention strategies can be fun and rewarding. An excellent manual on conducting health-education gatherings in the community to promote health in older persons was compiled by Goldzweig in 1996 (73). In such a model, educational forums, regular health assessments and incentives to patients practising healthy behaviours are all combined. Such multifaceted approaches can certainly be taken by chiropractors wishing to play an active role in promoting 'successful ageing' in their practices.

The motto of the British Geriatrics Society, 'Adding Life to Years', is useful to keep in mind when incorporating HPP activities into the care of older persons.[74] An older patient may not be particularly interested in adding years to their life, whereas a doctor's suggestions aimed at adding life to their later years may be more warmly embraced.

Summary

In this chapter, an overview of the most common health concerns in older patients has been presented, as well as the risk factors related to these health concerns and preventive measures that can be incorporated into chiropractic practice. Given the diversity of chiropractic practice styles and philosophical values that drive the chiropractic profession, some chiropractors may choose to leave prevention and health promotion (aside from the chiropractic adjustment) up to other providers. While this is a perfectly acceptable decision, it is the author's hope that this chapter has helped to raise the reader's awareness of the breadth of opportunities that exist in health-promotion practices. The author also hopes that this chapter has sparked some interest in empowering our patients, old and young, to take charge of their health by exploring natural alternatives to pharmaceutical and surgical interventions.

References

1 Department of Health and Human Services. A profile of older Americans. Administration on Aging and the Program Resources Department; American Association of Retired Persons, 1996.

2 Lubitz J, Beebe J, Baker C. Longevity and Medicare expenditures. N Engl J Med 1995; 332: 999–1003.

3 Hoffman C, Rice D, Sung HY. Persons with chronic conditions: their prevalence and costs. JAMA 1996; 276: 1473–1479.

4 Christensen MG, Kerkoff D, Kollasch MW. Job Analysis of Chiropractic 2000: A Project Report, Survey Analysis, and Summary of the Practice of Chiropractic within the United States. Greely, CO: National Board of Chiropractic Examiners, CO. 2000.

5 Rao JK *et al.* Use of complementary therapies for arthritis among patients of rheumatologists. Ann Intern Med 1999; 131: 409–416.

6 Killinger LZ, Azad A, Zapotocky B, Morschhauser EC. Development of a model curriculum in chiropractic geriatric education: process and content. J Neuromusculoskeletal Syst 1998; 6: 146–153.

7 Hawk CK, Killinger LZ, Zapotocky B, Azad A. Chiropractic training in the care of the geriatric patient: an assessment. J Neuromusculoskeletal Syst 1997; 5:15–25.

8 Bowers, L. Clinical assessment of geriatric patients: unique challenges. Top in Clin Chiropractic 1996; 3(2):10–22.

9 Fox PJ, Breur W, Wright JA. Effects of a health promotion program on sustaining health behaviors in older adults. Am J Prevent Med 1997; 13: 257–264.

10 Anderson RT *et al.* Issues of aging and adherence to health interventions. Control Clin Trials 2000; 21: 171S–183S.

11 Talarico LD. Preventive gerontology: strategies for optimal aging. Patient Care 1995; 15 May: 195–211.

12 Jamison J. Exploring the behavior of chiropractic patients. Chiropractic J Austr 2000; 30: 96–101.

13 US Department of Health and Human Services. Healthy People 2010. DHHS, 2000.

14 Hawk CK. Should chiropractic be a wellness profession? Top Clin Chiropractic 2000; 7(1): 23–26.

15 Hawk CK *et al.* Chiropractic care for patients aged 55 years and older: report from a practice-based research program. J Am Geriatr Soc 2000; 48: 534–545.

16 Rupert R *et al.* A survey of practice patterns and the health promotion and prevention attitudes of US chiropractors. Maintenance care: Part I. J Manipulative Physiol Ther 2000; 23: 1–9.

17 Rupert R *et al.* Maintenance care: health promotion services administered to US chiropractic patients aged 65 and older, Part II. J Manipulative Physiol Ther 2000; 23: 10–19.

18 Hawk CK, Dusio ME. A survey of 492 chiropractors on primary care and prevention related issues. J Manipulative Physiol Ther 1995; 18: 57–64.

19 Sawyer CE. The role of the chiropractic doctor in health promotion. Proceedings of the 1992 International Conference on Spinal Manipulation 1992; May 15–17: 216–217.

20 Kane RL. The public health paradigm. In: Hickey T, Speers M, Prohasta T, eds. Public Health and Aging. Baltimore, MD: Johns Hopkins University Press, 1997.

21 US Department of Health and Human Services, Office of Disease Prevention and Health Promotion. Clinician's Handbook on Preventive Services. 2nd edn. Washington, DC: US Government Printing Office, 1998.

22 Hickey T, Speers MA, Prohaska TR. Public Health and Aging. Baltimore, MD: Johns Hopkins Press,1997: 93–94.

23 Palmer BJ. It is as Simple as that. Davenport, Iowa: Palmer School of Chiropractic, reprinted 1994.

24 Palmer DD. The Chiropractic Adjuster: The Science, Art, and Philosophy of Chiropractic. Portland, OR: Portland Printing House, 1910.

25 Nelson C. Chiropractic scope of practice. J Manipulative Physiol Ther 1993; 16: 488–497.

26 Hawk CK. Chiropractic and primary care. In Advances in Chiropractic. Vol. 3. St Louis, MO: Mosby-Year Book, 1996.

27 Eisengerg DM *et al.* Unconventional medicine in the United States: Prevalence, costs, and patterns of use. N Engl J Med 1993; 328: 246–252.

28 Eisenberg DM *et al.* Trends in alternative medicine use in the United States, 1990–1997: results of a follow-up national survey. JAMA 1998; 280: 1569–1575.

29 Hurwitz EL *et al.* Use of chiropractic services from 1985–1991 in the United States and Canada. Am J Public Health 1998; 88: 771–776.

30 Meeker WC. Public demand and the integration of complementary and alternative medicine in the US health care system. J Manipulative Physiol Ther 2000; 23: 123–126.

31 Anon. The mainstreaming of alternative medicine. Consumer Reports 2000; May: 17–25.

32 Gonyea MA. The Role of the Doctor of Chiropractic in the Health Care System in Comparison with Doctors of Allopathic Medicine and Doctors of Osteopathic Medicine. Arlington, VA: Foundation for Chiropractic Education and Research, 1993.

33 Coulehan JL. Chiropractic and the clinical art. Soc Sci Med 1985; 21: 383–390.

34 Joseph JA *et al.* Age-related neurodegeneration and oxidative stress. Neurol Clin North Am 1998; 16: 747–755.

35 National Center for Health Statistics. Health, United States, 1998. Rockville, MD. Public Health Service, 1999.

36 De Lorgerill M *et al.* Mediterranean diet, traditional risk factors, and the rate of cardiovascular complication after myocardial infarction: final report of the Lyon Diet Heart Study. Circulation 1999; 99: 779–785.

37 Whelton PK, Apel LJ, Espelard MA *et al.* Sodium restriction and weight loss in the treatment of hypertension in older persons: a randomized controlled clinical trial of non-pharmacological interventions in the elderly (TONE). JAMA 1998; 279: 839–846.

38 Canadian Task Force on the Periodic Health Examination. Lowering the total blood cholesterol level to prevent coronary heart disease. In: The Canadian Guide to Clinical Preventive Health Care. Ottawa: Minister of Supply and Services, 1994: Chapter 54.

39 US Derpartment of Health and Human Services. Preventing and Controlling High Blood Pressure. National Heart, Lung, and Blood Institute, National Institutes of Health NIH, Publication No. 96-3655, Sept. 1996.

40 Hercberg S *et al.* The potential role of antioxidant vitamins in preventing cardiovascular diseases and cancers. Nutrition1998; 14: 513–520.

41 Stephens NG *et al.* Randomised controlled trial of vitamin E in patients with coronary disease: Cambridge Heart Antioxidant Study (CHAOS). Lancet 1996; 347: 781–786.

42 Russell RM, Rasmussen H, Lichenstein A. Modified food pyramid for people over 70 years of age. J Nutr 1999; 129: 751–753.

43 Jette AM *et al.* Exercise-it's never too late: the strong for life program. Am J Public Health 1999; 89(1): 66–72.

44 Killinger LZ. Trauma in the geriatric patient: a chiropractic perspective with a focus on prevention. Top Clin Chiropractic 1998; 5.

45 McCarthy KA. Management considerations in the geriatric patient. Top Clin Chiropractic 1996; 3(2): 66–75.

46 Manello DM. Osteoporosis: assessment and treatment options. Top Clin Chiropractic 1997; 4(3): 30–43.

47 Miller AL. Cardiovascular disease – toward a unified approach. Alt Med Rev 1996; 1: 132–147.

48 National Institute on Aging, National Institutes of Health. Exercise: a guide from the National Institute on Aging. NIH Publication No. NIH99-4258, 1999.

49 Solberg LI *et al.* A systematic primary care office-based smoking cessation program. J Fam Pract 1990; 30: 647–654.

50 Austin S. Recent progress in treatment and secondary prevention of breast cancer with supplements. Alt Med Rev 1997; 2: 4–11.

51 American Cancer Society. Colon cancer: what it is, and what you can do to prevent it. 1999.

52 Lee I, Paffenbarger RS. Physical activity and stroke incidence: the Harvard Alumni Health Survey. Stroke 1998; 29: 2049–2054.

53 Wannamethee G, Shaper AG. Physical activity and stroke in British middle aged men. BMJ 1992; 304: 597–601.

54 Gillium RF *et al.* Physical activity and stroke incidence in women and men: NHANES-1. Am J Epidemiol 1996; 143: 860.

55 Abbott RD *et al.* Physical activity in older middle-aged men and reduced risk of stroke: the Honolulu Heart Program. Am J Epidemiol 1994; 139: 881–883.

56 Sacco RL *et al.* Leisure time physical activity and ischemic stroke risk: the Northern Manhattan Stroke study. Stroke 1998; 29: 380–387.

57 Ascherio A, Rimm EB, Hernan MA *et al.* Intake of potassium, magnesium, calcium, and fiber, and risk of stroke among US men. Circulation 1998; 98: 1198–1204.

58 Serving K *et al.* Fish consumption and risk of stroke: the Zutpen study. Stroke 1994; 25: 328–334.

59 Davigus M *et al.* Dietary vitamin C, B, carotene, and 30 year risk of strokes: results from the Western Electric study. Neuroepidemiology 1997; 16: 69–79.

60 Hawker G. The epidemiology of osteoporosis. J Rheumatol Suppl 1996; 45(23): 2–5.

61 Souza T, Soliman S. Normal aging. Top Clin Chiropractic 1996; 3(2): 1–9.

62 Drugay M. Healthy People 2000. Breaking the silence: a health promotion approach to osteoporosis. J Gerontol Nurs 1997; 23(6): 36–43.

63 O'Connor DJ. Understanding osteoporosis and clinical strategies to assess, arrest, and restore bone loss. Alt Med Rev 1997; 2: 36–47.

64 Reid IR *et al*. Long term effects of calcium supplementation on bone loss and fractures in post-menopausal women, a randomized controlled trial. Am J Med 1995; 98: 331–335.

65 Dawson-Hughes B *et al*. A controlled clinical trial of the effect of calcium supplementation on bone density in post menopausal women. N Engl J Med 1990; 323: 878–883.

66 Harris SS, Dawson-Hughes B. Caffeine and bone loss in healthy post-menopausal women. Am J Clin Nutr 1994; 60: 573–578.

67 US National Institutes of Health. NIH Consensus Development Conference on Optimal Calcium Intake. Bethesda, MD: national Institutes of Health, 1994.

68 Petrovich, H, Masaki K, Rodriguez B. Pros and cons of post-menopausal hormone replacement therapy. Generations 1996–1997; 4 (winter): 7–12.

69 Rubinstein LZ. Update on preventive medicine for older people. Generations 1996–1997; 4 (Winter): 47–53.

70 DiMatteo MR. Adherence. In: Feldman MD, Christensen JF, eds. Behavioral Medicine in Primary Care: A Practical Guide. Stamford, CT: Appleton & Lange, 1997.

71 O'Connell D. Behavior change. In: Behavioral Medicine in Primary Care. Feinleib.

72 Chao D, Foy CG, Farmer D. Exercise adherence among older adult: Challenges and strategies. Control Clin Trials 2000; 21: 212S–217S.

73 Goldzweig IA. Creating a Community Health Forum: Health Promotion for Ethnic Minority Elderly. A manual produced with the support of the US Administration on Aging, the American Association of Retired Persons, the National Eldercare Institute on Health Promotion, and the Meharry Consortium Geriatric Education Center. Meharry Medical Center, 1996.

74 Singer C, Jones S, Ganzini L. Older patients. In: Feldman MD, Christensen JF. Behavioral Medicine in Primary Care: A practical guide. Stamford, CT: Appleton & Lange, 1997.

Appendix 30.1 Health promotion and prevention resources for older persons and geriatric caregivers

Alzheimer's Association
Tel: 1-800-438-4380
Website: www.alzheimers.org

American Cancer Society
Te: 1-800-ACS-2345
Website: www.cancer.org

American Association of Retired Persons
Website: www.aarp.org

American Heart Association
Tel: 1-800-AHA-USA1

American Society on Aging
Tel: +1-415-974-9600
Website: www.asa.org

Arthritis Foundation
Tel: 1-800-283-7800
Website: www.arthritis.org

Canadian Task Force on Periodic Health Examination
Tel: +1-519-682-4292, Ext. 2327

Mental Health Internet Resources
Website: www.mentalhealth.org

National Council on Aging
Tel: +1-202-479-1200
Website: www.ncoa.org

National Institute on Aging
Tel: 1-800-222-2225
Website: www.nih.gov/nia

National Institute of Health, Panel on Physical Activity and Cardiovascular Health
Tel: 888-NIH-CONSENSUS

National Osteoporosis Foundation
Tel: +1-202-223-2226
Website: www.nof.org

National Stroke Association
Tel: 1-800-Strokes
Website: www.stroke.org

US Preventive Services Task Force
Tel: +1-301-584-4015

31

Jurisprudence and geriatric care

Allan Freedman and Paul Carey

Growing old isn't so bad when you think of the alternatives.

Within the profession of chiropractic there are generalities and there are specifics. To explain this principle in further detail, consider that there are general rules concerning the conduct of a chiropractor as there are for all health-care professionals. There are statutory duties and there are duties that are established by common law.

In the event of a statutory breach of duty by a chiropractor there are sanctions that can be imposed. In the case of a common law breach of a standard there are repercussions resulting in awards of compensatory and possibly punitive damages.

For the most part, these two breaches, statutory and common law, are applicable to the conduct of chiropractors in any number of instances. However, there are instances in the professional practice of a chiropractor in which the general duty of care may be elevated or require different considerations. There are several circumstances in which an elevated standard of responsibility and care may be applied.

In the case of a specialty, as in the instance of a chiropractor who has achieved the status of 'clinical science's or 'radiologist', there is overtly or by implication a suggestion that the practitioner has attained a greater level of education and professional qualification, which requires a greater responsibility by the chiropractor as they are therefore held to a higher standard of care.

The actions of a chiropractor may elevate the standard to which the doctor must attain, as in the case of an advertisement by a practitioner indicating an aspect of the doctor's practice which implies or overtly suggests that the doctor has qualifications over and above those of the 'usual and customary' practitioner. The elevation of a practitioner's standard of care may involve claims to specialize in geriatric care, chronic conditions, or more gentle techniques and care for the elderly.

For the purposes of this review of the issue of chiropractic care of geriatric patients, the overriding principle relates to the general principle of law known as the 'thin skull rule'.[1] This 'rule' obligates a practitioner to assume a responsibility for a patient based upon the presumed frailties, specific quirks or nuances that may relate to such a patient. This may be a greater risk of fractures, strains or injury due to weaker muscle, bone and ligament tissues. Older patients are simply not as strong as younger patients. They have a greater risk of fractures due to osteoporosis. Geriatric patients are also at greater risk of injury from falls off treatment tables or just in the office itself. The chiropractor must be aware of this risk and offer help to patients moving over or off the treatment table as may be need. Is the office floor clear of clutter or loose carpeting, and so on? All of these circumstances may make the environment of the chiropractic practice more circumspect when dealing with the risks associated with care being provided to the elderly patient.

In obtaining consent and informed consent to treatment, the chiropractor not only is obliged to obtain such consent, but also must be confident that the patient understands the consent that is being provided to the doctor. It is imperative that the practitioner keep in mind that an elderly patient's eyesight and quite possibly reading skills may be limited. The elderly patient may be more easily confused than a younger patient. Thus, the chiropractor must proceed more slowly in their activity with such a patient, while ensuring that the patient hears and understands what the doctor is saying and doing. This is just as applicable to the issue of dealing with children, sports injuries or other situations that have some characteristics to suggest that it is not the 'usual and customary' situation. This situation is as applicable to the practice of other complementary and alternative health-care practices as it is with chiropractic or, for that matter, allopathic medicine.

This chapter reviews those issues involving the practice of the profession of chiropractic as it relates to the treatment of a geriatric patient. In particular, it is concerned with the following issues involving chiropractic care: consent to treatment, informed consent, substituted decision making, issues of misconduct, mandatory reporting and record keeping. All of the issues involved in the proper practice of the profession and compliance with general standards of practice are applicable to dealing with geriatric patients. This paper will be limited to those particular issues that are specific to the interaction of a practitioner with a geriatric patient.

Consent

It is trite and entrenched law that a health-care provider is obligated to obtain the consent of a patient before touching and treating a patient. This principle is set out, in some cases by the statutory obligations imposed upon the practitioners,[2] in other cases by the professional standards imposed by professions over and above the statutory obligations,[3] and in all cases by common-law decisions established by legal precedent.[4] If there are risks associated with the treatment (and treatment may include examinations) then not only must the patient provide his or her consent, but the practitioner must also receive an informed consent from the patient.

It must be remembered that consent is quite different and distinct from informed consent. Consent is the patient agreeing to examination or treatment in a broad sense. Informed consent is the patient agreeing to treatment or even examination where there are known material risks. Material risk is the risk of severe injury (e.g. stroke) or harm even though it may be infrequent, or a minor injury that may occur on a regular basis, such as rib fracture. The law assumes that the patient has a right to know and will want to know of these risks. The patient must be given the opportunity to accept or decline any such risk, either minor or severe.

As such, the issue of consent must be dealt with, whether or not it involves the matter of risk or no risk.

This becomes even more important in the event that any of the care which is provided to the patient, or any treatment regimen provided or suggested, including such matters as home exercise programmes, involve advice or treatment that is not customary and ordinary.[5]

For the purposes of ensuring that consent has been validly obtained, the patient must be in a position to provide the consent voluntarily, without duress and without misrepresentation. The consent may be personal to the practitioner and limited to a specific act. Even more importantly, the patient must have the mental capacity to provide the consent and not be under any constraints, whether legal, physical or mental.

It is the responsibility of the practitioner to be in a position to prove that the consent was obtained. As such, if the patient is elderly, living in a nursing home or under medication, or has a physical impediment (e.g. hearing or visual) the practitioner must ensure that the consent was dealt with in a manner appropriate to overcome the difficulties that affect the patient.

A doctor who is contemplating dealing with a geriatric patient would be wise to consider having an assistant present to observe the interaction between the patient and doctor, to ensure that the patient was capable of providing consent to the doctor. This issue takes on a further degree of importance if the patient is a resident in a nursing home and requires regular medication. In those situations where a patient is a resident of a nursing home, it is not enough for the practitioner to have merely received an initial consent to treatment from a caregiver. If the care requires ongoing dialogue and/or changes in treatment, the practitioner must ensure that he or she has received authority from the appropriate party in order to provide the continued treatment. If the patient suffers from Alzheimer's disease or dementia, he or she is unlikely to be in a position to provide consent. The issue of consent as it relates to geriatric patients is similar to that of dealing with consent as it relates to children. The issue requires further consideration than that required of the 'usual and customary patient'. Did the patient understand and agree to care? Can you prove it? Remember that this will only become a major issue if something goes wrong or there is a dispute.

Having regard to the particular limitations that may relate to a geriatric patient, it is also incumbent upon a health-care practitioner to ensure that he or she has provided adequate information to the patient, which the patient is capable of understanding. This may require further consideration to be given, if appropriate, to warnings concerning such matters as home exercise programmes, limitation of daily activities, including hobbies, sports or simple matters such as exercise or driving, and the possible risks associated with terminating health care or refusing a recommended referral. Patients may not be compliant for any length of time with respect to instructions for compliance outside the office, particularly concerning instructions with respect to exercise programmes to be undertaken at home. They forget or they feel they are not obligated to do these things, and often they will not tell the doctor of their non-compliance.

Substituted decisions

As might be expected, it is inevitable that if a doctor is treating geriatric patients, the matter of 'substituted decisions' or 'living wills' may arise. A geriatric practice will ultimately involve a number of patients who will not be able to make decisions on their own behalf. Again, the impediment may involve a physical or mental difficulty that may prohibit the patient from providing consent to the doctor. In such a case, either the patient will have designated an attorney to deal with matters of care, or alternatively a substituted decision maker will be appointed to act on behalf of the patient.[6] Failure to have a substituted decision maker designated or appointed is insufficient reason to fail to obtain consent from the patient. In addition, a practitioner must obtain valid informed consent from the substituted decision maker. They must understand and agree to care after they too have been fully informed.

Referrals

It is always a matter of professional responsibility for a health-care practitioner to refer a patient when necessary.[7] The circumstances for such a referral may include, but not be limited to, the following circumstances:

- The complaint of the patient was beyond the scope of the practitioners practice.
- The patient has received care from which he or she has not benefited.

- The practitioner requires a second opinion as to any portion of the care to be provided to the patient, including the diagnosis and/or the plan of management.
- The need sometimes to obtain further substantiation with respect to the need for care and ensuring consent and informed consent was properly given and received.
- The failure to provide a reasonable and timely referral may give rise to a claim of negligence.

As in the case of a geriatric patient, the obligation to refer may be heightened in the event that the care being provided to the patient gives rise to a suspicion that the patient requires additional care for ailments or complaints for which he or she had not initially presented to the doctor's office.

Record keeping

The standards relating to record keeping may well require further consideration when dealing with a patient whose mental or physical capacity is not consistent with a patient of normal or reasonable capabilities. It would be prudent for a practitioner to ensure that the doctor's file fully documents the history of the patient, any issues relating to substituted decision makers and the obtaining of consent. The need for signed informed consent becomes obvious. In addition to the specifics of the records which are to be maintained by the practitioner, the records should substantiate the following: that the treatment was rendered, and that it was therapeutically necessary, given in accordance with professional standards and not misrepresented. As might be anticipated, when dealing with an elderly patient, the potential for disagreement may well arise when considering that a patient may take exception to unique or unusual 'therapeutic practices', whether these involve the use of 'magnetic healing', nutrients, orthotics or modalities. This is not to indicate that such treatments are not worthwhile or therapeutically necessary. However, the doctor should be cautioned to take into account the age, frailty and mental and physical impairments of the patient. The onus will be on the practitioner to substantiate the treatment. The greater the deviation from the 'usual and customary' treatment, if any, the greater will be the onus on the doctor to validate the plan of management arising from the history taking, examination and diagnosis.

A practitioner may, in their records, fail to document the patient's comments, concurrent treatment or important life events (e.g. a death or a problem with family) of which they are made aware or should be aware. These can be a most important issue and need to be part of the patient records.

Should a subsequent debate arise over the validity of the plan of management, it is quite likely that it will not be the elderly patient who will be complaining. It is more likely that a third party, such as a family member, will have a concern over the care that was provided. The matter of health care is not a matter of contract but arises from a professional issue which requires the relationship to be dealt with by means of professional standards. Since these standards may be debated in the criminal, civil or administrative arenas, the complaint is not necessarily limited to the doctor and patient. As such, it is imperative that the records reflect what has occurred to an extent that will allow third parties an understanding of the dynamics of the relationship between the doctor and patient.

Much has been written about the length of time for which records concerning a patient must be maintained by a practitioner. There are statutory requirements that are generally delineated in legislation governing a profession. However, since the records also assist the doctor in providing information to third parties regarding the relationship of the doctor and patient, they should be retained for the maximum period wherein a review of the records might be undertaken. If the limitation period for instituting a cause of action against a practitioner is 1 year, as is the case for a chiropractor, a medical doctor or those governed under similar legislation, or 6 years, as is the case for naturopaths or homoeopaths who do not have specific limitation periods concerning the instituting of an action for negligence, then the records should not merely be retained for the period of 1 or 6 years. It may well be that the individual was unaware of the act of negligence for some time after the initial treatment. The limitation period does not generally start to run until the patient 'knew or ought to have known' that the practitioner was negligent. Quite simply, longer is better in retaining records as they more often protect rather than hurt or inconvenience the practitioner.

In the case of Novak v. Bond,[8] being a British Columbia action, the Supreme Court of Canada dealt with the issue of the limitation period affecting the commencement of an action by a patient with respect to a claim for negligence arising out of a treatment for breast cancer.

In this particular case, the patient had last seen the doctor on October 1, 1990, and commenced an action for negligence on April 9, 1996. The limitation period for such actions in British Columbia is governed by Section 6 of the Limitation Act, RSBC 1996, c. 266, and specifies a limitation period of 2 years. However, subsection 6(4)(b) allows the limitation period to be extended, as enunciated by the Court, 'until a reasonable person would consider that the plaintiff ought, in the person's own interests and taking the person's circumstances into account, to be able to bring an action'. Having regard to the fact that the Court was divided in its decision, with four Justices allowing the action to continue and three Justices opposing the continuation of the action, the issue is not necessarily settled outside the facts upon which the case at hand was decided.

As the issue regarding when a claim for compensation may be commenced by a patient is open to continued debate, as was raised in the Novak case, it is imperative that a practitioner ensure that he or she is knowledgeable about the limitation of actions which can be commenced with respect to care provided to a patient, and to ensure that patient files are maintained during any period during which an action may be commenced. This is to protect both the doctor and the patient.

Even more important is the fact that a claim for negligence may be commenced by a third party who has incurred some loss as a result of the negligence of the doctor as it relates to the elderly patient. The limitation period of this third party would not commence until the third party, if a minor, reaches the age of majority, e.g. 18 years of age. Finally, there is no limitation period with respect to a matter of a professional complaint to a regulatory board. It may be of little solace to the practitioner to indicate that the records of the doctor had been eliminated in accordance with the statutory obligations merely to maintain records for a period of, for example, 7 years from the last treatment date. The patient may well have access to records, whether personal or governmental (as in the case of provincial health-care payments), which may suggest that treatment was unreasonable or improper. The doctor will then be put in a position of having to substantiate his or her professional conduct solely on recollection, and in the face of a diametrically opposite position being maintained by the patient. The complaint may range from an allegation of a lack of consent or informed consent, through billing, to inappropriate treatment or inappropriate conduct by the doctor in terms of office protocols, comments or general decorum.

Misconduct rules

While a number of scenarios could give rise to a complaint of professional misconduct, most would be based upon an allegation that the doctor conducted himself or herself in a manner unbecoming a member of the College. There are specific allegations that may be applicable to a geriatric patient, e.g. Section 30 of the Regulations relating to Professional Misconduct pursuant to the Chiropractic Act of Ontario defines misconduct as 'influencing a patient to change his or her will or other testamentary instrument for the benefit of the member or anyone not at arm's length from the member'.[9] At least one regulatory body governing chiropractors has had to deal with at least one complaint involving a practitioner who was accused of 'influencing a patient to change his/her will'.[10] While such complaints may be rare, in the event that a patient has provided a gift in his or her will to a doctor, the practitioner may well come under scrutiny by the family of the patient.

While such conduct is applicable to the relationship between the practitioner and any adult patient, it is potentially more significant to the relationship between a doctor and a geriatric patient, having regard to the perceived imbalance of power which might be alleged to have existed between the doctor and patient, and/or the frailty of the patient at the time of the change having been made to the patient's last will and testament. If the patient wishes to make a bequest to the practitioner, the doctor must ensure that the patient obtains legal advice from his or her own legal counsel. The practitioner should also document that this was done. In addition, the doctor should be cautious in directing the patient to any lawyer for assistance, having regard to the conclusions that may be drawn from what might otherwise have been an innocent act of referral.

Mandatory reporting

There are at least three examples of mandatory reporting that can affect a health-care practitioner.

These are the reporting of child abuse, the reporting of a matter of sexual abuse of a patient by a healthcare practitioner and the reporting to the Registrar of Motor Vehicles of an individual who, in the opinion of the practitioner, should not be operating a motor vehicle.

In the instance of child abuse, the appropriate legislation in Ontario is dealt with pursuant to the Child and Family Services Act.[11] The legislation requires that 'a person who believes on reasonable grounds that a child is or may be in need of protection shall forthwith report the belief and the information upon which it is based to a society (children's aid society)'. It further establishes an obligation upon the practitioner that takes precedence to the statutory or common law duty of confidentiality, namely;

Despite the provisions of any other Act, a person referred to in subsection (4) who, in the course of his or her professional or official duties, has reasonable grounds to suspect that a child is or may be suffering or may have suffered abuse shall forthwith report the suspicion and the information on which it is based to a society. Subsection (4) defines those persons who are subject to Section 72(3), in addition to other individuals, the following: Subsection (3) applies to every person who performs professional or official duties with respect to a child, including, a health care professional, including a physician, nurse, dentist, pharmacist and psychologist … .

It should be noted that while subsection (3) makes mention of 'physician, nurse, dentist, pharmacist and psychologist', the list is not inclusive, having regard to the words '… including, a health care professional, including …'. A chiropractor, and those other healthcare practitioners who are dealing with a situation that could be the subject matter of an obligation pursuant to the Child and Family Services Act would be wise to ensure that his or her obligations are fully and timely performed.

It would be prudent of a health-care practitioner to ascertain whether there is a similar obligation placed upon a practitioner to report situations involving geriatric abuse. Unless the legislation in any particular jurisdiction authorizes the release of the information, or unless the patient gives appropriate consent to the release of the information by the practitioner, the situation must be maintained as confidential in accordance with the statutory obligations imposed upon the practitioner or the implied terms of the relationship which are established between the doctor and patient. At a minimum, it might be considered reasonable for a health-care practitioner, other than a 'legally qualified medical practitioner', to obtain the consent of the patient to discuss their state of health with their medical practitioner, if available. In this case, the medical practitioner may be required to file a report to the Registrar as set out by legislation.

In the situation involving the reporting of sexual abuse by a practitioner, the obligations are somewhat clearer. Pursuant to the Code enacted as part of the Regulated Health Professions Act, a practitioner is required to report an abuse by a member of a regulated health profession. As such, a chiropractor who becomes reasonably certain of an incident is obliged to report this to the appropriate authority.

With respect to the matter of reporting patients who may be incapable of operating a motor vehicle to the licensing authorities, the issue is not quite as clear as in the case of sexual abuse reporting. In Ontario, the Highway Traffic Act[12] sets out the following:

Every legally qualified medical practitioner shall report to the Registrar the name, address and clinical condition of every person sixteen years of age or over attending upon the medical practitioner for medical services who, in the opinion of the medical practitioner, is suffering from a condition that may make it dangerous for the person to operate a motor vehicle.

The Section of the Act specifically sets out the obligation to be applicable to a 'legally qualified medical practitioner'. As such, there would be no obligation upon other health-care practitioners, including, chiropractors, dentists, psychologists, optometrists, naturopaths or other complementary and alternative health-care practitioners. There may be situations in which a geriatric patient will choose to seek care from an alternative health-care practitioner in lieu of seeking care from a medical doctor in order to avoid the issue of reporting by the practitioner any suspicion that the patient is incapable of operating a motor vehicle safely. Consider the circumstance of a patient who attends at a practitioner's office and complains of dizziness, blurring vision and periods of nausea. In a medical doctor's office, such information might well lead to a reporting of the patient to the Registrar as instructed by the Highway Traffic Act. In the case of other health-care practitioners, the matter appears to be solely governed by the matter of confidentiality to which the practitioner is bound.

Use of forms

There is a sense of security in maintaining forms for use in a health-care practitioner's office which deal with any number of issues, such as personal history, consent to treatment, informed consent, examination results, plan of management, and exercise or home therapy programmes. The forms are useful for consistency and as a reminder of those matters that should be dealt with by the practitioner or by the patient. The use and maintenance of forms can be employed to substantiate the reasons for the care, and the providing of such care by the health practitioner.

However, just as the 'forms' will be a sense of security and part of a defence for a doctor at some time in the future, the forms may well cause concern for the doctor if they are maintained by the office but are not fully and accurately completed by the practitioner. If the forms are used or even maintained in the practitioner's office, they have importance, and when dealing with matters of importance regarding a patient, there will be little sympathy for a doctor who attempts to downplay the importance of any documentation in the office. What becomes even more difficult is the attempt by the health-care practitioner to justify the fact that the form was not completed at all, or not accurately and/or fully completed by the doctor. Any incident that leads to a criminal, civil or professional complaint will require a full and complete review of documentation, including the forms of the practitioner. The message is clear: if a practitioner uses forms, then the form must be completed when applicable in a proper fashion and to the extent that was clinically indicated. Any derivation from this principle will require justification by the practitioner which should be recorded in the patient's file.

Human rights issues

A health-care practitioner should be cognizant in the establishment and operation of a health-care facility that certain patients may require access and facilities that would not otherwise be required by the 'average' patient, as in the case of a patient who requires the use of a wheelchair or crutches, or is otherwise unable to walk up a flight of stairs or open a door which has a minimum of entry space.

The Ontario Human Rights Code[13] sets out that, 'Every person has a right to equal treatment with respect to services, goods and facilities, without discrimination because of race, ancestry, place of origin, colour, ethnic origin, citizenship, creed, sex, sexual orientation, age, marital status, family status or handicap'. A health-care practitioner should be cognizant of the legislation in his or her jurisdiction to ensure that he or she is complying with those obligations which require that the practitioner ensure that a geriatric patient is provided health-care services without regard to their age and any handicap that may exist on the part of the patient's state of health. There have been incidences of health-care practitioners having complaints lodged against them pursuant to the Code over human rights issues such as wheelchair accessibility. Such complaints have led to significant grief and costs.

Ethical issues

Throughout this chapter certain ethical and moral issues have been raised which transcend or, more importantly, fly in the face of statutory obligations. For example, in the case of 'mandatory reporting' it was noted that in some jurisdictions the obligation to report a patient who was not capable of operating a motor vehicle was limited to 'legally qualified medical practitioners'. However, what of the chiropractor or other health-care professional who is contacted by a patient who is a 70-year-old individual complaining about dizziness and blurred vision, and whose occupation is driving a school bus. The legislation does not afford protection to such practitioners, nor might the doctor be given consent by the patient to release such information.

As noted earlier, it may be left to the practitioner to refer the patient to a medical doctor or alternatively to receive permission from the patient to consent to discuss the patient's state of health with the medical practitioner. On failing to receive such a consent, the practitioner is faced with the dilemma of maintaining the confidentiality of such information or releasing the information in contravention of the practitioner's obligations. The issue of confidentiality, as it applies to the ethical issues facing the practitioner, is also applicable to the matter of physical abuse, from which the patient may suffer at the hands of family members. Again, the patient may not wish the information to be released and the practitioner may not have a statutory authority or its protection to release such informa-

tion. As such, the dilemma for the chiropractor may not be resolved or solvable at this time.

Summary

While each of the issues dealt with in this chapter may well be applicable to situations involving patients other than those who are elderly, the care of a geriatric patient takes on a potentially higher amount of vigilance and concern. A history taking may require additional time and investigation. Record keeping may have to set out documentation that would not otherwise be relevant to a 'usual and customary patient'. The practitioner may have to face legal and ethical issues relating to reporting of the abuse of an elderly patient, and ensure that the relationship between the doctor and patient does not compromise the relationship, and that the practitioner does not take advantage of the patient, particularly in relation to testamentary gifts.

In any situation in which the health-care practitioner presents himself or herself as having a greater expertise than that of a fellow practitioner, the standard of care of the practitioner will be expanded upon and the obligation of the practitioner in providing care, over and above that of the reasonable practitioner, will be imposed upon the doctor. This principle does not suggest that there will be a decreasing level of responsibility should the doctor not hold himself or herself out as a specialist in the area of geriatrics. As indicated previously, a doctor is expected to be knowledgeable in any field of care that they provide to the patient, whether it involves sports injuries, paediatrics or geriatric care.

References

1 Linden AM, Klar LN. Canadian Tort Law. 10th edn. Butterworths, 1994: 376.
2 Ontario Regulation 852/93, Section 3, Chiropractic Act. RSO, 1991: C.21.
3 Canadian Chiropractic Association.
4 Mason v. Forgie, New Brunswick Queens Bench.
5 Carey PF, Freedman AM, Moss JA. The other informed consent. J Can Chiropractic Assoc 2000; 44: 76.
6 Substitute Decisions Act of Ontario. SO, 1992: S.30.
7 Ontario Regulation 852/93, Section 13, Chiropractic Act. RSO, 1991: C.21.
8 Novak v. Bond I. SCR, 1999: 8089.
9 Ontario Regulation 852/93, Section 30, Chiropractic Act. RSO, 1991: C.2110.
10 Report of the Complaints Committee. Annual Report of the College of Chiropractors of Ontario, 1999: 11.
11 Child and Family Services Act. RSO, 1990: C.11, Section 72(2)12.
12 Highway Traffic Act. RSO, 1990: H.8, Section 203(1)13.
13 Human Rights Code. RSO, 1990: H.19, Section 1.

Appendix: Human genetics

Brian J Gleberzon

The human genome (the sum total of all genetic information) is organized into 23 pairs of chromosomes. Each set of chromosomes is provided by either the egg or sperm of a parent. Each human cell therefore contains 46 chromosomes in total, with the exception of the sex cell which contain only 23 chromosomes. Each chromosome is composed of millions of separate groups of genetic material, in a code determined by the sequence of four structures called *nucleotides*. These nucleotides are adenonine, guanine, thymine and cytosine. In the field of genetics, it is customary to refer to each nucleotide by the first letter of its name (A for adenonine, G for guanine, etc.). A and G are purines; C and T are pyrimidines.

In the 1950s, Watson and Crick determined that chromosomes are arranged in two strands or chains of nucleotides that twist around each other, forming a double helix. Along with the research of Erwin Chargaff, Watson and Crick determined that these strands align themselves in an antiparallel pattern. That is, the strands run in opposite directions. Researchers also determined that the chromosomes are bonded to each other in a particular manner. Specifically, A always bonds only with T, and C always bonds only with G.

At this biochemical level, the total pattern of these nucleotides is also referred to as deoxyribonucleic acid (DNA). Looked at another way, DNA is the specific pattern of four different nucleotides on a long string called a chromosome. A discrete section or bundle of a chromosome is called a *gene*. Each gene comes in at least two forms, called *alleles*. Each allele may result in a different physiological trait. One allele is provided by each biological parent. One way to envision this arrangement is to imagine a long string (the chromosome) with several million beads on it (the genes). This analogy is called the bead theory. This model supports four basic principles involving the gene:

1. The gene is a fundamental unit, indivisible by other interactions (such as crossing-over or *translocation*). The gene is the biological equivalent of the atom in quantum mechanics.
2. The gene is the fundamental unit of change or *mutation*. It changes from one allelic form to another, but no smaller component within it changes.
3. The gene is the basic unit of function.
4. The chromosome is merely a vector or transporter for genes.

A gene can be several hundred or several million nucleotides long. Each gene begins at a sequence of nucleotides that function as a *start* segment, and each gene ends at a sequence of nucleotides that function as a *stop* segment. To keep things simple, it is best to envision all information between the start and stop segments that comprise one gene as containing the information for the development of a particular physiological trait or *phenotype*.

Not all information between the start and stop segments is required for the eventual development of a physiological trait. The information that is not required and that is eventually edited out is termed an *intron* or intervening sequence. The genetic information that is important and preserved, and ultimately determines a phenotype, is termed an *extron*.

Each pair of alleles contains genetic information for the development of a different physiological outcome. Some genes control vital biological traits or characteristics. Other genetic information may be dormant, requiring a particular trigger to become active (as in the case of some *oncogenes* that result in cancer after exposure to certain viruses or toxins), or it may not be expressed at all. Such information may be an evolutionary remnant. Still other phenotypical traits, such as height, require the interaction of several different genes. Moreover, the ultimate determination of a trait such as height is mitigated by many different external forces, such as nutrition.

Alleles interact in certain ways. Generally speaking, one allele is *dominant, recessive, incompletely dominant* or *codominant* to its counterpart. If one allele is dominant to the other allele, only that information coded on the dominant allele is expressed in the person's phenotype. In the case of recessive modes of inheritance, a trait is only manifested if other forms of the gene are absent. Some alleles are codominant, meaning that both alleles are expressed in the individual's phenotype. If the alleles are incompletely dominant, both alleles are expressed, but neither one dominantly (a blended-type outcome).

Another important feature of human genetics is that gender is determined by the combination of the 23rd pair of chromosomes, referred to as the *sex chromosomes*. These chromosomes are in two types: X or Y. Males are XY, females are XX. Because men produce sperm with either X or Y chromosomes, and women produce eggs with only X chromosomes, offspring are either XX or XY. All chromosomes other than the sex chromosomes are referred to as *autosomal chromosomes*. Genes, therefore, are either on the sex chromosomes (*sex-linked*) or on the autosomal chromosomes.

There are a few biological processes that need to be reviewed at this time. When DNA is reproduced, the process is called *replication*. In all cells except for the sex cells, this occurs during the process of cellular division called *mitosis*. Mitosis results in each offspring cell containing all the genetic information of the parents. In the case of humans, this amounts to a total of 46 chromosomes. The sex cells, however, reproduce during a process called a *meiosis*. During this process, the amount of genetic information in the sex cells (or gametes) is reduced by one half, from 46 chromosomes to 23 chromosomes. During this reduction of genetic information, each resultant cell randomly contains one half of the genome. This phenomenon, whereby a gene pair randomly separates during meiosis such that one half of the sex cells carry one allele and the other half of the gametes carry the other allele, is called *Mendel's First Law of Genetics* (named after the father of genetic analysis, Gregor Mendel).

Not only did Mendel predict that an allele pair separates equally, *Mendel's Second Law* states that different gene pairs separate independently. As an example,

consider the case of a gene that has two allelic forms. We can designate one allele as upper case 'Q' and the other allele as lower case 'q'. In a heterozygous adult, the gene pair could be described as *Qq*. Mendel predicted that one half of the gametes would possess the *Q* allele and the other half would contain the *q* allele. This process can be applied to any number of paired alleles. For example, another set of genes with allelic forms *Jj* may exist in a person's genome. If an adult had a genetic composition of *QqJj*, the individual would produce gametes with the following genetic information in equal numbers: *QJ Qj qJ* and *qj* (the separation of each genetic pair is independent of the other).

A key question remains: what exactly do genes do? Among the more important hypotheses developed by geneticists to explain a gene's function is the *one-gene-one–enzyme hypothesis*. As the name implies, the hypothesis states that each gene is responsible for the production of a particular enzyme. A modern-day geneticist named Ingram concluded that the gene determines the primary structure (*sequence*) of amino acids of each enzyme. Or, looked at the other way, the amino acid sequence of an enzyme is a direct reflection of the linear sequence of nucleotides on the gene. Notice how well this fits with the second principle of gene interactions. A gene mutation may result in a different amino acid being inserted into the enzyme. This correlation between the location of a mutant site on a gene and the location of an amino acid substitution on a polypeptide chain such as an enzyme is called *collinearity*. The new enzyme may have different biochemical properties to the original enzyme. This may be the result of the new enzyme having a different three-dimensional architecture (recall that the spatial geometry or three-dimensional folding of an enzyme, termed the secondary, tertiary and quaternary structure, is vital for the 'lock and key' function of enzymes).

The next process to be explained is the process whereby the conversion of a nucleotide sequence into an amino acid sequence occurs. This conversion occurs during two cellular events called *transcription* and *translation*. DNA is not directly converted into an enzyme. Instead, DNA is *transcribed* into another molecule called ribonucleic acid (RNA). The RNA molecule exits the cell's nucleus, acting as a 'DNA messenger'. This molecule is called messenger or mRNA. RNA is very similar to DNA except for two features: (i) RNA is single stranded and (ii) RNA is composed of a nucleotide called uracil instead of thymine that always bonds only to adenine. It is during the conversion from DNA to RNA that the introns are deleted. Therefore, RNA is composed only of extrons.

The mRNA leaves the nucleus and enters a cellular structure called a *ribosome*. A ribosome is essentially a protein factory. Within the ribosome, RNA directs the production of a particular enzyme (a type of protein). This production of an enzyme inside the ribosome is accomplished by another molecule called transfer or tRNA.

The function of the tRNA molecule is to transfer specific amino acids within the ribosome and to attach each amino acid to the mRNA template in a specific order, thus forming a specific enzyme. To accomplish this goal, there are several dozen different tRNA molecules, each one carrying a particular amino acid. The stage during which the t-RNA 'reads' the sequence of mRNA and assembles the appropriate amino acid sequence is called *transcription*. The process of transcription is the last step in the production of the enzyme. Recall that mRNA is a sequence of nucleotides as determined from the DNA molecule (which acts as a *template*). Every three nucleotides on the mRNA are recognized by a complementary set of three nucleotides on the tRNA. This sequence of three nucleotides on the mRNA is called a *codon* and the corresponding sequence on the tRNA is called the *anticodon*. Over the years, geneticists cracked the 'codon code' and determined that each triplet of nucleotides on the mRNA directed the attachment of a particular tRNA, carrying with it a particular amino acid.

It is now possible to review the entire process from start to finish. DNA is transcribed into mRNA. The purine and pyrimidine sequence on the mRNA is complementary to the sequence of DNA nucleotides. Only that genetic information referred to as an extron is transcribed into mRNA. The mRNA strand enters the ribosome. Triplet sequences of the mRNA are each referred to as a codon. In the ribosome, dozens of different tRNA molecules, each carrying a particular amino acid, have a specific anticodon sequence. The tRNA attaches to the complementary mRNA molecule, matching the anticodon to the codon. Each mRNA is 'read' inside the ribosome by the tRNA, beginning with the start codon and ending with the stop codon. As the tRNA attaches to the complementary codon of the mRNA, the appropriate amino acid, attached to the

tRNA, is attached to other amino acids in a specific order along the polypeptide chain. This ultimately results in the formation of a specific enzyme.

At this juncture, several important genetic processes must be explained. If a chromosome is a long chain of nucleotides arranged in a specific order to create a particular polypeptide composed of amino acids, it logically follows that any change in the order of the nucleotide sequence will result in the formation of a different enzyme. For example, during replication or transcription, some information may be inadvertently lost. This is called *deletion*. Alternatively, the opposite may happen where a sequence is mistakenly repeated in a process called *duplication*. The information on the DNA can become twisted around (the total amount of DNA is unchanged, but the sequence is altered). This is called *inversion*. Lastly, two different strands of chromosomes may exchange nucleotide sequences in a process called *translocation*. Collectively, these genetic mutations are called *chromosomal rearrangements*.

At this point, two important genetic terms must be defined. *Expressivity* is the degree to which a phenotypical trait is observed in a person. For example, consider two patients with rheumatoid arthritis. While each individual demonstrates some characteristics of the condition, they may demonstrate symptoms to a different extent. This variability in the manifestation of a disease is called *expressivity*. If a disease is classified as having a high expressivity, this implies that the manifestations of the disease vary greatly between affected individuals. If a disease typically affects individuals to the same extent, such a disease is said to demonstrate low expressivity.

Alternatively, two individuals may have the same genetic composition that would cause the manifestations of a particular disease but one individual may show no signs of the condition whatsoever. This phenomenon, whereby individuals may or may not manifest any signs or symptoms of a disease, is referred to the gene's *penetrance*. Those genetic disorders that always result in physical manifestations are referred to as demonstrating complete penetrance. If a disease is demonstrated less frequently, despite the possession of the appropriate genetic composition, the genes that are responsible for the disease are said to demonstrate incomplete penetrance.

In summary, penetrance is the percentage of persons with a given genotype who exhibit the corresponding phenotype. The extent or degree of this phenotypical expression is described as the expressivity of a particular gene.

Now that the reader is equipped with a working knowledge of many of the key genetic concepts, an exploration of the different modes of inheritance can be provided, along with specific clinical examples of each process.

Autosomal dominant genetic traits

In the pattern of inheritance called autosomal dominant, at least one parent must always manifest a particular disease. Consider a disease that has two allelic forms, such as *Marfan's disease*, which is a disease of aberrant collagen formation. It is convenient to simplify the allelic forms as (*M*), which causes the disease, and (*m*), seen in non-Marfan individuals. The disease would manifest itself if a person was homozygous (same) dominant (*MM*), or heterozygous (mixed) (*Mm*). Notice that two different genotypes, MM and Mm, both result in the same phenotype. In those diseases that follow this mode of inheritance, the possession of the gene that produces the aberrant form of collagen is dominant to the gene that results in the production of normal collagen. Persons with a genome (*mm*) would be physiologically normal, as they do not possess any genetic information that results in aberrant collagen formation. The mode of inheritance of Marfan's disease can be understood using a genetic family tree called a *pedigree analysis*. For example, consider the scenario of a man afflicted with Marfan's who came from an entire family that had Marfan's for the past 10 generations (thus we may assume that he is homozygous for the disease) and who fathers a child with a women who does not have Marfan's disease. The genomes of each parent can be represented as follows:

Genotype	Phenotype	Genotype	Phenotype
Parents: Father (*MM*) Homozygous dominant Gametes: (*M*) or (*M*)	Marfan's	Mother (*mm*) Homozygous recessive (*m*) or (*m*)	Non-Marfan's

Children: All would be heterozygous (*Mm*) and display symptoms of Marfan's disease.

As a further exercise, a pedigree analysis can help to predict what the genotypical and phenotypical charac-

teristics would be if one of the offspring from the above scenario (genome of *Mm*, and displays signs of Marfan's disease) were to have children with a non-Marfan's individual (*mm*). One parent would be heterozygous (with the disease), and the other parent would be recessive for the trait (with no traces of the disease).

Parents:	(*Mm*) Marfan's gametes; (*M*) or (*m*)	and	(*mm*) Non-Marfan's (*m*) only

Children: Half would be (*Mm*) heterozygous, and display Marfan's disease
Half would be (*mm*) homozygous recessive, and not display any signs of Marfan's disease.

It can therefore be concluded that if a child has Marfan's, they must have had a parent with Marfan's. This is also the case for other diseases that follow an autosomal dominant mode of inheritance, such as Huntington's chorea, neurofibromatosis and ankylosing spondylitis.

Diseases that follow an autosomal dominant mode of inheritance are usually quite rare. This is because the disease is typically lethal, resulting in the afflicted person's death before an individual can reproduce. A notable exception to this general rule is Huntington's chorea. This is due to the fact that symptoms of Huntington's chorea usually are not noticeable until after the age of 40 years. By that time, the individual has probably already had children.

Sex-linked dominant genetic traits

This mode of inheritance is very rare. Geneticists think that the gene that controls hairy ear rims in humans follows a sex-linked dominant mode of inheritance, found only on the Y-chromosomes. In this scenario, the condition could only affect men. If a son displays the condition, his biological father must also have had the condition. For those conditions that are linked to the X-chromosome and are dominant, affected men would pass the disease on to all of their daughters and none of their sons.

Autosomal recessive genetic disorders

A disease that follows an autosomal recessive mode of inheritance manifests when the dominant genes are absent. Such diseases are observed in the children of phenotypically normal adults. An example of this is seen in *Tay–Sachs disease*.

In the normal human brain, biologically toxic byproducts called gangliosides are degraded by an enzyme called hexosaminodase-A. In the absence of this enzyme, these gangliosides accumulate, resulting in blindness, paralysis and death, usually before the age of 5 years. Individuals who are heterozygous produce only half the normal amount of the enzyme, but this is sufficient for normal function.

Because Tay–Sachs is fatal, individuals that possess the recessive allele of the gene do not survive long enough to reproduce. Phenotypically normal, homozygous (dominant) individuals would not produce gametes containing the fatal (recessive) allele. However, normal individuals who possess a heterozygous genome could produce a Tay–Sachs childs. Such individuals are called *carriers*. For example, consider the outcome if a phenotypically normal parent who is a carrier has a child with a phenotypical normal parent who is homozygous recessive, where Tay–Sachs (*T*) is the normal allele and (*t*) is the aberrant form of the gene.

	Genotype	Phenotype	Genotype	Phenotype
Parent:	(*Tt*)	Normal	(*Tt*)	Normal
	gametes: (*T*) or (*t*)		(*T*) or (*t*)	
Children:		(*T*)	(*t*)	
	(*T*)	(*TT*)	(*Tt*)	
	(*t*)	(*Tt*)	(*tt*)	

In the above example, three-quarters of the children would be phenotypically normal and one-quarter would manifest Tay–Sachs. Half of the children would be carriers. The chance of conceiving a child with Tay–Sachs increases if relatives have children. This is why such autosomal recessive diseases as Tay–Sachs are more commonly observed in cultures that encourage marriages within the same cultural groups (who are more likely to be closely related) such as Ashkanesi Jews (Jews from Western Europe).

Other disorders that follow an autosomal recessive mode of inheritance include phenylketonuria, galactosaemia, Niemann–Pick disease, thalassaemia, dysautonomia and cystic fibrosis. Most autosomal recessive disorders result in the lack or absence of the production of a necessary biological enzyme, causing an accumulation of toxins.

Cystic fibrosis is the most common lethal genetic disorder in Caucasians, occurring in 1 in 1600 live births. It is estimated that 1 in 20 people are carriers. Cystic fibrosis causes abnormal exocrine secretions, especially of the lung, resulting in a mucous, viscid substance.

Because of the severity of many of these disorders, many potential parents who are at higher risk to be carriers of a disease often seek *genetic counselling* to determine whether they are carriers. The results of the tests may heavily influence the decision of a couple as to whether or not to have children.

Codominant genetic traits

Culture, environment and genetics are often interwoven, as in the case of *sickle cell anaemia*. In central Africa, in areas of the Savannah, traditional agricultural use the 'slash and burn' technique. This technique allows for the clearance of large areas to plant crops. The problem, however, is that by removing the grasses and their root systems areas of stagnant water can develop. Such areas are breeding grounds for mosquitoes, especially the species of *Anopheles* that carries the parasite (*Plasmodium*) that causes malaria. As an adaptation to this parasite, some individuals have developed red blood cells that are less prone to infection. Such cells assume a 'sickle shape'. The individuals with sickle-shaped red blood cells were at a relative advantage compared with those who did not have such red blood cells, who would contract malaria and die. The mutant haemoglobin molecule, called haemoglobin-S, results in a single mutation (valine substituted for glutamic acid). It has been demonstrated by electrophoresis that the allele that produces normal haemoglobin (*HbA*) is codominant with the allele that produces sickle-shaped haemoglobin (*HbS*). Individuals who possess a *HbA HbA* genome produce normal haemoglobin, but have no resistance to malaria. People who are (*HbS HbS*) manifest severe anaemia. Individuals who are (*HbA HbS*) produce the sickle-cell trait, where up to 40% of total blood volume contains sickle-shaped cells. Such individuals are better protected from malaria. However, these people are endangered at high altitudes, which have lower concentrations of oxygen. Therefore, a genetic adaptation may be advantageous in one environment and deleterious in another.

Incomplete dominant genetic traits

For the sake of completeness, incomplete dominance is described. In plants, there is an allele that directs the colour of petals. One homozygous genotype of a plant produces white petals. Another homozygous genotype produces red petals. The heterozygous genotype produces pink petals. The heterozygous genotype therefore results in a 'blended' phenotype, wherein one allele is neither dominant over nor recessive to the other.

Sex-linked recessive genetic disorders

Haemophilia is inherited following a sex-linked recessive mode of inheritance. In this case, the gene that controls haemophilia is linked or attached to the X-chromosome. As an example, what would be the genomes of the parents of a haemophilic girl (*H* results in normal blood clotting and *h* results in haemophilia)?

The girl is XX and, because haemophilia is a recessive trait, her genotype must be *XhXh*. Because one half of the child's genetic information is derived from each parent, the father must have been *XhY* and haemophilic. The mother, however, could have been either heterozygous and non-haemophilic (*XHXh*) or homozygous recessive and haemophilic (*XhXh*). Most X-linked recessive disorders are observed in male children.

Multiple allelic genetic traits

To this point, only those gene loci with only two allele forms have been considered. However, many genes exhibit *multiple allelic forms*. An example is the *ABO blood type*. There are four major blood types: A, B, AB and O. There are three allelic forms of the blood type genes: *IA*, *IB* and *i*. The *IA* and *IB* alleles are codominant to each other and both are dominant to the *i* allele. A-type blood can be either *IAIA* or *IAi*. B-type blood is the genetic result of either *IBIB* or *IBi*. Individuals who are AB-type can only possess an *IAIB* genotype. O-type individuals can result from *ii* genotypes.

What is the parentage of a child with AB-type blood?

	Phenotype	Genotype
Child:	AB	I*AIB*

The parental gametes must have been *IA* and *IB*.
Therefore, one parent was either I*AIA* or I*Ai* (A-type blood) and the other parent was either I*BIB* or I*Bi* (B-type blood).

Chromosomal abnormalities

There are three main types of chromosomal abnormalities: deletions, translocations and non-dysjuction.

If a part of a chromosome is missing, the abnormality is called a deletion. For example, if part of chromosome 5 is missing, it results in a child with a disorder called *cris-du-chat*. Such children demonstrate severe mental retardation and a characteristic high-pitched cry.

Translocation is said to occur when two chromosomes exchange genetic information. For example, if chromosomes 9 and 22 trade genetic information, the result is what is called the *Philadelphia chromosome*. This chromosome is found in patients with chronic myelogenous leukaemia.

Non-dysjunction is a chromosomal abnormality that may occur during meiosis. If, during meiosis, the sex chromosomes do not segregate equally, some gametes may have both sex chromosomes, while other gametes have no sex chromosomes. This non-segregation is called *non-dysjunction*. For example, if one gamete has two X chromosomes and it joins with a gamete with a Y chromosome, the child would be *XXY*, and have *Klinefelter's syndrome*. These people are phenotypically male but have several developmental anomalies. If the gamete that did not possess any, sex chromosomes joined with a normal gamete containing an X chromosome, the child's genotype would be *XO*. Such individuals are said to have *Turner's syndrome*.

Similarly, some individuals possess additional Y chromosomes. The number of inmates in maximum security prisons with an *XYY* genotype is much higher than the number of such individuals in the general public. Some geneticists have therefore speculated that the Y chromosome dictates states of aggression. *XXX, XXXX* and *XXXXX* genomes also exist. Each additional X chromosome results in a child with more severe mental retardation.

Non-dysfunction may also occur among autosomal chromosomes. If chromosome 21 does not segregate into gametes equally, it could result in three 21 chromosomes in an individual's genome. *Trisomy 21* results in *Down's syndrome*, which is characterized by varying degrees of mental retardation, short stature, hypotonic muscles, hypermobile joints and distinct facial features of oblique palpebral fissures and epicanthic folds. Congenital heart defects are also more common, as is acute myelogenous leukaemia. The incidence of Down's syndrome increases with maternal age (1 in 30 live births to mothers over the age of 45 have Down's syndrome).

Autoimmune disorders

The purpose of the immune system is to differentiate those molecules that are 'self' from those that are 'non-self'. This differentiation is accomplished by the identification of genetic markers on cellular surfaces called *antigens*. The HLA (human leucocyte antigen) system of genes directs the formation of antigens. Foreign antigens are recognized and disabled by specific host-produced cells called lymphocytes. The lymphocytes are responsible for the detection and, if required, destruction of foreign antigenic molecules. Some lymphocytes direct the production of antigen-specific antibodies during the *humoral* response. After the initial exposure, the host can subsequently produce the specific antibody very quickly, using the original antibody as a template. Lymphocytes are also involved in the *cell-mediated* immune response.

The ability of the immune system to determine self-tissues from non-self or foreign tissues is predicated on the assumption that the body has a mechanism to produce only those lymphocytes to non-self antigenic molecules. This ability is the result of a process called the *clonal selection model*. This model posits that a lymphocyte recognizes only one specific antigenic marker, and produces only one specific attack cell. Of particular note is that this ability exists before any exposure to the stimulatory antigen.

Two fundamental questions must still be answered: (i) how is self-tissue identified, and (ii) how are specific immunological cells developed prior to the exposure to various antigens?

The answers to both questions lie within the development of immunogenic stem cells. Initially, during embryonic development, lymphocytic stem cells are able to produce all the possible variations of immunogenic attack cells. However, early in embryonic development, those cell lines or clones that produce self-antibodies are selected against or inhibited. Those stem cells that are selected against (that could produce lymphocytes to self-antigens) are called *forbidden clones*. Only immunogenic cells that produce lymphocytes against foreign (non-self) antigens can still be potentially produced.

An auto-immune disease is a disease in which a forbidden clone is activated. No longer inhibited, tissues containing self-antigens stimulate the production of lymphocytes that attack the host's tissues. The destruction of host tissue releases more stimulatory antigens, which produce still more lymphocytes, in an ever increasing, self-prepetuating cycle. Such autoimmune disorders include diabetes mellitus, rheumatoid arthritis and Hashimoto's thyroiditis.

Autoimmune, codominant, multiallelic, multifactorial disorder: type I diabetes mellitus

Type I diabetes (formerly known as insulin-dependent diabetes mellitus, or IDDM) can serve as a model to demonstrate several genetic concepts simultaneously. Consider that there are basically three ways to develop diabetes:

- Those cells of the pancreas that produce insulin could be destroyed.
- Insulin could be produced in sufficient amounts but the insulin is either ineffective or is destroyed.
- The receptor sites on peripheral cells for insulin are altered or destroyed.

Biochemical analysis has revealed many subtypes of type I diabetes. One form is characterized by antibodies to pancreatic cells. This form of diabetes is also associated with HLA-B8 and HLA-Dr3 alleles. Another form of diabetes has demonstrated high amounts of antibodies to exogenous insulin and is associated with HLA-B15 and HLA-Dr4. A hybrid form of diabetes, characterized by antibodies to both pancreatic cells and exogenous insulin, has also been identified and is associated with HLA-B8/15 and HLA-Dr3/4 alleles.

Some geneticists have proposed a three-allele (*S1, S2* and *s*) codominant model to account for all of these observations:

Allele form	HLA associations	Phenotype
S1S1 or *S1s*	HLA-B8 and -Dr3	Diabetic with antibodies to pancreatic cells
S2S2 or *S2s*	HLA-B15 and -Dr4	Diabetic and antibodies to exogenous insulin
S1S2	HLA-B8/15 and -Dr3/4	Features of both above
ss	No HLA association	Non-diabetic

In this model, (*S1*) and (*S2*) are codominant and are both dominant over the (*s*) allele. However, because the genes responsible for the development of diabetes display incomplete penetrance (not all individuals with the genes for diabetes develop diabetes), other factors are involved. As described in Chapter 12, epidemiologists have proposed several theoretical models for diabetic development.

In one model, individuals with a certain HLA complement are exposed to certain viruses (such as *Coxsackie B4*). In these individuals, the virus stimulates the production of forbidden clones that can produce antibodies that attack either the host's pancreatic cells or their exogenous insulin, or both.

The following is a comprehensive pathogenic model for type I diabetes:

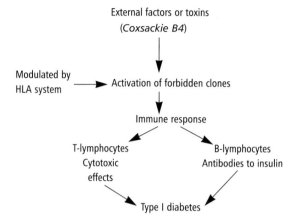

Index